D1452252

Multimodal Cardiovascular Imaging

Principles and Clinical Applications

NOTICE

Medicine is an ever-changing science. As new research and clinical experience broaden our knowledge, changes in treatment and drug therapy are required. The authors and the publisher of this work have checked with sources believed to be reliable in their efforts to provide information that is complete and generally in accord with the standards accepted at the time of publication. However, in view of the possibility of human error or changes in medical sciences, neither the authors nor the publisher nor any other party who has been involved in the preparation or publication of this work warrants that the information contained herein is in every respect accurate or complete, and they disclaim all responsibility for any errors or omissions or for the results obtained from use of the information contained in this work. Readers are encouraged to confirm the information contained herein with other sources. For example and in particular, readers are advised to check the product information sheet included in the package of each drug they plan to administer to be certain that the information contained in this work is accurate and that changes have not been made in the recommended dose or in the contraindications for administration. This recommendation is of particular importance in connection with new or infrequently used drugs.

Multimodal Cardiovascular Imaging

Principles and Clinical Applications

Olle Pahlm, MD, PhD
Professor of Clinical Physiology, Lund University
Senior Consultant, Center for Imaging and Physiology
Skåne University Hospital
Lund, Sweden

Galen S. Wagner, MD
Associate Professor of Medicine
Duke University Senior Faculty of the
Duke Clinical Research Institute
Duke University Medical Center
Durham, North Carolina, USA

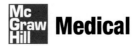

New York   Chicago   San Francisco   Lisbon   London   Madrid   Mexico City
Milan   New Delhi   San Juan   Seoul   Singapore   Sydney   Toronto

WG
141
.M962
2011

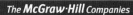
The McGraw-Hill Companies

Multimodal Cardiovascular Imaging: Principles and Clinical Applications

Copyright © 2011 by The McGraw-Hill Companies, Inc. All rights reserved. Printed in China. Except as permitted under the United States Copyright Act of 1976, no part of this publication may be reproduced or distributed in any form or by any means, or stored in a data base or retrieval system, without the prior written permission of the publisher.

1 2 3 4 5 6 7 8 9 0   CTP/CTP   14 13 12 11

Set ISBN 978-0-07-161346-0
Set MHID 0-07-161346-3
Book ISBN 978-0-07-161348-4
Book MHID 0-07-161348-X
DVD ISBN 978-0-07-161349-1
DVD MHID 0-07-161349-8

This book was set in Minion by Glyph International.
The editors were James Shanahan and Christine Diedrich.
The production supervisor was Phil Galea.
Project management was provided by Vipra Fauzdar, Glyph International.
The designer was Alan Barnett; the cover designer was Anthony Landi.
China Translation & Printing Services, Ltd. was printer and binder.

Cataloging-in-Publication Data is on file with the Library of Congress

McGraw-Hill books are available at special quantity discounts to use as premiums and sales promotions, or for use in corporate training programs. To contact a representative please e-mail us at bulksales@mcgraw-hill.com.

This book is dedicated to our wives, Elisabet and Marilyn, for providing the multimodal realities that balance our multimodal imaginations.

CONTENTS

Contributors ix

Acknowledgments xv

Introduction 01
Olle Pahlm, Galen Wagner, Nina Hakačova, and Ljuba Bacharova

SECTION I

Current Methods and Their Applications for Cardiovascular Multimodal Imaging

1. Echocardiography 07
Sebastian T. Palmeri, Liliana Cohen, and Daniel M. Shindler

2. Phonocardiography 41
Anna-Leena Noponen, Sakari Lukkarinen, and Raimo Sepponen

3. Myocardial Perfusion Single Photon Emission Computed Tomography and Positron Emission Tomography 50
Marcus Carlsson and Juhani Knuuti

4. Coronary Angiography 71
Kjell C. Nikus

5. Cardiac Computed Tomography. 81
Monvadi B. Srichai and João A. C. Lima

6. Cardiac Magnetic Resonance Imaging in Ischemic Heart Disease 104
Erik Hedström, Martin Ugander, and Håkan Arheden

7. Electrocardiography of Ischemic Heart Disease 128
Henrik Engblom and David G. Strauss

8. Electrophysiologic Mapping 146
Donald D. Hegland, Kevin P. Jackson, and James P. Daubert

9. Nuclear Cardiology Applied to Electrophysiology. 171
Philippe Chevalier, Roland Itti, and Laurence V. Bontemps

10. Optical Mapping of Electrical Activity 179
Jiashin Wu, Hiroshi Morita, and Douglas P. Zipes

11. Dipolar Electrocardiotopography Imaging . . 191
Ljuba Bacharova and Anton Mateasik

SECTION II

Foundations of Future Methods for Cardiovascular Multimodal Imaging

12. Electrocardiographic Imaging of Epicardial Potentials. 205
Fady Dawoud, John L. Sapp, John C. Clements, and B. Milan Horáček

13. Electromechanical Modeling Applied to Cardiac Resynchronization Therapy. 222
Jason Constantino, Viatcheslav Gurev, and Natalia A. Trayanova

14. Computational Cardiac Electrophysiology: Modeling Tissue and Organ. 233
Martin J. Bishop, Hermenegild J. Arevalo, Patrick M. Boyle, Natalia A. Trayanova, Edward Vigmond, and Gernot Plank

15. Cardiac Simulation for Education: The Electrocardiogram According to ECGSIM . . . 266
Adriaan van Oosterom and Thom F. Oostendorp

16. Graphical Analysis of Heart Rate Patterns to Assess Cardiac Autonomic Function. 284
Phyllis K. Stein and Panagiotis Pantazopoulos

17. Development of the Heart, with Particular Reference to the Cardiac Conduction Tissues 299
Robert H. Anderson, Aleksander Sizarov, and Antoon F. M. Moorman

SECTION III

Cardiovascular Multimodal Imaging in Key Clinical Problems

18. Congenital Heart Disease: Atrioventricular Septal Defect 315
Nina Hakačova

19. Right Ventricular Cardiomyopathies 322
Vincent L. Sorrell, Julia H. Indik, Nishant Kalra, and Frank I. Marcus

20. Ischemic Heart Disease 354

*Brian B. Ghoshhajra, Ricardo C. Cury, and
Richard D. White*

21. Acute Myocardial Infarction 360

*Joey F. A. Ubachs, Lia E. Bang, Jacob T. Lønborg,
Philip Hasbak, Nina Hakačova,
and Galen S. Wagner*

22. Diseases of the Aorta 368

Igor Mamkin and John F. Heitner

23. Peripheral Vascular Disease 392

Rajan Hundal, Anthony DeFrance, and Peter S. Fail

24. Pulmonary Vascular Disease 402

Stephen F. Crawley and Andrew J. Peacock

25. Atrial Fibrillation 420

Rob MacLeod and J. J. E. Blauer

Index 433

CONTRIBUTORS

Robert H. Anderson, BSc, MD, FRCPath
Visiting Professor
Institute of Human Genetics
University of Newcastle
London, United Kingdom

Hermenegild J. Arevalo, BS
Institute of Computational Medicine
Johns Hopkins University
Baltimore, Maryland, USA

Håkan Arheden, MD, PhD
Professor
Department of Clinical Physiology
Lund University
Skåne University Hospital
Lund, Sweden

Ljuba Bacharova, MD, PhD, MBA
Department of Biophotonics
International Laser Center
Bratislava, Slovak Republic

Lia E. Bang, MD, PhD
Department of Cardiology
Copenhagen University Hospital, The Heart Center
Copenhagen, Denmark

Martin J. Bishop, MPhys, DPhil
Wellcome Trust Postdoctoral Research Fellow
Computing Laboratory
University of Oxford
Oxford, United Kingdom

J. J. E. Blauer, BS
Department of Bioengineering
Comprehensive Arrhythmia Research and Management Center
Scientific Computing and Imaging Institute
Salt Lake City, Utah, USA

Laurence V. Bontemps, PhD
Assistant Professor
Department of Nuclear Medicine
Claude Bernard University Lyon 1
Hospices Civils de Lyon
Lyon, France

Patrick M. Boyle, BSc
PhD Candidate
Department of Electrical and Computer Engineering
University of Calgary
Calgary, Alberta, Canada

Marcus Carlsson, MD, PhD
Associate Professor
Department of Clinical Physiology
Lund University
Skåne University Hospital
Lund, Sweden

Phillippe Chevalier, MD, PhD
Head of Arrhythmia Unit
Hôpital Louis Pradel
Hospices Civils de Lyon
Lyon, France

John C. Clements, PhD
School of Biomedical Engineering
Dalhousie University
Halifax, Nova Scotia, Canada

Liliana Cohen, MD
Assistant Professor of Medicine
University of Medicine & Dentistry of New Jersey
Robert Wood Johnson Medical School
New Brunswick, New Jersey, USA

Jason Constantino, BS
Graduate Student
Department of Biomedical Engineering
Institute of Computational Medicine
Johns Hopkins University
Baltimore, Maryland, USA

Stephen F. Crawley, MBChB
Clinical Research Fellow
Scottish Pulmonary Vascular Unit
Golden Jubilee National Hospital
Glasgow, United Kingdom

Ricardo C. Cury, MD, FSCCT
Medical Director of Cardiac MRI and CT
Baptist Cardiac & Vascular Institute
Baptist Hospital of Miami
Miami, Florida, USA
Consultant Radiologist
Massachusetts General Hospital
Boston, Massachusetts, USA

James P. Daubert, MD
Professor of Medicine
Chief, Clinical Cardiac Electrophysiology
Duke University Medical Center
Durham, North Carolina, USA

Fady Dawoud, PhD
School of Biomedical Engineering
Dalhousie University
Halifax, Nova Scotia, Canada

Anthony DeFrance, MD
Clinical Associate Professor
Stanford University
Palo Alto, California, USA

Henrik Engblom, MD, PhD
Department of Clinical Physiology
Lund University
Skåne University Hospital
Lund, Sweden

Peter S. Fail, MD, FACC, FACP, FSCAI
Director of Cardiac Catheterization Laboratories
Interventional Research and CT Imaging
Cardiovascular Institute of the South
Houma, Louisiana, USA

Brian B. Ghoshhajra, MD, MBA
Instructor in Radiology
Harvard Medical School
Director, Cardiac MRI
Cardiac CT PET MR Program
The Massachusetts General Hospital
Boston, Massachusetts, USA

Viatcheslav Gurev, PhD
Associate Research Scholar
Department of Biomedical Engineering
Institute of Computational Medicine
Johns Hopkins University
Baltimore, Maryland, USA

Nina Hakačova, MD, PhD
Children's Heart Centre
Skåne University Hospital
Lund, Sweden

Philip Hasbak, MD, PhD
Chief Physician
Department of Clinical Physiology, Nuclear Medicine, & PET
Rigshospitalet, Copenhagen University Hospital
Copenhagen, Denmark

Erik Hedström, MD, PhD
Department of Clinical Physiology
Lund University
Skåne University Hospital
Lund, Sweden

Donald D. Hegland, MD
Medical Instructor
Duke University Medical Center
Durham, North Carolina, USA

John F. Heitner, MD
Director, Noninvasive Cardiology
Division of Cardiovascular Diseases
New York Methodist Hospital
Weill Cornell Medical College
Brooklyn, New York, USA

B. Milan Horáček, PhD
Professor
Department of Medicine
Dalhousie University
Halifax, Nova Scotia, Canada

Rajun Hundal, MD, MA
California Pacific Medical Center
San Francisco, California, USA

Julia H. Indik, MD, PhD
Associate Professor of Medicine
Sarver Heart Center
University Medical Center
Tucson, Arizona, USA

Roland Itti, MD, PhD
Professor, Department of Nuclear Medicine
Claude Bernard University Lyon 1
Hospices Civils de Lyon
Lyon, France

Kevin P. Jackson, MD
Clinical Cardiac Electrophysiology
Duke University Medical Center
Durham, North Carolina, USA

Nishant Kalra, MD
Imaging Fellow, Department of Internal Medicine
Division of Cardiology
University of Arizona
Tucson, Arizona, USA

Juhani Knuuti, MD, PhD
Professor and Director
Turku PET Center
Turku University Hospital
Turku, Finland

João A.C. Lima, MD, MBA
Professor of Medicine
Director, Cardiovascular Imaging
Division of Cardiology
Johns Hopkins University
Baltimore, Maryland, USA

Jacob T. Lønborg, MD
Catheterization Laboratory
Department of Cardiology
Rigshospitalet, Copenhagen University Hospital
Copenhagen, Denmark

Sakari Lukkarinen, MSc
Researcher
Department of Electronics
Helsinki University of Technology
Espoo, Finland

Rob MacLeod, PhD
Scientific Computing and Imaging Institute
University of Utah
Bioengineering Department
Comprehensive Arrhythmia Research & Management Center
Cardiovascular Research and Training Institute
Salt Lake City, Utah, USA

Igor Mamkin, MD
Associate Director
Cardiovascular Disease Fellowship Program
Division of Cardiology
New York Methodist Hospital
Brooklyn, New York, USA

Frank I. Marcus, MD
Professor Emeritus
Department of Medicine
Sarver Medical Center
University Medical Center
Tucson, Arizona, USA

Anton Mateasik, RNDr, PhD
Department of Biophotonics
International Laser Center
Bratislava, Slovak Republic

Antoon F. M. Moorman, PhD
Department of Anatomy, Embryology, & Physiology
Academic Medical Center
University of Amsterdam
Meibergdreef, Amsterdam, The Netherlands

Hiroshi Morita, MD, PhD
Assistant Professor
Department of Cardiovascular Medicine
Okayama University Graduate School of Medicine, Dentistry and Pharmaceutical Sciences
Okayama, Japan

Kjell C. Nikus, MD
Specialist in Internal Medicine
Senior Consultant in Cardiology
Heart Center
Tampere University Hospital
Tampere, Finland

Anna-Leena Noponen, MD, PhD
Pediatric Cardiology
Jorvi Hospital
Department of Pediatric and Adolescent Medicine
Helsinki University Central Hospital
Helsinki, Finland

Thom F. Oostendorp, MD
Donders Institute for Brain, Cognition, and Behavior
Radboud University Nijmegen Medical Center
Nijmegen, The Netherlands

Olle Pahlm, MD, PhD
Professor of Clinical Physiology, Lund University
Senior Consultant, Center for Imaging and Physiology
Skåne University Hospital
Lund, Sweden

Sebastian T. Palmeri, MD
Division of Cardiovascular Diseases
University of Medicine & Dentistry of New Jersey
Robert Wood Johnson Medical School
New Brunswick, New Jersey, USA

Panagiotis Pantazopoulos, MD, MS
Research Assistant
Cardiovascular Division
Washington University School of Medicine
St. Louis, Missouri, USA

Andrew J. Peacock, MD, FRCP
Director
Scottish Pulmonary Vascular Unit
University of Glasgow
Glasgow, United Kingdom

Gernot Plank, PhD
Associate Professor
Institute of Biophysics
Medical University of Graz
Graz, Austria
Oxford e-Research Centre
University of Oxford
Oxford, United Kingdom

John L. Sapp, MD
Queen Elizabeth II Hearts Sciences Centre
Department of Medicine (Cardiology)
Dalhousie University
Halifax, Nova Scotia, Canada

Raimo Sepponen, DSc
Professor
Department of Electronics
Helsinki University of Technology
Espoo, Finland

Daniel M. Shindler, MD, FACE
University of Medicine & Dentistry of New Jersey
Robert Wood Johnson Medical School
New Brunswick, New Jersey, USA

Aleksander Sizarov, MD
Department of Anatomy Embryology & Physiology
Academic Medical Center
University of Amsterdam
Meibergdreef, Amsterdam, The Netherlands

Vincent L. Sorrell, MD, FACC, FASE
Professor, Cardiology, Radiology, Pediatrics
The Allan C. Hudson & Helen Lovaas Chair of Cardiac Imaging
University of Arizona
Sarver Heart Center
Tucson, Arizona, USA

Monvadi B. Srichai, MD, FAHA, FACC
Assistant Professor
Departments of Radiology and Medicine
New York University School of Medicine
New York, New York, USA

Phyllis K. Stein, PhD
Research Associate Professor of Medicine
Cardiovascular Division
Director of Heart Rate Variability Laboratory
Washington University School of Medicine
St. Louis, Missouri, USA

David G. Strauss, MD, PhD
Division of Cardiology
Department of Medicine
Johns Hopkins University
Baltimore, Maryland, USA

Natalia A. Trayanova, PhD
Professor
Department of Biomedical Engineering
Institute of Computational Medicine
Johns Hopkins University
Baltimore, Maryland, USA

Joey F. A. Ubachs, MD
Department of Clinical Physiology
Lund University
Skåne University Hospital
Lund, Sweden

Martin Ugander, MD, PhD
Research Fellow, Cardiovascular MRI
Laboratory of Cardiac Energetics
National Heart, Lung, and Blood Institute
National Institutes of Health
Bethesda, Maryland, USA

Adriaan van Oosterom, PhD
Professor Emeritus
Radboud University
Nijmegen, The Netherlands

Edward Vigmond, PhD
Department of Electrical & Computer Engineering
University of Calgary
Calgary, Alberta, Canada

Galen S. Wagner, MD
Associate Professor of Medicine
Duke University Senior Faculty of the Duke Clinical
Research Institute
Duke University Medical Center
Durham, North Carolina, USA

Richard D. White, MD, FACR, FACC, FAHA, FSCCT
Professor and Chairman
Department of Radiology
University of Florida College of Medicine
Jacksonville, Florida, USA

Jiashin Wu, PhD
Director, Electrophysiology Core
College of Medicine
Department of Molecular Pharmacology and Physiology
University of South Florida
Tampa, Florida, USA

Douglas P. Zipes, MD
Distinguished Professor
Professor Emeritus of Medicine, Pharmacology, and Toxicology
Director Emeritus, Division of Cardiology
Krannert Institute of Cardiology
Indiana University School of Medicine
Indianapolis, Indiana, USA

ACKNOWLEDGMENTS

The idea for creating a book on cardiovascular multimodal imaging originated during a meeting between us and McGraw-Hill Editor Ruth Weinberg in Durham, North Carolina, in September 2007. We are very appreciative of Ruth for her initiative to look into the future of cardiovascular medicine to find new aspects that would be of increasing importance. During the planning phase of the manuscript, we were very fortunate to have several conversations with Professor Håkan Arheden, Clinical Physiology at Lund University, who has both clinical and scientific experience in the various cardiovascular imaging modalities. Håkan suggested the concept of developing a "matrix approach" by including both the individual modalities and the common clinical problems potentially addressed by multimodal imaging. Håkan recruited his Lund colleague, Dr. Martin Ugander, to think further with us about how the publication might best include electronic material in addition to print formats.

We also express appreciation to Drs. Ljuba Bacharova and Nina Hakačova for their many creative contributions at the various stages in the evolution of this publishing venture. They eagerly volunteered to develop key book chapters, coauthored the introductory chapter with us, and created the art for the book cover.

We are grateful to McGraw-Hill's Editor-in-Chief for Internal Medicine, Jim Shanahan, who assumed responsibility for the book, and to Christine Diedrich, Developmental Editor, who worked diligently with the authors in developing their chapters through the many "loose ends" required for book completion. Christine's courteous and firm communication with each of these experts has brought the various pieces of this enterprise together.

We express our great appreciation to the authors of these 25 chapters for their patience with us and their persistence with timely completion of responsibilities. We especially acknowledge their willingness to stretch their imagination in the newly emerging field of multimodal imaging.

We have known and worked with Beverly Perkins over many years in our various capacities in medical research and publishing and have observed her "magical" communication with the wide varieties of participating personalities. The success of the overall process was only possible because of her consistent management of all aspects of the production of this book.

Olle Pahlm and Galen Wagner

INTRODUCTION

Olle Pahlm, Galen S. Wagner, Nina Hakacova, and
Ljuba Bacharova

SECTIONS I AND II OVERVIEW / 1

SECTION III OVERVIEW / 1

CHALLENGES OF MMI / 3

STEPS IN MMI CONSIDERATION / 3
    Adding Information From Multiple Imaging Modalities / 3
    Side-by-Side Comparison of the Information from Different
        Imaging Modalities / 3
    Conversion of a One- or Two-Dimensional Imaging Modality
        Into Three-Dimensional Myocardial Anatomy / 3
    Converting an ECG Into an Image for Side-by-Side Comparison
        With Other Imaging Modalities / 3
    Fusion of Information from Multiple Imaging Modalities / 3

During the past several decades, many diagnostic cardiovascular modalities have been developed. Combining these into multimodal imaging (MMI) creates enhanced decision support for clinical management of patients with cardiovascular disease.

Progression from additive consideration of the primary data from different modalities, to side-by-side comparison of the different images, to superimposition of the structural and functional characteristics of the different images, provides the increased understanding required for optimal improvement of clinical diagnosis. Multimodal imaging is also a way to continually update and reevaluate paradigms of individual diagnostic methods.

In this book, a team of distinguished authors—clinicians as well as computer scientists, mathematicians, and physicists—has been brought together to provide a wide range of aspects important to the development and use of MMI. The authors have been requested to confine their chapters to their own area of interest and expertise and to include both their current experiences and future considerations.

The chapters are divided into three sections based on the perspectives of the authors. Sections I and II contain chapters that focus on a *single diagnostic modality* and its broad application in clinical cardiovascular conditions. Section III contains chapters that focus on a *single clinical condition* and how MMI can provide decision support. This format provides duplication of information in chapters in the sections of the book.

SECTIONS I AND II OVERVIEW

In Table I–1, the imaging modalities included in the 17 chapters in Sections I and II are presented as columns, and the general clinical conditions for which they provide diagnostic capability are presented as rows. The modalities are ordered according to the sequence of chapters and are numbered from 1 to 17 accordingly. Some of the modalities are considered in more than one chapter in Section I.

Chapters in Section I include many modalities that currently produce direct images of cardiovascular structures and their function (eg, coronary angiography, echocardiography, SPECT, and magnetic resonance imaging). Because the inexpensive and widely available electrocardiogram (ECG) is now being developed into an imaging modality, several chapters are devoted to considering the perspectives of standard scalar ECG, spatial dipolar electrocardiotopographic [DECARTO] imaging, the inverse problem of ECG (ie, deducing cardiac excitation patterns from body surface recordings), and autonomic modulation. Section II covers the emerging technologies that are leading to the creation of direct imaging of cardiac activation and recovery. This requires extensive mathematical modeling by physicists, engineers, and computer scientists in concert with the academic clinician-investigators who will ultimately use the methods for their diagnostic and therapeutic decision support. Three of the imaging modalities that exist as simulations or models, rather than as clinically available methods, are considered in dedicated chapters: "Cardiac Simulation for Education: Electromechanical Modeling Applied to Cardiac Resynchronization Therapy" (Chapter 13 by Constantino et al), "Computational Cardiac Electrophysiology: Modeling Tissue and Organ" (Chapter 14 by Bishop et al), and The Electrocardiogram According to ECGSIM" (Chapter 15 by van Oosterom et al). These methods are currently used to guide clinical investigators in the development and evaluation of new cardiovascular therapies and might be developed into clinically useful tools in the future.

Some explanations about the various modalities might be helpful. *Coronary angiography* refers only to radiographic visualization of intra-arterial contrast. The chapters on the common general clinical imaging methods (eg, echocardiography) include the many specific adaptations in which those methods are employed (eg, imaging of blood flow based on the Doppler principle; conventional precordial, transesophageal, and intracardiac imaging).

SECTION III OVERVIEW

In Table I–2, the eight chapters presenting the use of MMI for decision support in the various clinical conditions in Section III are presented in the seven columns, and the individual modalities are presented as rows. The clinical conditions are ordered according to the sequence of chapters, which are numbered from 18 to 25. Some of the clinical conditions listed in Table I–1 do not appear in Table I–2 because in Section III, no chapter dedicated to that condition (eg, valve disease) has been included. Also, some of the imaging modalities listed in Table I–1 do not appear in Table I–2 because none of the authors in Section III has elected to consider that modality (eg, optical imaging).

Chapters in Section III emphasize how MMI can be used for diagnosis and therapeutic decision support for various cardiac conditions (eg, congenital heart diseases, ventricular cardiomyopathies, myocardial ischemia/infarction). A broad spectrum of

TABLE I–1. Imaging Modalities in Sections I and II

	Echo-cardiography	Phono-cardiography	Nuclear Cardiology	Coronary Angiography	CT	MRI	ECG	Optical Mapping	Modeling	Simulation	Fetal Development
Congenital Heart Disease	1	2			5					15	17
Cardiomyopathies	1		3, 9				11, 16		13		
Valvular Heart Disease	1	2									
Ischemic Heart Disease	1		3, 6	4	5	6, 7, 8	7,9, 11,16			15	
Aortic Disease					5						
Pulmonary Vascular Disease					5	8					
Tachyarrhythmias	1, 8		8, 9		8	8	8,12	10	14		
Pericardial Disease	1				5						
Cardio-Neurological Disorders			9				16				
Cardiac Masses					5						

CT, computed tomography; ECG, electrocardiography; MRI, magnetic resonance imaging.

cardiovascular conditions has been included with no attempt to fit the size of the chapters to the clinical importance of the conditions. Rather, the authors selected the breadth to include in their chapter based on both interest and expertise.

Some chapters provide case reports of how academic clinicians/scientists are currently using MMI modalities to improve their clinical therapeutic decision support (eg, Chapter 21 by Ubachs et al).

TABLE I–2. Clinical Conditions in Section III

	Congenital Heart Disease	Cardiomyopathies	Ischemic Heart Disease	Aortic Disease	Peripheral Vascular Disease	Pulmonary Vascular Disease	Tachyarrhythmias
Echocardiography	18	19	20	22		24	25
Nuclear Cardiology		19	20, 21			24	
Coronary Angiography		19	20, 21	22			
CT		19	20	22	23	24	
MRI	18	19	20, 21	22	23	24	25
ECG	18		21			24	25
Fetal Development	18						

CT, computed tomography; ECG, electrocardiography; MRI, magnetic resonance imaging.

CHALLENGES OF MMI

It should be emphasized that the pathway toward successful integration of information from multiple imaging modalities is challenging. A common question is how to consider discordant results when performing combination imaging. The MMI approach extends beyond the traditional concept where one method is compared with a gold standard method to the new concept that each modality provides unique diagnostic information. Traditionally, when discrepancies with the gold standard modality occur, the term "false" is often used. The discrepant results are assigned as *false negative* or *false positive*, and these false results may diminish the perceived value of a certain modality in the diagnostic decision making. The alternative consideration in MMI is that different diagnostic imaging modalities are based on different biophysical principles. Therefore, they each provide different information and visualize different specific characteristics of the same structures or functions. Thus, both agreements and disagreements between the results of particular modalities may have their own specific diagnostic value.

STEPS IN MMI CONSIDERATION

The perspective of a step-wise approach to the means of combining several imaging modalities to provide understanding of cardiovascular pathophysiologic processes is presented in Figure I–1 and described in the following sections.

■ ADDING INFORMATION FROM MULTIPLE IMAGING MODALITIES

Each modality provides its own means of displaying primary information about the heart, and each method is interpreted separately. Selected aspects of the result of applying the various individual modalities are then sequentially related. For example, to the information about cardiac dysfunction by echocardiography, a myocardial scintigram may add the information that the dysfunction is caused by reduced myocardial perfusion.

■ SIDE-BY-SIDE COMPARISON OF THE INFORMATION FROM DIFFERENT IMAGING MODALITIES

This approach provides a tool to test the accuracy of a more available method comparing it to the less available method considered as a reference. As pointed out earlier, it needs to be kept in mind that different diagnostic imaging methods are often based on different biophysical principles and thus provide more or less different information and visualize

different specific characteristics of the same structures or functions. Disagreements between the results of particular methods may therefore have their own specific diagnostic value.

■ CONVERSION OF A ONE- OR TWO-DIMENSIONAL IMAGING MODALITY INTO THREE-DIMENSIONAL MYOCARDIAL ANATOMY

Using sophisticated methods of image processing, the recordings of one imaging modality can be transformed into three-dimensional (3D) images. This conversion can provide better understanding of the structure and function of the heart in an individual patient. An example is the conversion of the two-dimensional echocardiographic images of the heart valves into 3D images.

■ CONVERTING AN ECG INTO AN IMAGE FOR SIDE-BY-SIDE COMPARISON WITH OTHER IMAGING MODALITIES

An ECG can be projected onto a 3D image of a digital heart model and then compared with information from other imaging methods. This provides a strong tool for understanding electrofunctional and anatomic characteristics of the heart. An example is the projection of an ECG showing infarction into a DECARTO plot that indicates size and localization of the infarcted area. The DECARTO plot can then be directly compared with a method for assessment of myocardial perfusion (eg, SPECT imaging).

■ FUSION OF INFORMATION FROM MULTIPLE IMAGING MODALITIES

Fusion of images may make the resulting image more informative than any of the input images. An example is the superimposition of the 3D model of the infarcted area by one modality onto an initially ischemic area by another modality for assessment of myocardial salvage.

Rapid development of new imaging modalities is opening extensive opportunities in imaging the cardiovascular system from anatomic, pathophysiologic, and electrophysiologic perspectives. McGraw-Hill publishes the cardiovascular text *Hurst's The Heart*, and this book on cardiovascular MMI can be considered as a complementary volume. The mission of this book is to introduce several levels of integration of multimodality information—with the patient both at the beginning and at the end of the MMI chain.

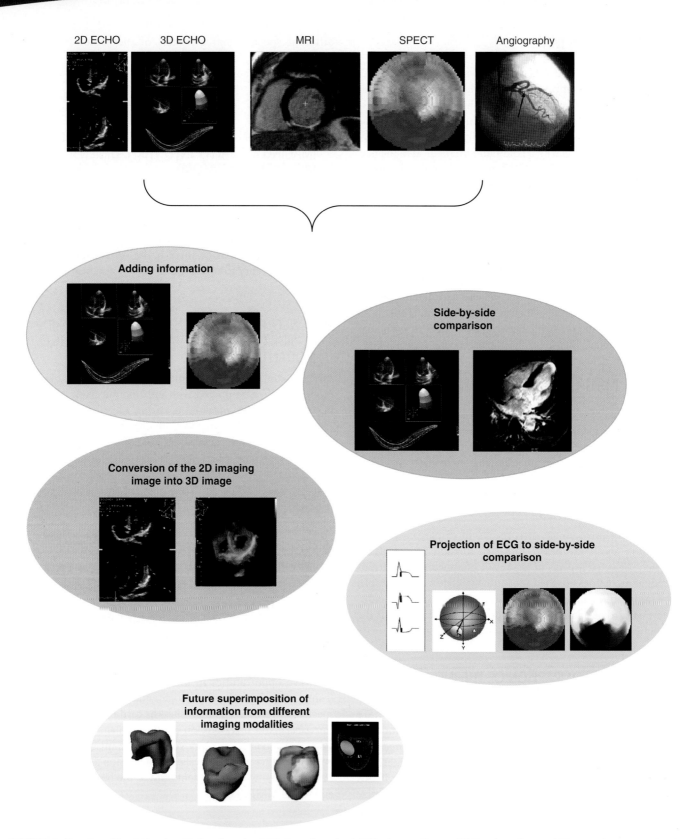

FIGURE I–1. Steps in multimodal imaging. 2D, two dimensional; 3D, three dimensional; ECG, electrocardiogram; ECHO, echocardiogram; MRI, magnetic resonance imaging; SPECT, single photon emission computed tomography. Reprinted from *Journal of Electrocardiology,* 42(2), Hakacova N, Cardiac imaging of anatomy and electrocardiology–hand in hand in future steps, Copyright March-April 2009, with permission from Elsevier.

SECTION I

Current Methods and Their Applications for Cardiovascular Multimodal Imaging

1. Echocardiography 7

2. Phonocardiography 41

3. Myocardial Perfusion Single Photon Emission Computed Tomography and Positron Emission Tomography 50

4. Coronary Angiography 71

5. Cardiac Computed Tomography 81

6. Cardiac Magnetic Resonance Imaging in Ischemic Heart Disease 104

7. Electrocardiography of Ischemic Heart Disease 130

8. Electrophysiologic Mapping 146

9. Nuclear Cardiology Applied to Electrophysiology 171

10. Optical Mapping of Electrical Activity 179

11. Dipolar Electrocardiotopography Imaging 191

CHAPTER 1
ECHOCARDIOGRAPHY

Sebastian T. Palmeri, Liliana Cohen, and Daniel M. Shindler

INTRODUCTION / 7

PHYSICS / 7
Sound / 7
Echocardiography Systems / 7
Doppler Principles / 8
Color Flow Doppler / 9

NORMAL CARDIAC ECHO DOPPLER EXAMINATION / 9
Standard Imaging Views / 9

ASSESSMENT OF LEFT VENTRICULAR SYSTOLIC AND
DIASTOLIC FUNCTION / 14
Left Ventricular Systolic Function / 14
LV Diastolic Function / 15
Stress Echocardiography / 19

CLINICAL CASE STUDIES / 20
Case 1: Congestive Heart Failure / 20
Case 2: Hypertension / 21
Case 3: Arrhythmias / 22
Case 4: Mitral Regurgitation / 23
Case 5: Cerebrovascular Accident/Syncope / 25
Case 6: Heart Murmurs / 28
Case 7: Chest Pain / 33
Case 8: Acute Pericarditis / 35
Case 9: Infective Endocarditis / 36
Case 10: Routine Screening / 37

CONCLUSION / 38

INTRODUCTION

Since the 1950s when Edler and Hertz[1,2] in Lund, Sweden, recorded ultrasonic images of the heart walls and normal and rheumatic mitral valves, echocardiography has assumed a central role in the diagnosis and management of most cardiac disorders.

The purpose of this chapter is to examine the role of modern echocardiography from the perspective of the general practitioner. After a brief summary of the salient technical aspects of echocardiography and the elements of a normal echocardiographic examination, 10 clinical vignettes will be presented to illustrate the central role of echocardiography in contemporary medicine.

PHYSICS

■ SOUND

Sound is a mechanical phenomenon involving the transfer of energy through a medium. Ultrasound occurs in nature as illustrated by certain bat species that use ultrasound to navigate and to identify prey. The dog whistle is an example of a simple man-made ultrasound device.

A sound wave is generally depicted as a sine wave. Sound is defined by its amplitude, wavelength (λ) (the distance between cycles), and its frequency (f), the number of cycles in a given period of time (Fig. 1–1). Velocity ($v = f \times \lambda$) is the speed at which a sound wave travels through a particular medium or body tissue. Velocity is dependent on the physical properties of the tissue and its acoustic impedance, which is primarily determined by the tissue's density.

The frequency of a sound wave is measured in hertz (Hz). One cycle per second is 1 Hz. Ultrasound is sound above the audible range, having a frequency greater than 20,000 cycles per second (20 kHz). In clinical medicine, transducers create ultrasound waves with much higher frequencies, ranging from 2 to 15 MHz. Higher frequency transducers give superior near-field resolution but have less tissue depth penetration.

A sound wave will travel in a relatively straight line through a homogeneous medium with some attenuation due to absorption and scatter until it reaches an interface between media with different densities. At the interface, the sound wave will undergo reflection and refraction proportional to the different densities of the two tissues (Fig. 1–2).

■ ECHOCARDIOGRAPHY SYSTEMS

Modern commercial ultrasound systems are comprised of three basic components: a transducer that serves as a sound originator and as a receiver, a computer, and a display monitor. The ultrasound transducer contains piezoelectric elements, which were originally quartz but are now complex ceramics.

The piezoelectric effect was described by the brothers Jacques and Pierre Curie in 1880.[3-5] The brothers discovered that mechanical stress caused certain crystals to alter their shape and produce an electrical charge proportional to the mechanical stress (Fig. 1–3). This property is now referred to as reverse piezoelectricity. Commercial uses of piezoelectric elements include the igniters in gas grills and triggers for automobile air bags.

Piezoelectric elements also have the property of changing shape when placed in an electric field creating ultrasonic sound waves (Fig. 1–4). When functioning as a transducer as part of an ultrasound system, the piezoelectric elements are placed in an electric current, causing them to change shape and emit an ultrasonic wave.

Modern phased array ultrasound transducers contain several thousand piezoelectric elements that are focused electronically. This allows for some of the piezoelectric elements to transmit sound waves, while other elements are simultaneously receiving the returning sound waves, thereby creating continuous wave systems.

When functioning as a receiver of the reflected sound waves, the echoes, the piezoelectric elements change shape and create electrical pulses. The computer signal processor knows the amount of time from the moment that the transducer emitted the ultrasonic wave until it received the returning echo sound wave. Knowing the speed of ultrasonic waves through tissue (sound travels through water, the primary constituent of human soft tissue, at approximately 1540 m/s), the computer can then calculate the distance of the reflecting tissue from the transducer (Fig. 1–5).

Although the electronics are complex, the principles are simple. With this distance information, the computer creates visual analog or digital displays. Displaying the points over time allows

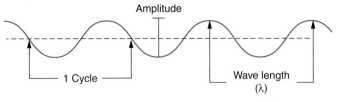

A: Sound wave elements.

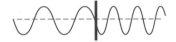

B: Sound waves with similar amplitudes but different frequencies.

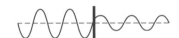

C: Sound waves with similar frequencies but different amplitudes.

FIGURE 1–1. Sound waves. **A.** Sine wave display of a sound wave. **B.** Two sound waves with similar amplitudes but different frequencies. **C.** Two sound waves with similar frequencies but different amplitudes.

for the graphic depiction of the heart, creating M-mode (time motion), and two-dimensional echocardiograms (Fig. 1–6).

■ DOPPLER PRINCIPLES

In 1842, the Austrian mathematician, Christian Doppler, presented a treatise entitled "On the Colored Light of Binary Stars and Certain Other Stars of the Heavens," in which he postulated that the perceived color of the light waves emanating from stars was affected by the motion of the stars. In 1845, the Dutch chemist and meteorologist Buys Ballot demonstrated the acoustic principles of the Doppler effect in a now classic experiment using musicians on a moving train to explain the

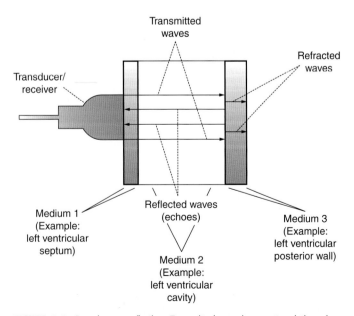

FIGURE 1–2. Sound wave reflection. Transmitted sound waves travel through a medium of one density until they come in contact with a medium of a different density at which the sound waves are reflected back toward their source.

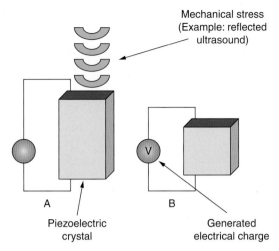

FIGURE 1–3. Reverse piezoelectricity. **A.** A piezoelectric element is struck by a mechanical force, in this case a reflected sound wave. **B.** When the piezoelectric element is struck by the mechanical force, it changes its shape and generates a proportional electric current.

perceived changes in a sound's pitch when it is emitted from a moving source.[6] To the stationary observer, the sound appears to increase in frequency (pitch) as the source approaches due to compression of the sound wave and to diminish in frequency as the source recedes (Fig. 1–7).

In echocardiography, the Doppler effect or shift is the difference between the frequency of the original transmitted sound wave compared with the frequency of the received sound waves caused by the motion of the reflecting tissue. The computer measures the Doppler shift and then uses this information to calculate the velocity of the moving reflecting target. In cardiac Doppler, the moving target has been red blood cells. Therefore, the Doppler shift can be used to provide the indirect assessment of the direction and velocity of blood, which in turn serve as the basis for echocardiographic-derived hemodynamic measurements. More contemporary tissue Doppler techniques assess the movement of actual cardiac structures, for example, the mitral valve annulus.

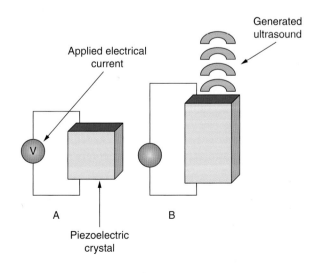

FIGURE 1–4. Piezoelectricity. **A.** An electric current is applied to a piezoelectric element causing it to change its shape. **B.** When the piezoelectric element changes its shape, it emits an ultrasound wave.

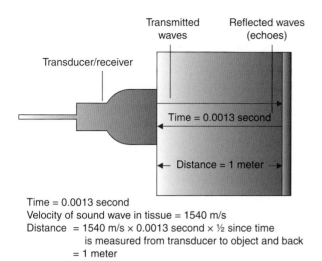

FIGURE 1–5. Distance calculations. Echocardiographic method of determining an object's distance from the transducer. In this example, the object is 1 meter from the transducer as calculated from the time for the transmitted sound wave to strike the distant object and be reflected back to the transducer. The distance information is used to construct structural images.

Time = 0.0013 second
Velocity of sound wave in tissue = 1540 m/s
Distance = 1540 m/s × 0.0013 second × ½ since time
is measured from transducer to object and back
= 1 meter

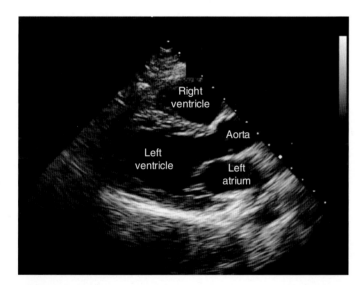

FIGURE 1–6. Parasternal long axis view. A two-dimensional parasternal long axis image of a normal heart.

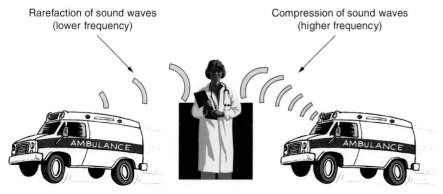

FIGURE 1–7. The Doppler shift principle. The sound heard by the observer is perceived to be of a higher pitch as the originating source approaches the observer and of a lower pitch as the source moves away from the observer.

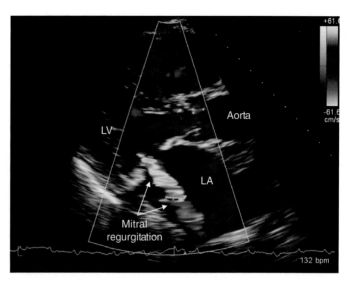

FIGURE 1–8. Color flow Doppler image. Parasternal long-axis color flow image of mitral valve regurgitation. LA, left atrium; LV, left ventricle.

An important practical point in clinical ultrasound imaging is that the angle between the transmitted sound waves and the path of the moving target is critical to the mathematical calculations. The more parallel the transmitted ultrasound is to the moving target, the more accurate the calculation of the target's velocity. At an angle of 90°, the Doppler shift cannot be recorded.

The opposite is true in two-dimensional echocardiography, in which the quality of the images is optimized when the structures are perpendicular to the transmitted ultrasound.

■ COLOR FLOW DOPPLER

Color flow Doppler provides a spatial display of blood flow velocity and direction. This is accomplished by having the transducer simultaneously transmit multiple sound waves in a predetermined sector. By measuring the Doppler frequency shift, blood flow velocity and direction are determined and displayed in two-dimensional space as a color map. This information is continuously updated during the cardiac cycle, providing real-time depictions of intracardiac blood flow velocity and direction. For example, a mitral regurgitant blood flow jet becomes recognizable when the Doppler color flow information is displayed superimposed on the real-time two-dimensional images of the mitral valve (Fig. 1–8).

NORMAL CARDIAC ECHO DOPPLER EXAMINATION

■ STANDARD IMAGING VIEWS

The standard cardiac echo Doppler clinical examination includes four basic transducer positions (Fig. 1–9) to obtain the following nine views:

1. Parasternal long axis

2. Right ventricular inflow/right ventricular outflow

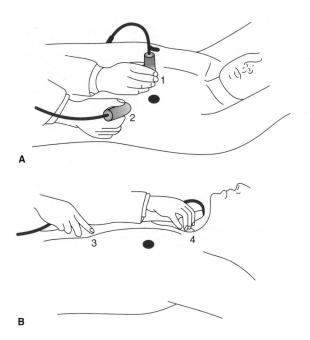

A

B

FIGURE 1–9. Transducer positions. Illustration of the four basic transducer positions for obtaining the standard transthoracic echocardiographic views. The patient is on his left side for transducer positions 1 (parasternal long axis) and 2 (apical) and flat on his back for positions 3 (subcostal) and 4 (suprasternal). Reproduced from Oh J, et al. *The Echo Manual.* Third Edition, 2006. By permission of Mayo Foundation for Medical Education and Research. All rights reserved.

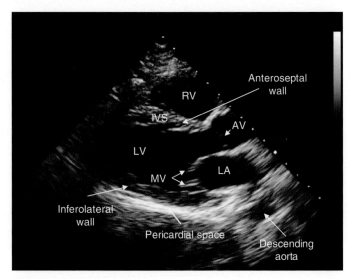

FIGURE 1–10. Parasternal long axis view. A parasternal long axis image is obtained with the patient lying on his left side; the transducer is positioned in the patient's fourth left intercostal space. AV, aortic valve; IVS, interventricular septum; LA, left atrium; LV, left ventricle; MV, mitral valve; RV, right ventricle.

3. Parasternal short axis
4. Apical four-chamber
5. Apical five-chamber
6. Apical two-chamber
7. Apical three-chamber
8. Subxiphoid four-chamber/short axis
9. Suprasternal notch

Each view typically includes a two-dimensional recording followed by M-mode, color flow, and Doppler recordings. The following sections and tables outline the cardiac structures and the most common two-dimensional and Doppler abnormalities for each of the echocardiographic views.

Parasternal Long Axis

With the patient lying on his or her left side, the transducer is placed at the left parasternal border in the fourth left intercostal space (position 1) (Fig. 1–10; Table 1–1).

Right Ventricular Inflow

Without changing the transducer's position on the patient's chest (position 1), the transducer is tilted inferiorly and angled medially to visualize the right atrium and the right ventricle (Fig. 1–11; Table 1–2).

TABLE 1–1. Cardiac Structures and Echo Doppler Abnormalities Evident in the Parasternal Long Axis View

Cardiac Structures	Echocardiographic Abnormalities	Doppler Abnormalities
Right ventricle	Dimensions Hypertrophy Ebstein anomaly Arrhythmogenic right ventricle	Ventricular septal defects
Aortic root	Dimensions Dissection	
Aortic valve	Leaflet thickness vegetations	Outflow obstruction • Aortic stenosis • Hypertrophic cardiomyopathy • Aortic insufficiency
Mitral valve	Leaflet appearance Mitral valve prolapse/flail Systolic anterior motion Mitral valve vegetations Mitral annular calcification	Stenosis Regurgitation
Left ventricle	Dimensions Hypertrophy Wall motion: anteroseptal and inferolateral walls	Muscular ventricular septal Defects
Septum	Atrial septal defects Atrial septal aneurysm	Intra-cardiac shunt
Pericardium	Effusion Tumors Cysts	

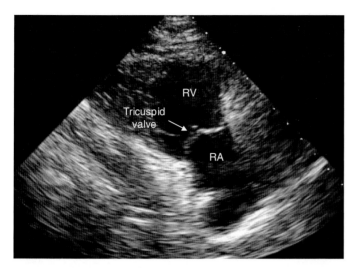

FIGURE 1–11. Right ventricular inflow view. A right ventricular inflow image is obtained with the patient and transducer positioned as in the parasternal long axis view. The transducer is tilted inferiorly and angled medially to provide images of the right atrium, the right ventricle, and the tricuspid valve. RA, right atrium; RV, right ventricle.

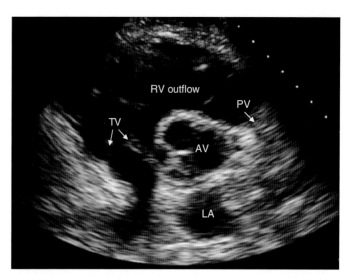

FIGURE 1–12. Parasternal short axis view. A parasternal short axis image is obtained by rotating the transducer 90° clockwise. Parasternal short axis views are generally obtained at the levels of the cardiac base, the mitral valve, the mid cavity, and the LV apex. This is a short axis image at the cardiac base. AV, aortic valve; LA, left atrium; PV, pulmonic valve; TV, tricuspid valve.

Right Ventricular Outflow

Without changing the transducer's position on the patient's chest (position 1), the transducer is tilted superiorly and angled laterly to visualize the pulmonary artery and the outflow of the right ventricle.

Parasternal Short Axis

Without changing the transducer's position on the patient's chest (position 1), the transducer is rotated 90° clockwise, and the heart is scanned from base to apex (Figs. 1–12 and 1–13; Table 1–3).

Apical Four-Chamber

The transducer is positioned at the patient's apex or point of maximal impulse. The ultrasound beam is directed toward the patient's right shoulder (position 2) (Fig. 1–14; Table 1–4).

Apical Five-Chamber

The transducer is angulated slightly anteriorly to bring the left ventricular outflow tract and the aortic valve into better definition (Fig. 1–15; Table 1–5).

Apical Two-Chamber

The transducer is positioned at the patient's cardiac apex as it is in the apical four-chamber and five-chamber views, but it is rotated 90° counterclockwise (Fig. 1–16; Table 1–6).

TABLE 1–2. Cardiac Structures and Echo Doppler Abnormalities Evident in the Right Ventricular Inflow View

Cardiac Structures	Echocardiographic Abnormalities	Doppler Abnormalities
Right atrium	Dimensions Masses Chiari network Eustachian valve	Membrane in the right atrium
Tricuspid valve	Leaflet thickness Vegetations	Stenosis Regurgitation
Right ventricle	Dimensions Wall thickness Contractility	

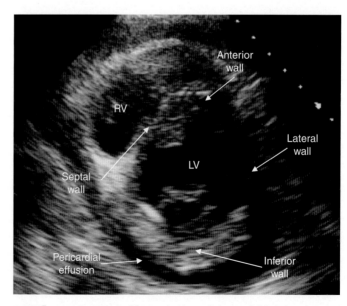

FIGURE 1–13. Parasternal mid LV cavity short axis image slightly below the mitral valve. LV, left ventricle; RV, right ventricle.

TABLE 1–3. Cardiac Structures and Echo Doppler Abnormalities Evident in the Parasternal Short Axis View

Cardiac Structures	Echocardiographic Abnormalities	Doppler Abnormalities
Proximal aorta	Aortic valve morphology	Membranous and supracristal ventricular septal defects
Right venricular outflow track	Infundibular stenosis	
Pulmonic valve	Appearance vegetations	Stenosis Regurgitation
Tricuspid valve	Appearance vegetations	Stenosis Regurgitation
Mitral valve	Appearance vegetations	Stenosis Regurgitation
Left ventricle: • Base • Mid cavity • Apex	Wall motion: anterior; septal; anteroseptal; lateral and inferior walls	

TABLE 1–4. Cardiac Structures and Echo Doppler Abnormalities Evident in the Apical Four-Chamber View

Cardiac Structures	Echocardiographic Abnormalities	Doppler Abnormalities
Left atrium	Dimensions Pulmonary veins	Atrial septal defects Patent foramen ovales Pulmonary blood flow
Left ventricle	Dimensions wall motion: inferoseptum; apex; and anterolateral walls Aneurysms Mural thrombus	
Right atrium	Dimensions Chiari network Eustachian valve	
Right ventricle	Dimensions Arrhythmogenic right ventricle	Ventricular septal defects
Mitral valve	Appearance	Stenosis Regurgitation
Tricuspid valve	Appearance Location	Stenosis insufficiency
Pericardial space	Effusion Tamponade: right atrial/right ventricular collapse	Tamponade: abnormal mitral inflow respiratory variation

Apical Three-Chamber

The transducer remains positioned at the patient's cardiac apex as it is in the apical four-chamber and five-chamber views, but it is rotated 180° counterclockwise (Fig. 1–17; Table 1–7).

Subxiphoid

The transducer is located in the patient's right upper quadrant directly below the xiphoid process (position 3). The ultrasound beam is directed at the patient's left shoulder. From this position,

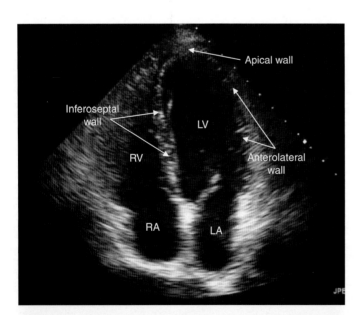

FIGURE 1–14. Apical four-chamber view. An apical four-chamber image is obtained with the patient lying flat or on his left side with the transducer positioned at the patient's point of maximal impulse and directed at his right shoulder. LA, left atrium; LV, left ventricle; RA, right atrium; RV, right ventricle.

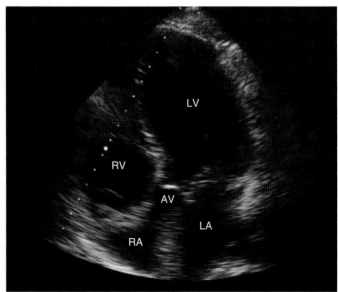

FIGURE 1–15. Apical five-chamber view. An apical five-chamber image is obtained with the patient and the transducer similarly positioned to the apical four-chamber view with slight anterior angulation to bring the left ventricular outflow tract into the plane of view. AV, aortic valve; LA, left atrium; LV, left ventricle; RA, right atrium; RV, right ventricle.

TABLE 1–5. Cardiac Structures and Echo Doppler Abnormalities Evident in the Apical Five-Chamber View

Cardiac Structures	Echocardiographic Abnormalities	Doppler Abnormalities
Left atrium	Dimensions	Atrial septal defects Patent foramen ovales
Left ventricle	Dimensions Wall motion: inferoseptum; apex; and lateral walls Aneurysm Mural Thrombus	
Right atrium	Dimensions	
Right ventricle	Dimensions	
Mitral valve	Appearance	Stenosis Regurgitation
Tricuspid valve	Appearance Location	Stenosis Regurgitation
Left ventricular outflow tract	Sub/supravalvular membranes	Obstruction Regurgitation

TABLE 1–6. Cardiac Structures and Echo Doppler Abnormalities Evident in the Apical Two-Chamber View

Cardiac Structures	Echocardiographic Abnormalities	Doppler Abnormalities
Left atrium	Dimensions Left atrial appendage	Atrial septal defect Patent foramen ovale
Left ventricle	Dimensions Wall motion: anterior; apex; and inferior walls	

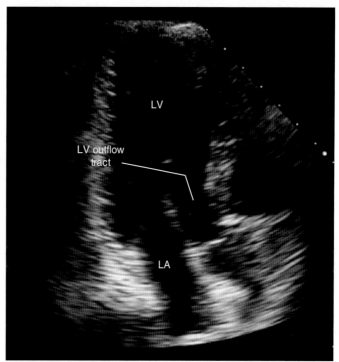

FIGURE 1–17. Apical three-chamber view. An apical three-chamber view is obtained with the patient and the transducer similarly positioned to the apical four-chamber view with the transducer rotated 180° counterclockwise. LA, left atrium; LV, left ventricle.

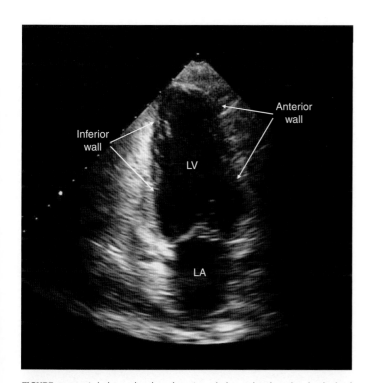

FIGURE 1–16. Apical two-chamber view. An apical two-chamber view is obtained with the patient and the transducer similarly positioned to the apical four-chamber view with the transducer rotated 90° counterclockwise. LA, left atrium; LV, left ventricle.

TABLE 1–7. Cardiac Structures and Echo Doppler Abnormalities Evident in the Apical Three-Chamber View

Cardiac Structures	Echocardiographic Abnormalities	Doppler Abnormalities
Left atrium	Dimensions	Atrial septal defect Patent foramen ovale
Left ventricle	Dimensions wall motion: anteroseptal; apex; and inferolateral	
Left ventricular outflow tract		

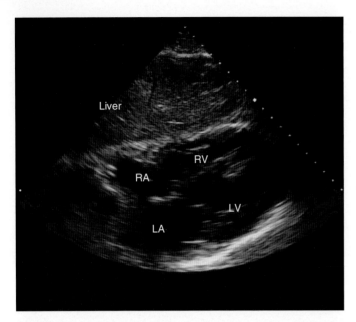

FIGURE 1–18. Subxiphoid/subcostal view. A subxiphoid/subcostal image is obtained with the patient lying flat with the transducer positioned below the patient's xiphoid process. The transducer is directed to the patient's left shoulder. LA, left atrium; LV, left ventricle; RA, right atrium; RV, right ventricle.

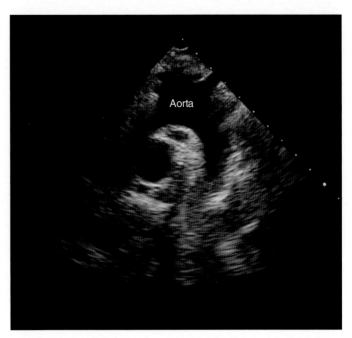

FIGURE 1–19. Suprasternal view. A suprasternal image is obtained with the patient lying flat and the transducer positioned in the patient's suprasternal notch. The ultrasound beam is directed anteriorly to image the ascending aorta and posteriorly and to the left to image the descending aorta.

the ultrasound waves travel through the patient's liver, a solid structure. This will often provide superior images in patients with severe chronic obstructive pulmonary disease (COPD) or morbid obesity in whom imaging in the standard parasternal positions often provides suboptimal images (Fig. 1–18; Table 1–8).

Suprasternal Notch

The transducer is positioned in the patient's suprasternal notch (position 4). The ultrasound beam is directed anteriorly and to

the right to image the ascending aorta and posteriorly and to the left to image the descending aorta (Fig. 1–19; Table 1–9).

ASSESSMENT OF LEFT VENTRICULAR SYSTOLIC AND DIASTOLIC FUNCTION

■ LEFT VENTRICULAR SYSTOLIC FUNCTION

The most common clinical indication for echocardiographic imaging is an assessment of left ventricular (LV) function. There are four methods of assessing LV systolic function:

- Visual inspection
- Contrast enhancement
- Regional wall motion scoring
- Quantitative methods
  - Fractional shortening
  - Simpson method

TABLE 1–8. Cardiac Structures and Echo Doppler Abnormalities Evident in the Subxiphoid/Subcostal View

Cardiac Structures	Cardiac Abnormalities	Doppler Abnormalities
Left atrium	Dimensions	Atrial septal defects Patent foramen ovale
Left ventricle	Dimensions Wall motion	
Right atrium	Dimensions	
Right ventricle	Dimensions Hypertrophy	Ventricular septal defects
Mitral valve	Appearance	Stenosis Regurgitation
Tricuspid valve	Appearance Location	Stenosis Regurgitation
Pericardial space	Effusion/tamponade	Tamponade
Inferior vena cava	Hepatic vein respiratory variation	Hepatic vein blood flow

TABLE 1–9. Cardiac Structures and Echo Doppler Abnormalities Evident in the Suprasternal View

Cardiac Structures	Echocardiographic Abnormalities	Doppler Abnormalities
Aorta	Atherosclerosis Aneurysmal dilatation Dissection	Aortic insufficiency Coarctation Patent ductus arteriosus
Pulmonary artery	Dimensions Pulmonary emboli	

TABLE 1–10. Visual Assessment of Global Left Ventricular Systolic Function

Visual Assessment	Approximate Left Ventricular Ejection Fraction (%)
Increased	>75
Normal	55-75
Mildly reduced	45-55
Moderately reduced	35-45
Severely reduced	<35

An accurate assessment of LV systolic function depends on the identification of the endomyocardial surface in each of the transducer positions.

Visual Inspection

Visual inspection provides a qualitative and a semiquantitative assessment of LV systolic function LV ejection fraction (LVEF) (Table 1–10).

Contrast Enhancement

In patients in whom the endomyocardial border is not well defined, for example for patients with COPD or morbid obesity, better definition of the endomyocardial borders (ie, the LV cavity) can be obtained with the injection of intravenous contrast material. This contrast is comprised of gas-filled microbubbles or microspheres to opacify the LV chamber and thereby better define the borders, shape, and regional and global wall motion of the left ventricle (Fig. 1–20).

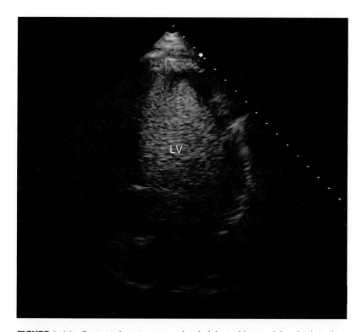

FIGURE 1–20. Contrast. A contrast agent is administered in a peripheral vein to better define the LV cavity, the LV endomyocardial borders, LV regional and global wall motion, and possible LV filling defects. LV, left ventricle

Regional Wall Motion Scoring

Regional wall motion scoring is a semiquantitative method in which 17 discrete segments of the LV chamber are identified, each of which is given a score (normal or hyperkinesis = 1, hypokinesis = 2, akinesis [negligible thickening] = 3, dyskinesis [paradoxical systolic motion] = 4, and aneurysmal [diasystolic deformation] = 5) (Fig. 1–21).[7]

The wall motion score index (WMSI) is obtained by dividing the sum of the wall motion scores by the number of satisfactorily visualized segments:

$$\underset{(\text{normal} = 1.0)}{\text{WMSI}} = \frac{\text{Sum of the individual segment scores}}{\text{Number of segments scored}}$$

The wall motion score (WMS) LVEF is obtained by dividing the sum of the regional wall motion scores by the number of segments scored and then multiplying by 30 (normal = 2, hypokinesis = 1, akinesis = 0, and dyskinesis = -1) (Table 1–11):

$$\underset{(\text{normal} \geq 60\%)}{\text{WMS LVEF}} = \frac{\text{Sum of the individual segment scores}}{\text{Number of segments scored}} \times 30\%$$

Quantitative Methods

Fractional Shortening Fractional shortening is the classic M-mode method to estimate LV systolic function. The LV end-diastolic (LVED) and end-systolic (LVES) dimensions are measured in either the parasternal long axis or short axis view:

$$\underset{(\text{normal} > 27\%)}{\text{Fractional shortening}} = \frac{\text{LVED} - \text{LVES}}{\text{LVED}} \times 100\%$$

Fractional shortening is based on a single plane creating a limited "keyhole" view of the left ventricle (Fig. 1–22). Therefore, it is only useful for normal ventricles and in patients with dilated cardiomyopathies without regional wall motion abnormalities.

Simpson Method When there are regional wall motion abnormalities, the more reliable quantitative system of determining LV volumes and LVEF is based on the Simpson method (Figs. 1–23 and 1–24). In either the apical four-chamber or two-chamber view, the endocardial border is traced in end-diastole and end-systole. The LV is then divided into a number of cylinders or discs, generally 20, of equal height. Individual volumes are calculated to yield the overall LV volume and LVEF.

■ LV DIASTOLIC FUNCTION

Diastole is an energy-dependent process with four phases:

1. The isovolumic relaxation time (IVRT) during which LV pressure drops but the mitral valve remains closed.

2. Early rapid LV filling begins when LV pressures fall below left atrial pressures and the mitral valve opens. Transmitral blood flow in this early phase is due to a combination of myocardial relaxation and elastic recoil, which in effect sucks blood into the left ventricle. The E wave depicts early diastolic mitral inflow velocity. It is a measure of LV relaxation.

3. The diastasis period is the mid-diastolic period during which transmitral blood flow is minimal.

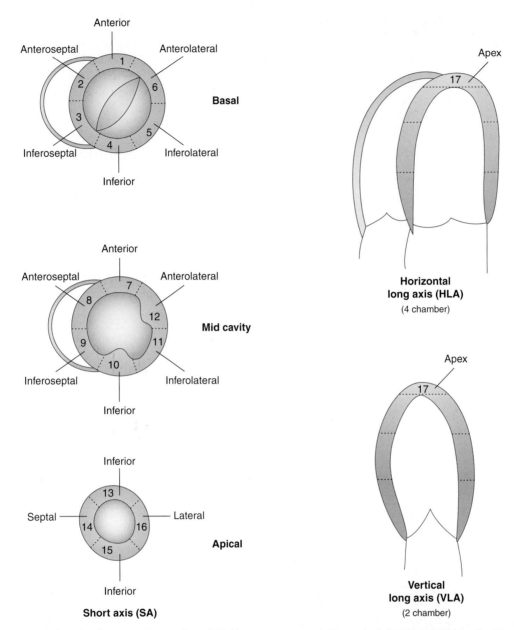

FIGURE 1–21. Left ventricular (LV) wall segments. The LV walls are divided into 16 segments to provide a method of semiquantitatively grading LV regional and global systolic function. LAX, parasternal long axis; 4C, apical four-chamber; 2C, apical two-chamber; SAX, parasternal short axis; MV, mitral valve level; PM, papillary muscle level; AP, apex. Reprinted with permission. *Circulation*. 2002;105:539-542. © 2002 American Heart Association, Inc.

TABLE 1–11. Visual Assessment of Regional Left Ventricular Wall Motion

Wall Motion Score Index	Wall Motion Score Left Ventricular Ejection Fraction
1 = Normal	3 = Increased
2 = Hypokinetic	2 = Normal
3 = Akinetic	1 = Hypokinetic
4 = Dyskinetic	0 = Akinetic
5 = Aneurysmal	−1 = Dyskinetic

4. End-diastole is the final phase during which there is an increase in transmitral flow resulting from left atrial contraction. In normals, approximately 15% to 20% of LV filling occurs during this phase. End-diastole is depicted by the A wave.

Doppler diastolic indices are affected by a patient's age, heart rate and rhythm, conduction abnormalities, and the loading conditions of the heart. Figure 1–25 illustrates normal and abnormal mitral inflow diastolic filling patterns.

Normal LV Diastolic Function

When assessing LV diastolic function, the Doppler sample volume is positioned at the tips of the mitral valve leaflets in the apical four-chamber view. Doppler measurements are made of

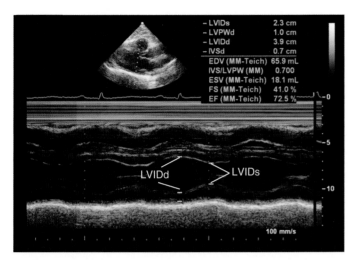

FIGURE 1–22. Fractional shortening. A parasternal long axis M-mode image with an end-diastolic dimension of 3.9 cm, an end-systolic dimension of 2.3 cm, and normal calculated left ventricular fractional shortening of 41.0% (normal >27%), and normal left ventricular ejection fraction of 72.5% (normal ≥55%). EF, ejection fraction; FS, fractional shortening; LVIDd, left ventricular end-diastolic dimension; LVIDs, left ventricular end-systolic dimension.

the IVRT, the E wave, the E wave deceleration time, and the A wave (Fig. 1–26).[8]

Due to normally rigorous myocardial contraction and brisk LV elastic recoil, approximately 80% of LV filling occurs during the early phase of diastole. This results in the E wave velocity being 1.0 to 1.5 times greater than that of the A wave, a deceleration time >140 ms, septal E′ >10 cm/s, and E/E′ <8 (see "Tissue Doppler Imaging" below).

Abnormal LV Diastolic Function

Grade 1: Mild LV Diastolic Dysfunction Due to impaired myocardial relaxation, the E wave velocity is reduced, and the deceleration time is prolonged. This results in more filling in late diastole, which is reflected in an increase in the A wave velocity and an E/A ratio of <1.0 (Fig. 1–27).

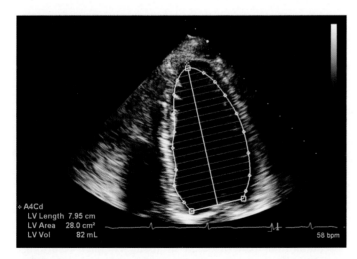

FIGURE 1–23. Simpson method. In the apical four-chamber view, the left ventricular (LV) cavity is divided into 20 cylinders or discs at end-diastole, and the LV volume and global LV ejection fraction are calculated.

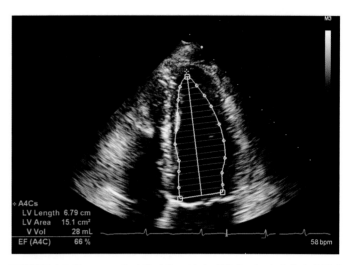

FIGURE 1–24. Simpson method. The left ventricular (LV) chamber is similarly divided in end-systole, and the LV ejection fraction (EF) is calculated.

Grade 2: Moderate LV Diastolic Dysfunction (Pseudonormal) Impaired myocardial relaxation is combined with a mild to moderate increase in left atrial pressures, which results in a pseudonormalized LV filling pattern, ie an E > A wave pattern.

There are several methods of differentiating normal from pseudonormal LV diastolic function, including (1) identification of diastolic flow abnormalities in the pulmonary veins, (2) use of the Valsalva maneuver, and (3) use of tissue Doppler imaging.

Grade 3: Severe LV Diastolic Dysfunction (Reversible) Impaired myocardial relaxation combined with a marked increase in left atrial pressures causes a shortened IVRT, which results in rapid but shortened early filling as reflected by an increase in E wave velocity and a shortened deceleration time. The A wave velocity and duration are reduced because of rapidly increasing pressures in the noncompliant left ventricle. This results in a "restrictive pattern" of transmitral filling with an E/A ratio >1.5 and a deceleration time of <140 ms.

Grade 4: Severe LV Diastolic Dysfunction (Irreversible) The resting transmitral filling patterns are similar to the grade 3 pattern; however, the patterns differ during a Valsalva maneuver.

Valsalva Maneuver

The Valsalva maneuver can help differentiate between a normal filling pattern and a grade 2 "pseudonormalized" pattern seen in patients with impaired relaxation combined with a mild-moderate increase in filling pressures.

During phase 2 of a Valsalva maneuver, there is decreased venous return with a resultant decrease in the heart's preload. If the Valsalva maneuver is maintained, there will be a resultant decrease in stroke volume and systemic blood pressure. In normals, a Valsalva maneuver will result in a decrease in both the E and A waves. Therefore, the normal E > A ratio is preserved. However, in patients with LV diastolic dysfunction and a grade 2 "pseudonormalized" pattern of their resting diastolic filling, the Valsalva maneuver will cause a decrease in the E wave and an increase in the A wave, thereby causing an abnormal A > E wave pattern and the unmasking of the diastolic dysfunction.

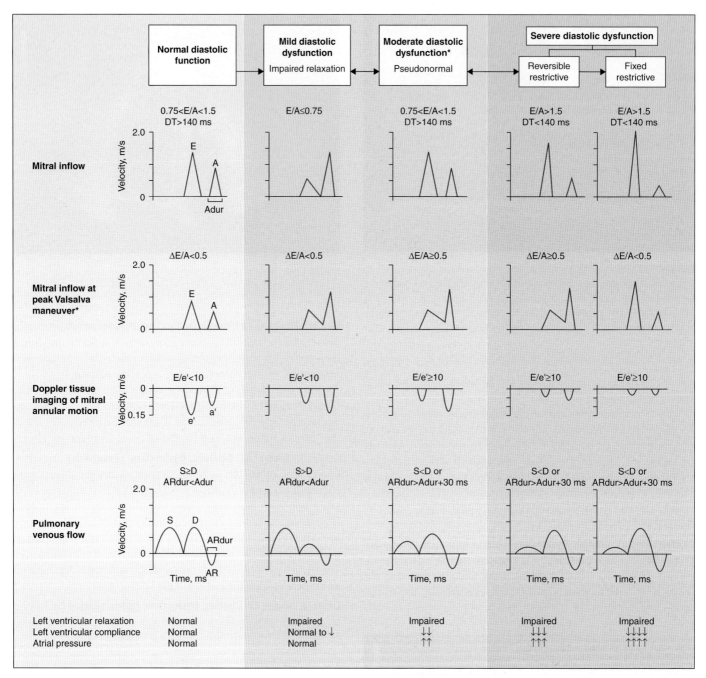

FIGURE 1–25. Left ventricular (LV) diastolic inflow patterns. Normal and abnormal diastolic transmitral inflow and pulmonary venous flow patterns are illustrated. A, velocity at atrial contraction; a′, velocity of mitral annular motion with atrial systole; Adur, A duration; AR, pulmonary venous atrial reversal flow; ARdur, AR duration; D, diastolic forward flow; DT, deceleration time; E, peak early filling velocity; e′, velocity of mitral annulus early diastolic motion; S, systolic forward flow; *, corrected for E/A fusion. Reproduced with permission from Redfield M, et al. Burden of systolic and diastolic ventricular dysfunction in the community. *JAMA*. 2003;289:194-202. Copyright 2003 American Medical Association. All rights reserved.

Tissue Doppler Imaging

Tissue Doppler imaging focuses on the motion of cardiac structures, specifically the septal and lateral regions of the mitral annulus, to assess myocardial relaxation. The same Doppler principles are used to measure the relatively slower velocity but higher amplitude of the motion and direction of myocardial tissue in the same way that the velocity and direction of blood flow are measured.

The E′ wave velocity, when measured at the medial or septal portion of the mitral annulus, is normally ≥10 cm/s; when the

E′ wave velocity is measured at the lateral portion of the mitral annulus, it is generally higher, normally ≥15 cm/s (Figs. 1–28 and 1–29).

The E′ wave reflects myocardial relaxation. It is depressed in all stages of diastolic dysfunction. Therefore, there is no "pseudonormal pattern" seen in tissue Doppler recordings. Also, because the E wave increases with higher filling pressures, the E/E′ ratio correlates well with LV filling pressures.

Patients with normal LV diastolic relaxation and filling pressures will a have septal E′ wave velocity >10 cm/s and an E/E′

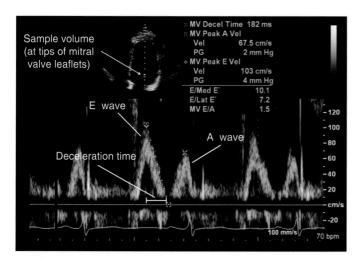

FIGURE 1–26. Normal left ventricular diastolic mitral inflow. With the sample volume placed at the tips of the mitral valve (MV) leaflets, a normal mitral inflow pattern is illustrated with an early rapid E wave velocity of 103 cm/s, a late A wave velocity following atrial contraction of 67.5 cm/s, an E/A ratio of 1.5 (normal >1.0), and a deceleration time of 182 ms.

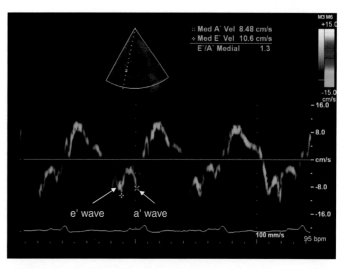

FIGURE 1–28. Tissue Doppler. By placing the sample volume at the medial/septal or lateral aspect of the mitral valve annulus, the relatively slower velocity but higher amplitude of the heart itself can be assessed. In this example, at the medial aspect of the mitral annulus, the velocity of the e′ wave is 10.6 cm/s, lowerset, the a′ wave velocity is 8.48 cm/s, and E′/A′ ratio is 1.3.

ratio of <8. Patients with grade 2 pseudonormalized LV filling patterns will have an E′ wave velocity of <7 cm/s and an E/E′ ratio of >15 due to their increased filling pressures.

■ STRESS ECHOCARDIOGRAPHY

For patients who are unable to exercise, dobutamine stress echocardiography is a clinically useful alternative to pharmacologic nuclear stress testing. Unlike the vasodilating agents used in nuclear imaging, dobutamine stimulates the adrenergic receptors causing an increase in myocardial contractility, heart rate, and blood pressure and, as a consequence, an increase in myocardial oxygen demand.

Dobutamine stress echocardiography is recommended for the intermediate-risk patient or to assess the hemodynamic significance of a known angiographic borderline coronary lesion.

A *normal response* is normal global and regional wall motion at rest and during dobutamine stress (Fig. 1–30).

An *ischemic response* is normal regional wall motion at rest that becomes hypokinetic or akinetic during dobutamine infusion.

Dobutamine stress echocardiography can also be used in patients who present with congestive heart failure. A biphasic response is suggestive of an ischemic etiology for the patient's congestive heart failure, as well as myocardial stunning or hibernation, and therefore potential myocardial viability.

In a *biphasic response*, the resting regional wall is hypokinetic or akinetic.

Phase 1: At a mid-dobutamine dose range, the ischemic but viable myocardium is stimulated to contract.

Phase 2: The ischemic but viable myocardium becomes more ischemic and then akinetic.

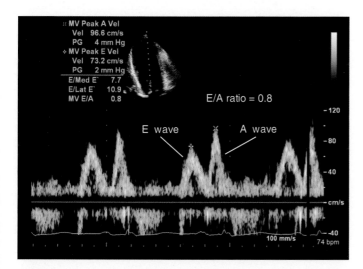

FIGURE 1–27. Grade 1 abnormal left ventricular diastolic mitral inflow. In this example, the E wave velocity is decreased (73.2 cm/s), the A wave velocity is increased (96.6 cm/s), and the E/A ratio is reversed (0.8). MV, mitral valve.

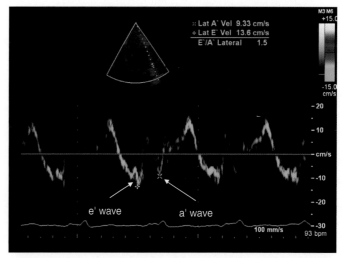

FIGURE 1–29. Tissue Doppler. In this example, at the lateral aspect of the mitral annulus, the velocity of the e′ wave is 13.6 cm/s, and that of the a′ wave is 9.33 cm/s.

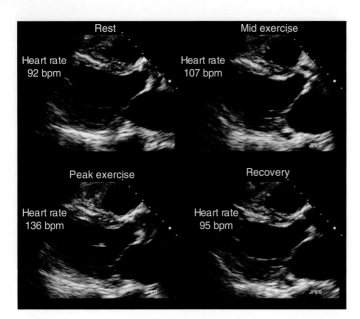

FIGURE 1–30. Stress echocardiography. Illustrated is a parasternal long axis "quad plot" comprised of continuous loop recordings obtained at rest, at the midpoint of the stress, at peak stress, and in recovery after stress. bpm, beats per minute.

Failure to demonstrate phase 1 signifies nonischemic nonviable myocardium. Because revascularization, therefore, would no longer be an option, further costly diagnostic testing may not be needed.

In 2003, the American College of Cardiology (ACC), the American Heart Association (AHA), and the American Society of Echocardiography (ASE) issued guidelines on the use of echocardiography in clinical medicine.[9] The ACC/AHA/ASE use the following classification scheme:

Class I: Conditions for which there is evidence and/or agreement that a given procedure is useful and effective.

Class II: Conditions for which there is conflicting evidence and/or a divergence of opinion.

Class III: Conditions for which there is evidence and/or general agreement that a procedure is not useful or effective.

Stress Echocardiography Guidelines

Class I

- Diagnosis of myocardial ischemia in patients with an intermediate likelihood of coronary artery disease with baseline electrocardiogram (ECG) abnormalities including ST-segment depression, LV hypertrophy (LVH), left bundle branch block, Wolff-Parkinson-White syndrome, or digoxin use.
- Assessment of the functional significance of a coronary lesion prior to possible revascularization.
- Assessment of myocardial viability prior to possible revascularization.

Class III

- Screening of asymptomatic patients with a low likelihood of coronary artery disease.

CLINICAL CASE STUDIES

The vignettes that follow were selected to illustrate the role of echocardiography in common clinical cases. Included in the discussion of each case are the salient guidelines from the ACC/AHA/ASE 2003 Task Force.[9]

■ CASE 1: CONGESTIVE HEART FAILURE

Case

A 75-year-old white man presents with a history of a myocardial infarction but no recent chest pain, easy fatigability, progressive dyspnea on exertion, dependent edema, nocturia, and a 20-pound weight gain.

Physical examination reveals distended jugular veins, bilateral rales, S_3 and S_4 gallops, abdominal swelling, and 3+ pretibial edema. ECG results are as follows: sinus rhythm; rate = 88 bpm; QRS = 130 ms; and poor precordial R wave progression.

ACC/AHA/ASE Guidelines: Patients With Dyspnea, Edema, or Cardiomyopathy

Class I

- In patients with clinical diagnosis of heart failure
- In patients with edema and suspected heart disease
- In patients with dyspnea and signs of heart failure
- In patients with suspected cardiomyopathy
- In patients exposed to cardiotoxic agents

Overview

Heart failure is a common clinical syndrome and one of the most common indications for echocardiography. Approximately five million people in the United States have clinical heart failure, with more than 500,000 new cases of heart failure diagnosed annually.[10] The presence of heart failure continues to increase with the overall aging of our population. Heart failure is the leading hospital discharge diagnosis for patients over the age of 65 years. Patients with clinical heart failure can have impaired LV systolic function and/or LV diastolic dysfunction.

Echocardiography is useful in differentiating between the various etiologies of heart failure such as coronary artery disease, hypertension, valvular heart disease, and primary cardiomyopathies. Echocardiography is also useful in ruling out the nonmyocardial disorders that can present as heart failure such as pericardial disease and hypovolemic shock.

Doppler allows for the quantification of the severity of valvular abnormalities, an estimate of pulmonary pressures, and an assessment of LV diastolic function.

Most adult patients who present with heart failure have an ischemic cardiomyopathy, hypertensive heart disease, or valvular abnormalities. Less common are primary disorders of the myocardium, which have been classified by the World Health Organization into five broad categories: dilated, hypertrophic, restrictive, arrhythmic right ventricular (RV), and unclassified, each of which has distinguishing echocardiographic features (Table 1–12).[11]

TABLE 1–12. World Health Organization/International Society and Federation of Cardiology: Classification of Cardiomyopathies

Cardiomyopathy	LV Chamber Size	LV Wall Thickness	LV Systolic Function	LV Diastolic Function
Dilated	Dilated (RV may be dilated)	Normal or thinned	Reduced (regional or global)	Abnormal
Hypertrophic	Normal	Increased (concentric or asymmetric)	Normal	Abnormal (LVOT obstruction)
Restrictive	Small	Normal	Normal	Abnormal
Arrhythmogenic right ventricular dysplasia	RV dilated	Normal	RV reduced (LV may be reduced)	Abnormal

LV, left ventricular; LVOT, left ventricular outflow tract; RV, right ventricular.

Dilated Cardiomyopathy

Patients with a dilated cardiomyopathy will often have spherical LV chamber dilatation. The LV wall motion is most typically globally reduced; however, regional wall motion abnormalities are not uncommon. Echocardiography can provide accurate measurements of LV dimensions, volumes, pressures, and LV systolic and diastolic function (Figs. 1–31 to 1–33).

As previously described, dobutamine stress echocardiography can give important additional information regarding the etiology of the dilated cardiomyopathy. An inducible wall motion abnormality would suggest coronary artery disease. Another indicator of ischemia would be an akinetic or hypokinetic "hibernating" wall that contracts more normally when stimulated.

Cardiac Resynchronization Therapy

Tissue Doppler imaging is used in cardiac resynchronization therapy, which is the use of multiple lead/biventricular pacing to help optimize LV systolic function and improve morbidity and mortality in patients with severe LV systolic impairment.[12-14]

■ CASE 2: HYPERTENSION

Case

A 62-year-old African American man presents with a long history of poorly controlled hypertension, increasing exercise intolerance, and chronic renal insufficiency.

Physical examination reveals a sitting blood pressure of 176/94 mm Hg, clear lungs, prominent point of maximal intensity (PMI), and an S_4 gallop. ECG results are as follows: normal sinus rhythm; left axis deviation; and LVH with repolarization changes.

ACC/AHA/ASE Guidelines: Patients With Hypertension

Class I

• To asses resting LV function and LVH

Class IIa

• Identification of LV diastolic filing abnormalities

Class III

• Reevaluation to assess LV mass or function to guide antihypertensive therapy

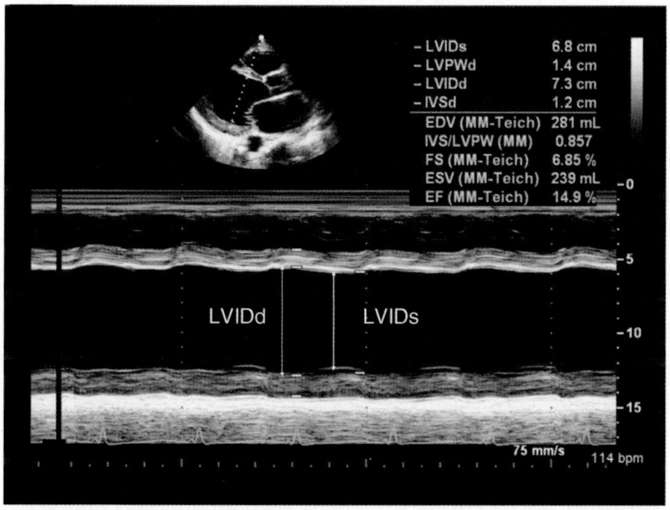

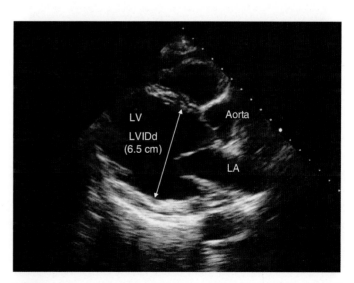

FIGURE 1–31. Dilated cardiomyopathy. Parasternal long axis M-mode images of a dilated left ventricle (normal LVId < 6.0 cm) with a severely reduced left ventricular systolic function and fractional shortening of 6.85% (normal >27%). EF, ejection fraction; FS, fractional shortening; LVIDd, left ventricular internal dimension in end-diastole; LVIDs, left ventricular internal dimension in end-systole.

FIGURE 1–32. Dilated cardiomyopathy. Parasternal long axis image of a dilated LV chamber with an end-diastolic dimension of 6.5 cm (normal <6.0 cm). LA, left atrium; LV, left ventricle; LVIDd, left ventricular internal dimension in end-diastole.

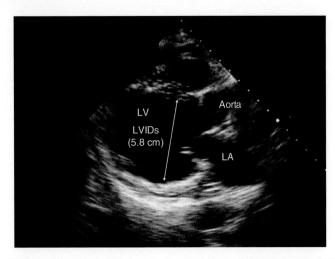

FIGURE 1–33. Dilated cardiomyopathy. Parasternal long axis image of a dilated LV chamber with an end-systolic dimension of 5.8 cm (normal < 4.0 cm). LA, left atrium; LV, left ventricle, LVIDs, left ventricular internal dimension in end-systole.

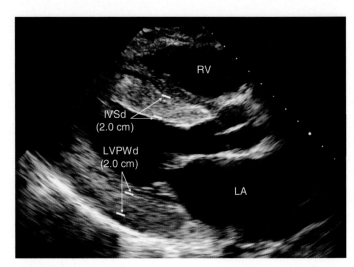

FIGURE 1–35. Hypertensive heart disease. Parasternal long axis image illustrating marked concentric left ventricular hypertrophy, approximately 2.0 cm (normal <1.1 cm), with a normal left ventricular chamber size, normal left ventricular fractional shortening, and left atrial dilatation. IVSd, interventricular septal wall thickness; LA, left atrium; LVPWd, left ventricular posterior wall thickness; RV, right ventricle.

Overview

Approximately one-third of the adult US population, 40% of African Americans, and more than two-thirds of people over the age of 65 have hypertension.[10] Although hypertension is a significant factor in the development of atherosclerotic vascular disease, it is the principal contributing factor to developing LVH.

The Framingham Heart Study demonstrated the prognostic value of electrocardiographically determined LVH.[15] Subsequently, the Framingham Heart Study investigators and others have demonstrated the superiority of echocardiographically determined LV mass and hypertrophy predicting coronary heart disease, strokes, and increased mortality (Figs. 1–34 and 1–35).[16,17]

Heart Failure With Preserved LV Systolic Function

Hypertension is also the principal etiology for preserved systolic function heart failure (ie, diastolic heart failure). In the

Framingham Heart Study, 75% of patients with heart failure had a history of hypertension, and mild hypertension doubled the lifetime risk of developing heart failure.[18]

In the Mayo Clinic's report from Olmsted County, approximately 40% of the heart failure patients had diastolic heart failure with preserved LV systolic function.[19] In the Framingham Heart Study, 51% of patients with heart failure and preserved LV systolic function had an annual mortality rate of 8.7%, which was approximately four times that of the age-matched controls.[20]

The four elements of diastolic heart failure are:

- Symptoms suggestive of heart failure
- Normal LV systolic function, LVEF ≥45%
- Abnormal myocardial relaxation
- Increased filling pressures

The optimal management of diastolic heart failure with preserved systolic function is the subject of several ongoing clinical trials.

■ CASE 3: ARRHYTHMIAS

Case

A 29-year-old man with no known heart disease presents with the sudden onset of rapid palpitations and near syncope.

Physical examination is normal with the exception of a rapid irregularly irregular pulse. ECG results are as follows: atrial fibrillation with a ventricular response rate averaging 170 bpm.

ACC/AHA/ASE Guidelines: Patients With Palpitations and Arrhythmias

Class I

- Patients with suspected structural heart disease
- Evaluation of patients prior to radiofrequency ablation

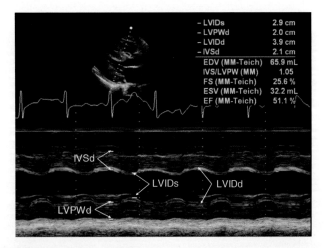

FIGURE 1–34. Hypertensive heart disease. Parasternal long axis M-mode image illustrating markedly increased left ventricular wall thickness of approximately 2.0 cm (normal <1.1 cm), with a normal left ventricular chamber size and normal left ventricular fractional shortening. IVSd, interventricular septal wall thickness; LVIDd, left ventricular internal dimension in end-diastole; LVIDs, left ventricular internal dimension in end-systole; LVPWd, left ventricular posterior wall thickness.

Class III

- Palpitations without arrhythmia or other cardiac signs or symptoms
- Isolated premature ventricular beats without suspicion of heart disease

Overview

Arrhythmias can occur in the presence or absence of structural heart disease. Echocardiography can identify common cardiac abnormalities associated with arrhythmias, thereby providing the clinician with important prognostic and therapeutic useful information.

Ventricular Arrhythmias/Sudden Death

For patients who present with ventricular arrhythmias, in the absence of a history of sudden death, the best predictor of a future sudden death event is the severity of the LV systolic dysfunction. In addition to providing quantitative information regarding LV systolic and diastolic function, echocardiography also provides information regarding RV size and function.

Arrhythmogenic RV dysplasia (ARVD) is due to progressive myocardial atrophy with fibrofatty infiltration of the right ventricle. ARVD can be inherited as an autosomal dominant trait and has been reported as a cause of sudden death in the young.[21] The resting ECG shows RV conduction delay and characteristic epsilon waves–terminal notching of the QRS in leads V_1 to V_3. The morphology of the ventricular tachycardia is left bundle branch block because it originates in the right ventricle. Echocardiographic changes can appear late and generally include RV outflow and inflow dilatation and RV global or regional hypokinesis. Dilatation of the RV outflow tract >30 mm in the parasternal long axis view has been reported to be the most sensitive and specific sign of ARVD.[22] LV dilatation and hypokinesis occur in approximately 50% of patients with ARVD.

Atrial Fibrillation

Echocardiography plays a central role in the workup and treatment of patients with supraventricular arrhythmias, in particular, atrial fibrillation.[23] The prevalence of atrial fibrillation in the United States now exceeds two million, and atrial fibrillation results in more than 500,000 hospital admissions annually.[10] This increased prevalence and incidence reflects the aging of our population. Approximately 1% of people over the age of 60 years, 5% over the age of 70 years, and 10% over the age of 80 years have atrial fibrillation.[24] Ten percent of patients with heart failure have atrial fibrillation.

Echocardiographically demonstrated moderate to severe LV systolic dysfunction has been shown to predict a greater than two-fold increase in the rate of stroke.[25] Of note, atrial fibrillation occurs in 10% to 30% of patients in the absence of underlying disease and is called *lone atrial fibrillation*.[26]

Atrial fibrillation is responsible for up to 20% of all strokes. Patients with atrial fibrillation have an annual stroke rate of 5% and a two-fold increase in the risk of recurrent stroke.[27-29] In addition, patients in atrial fibrillation have an increase in heart failure and total mortality compared with people in sinus rhythm.

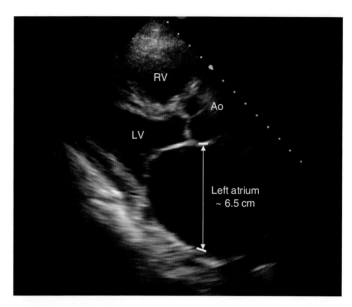

FIGURE 1–36. Parasternal long axis image demonstrating left atrial enlargement of 6.5 cm (normal <4.0 cm) with normal LV chamber size and LV wall thickness. Ao, aorta; LV, left ventricle; RV, right ventricle.

Cardioversion In recognition of the long-term deleterious effects of atrial fibrillation, clinicians are becoming more aggressive in their attempts to restore sinus rhythm before left atrial remodeling and scarring become irreversible.

Traditionally, echocardiographic measures of left atrial size and LV systolic function have been used to predict a patient's stroke risk and the outcome of cardioversion (Fig. 1–36).[29,30] Echocardiography is also being used more frequently to determine the timing of cardioversion.

In the absence of 3 to 4 weeks of anticoagulation, the incidence of a cardioembolic complication following cardioversion is up to 5%, depending on the severity of the underlying heart disease. The left atrial appendage is the source of most of the embolic events. Although not visible by transthoracic echocardiography, the left atrial appendage is visible in most patients by transesophageal echocardiography (Fig. 1–37). Using transesophageal echocardiography to screen patients for stasis or visible thrombi in the left atrial appendage, the incidence of acute neurologic events following cardioversion has been demonstrated to be <0.1%, which is comparable to the incidence in patients on long-term anticoagulation.[31]

Radiofrequency Ablation Echocardiographic-derived measures of left atrial size and volume are also being used in decision making regarding radiofrequency ablation. Increasingly, transesophageal echocardiography, intracardiac ultrasound, and three-dimensional echocardiography are being used in new catheter-based interventions, including radiofrequency ablation of sinus node dysfunction, atrial fibrillation, and left-sided accessory atrioventricular pathways.[32-35]

■ CASE 4: MITRAL REGURGITATION

Case

A 72-year-old man presents with increasing dyspnea on exertion and exercise intolerance.

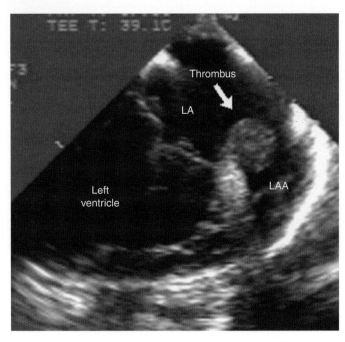

FIGURE 1–37. Left atrial thrombus. Transesophageal echocardiographic image of a dilated left atrium and large left atrial thrombus. LA, left atrium; LAA, left atrial appendage.

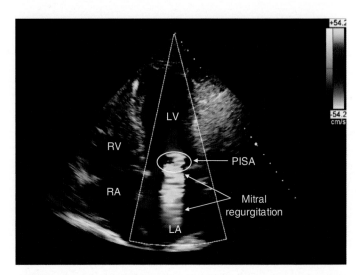

FIGURE 1–38. Mitral regurgitation. Apical four-chamber color flow Doppler image of severe mitral regurgitation with prominent PISA. LA, left atrium; LV, left ventricle; PISA, proximal isovelocity surface area; RA, right atrium; RV, right ventricle.

Physical examination reveals distended neck veins, basilar rales, an enlarged displaced PMI, and a grade 4/6 holosystolic murmur at the cardiac apex radiating to the anterior axillary line. ECG results are as follows: atrial fibrillation; normal QRS; and nonspecific ST-T wave changes.

ACC/AHA/ASE Guidelines: Patients With Native Valvular Regurgitation

Class I

- Assess LV and RV size and function and/or hemodynamics
- Reevaluate patients with mild or moderate regurgitation and changing symptoms
- Periodic reevaluation of asymptomatic patients with severe regurgitation
- Periodic reevaluation of asymptomatic patients with mild or moderate regurgitation and LV dilatation
- Assessment of medical therapy
- During pregnancy
- Patients with a history of anorectic drug use who are symptomatic or have cardiac murmurs

Class III

- Routine reevaluation of asymptomatic patients with mild mitral or aortic regurgitation with normal LV size and function

Overview

Valvular regurgitation is a common echocardiographic finding. In the absence of other cardiac abnormalities, trace or mild mitral, tricuspid, or pulmonic regurgitation can be a normal finding, whereas aortic regurgitation is never considered normal. Mild or moderate mitral or aortic regurgitation can also be missed when auscultation is performed by an inexperienced or distracted observer.

Mitral Regurgitation

Mitral regurgitation can be congenital or acquired, which can be acute or chronic. Common etiologies of chronic mitral regurgitation include degenerative disorders including mitral valve prolapse and mitral annular calcification; structural due to ischemia or LV dilatation; infectious endocarditis; and inflammation due to rheumatic or connective tissue disorders.

Two-dimensional echocardiography provides important structural information regarding the possible etiology of the mitral regurgitation including leaflet prolapse, flail leaflets, ruptured chordae tendineae, vegetations, and LV chamber size and function. Doppler indices provide a direct assessment of the hemodynamic significance of valvular regurgitant and stenotic abnormalities.

Figure 1–38 demonstrates moderately severe (3+) mitral regurgitation, as evident by the left atrial enlargement, mitral regurgitant jet, LV dilatation, and global LV hypokinesis.

Natural history studies have demonstrated that the onset of symptoms occurs late in the course of patients with chronic mitral insufficiency.[36] Current echocardiographic indications for mitral valve surgery on asymptomatic patients include LV chamber dilatation and/or LV systolic dysfunction and Doppler evidence of pulmonary hypertension.[37] Newer Doppler indices include an assessment of the regurgitant jet's length, area, and width; the width of the vena contracta; the effective regurgitant orifice area (EROA); regurgitant volume using the proximal isovelocity surface area; right-sided pressures; and pulmonary venous flow reversal (Table 1–13).[38-41]

Proximal Isovelocity Surface Area

The proximal isovelocity surface area (PISA) method is based on the principle that flow will converge at the site of an orifice at symmetrical velocities, equal to the flow rate through the orifice. By

TABLE 1–13. Echo Doppler Assessment of the Severity of Mitral Regurgitation

Severity	LA/LV Size	MR Jet Area	MR Jet Volume (ML/Beat)	MR Jet Fraction (%)	EROA (cm²)	Pisa Radius (mm)
Mild (1+)	Normal	Small <20% LA	<30	<30	<0.20	<4
Moderate (2+)	Mildly increased	Moderate	30-44	30-39	0.20-0.29	4-7
Moderate-severe (3+)	Dilated	Large	45-59	40-49	0.30-0.39	8-10
Severe (4+)	Dilated	Large >40% LA	>60	>50	>40	>10

EROA, effective regurgitant orifice area; LA, left atrial; LV, left ventricular; MR, mitral regurgitation; PISA, proximal isovelocity surface area.

measuring the distance from the first aliased color flow velocity at the regurgitant orifice, the blue-red interface, calculations can be made of the EROA and the regurgitant volume (see Fig. 1–38).

Mitral Valve Prolapse

Mitral valve prolapse was once considered a common congenital abnormality. It is now believed to be primarily a degenerative abnormality related either to a systemic connective tissue disorder or aging, occurring in approximately 2% of the general population.[42-44]

Traditionally, the diagnosis of mitral valve prolapse has depended on the auscultatory findings of a mid-systolic click followed by a mid-systolic mitral regurgitant murmur.

Echocardiographic criteria for mitral valve prolapse include thickened mitral leaflets (>5 mm), redundant with pan- or mid-systolic posterior motion (prolapse) of the anterior and/or posterior leaflets 2 mm or more beyond the plane of the mitral annulus in the parasternal long axis view (Figs. 1–39 to 1–41).

Transesophageal echocardiography has become an important part of the preoperative evaluation of patients with mitral regurgitation to help determine the feasibility of the clinically superior repair of the mitral valve rather than replacing it with a mechanical prosthesis or bioprosthesis.[45]

ACC/AHA/ASE Guidelines: Patients With Mitral Valve Prolapse

Class I

• Diagnosis in patients with physical signs of mitral valve prolapse

Class III

• Routine repetition in patients with mitral valve prolapse with no or mild regurgitation and no change in clinical signs or symptoms

■ CASE 5: CEREBROVASCULAR ACCIDENT/SYNCOPE

Case

An 83-year-old white woman presents with sudden onset of dysphasia and left-sided hemiparesis.

Physical examination reveals a blood pressure of 160/90 mm Hg, clear lungs, regular rhythm, S₄ gallop, no edema, and right-sided

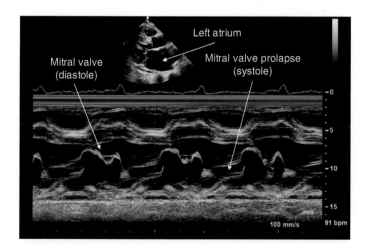

FIGURE 1–39. Mitral valve prolapse. Parasternal long axis M-mode image demonstrating pansystolic posterior ballooning of the posterior mitral valve leaflet.

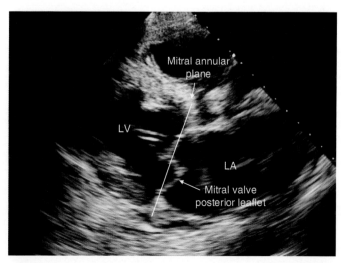

FIGURE 1–40. Mitral valve prolapse. Parasternal long axis image demonstrating systolic ballooning of the posterior mitral valve leaflet approximately 7 mm beyond the plane of the mitral annulus into the left atrium. LA, left atrium; LV, left ventricle.

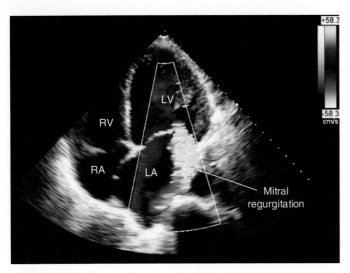

FIGURE 1–41. Mitral regurgitation. Apical four-chamber color flow image demonstrating severe eccentric mitral regurgitation. LA, left atrium; LV, left ventricle; RA, right atrium; RV, right ventricle.

upper and lower extremity weakness. ECG results are as follows: atrial fibrillation; LVH; and old inferior wall myocardial infarction.

ACC/AHA/ASE Guidelines: Patients With Neurologic Events

Class I

• Abrupt occlusion of any major peripheral or visceral artery

Overview

Every year, approximately 800,000 Americans suffer an acute cerebrovascular accident.[8] Stroke is the third leading cause of death in the United States, behind heart disease and cancer. It is currently estimated that approximately 20% of strokes are due to cardiac emboli, with higher rates in younger patients who do not have coexistent vascular disease.

Echocardiography has become an integral part of the workup of every patient admitted to a hospital with a cerebrovascular accident or transient ischemic attack. In addition to information relevant to an arrhythmia workup, LV function and valvular lesions, echocardiography provides valuable information to rule out a possible cardiac source of emboli (Table 1–14).

Transesophageal echocardiography provides superior spatial resolution for identifying vegetations as well as other potential

TABLE 1–14. Potential Cardiac Sources of Emboli Causing Neurovascular Events

Congenital	Valvular	Ventricular
Atrial septal defects	Rheumatic	Dilated with reduced left ventricular ejection fraction
Atrial septal aneurysm	Mitral annular calcification	Aneurysm
Patent foramen ovale	Prosthetic bacterial endocarditis	Mural thrombus

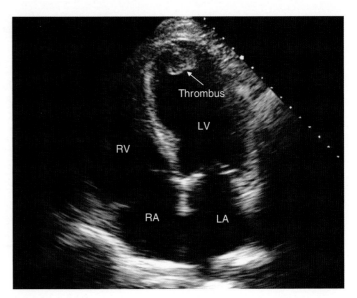

FIGURE 1–42. Left ventricular mural thrombus. Apical four-chamber image demonstrating a large, 2 cm × 2 cm left ventricular apical filling defect consistent with a mural thrombus. LA, left atrium; LV, left ventricle; RA, right atrium; RV, right ventricle.

cardiovascular sources of emboli including papillary fibroelastomas and aortic atheroma.

Atrial Fibrillation

The role of echocardiography in the workup, risk stratification, and management of atrial fibrillation in the prevention of cardiac embolic events was discussed earlier in Case 3.

LV Mural Thrombus

Prior to the era of reperfusion and the widespread use of antiplatelet and antithrombin agents, LV mural thrombi occurred in up to 50% of patients with large anterior wall myocardial infarctions. Contributing factors include the hypercoagulable postinfarction state, localized endocardial inflammation, and regional akinesis or dyskinesis. An estimated 10% of mural thrombi result in thromboembolic events (Fig. 1–42).[46] Figure 1–42 demonstrates a dilated left ventricle with apical akinesis/dyskinesis and an apical LV filling defect consistent with a mural thrombus.

Atrial Septal Defect/Patent Foramen Ovale

Atrial septal defects occur in approximately 5% to 10% of children with congenital heart disease. Secundum atrial septal defects are the most common. They are located in the central portion of the atrial septum and encompass the region of the foramen ovale. The degree of the left-to-right shunt is dependent on the size of the atrial septal defect. Large defects result in diastolic volume overload of the right ventricle and increased pulmonary blood flow.

In the apical four-chamber view, two-dimensional echocardiography can identify right atrial and RV dilatation and atrial septal wall echo dropout, which is a nonspecific finding. Diastolic flattening of the intraventricular septum can be seen in the parasternal short axis view. Doppler recordings can demonstrate elevated right-side pressure.

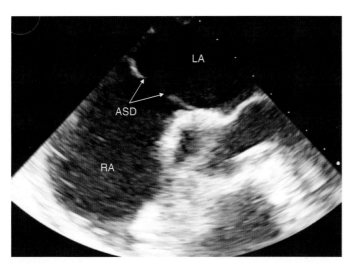

FIGURE 1–43. Atrial septal defect. Transesophageal echocardiogram demonstrating a right atrial enlargement and a 1-cm secundum-type atrial septal defect. ASD, atrial septal defect; LA, left atrium; RA, right atrium.

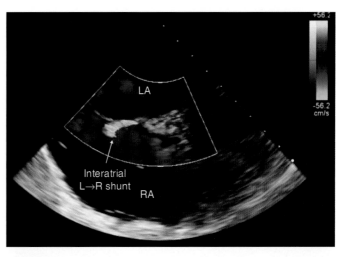

FIGURE 1–45. Patent foramen ovale. Transesophageal color flow image demonstrating a left to right (L → R) interatrial shunt from the left atrium across the patent foramen ovale to the right atrium. LA, left atrium; RA, right atrium.

A patent foramen ovale has been reported to occur in approximately 30% of the general population.[47]

In addition to routine transthoracic echocardiography, patients who present with a cerebrovascular accident frequently undergo contrast studies to rule out paradoxical shunts due to an intracardiac shunt.

Transesophageal echocardiography with intravenous injection of agitated saline with or without simple physiologic maneuvers such as coughing or Valsalva enhances the detection of shunts due to either an atrial septal defect (Figs. 1–43 and 1–44) or a patent foramen ovale (Figs. 1–45 and 1–46).

The presence of an atrial septal defect or a patent foramen ovale in the presence of an atrial septal aneurysm has been associated with an increased incidence of acute neurologic deficits.[48] Intracardiac echocardiographic imaging and three-dimensional echocardiography are new technologies that are being used to facilitate the implantation of percutaneous vascular closure devices.[48-50]

An association between patent foramen ovale and migraine headaches remains controversial.[51,52] A recently concluded prospective, randomized clinical trial showed no utility for the percutaneous closure of patent foramen ovale in treating migraines.[53]

Myxoma

Atrial myxomas are the most common tumors of the heart. Myxomas appear as pedunculated masses most commonly located in the left atrium attached to the atrial septum in the

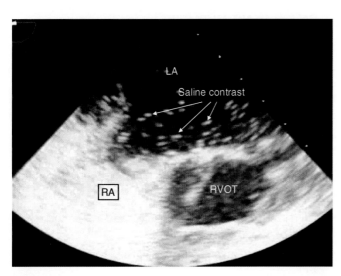

FIGURE 1–44. Atrial septal defect. Transesophageal echocardiogram with saline contrast opacifying the right atrium and demonstrating a right to left (R → L) interatrial shunt of contrast bubbles into the left atrium. LA, left atrium; RA, right atrium; RVOT, right ventricular outflow tract.

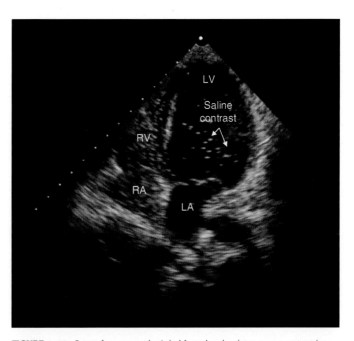

FIGURE 1–46. Patent foramen ovale. Apical four-chamber intravenous contrast image demonstrating right to left interatrial shunt with bubbles appearing in the left atrium and the left ventricle. LA, left atrium; LV, left ventricle; RA, right atrium; RV, right ventricle.

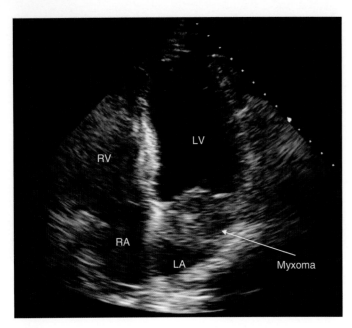

FIGURE 1–47. Myxoma. Parasternal long image view demonstrating a large, 3 cm × 4 cm left atrial myxoma. LA, left atrium; LV, left ventricle; RA, right atrium; RV, right ventricle.

area of the foramen ovale, and less commonly located in the right atrium, right or left ventricles, pulmonary veins, or vena cava. In addition to presenting as an acute thromboembolic event, a large, mobile, atrial myxoma can cause syncope by obstructing diastolic mitral inflow (Figs. 1–47 to 1–49).

Syncope

Syncope is a common clinical problem for patients of all ages but occurs most frequently in the elderly, who have an approximate 6% annual rate.[54] Cardiac causes for syncope are most common in the elderly. However, in the absence of a preexisting cardiac history or symptoms or abnormalities

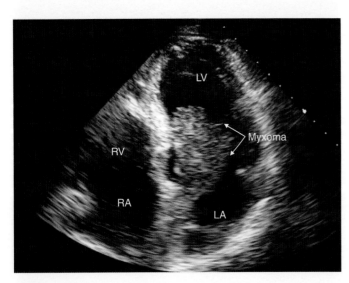

FIGURE 1–48. Myxoma. Parasternal long axis image demonstrating prolapse of a large left atrial myxoma across the mitral valve orifice into the left ventricle. LA, left atrium; LV, left ventricle; RA, right atrium; RV, right ventricle.

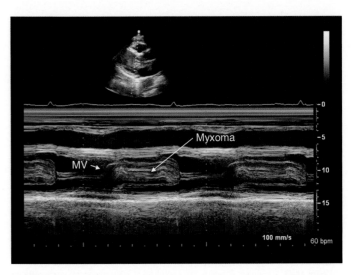

FIGURE 1–49. Myxoma. Parasternal long M-mode image demonstrating an echo-dense mass filling the mitral valve orifice from mid to late diastole. MV, mitral valve.

evident on physical examination or ECG, the incidence of unsuspected echocardiographic abnormalities is low. Current AHA/ACC guidelines recommend echocardiography as part of the workup of all patients with unexplained syncope.[55]

ACC/AHA/ASE Guidelines: Patients With Syncope

Class I

- In patients with suspected heart disease
- In patients with periexertional syncope

Class IIa

- In patients in high-risk occupations

Class III

- In patients with classic neurogenic syncope

■ CASE 6: HEART MURMURS

Case

A 26-year-old active woman presents with no cardiopulmonary complaints.

Physical examination reveals normal vital signs. Cardiac auscultation reveals normal S_1 and physiologically split S_2 and a grade 1/6 short systolic murmur at the left sternal border without appreciable clicks or gallops. ECG results are normal.

ACC/AHA/ASE Guidelines: Patients With a Heart Murmur

Class I

- Patients with a heart murmur and cardiorespiratory symptoms
- Asymptomatic patients with suspected structural heart disease

Class III

- Asymptomatic adults with innocent or functional heart murmurs

Overview

Echocardiography plays a central role, along with a careful history, cardiac auscultation, and ECG, in the assessment of patients who present with heart murmurs.

Innocent Murmurs

Not all murmurs reflect significant underlying cardiac abnormalities. Murmurs with the characteristics of this case are "innocent" functional flow murmurs often heard in children, adolescents, and young lean adults. Trace or mild mitral, tricuspid, and/or pulmonic regurgitation are common and can be considered normal in the otherwise normal heart. Soft systolic ejection murmurs due to aortic leaflet thickening/sclerosis are a degenerative process common in the elderly and, in the absence of an increase in the LV outflow velocity, are of no clinical significance.

Calcific Aortic Stenosis

Calcific aortic stenosis due to congenital bicuspid aortic valves or rheumatic heart disease generally presents in a patient's sixth decade, whereas degenerative aortic stenosis occurs one or two decades later. Unlike the patient who presents with an innocent flow murmur or aortic leaflet sclerosis, the characteristics of a hemodynamically significant aortic stenosis include diminished carotid pulses with a palpable thrill and audible transmitted cardiac murmurs; a prominent PMI; a precordial thrill; and a long late-peaking systolic murmur at the left sternal border with a diminished, absent, or paradoxically split S_2.

The severity of the aortic stenosis can be assessed echocardiographically by visual inspection of M-mode and two-dimensional recordings (Figs. 1–50 to 1–54). In the parasternal echocardiographic view, normal aortic leaflets will appear thin (ie, less thick than the walls of the aorta). Normal aortic leaflets are freely mobile. During ventricular systole, the leaflets will separate a minimum of 2 cm, opening the full width of the aortic root. Newer three-dimensional imaging technologies provide improved spatial, structural, and functional information (Fig. 1–55).

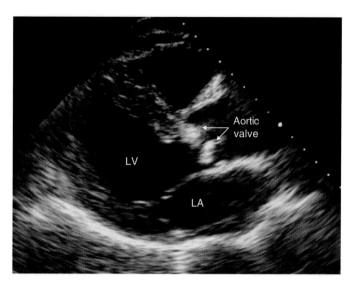

FIGURE 1–51. Aortic stenosis. Parasternal short axis image demonstrating heavily calcified aortic valve leaflets and mild concentric left ventricular hypertrophy. LA, left atrium; LV, left ventricle.

The severity of the aortic stenosis can be more accurately assessed by Doppler-derived peak and mean transvalvular gradients using the modified Bernoulli equation and by calculation of the aortic valve area using the continuity equation (Table 1–15).

Bernoulli Equation The Bernoulli equation is used to calculate pressures in the cardiac chambers, across valves, and across intracardiac and vascular shunts. The Bernoulli equation is based on the principle that the total energy in a closed system is constant. Therefore, the energy flowing into the system must be equal to the energy flowing out of the system.

Flow is dependent on pressure differences between two locations. In the presence of a narrowing, the velocity distal to the narrowing must be increased to maintain the energy in the

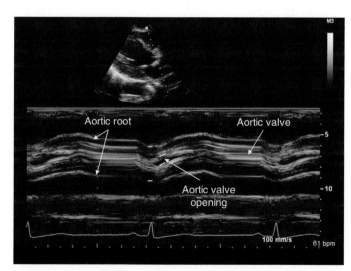

FIGURE 1–50. Aortic stenosis. Parasternal long axis M-mode image demonstrating thickened aortic valve leaflets with diminished systolic opening.

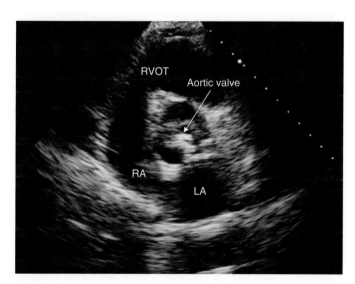

FIGURE 1–52. Aortic stenosis. Parasternal short axis image showing heavily calcified aortic valve leaflets. LA, left atrium; RA, right atrium; RVOT, right ventricular outflow tract.

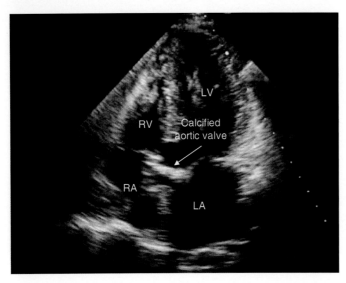

FIGURE 1–53. Aortic stenosis. Apical five-chamber image of heavily calcified aortic valve leaflets. RA, right atrium; RV, right ventricle; LA, left atrium; LV, left ventricle.

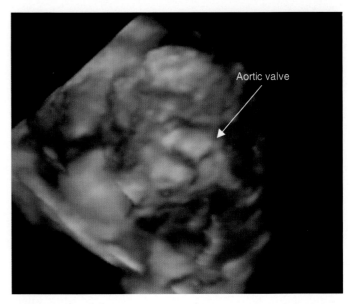

FIGURE 1–55. Aortic stenosis. Three-dimensional illustration of calcific aortic stenosis.

system. Because velocity and pressure are inversely proportional, the pressure distal to the narrowing must be decreased relative to the pressure proximal to the narrowing.

The pressure difference proximal and distal to the narrowing is measured by the Bernoulli equation: $\Delta P = 4V^2$.

Continuity Equation The continuity equation is also dependent on the principle of conservation of mass (ie, in a closed system, what flows in must flow out). To maintain flow within a system, the flow velocities at a stenotic orifice must be greater than the flow velocities proximal and distal to the stenosis. Because the flow rate is the product of the area and mean flow velocity, valve areas can be calculated from flow and velocity measurements.

The continuity equation uses these measurements to calculate valve areas, regurgitant volumes and regurgitant fractions, regurgitant orifice areas (EROA), and intracardiac shunt areas.

The continuity equation is as follows: $CSA^1 \times V^1 = CSA^2 \times V^2$. CSA^1 is the cross-sectional area proximal to the stenosis; V^1 is the velocity proximal to the stenosis; CSA^2 is the cross-sectional area of the stenotic area, and V^2 is the velocity at the stenosis. Because blood flow in the heart is pulsatile, the velocity time integral is substituted for mean velocity for calculation of valve areas.

Confounding factors in the echocardiographic assessment of the severity of aortic stenosis include the presence of coexistent subvalvular LV outflow tract obstruction due to hypertrophic cardiomyopathy, moderate or severe aortic valve regurgitation, and significantly reduced LV systolic function.

Low-Flow/Low-Gradient Aortic Stenosis Doppler imaging during dobutamine administration can help differentiate patients with severe aortic stenosis from patients who have only mild or moderate aortic stenosis with severe LV dysfunction.

Dobutamine should cause an increase in LV contractility with a resultant increase in stroke volume. In patients with mild to moderate aortic stenosis and LV dysfunction, dobutamine infusion will increase the stroke volume, with a resultant increase in the calculated aortic valve area (>0.2 cm²) with no change in the outflow gradient. In patients with severe aortic stenosis and a relatively fixed valve area, dobutamine infusion will result in an increase in the calculated LV outflow gradient.

Lack of contractile or inotropic reserve is defined as failure of dobutamine to increase the patient's stroke volume by >20%. These patients generally have a poor prognosis whether treated medically or surgically.[56]

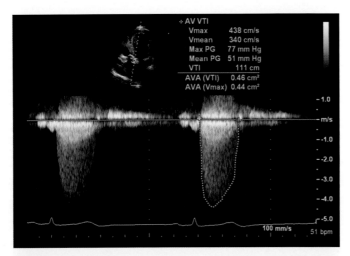

FIGURE 1–54. Aortic stenosis. Apical five-chamber Doppler display demonstrating high-velocity turbulent flow. The transvalvular gradients were calculated using the Bernoulli equation, and the aortic valve area was calculated using the continuity equation. AV, aortic valve; AVA, aortic valve area; PG, pressure gradient; V, velocity; VTI, velocity time integral.

ACC/AHA/ASE Guidelines: Native Valvular Stenosis

Class I

- Initial diagnosis with an assessment of chamber dimensions and hemodynamic severity

- Reevaluation in patients with worsening symptoms

- Reevaluation during pregnancy

TABLE 1-15. Echo Doppler Assessment of the Severity of Aortic Stenosis

Severity	LV Wall Thickness	Aortic Valve Area (cm²)	Mean Pressure Gradient[a] (mm Hg)	Peak Pressure Gradient[a] (mm Hg)	Peak Aortic Velocity (m/s)
Normal	Normal	>2			≤2.5
Mild	Normal	1.5- 2.0	<20	16-36	2.6-3
Moderate	Hypertrophy	1.0-1.5	20-40	36-50	3-4
Moderate-severe	Hypertrophy	0.7-1.0		50-64	
Severe	Hypertrophy	<0.7	>40	>64	>4

[a]Dependent on left ventricular systolic function.

LV, left ventricular.

Class III

- Routine reevaluation of stable asymptomatic adults with mild aortic stenosis
- Routine reevaluation of stable asymptomatic adults with mild to moderate mitral stenosis

Chronic Aortic Regurgitation

Aortic valve regurgitation can be the result of an abnormality of the aortic valve, including congenital, degenerative, or infectious abnormalities, or the result of diseases affecting the aortic root, such as acute aortic dissection, Marfan syndrome, syphilis, or trauma.

Natural history studies have demonstrated the predictive value of echocardiographic indices of LV size and systolic function.[57-59] Several newer Doppler and color flow imaging parameters have been correlated to angiographically assessed aortic regurgitation including (Figs. 1–56 to 1–58; Table 1–16):

- Length of the aortic regurgitant jet
- Width of the aortic regurgitant jet at its origin

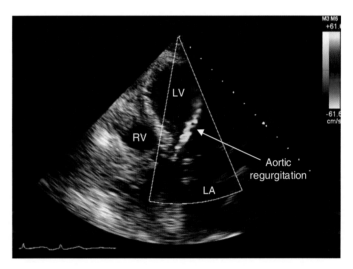

FIGURE 1–57. Aortic regurgitation. Apical five-chamber color flow image of aortic valve regurgitation. LA, left atrium; LV, left ventricle; RV, right ventricle.

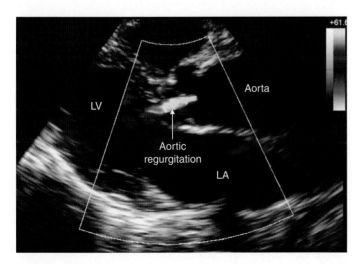

FIGURE 1–56. Aortic regurgitation. Parasternal long axis color flow image of aortic valve regurgitation. LA, left atrium; LV, left ventricle.

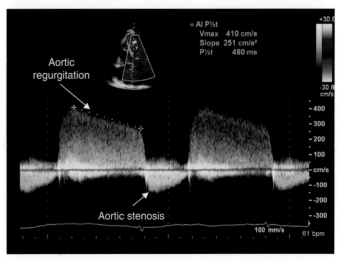

FIGURE 1–58. Aortic regurgitation. Apical five-chamber Doppler display of aortic valve regurgitation with a pressure half-time of 480 ms. P½t, pressure half-time.

TABLE 1–16. Echo Doppler Assessment of the Severity of Aortic Regurgitation

Severity	Jet Length	AR Jet Width (mm)	AR Jet Width ÷ LVOT Width (%)	AR Jet Fraction(%)	Pressure Half Time (ms)	EROA (cm²)
Mild (1+)	Minimal	< 4	<25	<30	>500	<0.10
Moderate (2+)	To leaflet tips	4-7	25-46	30-39	350-500	0.10-0.19
Moderate-severe (3+)		8-10	47-64	40-49	200-350	0.20-0.29
Severe (4+)	Papillary muscle	>10	>65	>50	<200	>30

AR, aortic regurgitation; EROA, effective regurgitant orifice area; LVOT, left ventricular outflow tract.

- Width of the aortic regurgitant jet relative to the width of the LV outflow tract
- Diastolic dysfunction including decreasing pressure half-times, a restrictive mitral inflow pattern due to increasing LV pressure, and EROA

Mitral Stenosis

Rheumatic mitral stenosis is rare in the United States; however, the increasing aging of the population has led to more degenerative valvular disease. When coupled with heavy mitral annular calcification, the patient can present with symptoms and hemodynamic features similar to mitral stenosis but is not as amendable to surgical repair (Figs. 1–59 to 1–62).

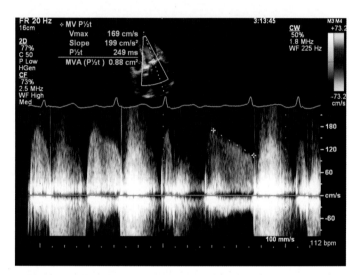

FIGURE 1–60. Mitral stenosis. Apical four-chamber Doppler display of severe mitral valve stenosis with a pressure half-time of 249 ms and a mitral valve area of 0.88 cm². P½ t, pressure half-time; MVA, mitral valve area.

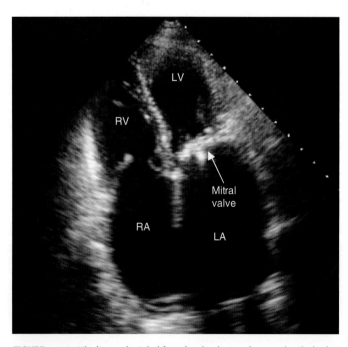

FIGURE 1–59. Mitral stenosis. Apical four-chamber image of a stenotic mitral valve. LA, left atrium; LV, left ventricle; RA, right atrium; RV, right ventricle.

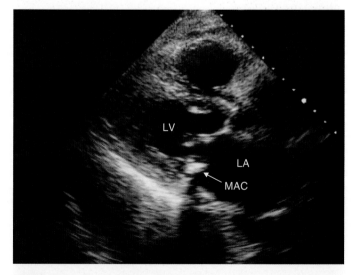

FIGURE 1–61. Mitral annular calcification. Parasternal long axis image of a mildly thickened anterior mitral valve leaflet and heavy posterior mitral annular calcification. LA, left atrium; LV, left ventricle; MAC, mitral annular calcification.

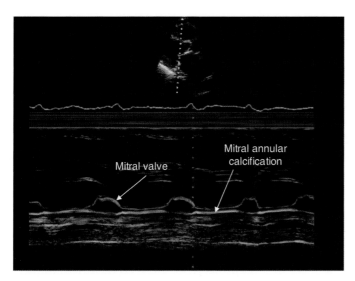

FIGURE 1–62. Mitral annular calcification. Parasternal long axis M-mode recording showing normal anterior mitral valve leaflet thickness, a decreased E → F slope, and mitral annular calcification.

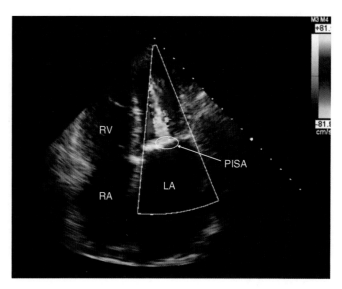

FIGURE 1–63. Mitral stenosis. Apical four-chamber color flow image showing turbulent flow across the mitral valve orifice. LA, left atrium; PISA, proximal isovelocity surface area; RA, right atrium; RV, right ventricle.

Mitral valve area can be estimated by the mean transmitral pressure gradient or by the proximal isovelocity surface area method (Fig. 1–63; Table 1–17). However, the mean transmitral pressure gradient can underestimate the severity of mitral stenosis in the setting of a low cardiac output and overestimate the severity of the mitral stenosis in the setting of mitral regurgitation. Because the pressure half-time method is independent of cardiac output and mitral regurgitation, it is preferred in the setting of heart failure or significant mitral regurgitation.

Pressure Half-Time The pressure half-time (PHT) is the time for a pressure gradient to decay to half its peak value. The PHT is proportional to the deceleration time, the time from the peak mitral inflow E wave velocity to return to the baseline. PHT equals 0.29 times the deceleration time. The mitral valve area (MVA) can be estimated using the following simple equation: MVA = 220 ÷ PHT.

Hypertrophic Cardiomyopathy

Family history, symptoms, ECG abnormalities, and the classic auscultatory findings of a nonradiating systolic murmur that increases after ventricular premature contractions, standing, during Valsalva, or after amyl nitrite administration are the hallmarks of obstructive hypertrophic cardiomyopathy.

Echocardiography confirms the clinical diagnosis of hypertrophic cardiomyopathy by identifying the location and severity of the LVH, which can be concentric or localized to the septum as in asymmetric septal hypertrophy (ASH), the apex, or the lateral free wall. Patients with obstructive hypertrophic cardiomyopathy also have abnormal systolic anterior mitral leaflet motion (SAM) and premature, mid-systolic aortic valve closure (Fig. 1–64).

Doppler provides quantitative information regarding a possible subvalvular LV outflow or intraventricular cavity gradients both at rest and with provocation, LV diastolic abnormalities, and common associated abnormalities such as mitral regurgitation.

ACC/AHA/ASE Guidelines: Patients With Cardiomyopathy

Class I

• Suspected hypertrophic cardiomyopathy based on family history, abnormal physical examination, or ECG

■ CASE 7: CHEST PAIN

Case

A 65-year-old white man presents with the acute onset of severe substernal chest pain.

TABLE 1–17. Echo Doppler Assessment of the Severity of Mitral Stenosis

Severity	Left Atrial Size	Mitral Valve Area (cm²)	Mean Pressure Gradient (mm Hg)	Pressure Half-Time (ms)	Pulmonary Artery Pressure (mm Hg)
Normal	Normal	>4		30-60	
Mild	Mildly increased	1.5-2.5	<5	90-150	<30
Moderate	Dilated	1.0-1.5	5-10	150-219	30-50
Severe	Dilated	<1.0	>10	>220	>50

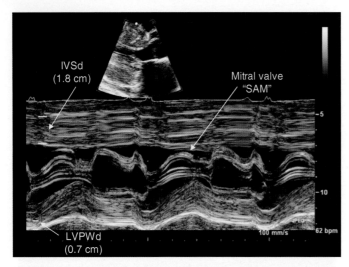

FIGURE 1–64. Hypertrophic cardiomyopathy. Parasternal long axis M-mode recording asymmetric left ventricular septal wall thickening, asymmetric septal hypertrophy, and systolic anterior motion of the anterior mitral valve leaflet. IVSd, interventricular septal wall dimension; LVPWd, left ventricular posterior wall dimension; SAM, systolic anterior motion.

TABLE 1–18. Potential Cardiovascular Causes of Acute Chest Pain

Etiology	Echo Doppler Findings
Ischemic	Abnormal regional wall motion
Aortic stenosis	Calcified leaflets with a significant left ventricular outflow gradient
Aortic dissection	Dilated aortic root; possible dissection flap; aortic regurgitation
Left ventricular hypertrophy; hypertrophic cardiomyopathy	Hypertrophy with or without left ventricular outflow obstruction
Pulmonary embolism	Right-sided dilatation; elevated right-sided pressures

Physical examination reveals normal vital signs, mild bibasilar rales, a regular rhythm, grade 2/6 apical systolic murmur, and an S_3 gallop. ECG results are as follows: normal sinus rhythm and T wave inversion in precordial leads V_2 to V_4.

ACC/AHA/ASE Guidelines: Patients With Chest Pain

Class I

- Patients with structural heart disease
- Patients with suspected myocardial ischemia during pain
- Patients with hemodynamic instability
- Patients with suspected aortic dissection

Overview

Chest pain is one of the leading complaints of patients who present to emergency departments. When the physical examination, ECG, and cardiac enzymes are nondiagnostic, echocardiography can provide valuable information that can be available immediately to help determine the etiology of the patient's chest pain (Table 1–18).

Coronary heart disease remains the number one killer in the United States. Each year, approximately 800,000 Americans are hospitalized with acute coronary syndromes, ST-segment elevation and non–ST-segment elevation myocardial infarction, or unstable angina.

ACC/AHA/ASE Guidelines: Patients With Acute Coronary Syndromes

Class I

- Diagnosis of acute coronary syndrome not evident by standard means
- Measurement of baseline LV function/infarct size

- Assessment of the extent of jeopardized myocardium
- Assessment of myocardial viability
- In patients with inferior wall infarction and suspected RV infarction
- When mechanical complications and/or mural thrombus are suspected

Acute Coronary Syndromes

In the setting of an acute coronary syndrome, echocardiography can:

- Confirm the diagnosis
  - Transient regional wall motion abnormalities associated with ECG changes and/or episodes of chest pain
- Contribute to the initial risk assessment
  - Based principally on overall LV function
- Assess possible complications
  - Acute mitral regurgitation
  - LV remodeling
  - Ventricular septal rupture
  - LV free wall rupture
  - Mural thrombi
  - RV infarction
  - Pericardial effusion
- Help assess the efficacy of the acute treatment
- Contribute to the predischarge risk assessment
  - LV function
  - Stress echocardiography

A regional wall motion abnormality evident on two-dimensional echocardiography is suggestive but not diagnostic of ischemic heart disease unless the wall motion abnormality is transiently associated with the patient's chest pain or ECG changes. On the other hand, normal regional and global wall motion in the setting of ongoing chest discomfort has an excellent negative predictive value for coronary artery disease.

Stress Echocardiography For patients unable to exercise, pharmacologic dobutamine stress echocardiography can give important information regarding the presence of jeopardized myocardium either in the area of the acute infarct or in remote regions supplied by other coronary arteries.

Aortic Dissection

Proximal aortic dissection is a life-threatening condition that needs to be considered in patients who present to the emergency department with chest pain and have nondiagnostic ECGs and negative cardiac enzymes. Classically, these patients will have a history of hypertension and the sudden onset of severe chest pain that radiates to their backs.

Two-dimensional transthoracic echocardiographic demonstration of aortic valve incompetence in the setting of dilatation of the aortic root and possibly an intimal flap is highly predictive of an acute proximal aortic dissection.[60] Either a transesophageal echocardiogram or chest computed tomography with contrast would be warranted pending emergent surgical evaluation (Fig. 1–65).[61,62]

■ CASE 8: ACUTE PERICARDITIS

Case

A 56-year-old college professor presents 6 weeks following an upper respiratory viral infection with shortness of breath and constant diffuse chest discomfort exacerbated by lying flat and deep inspiration.

Physical examination reveals a temperature of 100°F, clear lung fields, diminished heart sounds, and a three-component pericardial rub. ECG results are as follows: normal sinus rhythm, low QRS amplitude, and depressed PR segments in multiple leads.

ACC/AHA/ASE Guidelines: Patients With Pericardial Disease

Class I

- Patients with suspected pericardial disease
- Follow-up of patients with known pericardial disease
- Postinfarction patients with pericardial friction rubs accompanied by symptoms such as persistent pain, hypotension, and nausea

Class III

- Routine follow-up of small pericardial effusions in stable patients
- Routine follow-up in terminally ill patients
- Pericardial rubs following uncomplicated myocardial infarction or open heart surgery

Overview

Acute pericarditis is an inflammatory reaction to a variety of infectious and systemic abnormalities, the most common being viral, metabolic, oncologic, and systemic connective diseases and large transmural myocardial infarctions.

Pericardial Effusion

One of the earliest clinical uses for echocardiography was in diagnosing pericardial effusions.[62] Echocardiography can establish or confirm the presence of the pericardial effusion and provide a semiquantitative assessment of its size (Figs. 1–66 and 1–67; Table 1–19).

Pericardial Tamponade

The diagnosis of pericardial tamponade is based on classical physical findings and intracardiac pressure recordings. Increased intrapericardial pressure results in decreased right-sided filling, which may ultimately compromise left-sided filling and cardiac output. Echocardiography can provide confirmatory information regarding the size and hemodynamic effects

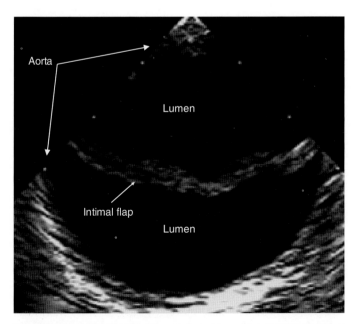

FIGURE 1–65. Aortic dissection. Transesophageal image demonstrating an intimal flap separating two aortic lumina. The true versus the false lumen cannot be determined by this single image.

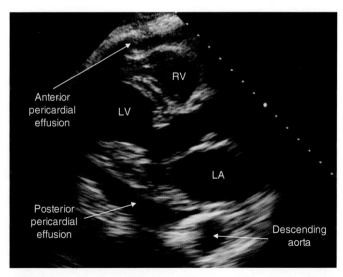

FIGURE 1–66. Pericardial effusion. Parasternal long axis image of a moderate-sized pericardial effusion, approximately 1.5 cm. LA, left atrium; LV, left ventricle; RV, right ventricle.

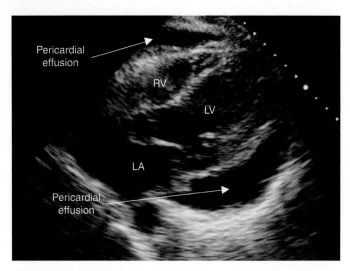

FIGURE 1–67. Pericardial effusion. Subxiphoid/subcostal image of a large pericardial effusion, approximately 2.0 cm. LA, left atrium; LV, left ventricle; RV, right ventricle.

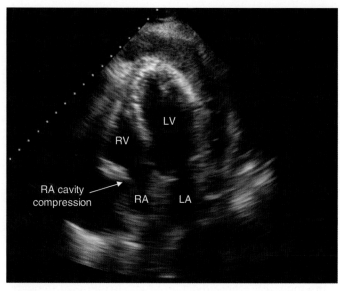

FIGURE 1–68. Pericardial tamponade. Apical four-chamber view demonstrating a large circumferential pericardial effusion with right atrial collapse. LA, left atrium; LV, left ventricle; RA, right atrium; RV, right ventricle.

of a pericardial effusion (Fig. 1–68). Echocardiographic signs of pericardial tamponade include:

- A large circumferential pericardial effusion. In some cases, smaller rapidly accumulating effusions following traumatic myocardial perforation and loculated effusions following open heart surgery may be hemodynamically significant.
- Concave right atrial free wall with late diastolic or early systolic cavity collapse.
- Concave RV free wall with early diastolic collapse.
- Abnormal septal motion due to respiratory variation in LV filling.
- Distension of the inferior vena cava unchanged by deep inspiration or sniffing.

A Doppler sign of pericardial tamponade includes >25% respiratory variation in transmitral flow velocity.

Pericardiocentesis

The presence of pericardial tamponade requires emergent percutaneous or surgical pericardiocentesis. Echocardiographic-guided percutaneous pericardiocentesis has greatly reduced the procedural complications including myocardial and/or coronary laceration, pneumothorax, arrhythmias, and death.[63,64]

■ CASE 9: INFECTIVE ENDOCARDITIS

Case

A 27-year-old intravenous drug user presents with arthralgias, myalgias, fevers, sweats, and shaking chills.

Physical examination reveals an agitated patient with a resting tachycardia and temperature of 101°F. The patient's lung fields are clear. Cardiac auscultation reveals a grade 3/6 diastolic blowing murmur at the lower left sternal border. Abdominal examination reveals left upper quadrant fullness and tenderness. Peripheral signs include oral petechiae and digital splinter hemorrhages and Osler nodes. ECG results are as follows: sinus tachycardia and nonspecific ST-T wave changes.

ACC/AHA/ASE Guidelines: Patients With Native Valve Endocarditis

Class I

- Diagnosis and assessment of hemodynamic severity
- Detection of associated abnormalities
- Reevaluation in patients with complex endocarditis including persistent fever or bacteremia or clinical deterioration

Overview

Infective endocarditis can involve any endocardial surface of the heart. Preexisting conditions such as congenital heart disease, rheumatic heart disease, mitral valve prolapse, and degenerative valve disease can be identified in approximately half of patients with infectious endocarditis. Predisposing vascular abnormalities include patent ductus arteriosus, coarctation of the aorta

TABLE 1–19. Echocardiographic Assessment of Pericardial Effusion Volume

Severity	Size[a]	Location	Volume
Physiologic	Echo-free space only in systole	Posterior	Trace (<25 cc)
Small	<1 cm	Posterior	<100 cc
Medium	1–2 cm	Anterior and posterior	100-500 cc
Large	>2 Cm	Circumferential	>500 cc

[a]Parasternal and subxiphoid transducer positions.

and atrioventricular shunts, as well as indwelling catheters or pacing wires.

The diagnostic criteria for infective endocarditis include classic clinical signs and symptoms coupled with two positive blood cultures and the following echocardiographic findings:

- An oscillating mobile mass or vegetation on a valve or chordae, in the path of a regurgitant jet or on an implanted device or wire

- A new regurgitant lesion

- An annular abscess

- Dehiscence of a prosthetic valve

The identification of a vegetation is the hallmark echocardiographic finding of infectious endocarditis (Figs. 1–69 and 1–70). Vegetations are generally characterized as mobile amorphous masses that begin as a composite of fibrous material and platelets and become secondarily infected following a bacteremia.[65] The sensitivity of transthoracic echocardiography for visualizing vegetations in proven native valve infectious endocarditis is <75% and is only approximately 25% in prosthetic valve endocarditis.[66,67] Therefore, infectious endocarditis cannot be ruled out by transthoracic echocardiography.

Transesophageal echocardiography is not recommended in patients with uncomplicated native valve endocarditis who have unambiguous transthoracic echocardiograms. However, because of its superior spatial resolution, transesophageal echocardiography is recommended in the following situations:

- When the transthoracic echocardiogram is technically limited or negative in the setting of a high clinical likelihood of endocarditis such as persistent unexplained fevers or positive blood cultures

- In the setting of preexisting native valve disease, for example, calcific aortic stenosis

- In patients with prosthetic valves

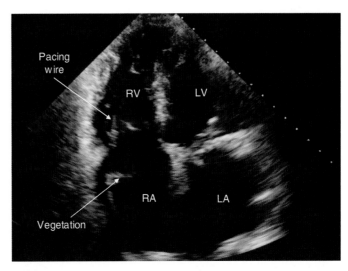

FIGURE 1–70. Infective endocarditis. Apical four-chamber image of a linear echo bright density attached to a pacing wire representing either a vegetation or thrombus. RA, right atrium; RV, right ventricle; LA, left atrium; LV, left ventricle.

The identification of a vegetation does not independently establish the diagnosis of active infectious endocarditis because vegetations may persist after the treatment of the acute illness.[68] The presence of a vegetation and its size and evolution have been correlated with clinical outcome; however, this remains controversial, and the mere detection of a vegetation is not an indication for surgery.[69,70]

Echocardiography can help in the assessment of the complications of infectious endocarditis, which include embolic events, native valve destruction and dysfunction, prosthetic valve dehiscence, abscess formation, conduction abnormalities, and acute decompensated heart failure.

■ CASE 10: ROUTINE SCREENING

Case

An 18-year-old man experiences transient dizziness while participating in a summer preseason football camp. The athlete had no prior cardiopulmonary signs or symptoms. His symptoms were quickly relieved with rest and fluids.

Physical examination revealed a mildly diaphoretic agitated young adult. Supine pulse was 96 bpm and regular. Blood pressure was 90/60 mm Hg with orthostatic changes. Cardiac auscultation revealed an innocent short 2/6 systolic ejection murmur. ECG results were normal.

Student Athlete

The majority of nontraumatic, nonheat or drug-related episodes of sudden death in young athletes are due to cardiovascular diseases. The most common cardiovascular disorders are hypertrophic cardiomyopathy, coronary anomalies, and myocarditis. However, the prevalence of significant underlying cardiovascular disease is ≤1/200 of approximately 12 million student athletes in the United States.[71]

Although recognizing the limits of current screening procedures, because the incidence of significant congenital and

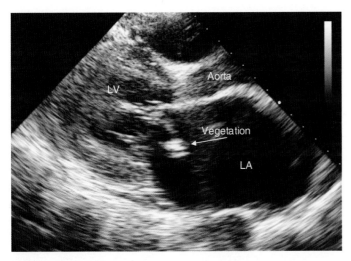

FIGURE 1–69. Infective endocarditis. Parasternal long axis image of a large, 1 cm × 1 cm, echo bright density attached to the anterior mitral valve leaflet. LA, left atrium; LV, left ventricle.

acquired abnormalities is low in the asymptomatic student athlete, current guidelines continue to recommend only a preparticipation history, physical examination, and ECG.[72] Two-dimensional echocardiography is recommended in symptomatic student athletes in whom a cardiovascular disorder is suspected.

Coronary Artery Disease

Older athletes with known coronary artery disease should have an LV function test and a maximal exercise stress test before competing in competitive or rigorous physical activity. Individuals with LVEFs ≥50%, normal age-adjusted exercise capacity, and no inducible ischemia can be considered to be at only mildly increased risk. Routine preparticipation screening is not recommended in asymptomatic adults.

The role of routine screening echocardiography in the asymptomatic young athlete or in the asymptomatic older individual who participates in strenuous physical exertion has not been established.

ACC/AHA/ASE Guidelines: Screening for Cardiovascular Disease

Class I

- Patients with a family history or first-degree relatives with genetically transmitted cardiovascular disease such as idiopathic dilated cardiomyopathies, hypertrophic cardiomyopathy, or ARVD
- Patients with Marfan syndrome or connective tissue diseases
- Baseline and follow-up in patients receiving cardiotoxic agents
- Potential donors for cardiac transplantation

Class III

- The general population
- Routine screening before competitive sports in patients with a normal cardiovascular history, physical examination, and ECG

CONCLUSION

Echocardiography is an exciting and rapidly evolving cardiac imaging modality. Echocardiography is safe and noninvasive, and it is virtually universally available in hospitals, offices, and clinics. New hand-held devices promise even greater availability and utility.

Echocardiography plays an important role in the diagnosis of many common clinical problems. Both transthoracic and transesophageal echocardiography have expanding roles in interventional cardiology. Digitally acquired echocardiographic studies can be transmitted electronically for remote expert interpretation.

Emerging three-dimensional, tissue Doppler, and intracardiac imaging technologies ensure greater future clinical applicability of echocardiography.

REFERENCES

1. Edler I, Hertz CH. The use of the ultrasonic reflectoscope for the continuous recording of movement of heart walls. *Kungl Fysiogr Sallsk i Lund Forhandl.* 1954;24:5.
2. Edler I, Hertz CH. Ultrasound cardiogram in mitral valvular diseases. *Acta Chir Scand.* 1956;111:230.
3. Curie J, Curie P. Développement, par pression, de l'électricité polaire dans les cristaux hémièdres à faces inclinées. *CR Acad Sci Gen.* 1880;91:294-295.
4. Curie J, Curie P. Sur l'électricité' polaire dans les cristaux hemièdres à faces inclinées. *CR Acad Sci Gen.* 1880;91:383-386.
5. Curie J, Curie P. Contractions et dilatations produites par des tensions dans les cristaux hémièdres à faces inclinées. *CR Acad Sci Gen.* 1880;93:1137-1140.
6. Houdas Y. Doppler, Buys-Ballot, Fizeau. Historical note on the discovery of the Doppler's effect. *Ann Cardiol Angeiol (Paris).* 1991;40:209-213.
7. Cerqueira MD, Weissman NJ, Dilsizian V, et al. Standardized myocardial segmentation and nomenclature for tomographic imaging of the heart. A statement for healthcare professionals from the Cardiac Imaging Committee of the Council on Clinical Cardiology of the American Heart Association. *Circulation.* 2002;105:539-542.
8. Redfield MM, Jacobsen SJ, Burnett JC, et al. Burden of systolic and diastolic ventricular dysfunction in the community. Appreciating the scope of the heart failure epidemic. *JAMA.* 2003;289:194-202.
9. Cheitlin MD, Armstrong WF, Aurigemma GP, et al. ACC/AHA/ASE 2003 Guideline Update for the Clinical Application of Echocardiography. A report of the American College of Cardiology/American Heart Association Task Force on Practice Guidelines. (ACC/AHA/ASE Committee to Update the 1997 Guidelines for the Clinical Application of Echocardiography). *J Am Soc Echocardiogr.* 2003;16:1091-1110.
10. Rosamond W, Flegal K, Furie K, et al. Heart Disease and Stroke Statistics–2008 Update. A Report from the American Heart Association Statistics Committee and Stroke Statistics Subcommittee. *Circulation.* 2008;117:e25-e146.
11. Richardson P, McKenna W, Bristow M, et al. Report of the 1995 World Health Organization/International Society and Federation of Cardiology Task Force on the Definition and Classification of Cardiomyopathies. *Circulation.* 1996;93:841-842.
12. Gregoratos G, Abrams J, Epstein AE, et al. American College of Cardiology/American Heart Association Task Force on Practice Guidelines/North American Society for Pacing and Electrophysiology Committee to Update the 1998 Pacemaker Guideline. ACC/AHA/NASPE 2002 guideline update for implantation of cardiac pacemakers and antiarrhythmia devices: summary article: a report of the American College of Cardiology/American Heart Association Task Force on Practice Guidelines. (ACC/AHA/NASPE Committee to Update the 1998 Pacemaker Guidelines). *Circulation.* 2002;106:2145-2161.
13. Abraham WT, Fisher WG, Smith AL, et al. Cardiac resynchronization in chronic heart failure. *N Engl J Med.* 2002;346:1845-1853.
14. Cleland JGF, Daubert JC, Erdmann E, et al. The effect of cardiac resynchronization on morbidity and mortality in heart failure. *N Engl J Med.* 2005;352:1539-1549.
15. Kannel WB, Gordon T, Offutt D. Left ventricular hypertrophy by electrocardiogram: prevalence, incidence, and mortality in the Framingham Study. *Ann Intern Med.* 1969;71:89-105.
16. Levy D, Anderson KM, Savage DD, et al. Echocardiographically detected left ventricular hypertrophy: prevalence and risk factors. *Ann Intern Med.* 1988;108:7-13.
17. Benjamin E, Levy D. Why is left ventricular hypertrophy so predictive of morbidity and mortality? *Am J Med Sci.* 1999;317:168-175.
18. Lloyd-Jones DM, Larson MG, Leip EP, et al. Lifetime risk for developing congestive heart failure: the Framingham Heart Study. *Circulation.* 2002;106:3068-3072.
19. Bursi F, Weston SA, Redfield MM, et al. Systolic and diastolic heart failure in the community. *JAMA.* 2006;296:2209-2216.
20. Vasan RS, Larson MG, Benjamin EJ, et al. Congestive heart failure in subjects with normal versus reduced left ventricular ejection fraction: prevalence and mortality in a population-based cohort. *J Am Coll Cardiol.* 1999;33:1948-1955.

21. Thiene G, Nava A, Corrado D, et al. Right ventricular cardiomyopathy and sudden death in young people. *N Engl J Med.* 1988;318:129-133.

22. Yoerger DM, Marcus F, Sherrill D, et al. Echocardiographic findings in patients meeting task force criteria for arrhythmogenic right ventricular dysplasia: new insights from the Multidisciplinary Study of Right Ventricular Dysplasia. *J Am Coll Cardiol.* 2005;15:860-865.

23. Fuster V, Rydén LE, Cannom DS, et al. ACC/AHA/ESC 2006 guidelines for the management of patients with atrial fibrillation: a report of the American College of Cardiology/American Heart Association Task Force on Practice Guidelines and the European Society of Cardiology Committee for Practice Guidelines. *J Am Coll Cardiol.* 2006;48:854-906.

24. Go AS, Hylek EM, Phillips KA, et al. Prevalence of diagnosed atrial fibrillation in adults: national implications for rhythm management and stroke prevention: the AnTi-coagulation and Risk Factors in Atrial Fibrillation (ATRIA) Study. *JAMA.* 2001;285:2370-2375.

25. Atrial Fibrillation Investigators. Echocardiographic predictors of stroke in patients with atrial fibrillation: a prospective study of 1066 patients from 3 clinical trials. *Arch Intern Med.* 1998;158:1316-1320.

26. Brand FN, Abbott RD, Kannel WB, et al. Characteristics and prognosis of lone atrial fibrillation. 30-year follow-up in the Framingham Study. *JAMA.* 1985;254:3449-3453.

27. Gage BF, Waterman AD, Shannon W, et al. Validation of clinical schemes for predicting stroke: results from the National Registry of Atrial Fibrillation. *JAMA.* 2001;285:2864-2870.

28. Penado S, Cano M, Acha O, et al. Atrial fibrillation as a risk factor for stroke recurrence. *Am J Med.* 2003;114:206-210.

29. The Stroke Prevention in Atrial Fibrillation Investigators. Predictors of thromboembolism in atrial fibrillation: II. Echocardiographic features of patients at risk. *Ann Intern Med.* 1992;116:6-12.

30. Singer DE, Albers GW, Dalen JE, et al. Antithrombotic therapy in atrial fibrillation. American College of Chest Physicians Evidence-Based Clinical Practice Guidelines (8th Edition). *Chest.* 2008;133(Suppl 6):546s-592s.

31. Klein AL, Grimm RA, Murray RD, et al. Assessment of cardioversion using transesophageal echocardiography investigators. Use of transesophageal echocardiography to guide conversion in patients with atrial fibrillation. *N Engl J Med.* 2001;344:1411-1420.

32. Tucker KJ, Curtis AB, Murphy J, et al. Transesophageal echocardiographic guidance of transseptal left heart catheterization during radiofrequency ablation of left-sided accessory pathways in humans. *Pacing Clin Electrophysiol.* 1996;19:272-281.

33. Kalman JM, Lee RJ, Fisher WG, et al. Radiofrequency catheter modification of sinus pacemaker function guided by intracardiac echocardiography. *Circulation.* 1995;92:3070-3081.

34. Chu E, Fitzpatrick AP, Chin MC, et al. Radiofrequency catheter ablation guided by intracardiac echocardiography. *Circulation.* 1994;89:1301-1305.

35. Smith SW, Light ED, Idriss SF, Wolf PD. Feasibility study of real-time three-dimensional intracardiac echocardiography for guidance of interventional electrophysiology. *Pacing Clin Electrophysiol.* 2002;25:351-357.

36. Rosen SE, Borer JS, Hochreiter C, et al. Natural history of the asymptomatic/minimally symptomatic patient with severe mitral regurgitation secondary to mitral valve prolapse and normal right and left ventricular performance. *Am J Cardiol.* 1994;74:374-380.

37. Rosenhek R, Rader F, Klaar U, et al. Outcome of watchful waiting in asymptomatic severe mitral regurgitation. *Circulation.* 2006;113:2238-2244.

38. Enriquez-Sarano M, Tajik AJ, Schaff HV, et al. Echocardiographic prediction of survival after surgical correction of organic mitral regurgitation. *Circulation.* 1994;90:830-837.

39. Zoghbi WA, Enriquez-Sarano M, Foster E, et al. Recommendations for evaluation of the severity of native valvular regurgitation with two-dimensional and Doppler echocardiography. *J Am Soc Echocardiogr.* 2003;16:777-802.

40. Enriquez-Sarano M, Avierinos JF, Messika-Zeitoun D, et al. Quantitative determinants of the outcome of asymptomatic mitral regurgitation. *N Engl J Med.* 2005;352:875-883.

41. Kang DH, Kim JH, Rim JH, et al. Comparison of early surgery versus conventional treatment in asymptomatic severe mitral regurgitation. *Circulation.* 2009;119:797-804.

42. Nishimura RA, McGoon MD, Shub C, et al. Echocardiographically documented mitral-valve prolapse: long-term follow-up of 237 patients. *N Engl J Med.* 1985;313:1305-1309.

43. Marks AR, Choong CY, Sanfilippo AJ, et al. Identification of high-risk and low-risk subgroups of patients with mitral-valve prolapse. *N Engl J Med.* 1989;320:1031-1036.

44. Freed LA, Levy D, Levine RA, et al. Prevalence and clinical outcome of mitral valve prolapse. *N Engl J Med.* 1999;341:1-7.

45. Smith MD, Cassidy JM, Gurley JC, et al. Echo Doppler evaluation of patients with acute mitral regurgitation: superiority of transesophageal echocardiography with color flow imaging. *Am Heart J.* 1995;129:967-974.

46. Keeley EC, Hillis LD. Left ventricular mural thrombus after acute myocardial infarction. *Clin Cardiol.* 1996;19:83-86.

47. Hagen PT, Scholz DG, Edwards WD. Incidence and size of patent foramen ovale during the first 10 decades of life: an autopsy study of 965 normal hearts. *Mayo Clin Proc.* 1984;59:17-20.

48. Von Bardeleben RS, Richter C, Otto J, et al. Long term follow up after percutaneous closure of PFO in 357 patients with paradoxical embolism: difference in occlusion systems and influence of atrial septum aneurysm. *Int J Cardiol.* 2009;134:33-41.

49. Hijazi Z, Wang Z, Cao Q, et al. Transcatheter closure of atrial septal defects and patent foramen ovale under intracardiac echocardiographic guidance: feasibility and comparison with transesophageal echocardiography. *Catheter Cardiovasc Interv.* 2001;52:194-199.

50. Mullen MJ, Dias BF, Walker F, et al. Intracardiac echocardiography guided device closure of atrial septal defects. *J Am Coll Cardiol.* 2003;41:285-292.

51. Kurth T, Tzourio C, Bousser MG. Migraine a matter of the heart? *Circulation.* 2008;118:1405-1407.

52. Rundek T, Elkind MS, DiTullio MR, et al. Patent foramen ovale and migraine. A cross-sectional study from the Northern Manhattan Study (NOMAS). *Circulation.* 2008;118:1419-1424.

53. Dowson A, Mullen MJ, Peatfield R, et al. Migraine Intervention With STARFlex Technology (MIST) trial: a prospective, multicenter, double-blind, sham-controlled trial to evaluate the effectiveness of patent foramen ovale closure with STARFlex septal repair implant to resolve refractory migraine headache. *Circulation.* 2008;117:1397-404.

54. Kapoor W. Evaluation and management of syncope. *JAMA.* 1992;268:2553-2560.

55. Strickberger SA, Benson DW, Biaggioni I, et al. AHA/ACCF Scientific Statement on the evaluation of syncope: from the American Heart Association Councils on Clinical Cardiology, Cardiovascular Nursing, Cardiovascular Disease in the Young, and Stroke, and the Quality of Care and Outcomes Research Interdisciplinary Working Group; and the American College of Cardiology Foundation: in collaboration with the Heart Rhythm Society: endorsed by the American Autonomic Society. *Circulation.* 2006;113:316-327.

56. Monin JL, Quere JP, Monchi M, et al. Low-gradient aortic stenosis: operative risk stratification and predictors for long-term outcome: a multicenter study using dobutamine stress hemodynamics. *Circulation.* 2003;108:319-324.

57. Henry WL, Bonow RO, Border JS, et al. Observations on the optimum time for operative intervention for aortic regurgitation. I. Evaluation of the results of aortic valve replacement in symptomatic patients. *Circulation.* 1980;61:471-483.

58. Henry WL, Bonow RO, Rosing DR, Epstein SE. Observations on the optimum time for operative intervention for aortic regurgitation. II. Serial echocardiographic evaluation of asymptomatic patients. *Circulation.* 1980;61:484-492.

59. Bonow RO, Picone AL, McIntosh CL, et al. Survival and functional results after valve replacement for aortic regurgitation from 1976 to 1983: impact of preoperative left ventricular function. *Circulation.* 1985;72:1244-1256.

60. Khandheria BK, Tajik AJ, Taylor CL, et al. Aortic dissection: review of value and limitations of two-dimensional echocardiography in a six year experience. *J Am Soc Echocardiogr.* 1989;2:17-24.

61. Moore AG, Eagle KA, Bruckman D, et al. Choice of computed tomography, transesophageal echocardiography, magnetic resonance imaging, and aortography in acute aortic dissection: International Registry of Acute Aortic Dissection (IRAD). *Am J Cardiol.* 2002;89:1235-1238.

62. Feigenbaum H, Waldhausen JA, Hyde LP. Ultrasound diagnosis of pericardial effusion. *JAMA.* 1965;191:711-714.

63. Callahan JA, Seward JB, Nishimura RA, et al. Two-dimensional echocardiographically guided pericardiocentesis: experience in 117 consecutive patients. *Am J Cardiol.* 1985;55:476-479.

64. Tsang TS, Sarano ME, Freeman W, et al. Consecutive 1127 therapeutic echocardiographically guided pericardiocenteses: clinical profile, practice patterns, and outcomes spanning 21 years. *Mayo Clin Proc.* 2002;77:429-436.

65. Wilson W, Taubert KA, Gewitz M, et al. Prevention of infective endocarditis: guidelines from the American Heart Association: a guideline from the American Heart Association Rheumatic Fever, Endocarditis and Kawasaki Disease Committee, Council on Cardiovascular Disease in the Young, and the Council on Clinical Cardiology, Council on Cardiovascular Surgery and Anesthesia, and the Quality of Care and Outcomes Research Interdisciplinary Working Group. *Circulation.* 2007;116:1736-1754.

66. Lindner JR, Case RA, Dent JM, et al. Diagnostic value of echocardiography in suspected endocarditis: an evaluation based on the pretest probability of disease. *Circulation.* 1996;93:730-736.

67. Shively BK, Gurule FT, Roldan CA, et al. Diagnostic value of transesophageal compared with transthoracic echocardiography in infective endocarditis. *J Am Coll Cardiol.* 1991;18:391-397.

68. Vuille C, Nidorf M, Weyman AE, Picard MH. Natural history of vegetations during successful medical treatment of endocarditis. *Am Heart J.* 1994;128:1200-1209.

69. Sanfilippo AJ, Picard MH, Newell JB, et al. Echocardiographic assessment of patients with infectious endocarditis: prediction of risk for complications. *J Am Coll Cardiol.* 1991;18:1191-1199.

70. Bayer AS, Bolger AF, Taubert KA, et al. Diagnosis and management of infective endocarditis and its complications. *Circulation.* 1998;98:2936-2948.

71. Maron BJ. Sudden death in young athletes. *N Engl J Med.* 2003;349:1064-1075.

72. Maron BJ, Zipes DP. 36th Bethesda Conference: eligibility recommendations for competitive athletes with cardiovascular abnormalities. *J Am Coll Cardiol.* 2005;45:1313-1375.

CHAPTER 2
PHONOCARDIOGRAPHY

Anna-Leena Noponen, Sakari Lukkarinen, and Raimo Sepponen

IINTRODUCTION / 41

BASICS OF PHONOCARDIOGRAPHY / 41
Clinical Auscultation / 41
Conventional Phonocardiography / 41
Digital Phonocardiography / 41

HEART SOUND ANALYSIS / 41
Heart Sound Analysis in Children / 41
Heart Sound Analysis in Adults / 42
Examples of Heart Sound Analysis / 42
Limitations of Phonocardiography / 43
Heart Sound Analysis in Telemedicine / 47

COMPARISON OF PHONOCARDIOGRAPHY WITH OTHER HEART SOUND IMAGING METHODS / 47
Clinical Auscultation / 47
Fetal Heart Sound Doppler Recording / 47
Laser Doppler Vibrometry / 47

COMBINATION WITH OTHER IMAGING METHODS / 48
Electrocardiography and Phonocardiography / 48
Cardiac Catheterization and Phonocardiography / 48
Echocardiography and Phonocardiography / 48
Magnetic Resonance Imaging and Phonocardiography / 48

THE FUTURE OF PHONOCARDIOGRAPHY / 48

INTRODUCTION

Cardiac auscultation is an important and basic component of a physical examination in clinical practice. For the experienced listener, auscultation provides quick and reliable diagnostic information about the state of the heart. Phonocardiography systems allow the listener to record these findings. Spectral phonocardiographic studies, introduced as early as 1955 by McKusick et al,[1] accurately characterize the quality of heart sounds and cardiac murmurs by creating a graphic record. Recording heart sounds and phonocardiograms enables building heart sound libraries and teaching material.[2-4] Dr. Proctor Harvey's audio tapes are classics in adult cardiology.

The significant improvements in personal computers over the past few decades have made it possible to design new highly capable phono-spectrocardiographic devices with digital signal analysis. Published studies have demonstrated the clinical validity of this method of recording and analyzing cardiac sounds.[5-9] Digital signal processing allows the combination of phonocardiography with other imaging modalities.

BASICS OF PHONOCARDIOGRAPHY

■ CLINICAL AUSCULTATION

Heart sounds provide information about both normal and pathologic physical events in the heart. The movement of blood and the movement and vibration of the heart structures produce audible sounds and murmurs. The causes of vibratory movement in the cardiovascular system can be categorized into two general mechanisms: (1) rapid acceleration and deceleration of blood flow or (2) continuous turbulence in blood flow. The sudden sounds caused by acceleration and deceleration of blood flow are called *heart sounds*, and the sounds produced by turbulent blood flow are labeled *murmurs*.

■ CONVENTIONAL PHONOCARDIOGRAPHY

Phonocardiography is a diagnostic technique that graphically records cardiac acoustic phenomena.[10] Visualization of heart sounds may help in understanding cardiac events (Fig. 2–1). A visual record may also help an inexperienced listener recognize and classify auscultatory findings. The essential elements of the phonocardiographic system are a transducer (microphone), an amplifier, a filter, and recording, analyzing, and transcription systems. In the past, all of the parts, including those needed for recording and transcription, were analog.

■ DIGITAL PHONOCARDIOGRAPHY

Today, recording and analysis are done digitally using personal computers and specialized software or by using custom electronic devices specially designed for this purpose. In addition, sophisticated analysis software, feature extraction, and classification algorithms (such as neural networks) may be used for further interpretation of sounds.[11,12]

A visual presentation provides an opportunity to study the timing, frequency, and intensity of different heart sound and murmur components. Spectral phonocardiography combined with traditional phonocardiographic tracing simultaneously depicts all of these features. Digital signal processing allows accurate fine-tuning of the visual representation in terms of various frequencies, intensities, and timing.

HEART SOUND ANALYSIS

■ HEART SOUND ANALYSIS IN CHILDREN

Over 90% of heart murmurs in children are physiologic and benign. Moreover, 75% of these murmurs are innocent vibratory murmurs.[13] Visual analysis of the phono-spectrocardiographic record enables differentiation between pathologic and physiologic pediatric murmurs. Simple quantitative criteria applied to the phono-spectrocardiographic record may significantly improve the diagnostic accuracy of any screener to the level of a subspecialist.[9] Advanced signal processing and pattern recognition tools have yielded even better diagnostic accuracy.[14] Artificial neural network–based screening has been reported to

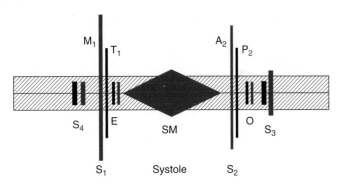

FIGURE 2–1. Heart sound events represented graphically. The red bars represent left-side events, and the black bars represent right-side events. The gray area is normally inaudible. The first heart sound (S_1) contains two components: the mitral valve closure sound (M_1) and the tricuspid valve closure sound (T_1). The second heart sound (S_2) contains two components: the aortic valve closure sound (A_2) followed by the pulmonary valve closure sound (P_2). The presystolic (atrial) gallop sound (S_4) is normally inaudible. The prodiastolic (ventricular) gallop (S_3) may be audible and is normal in children. Innocent systolic murmur (SM) is a common normal finding, especially in children. Ejection sounds (E) are normally inaudible. Opening snaps (O), if audible, indicate some level of pathology. Adapted from Leatham.[10]

have higher sensitivity and specificity than other signal processing methods.[8,12]

HEART SOUND ANALYSIS IN ADULTS

Phono-spectrocardiographic signal analysis is a promising clinical application in the assessment of the severity of aortic or carotid arterial stenosis.[2,5,6] Furthermore, as in children, it can be used to differentiate between pathologic and innocent murmurs. Traditional phonocardiography combined with spectral digital analysis, also known as acoustic cardiography, has been used to recognize and quantify heart sounds S_3 and S_4.[15-18] Changes in the recorded magnitude of S_3 and/or S_4 can perhaps be used to determine whether the patient's hemodynamic status is improving or worsening (Fig. 2–2).

EXAMPLES OF HEART SOUND ANALYSIS

The following examples of heart sound analysis are from pediatric patients, and they demonstrate the validity of modern phono-spectrocardiographic imaging techniques. The software used includes corresponding audio recordings and marker measures (Fig. 2–3).

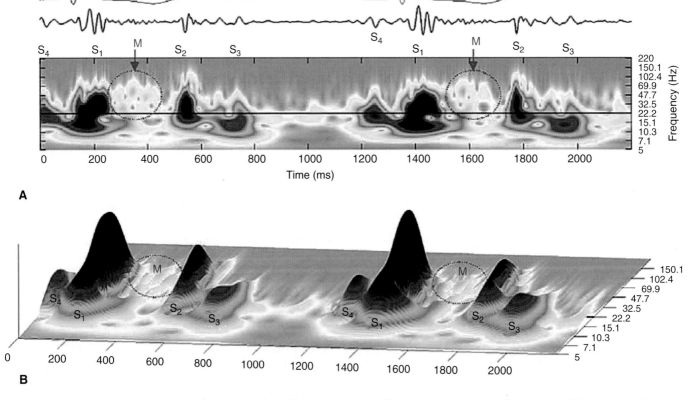

FIGURE 2–2. Acoustic cardiography report and time-frequency analysis of heart sounds from a subject with a systolic murmur. The upper panel (**A**) shows a two-dimensional acoustic cardiography report for a subject with a systolic murmur (M) and the panels below (**B**) illustrate the three-dimensional scalogram views of a two beats from the acoustic cardiography rhythm strip shown above. Because murmurs have higher frequency components than diastolic heart sounds, they do not have to be high in intensity to be detected by the human ear. Thus, in this case, it is easier for the human ear to detect the murmur than the low-frequency third and fourth heart sound. Adapted from Erne.[18]

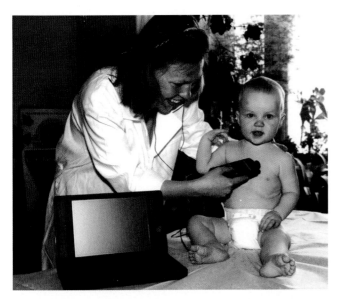

FIGURE 2–3. Heart sound recording system with a hand-held electronic stethoscope. Image courtesy of Dr. Anna-Leena Noponen.

In these phono-spectrograms (Figs. 2–4 to 2–11), timing is read from the time scale (at the bottom of the figures) by visually examining both the phonocardiogram and the spectrogram and then deciding the duration of a sound event or murmur and dragging the marker over the selected time segment. The intensities of S_1, S_2, and murmurs are read from the scale (to

the right in the figures, percentages of the recording capacity of the stethoscope) by positioning the marker over the phonocardiogram. The loudness of a murmur is estimated from the phonocardiogram by comparing the maximum amplitude of the murmur to the average value of the maximum amplitude of the first and second heart sounds. Finally, the frequencies (in hertz) are read by moving the marker over the spectrogram. The intensity level (on the left of the figures, the color scale) of the marked and nonmarked frequency limits of the sounds is between 45 and 50 dB (yellow color in the figures).

Hence, this system is able to display and reproduce cardiovascular sound events. For example, a musical murmur caused by harmonic movements of the heart and vasculature, such as an innocent vibratory murmur (Still's murmur) is usually visualized as a well-defined area or line on the spectrogram. Innocent systolic murmurs appear to have a lower peak frequency (below 200 Hz) and a shorter duration (below 80% of the duration of "audible systole" from the end of S_1 to the beginning of S_2) compared with recordings of pathologic murmurs. Also, innocent systolic murmurs always fade before the second heart sound. In contrast, the higher velocity blood flow of a pathologic cardiac lesion produces a more intense murmur and a wider frequency scale (in hertz). This phenomenon is clearly demonstrated on the spectrographic recordings.

■ LIMITATIONS OF PHONOCARDIOGRAPHY

Background noise can be eliminated with filtering systems, but phonocardiography still has limitations. The intensity of heart

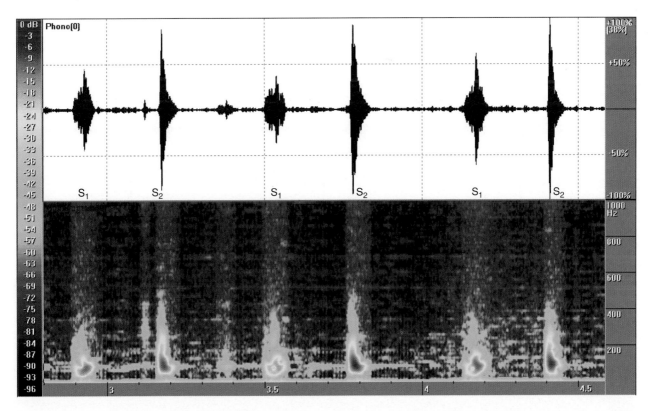

FIGURE 2–4. Normal heart auscultation in a 3-year-old child. The first (S_1) and second (S_2) heart sounds are clearly distinctive. There are no systolic or diastolic murmurs. The rapid breathing sound produces an irregular cloud on the third heart cycle.

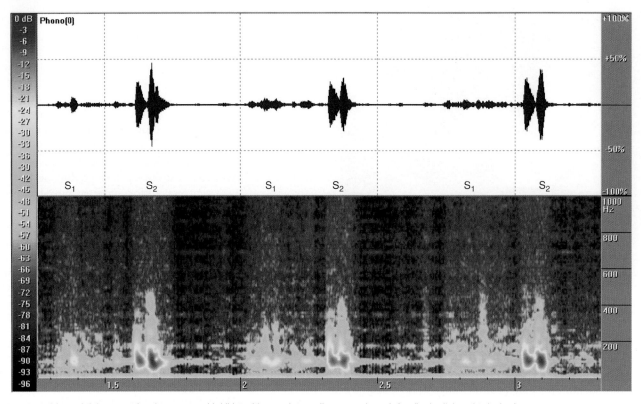

FIGURE 2–5. Atrial septal defect secundum in a 12-year-old child. In this case, the systolic murmur is weak, but fixed splitting of S_2 is clearly seen.

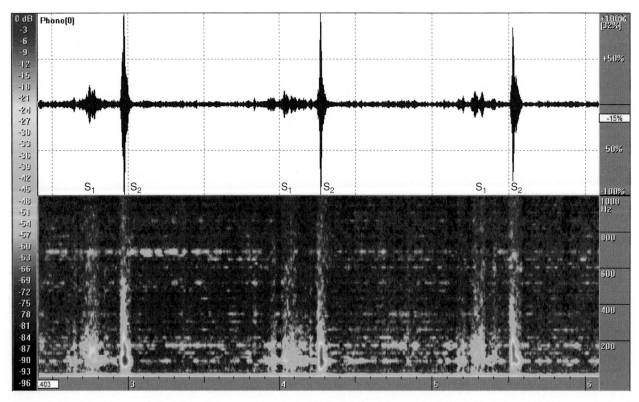

FIGURE 2–6. Pulmonary hypertension in a young adult with Down syndrome. The patient has an atrioventricular septal defect and Eisenmenger syndrome. Note the loud single S_2.

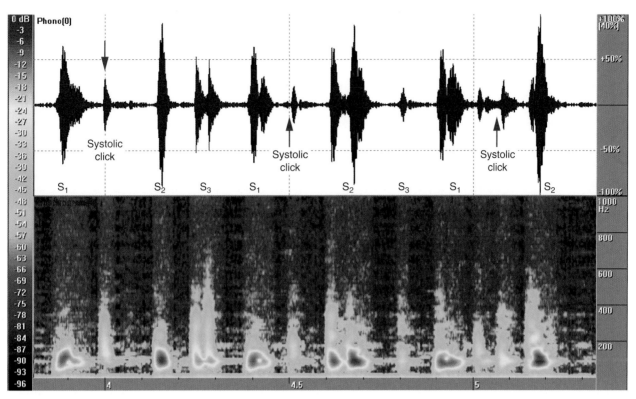

FIGURE 2–7. Mitral valve prolapse in an asymptomatic 8-year-old child. The cardiac echo demonstrated a mitral prolapse without regurgitation. Both the phonogram and spectrogram show a systolic mitral click and a diastolic S_3 prominent during inspiration.

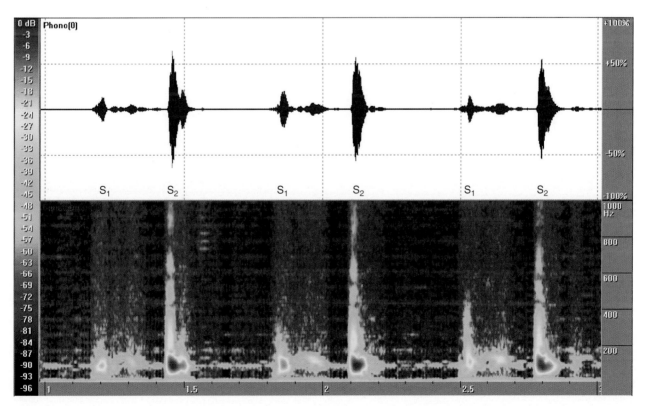

FIGURE 2–8. Innocent vibratory murmur (Still's murmur) in a 7-year-old child. On auscultation, a typical early and mid-systolic low-frequency musical murmur is heard at the left fourth intercostal space and the apex. The phonogram shows a rising and falling early mid-systolic murmur, and the spectrogram shows a typical dense configuration and a decreasing frequency, with a maximum gradient of approximately 150 Hz.

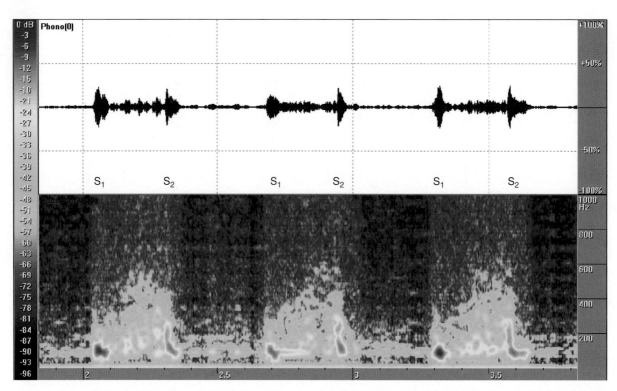

FIGURE 2–9. Ventricular septal defect (VSD) in a 6-year-old child. This is a perimembranous mild-to-moderate VSD. The size of the shunt was such that the benefits of surgery were not obvious. On echocardiography, the flow through the VSD is 5 m/s. On auscultation, a grade 4 pansystolic murmur is heard in the precordium. The phonogram shows a pansystolic, rather even murmur, and the spectrogram shows high frequencies suggesting high flow velocity. As the heart contracts, the size of the shunt is reduced, causing increased flow velocity and thus also increased frequencies toward end-systole.

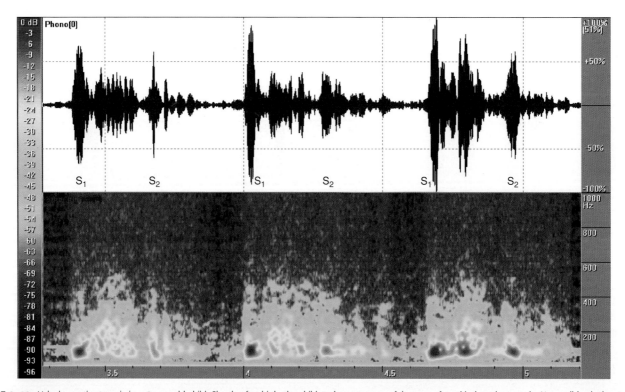

FIGURE 2–10. Valvular aortic stenosis in a 2-year-old child. Shortly after birth, the child underwent successful surgery for critical aortic stenosis. Now mild valvular stenosis is detected; the flow gradient is 25 mm Hg. Narrow-based regurgitation of aortic valve is also found. On auscultation, the child has a coarse grade 3 systolic murmur and also a short grade 1 early diastolic regurgitation murmur. The phonogram shows a diamond-shaped recording characteristic of a stenotic lesion. The aortic click is not visualized. This could be due to the mild stenosis and the child's young age. Poststenotic dilatation of the ascending aorta has not yet developed. A silent early diastolic flow murmur is also seen. The spectrogram shows a descending contour that supports stenosis; the maximum frequency is slightly over 500 Hz.

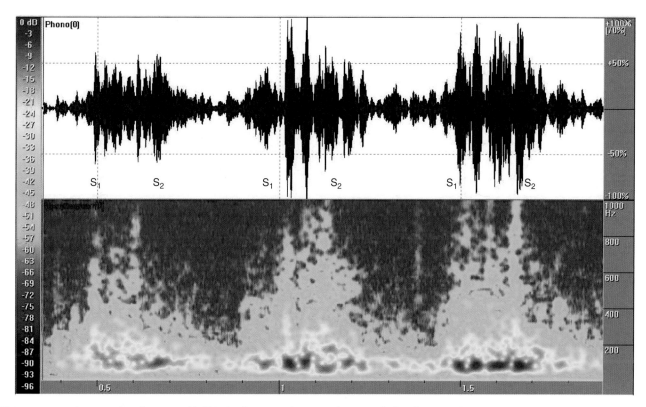

FIGURE 2–11. Patent ductus arteriosus in a 2-year-old child. The phonogram shows a consistent systolic-diastolic murmur that becomes louder toward end-systole and is quieter in diastole. The flow is rapid in systole, which is when the spectrogram shows the highest frequencies.

sounds varies between different auscultation areas and different persons. The loudness of heart sounds (in dB) is difficult to illustrate with the phonocardiographic method. Spectrograms may give more reliable information about the quality of a heart murmur, as seen in the examples in Figs. 2–4 to 2–11.

HEART SOUND ANALYSIS IN TELEMEDICINE

Telemedicine is a rapidly developing application area in clinical medicine. It allows the specialist to work in a wider geographical area and to offer services in rural areas. Today, data can be conveniently stored on personal computers or hand-held devices and transferred through communication networks, like the Internet or mobile phone networks, assuming such networks are available. Heart sound signals can be remotely monitored in real time in teleconsultations, the examination can be done interactively, or the signals can be stored and forwarded for more detailed analysis and consultation purposes.[19-21]

COMPARISON OF PHONOCARDIOGRAPHY WITH OTHER HEART SOUND IMAGING METHODS

CLINICAL AUSCULTATION

The acoustic information of phonocardiography visualizes the auditory events of the heart. Spectral phonocardiography emulates the ear and can be used during a teaching session. In clinical practice, observation of spectrograms or digital analysis of recorded heart sounds compensates for the inexperience of the listener. However, it must be kept in mind that this method is only a part of the clinical examination. It should never remain as the only criterion of a child's cardiac defect. The method may eliminate unnecessary consultations or echo examinations, but it should never replace echo examinations.

FETAL HEART SOUND DOPPLER RECORDING

Fetal heart rate monitoring using the Doppler shift resulting from the movements of the fetal heart is a standard examination in most obstetrical wards. Ultrasound-based instruments are not suitable for long-term surveillance of the unborn. Heart sound monitoring with an electronic stethoscope is noninvasive, and digital phonocardiography has proved to be a useful method for prenatal heart sound follow-up and screening of fetal heart murmurs.[22-24]

LASER DOPPLER VIBROMETRY

Laser Doppler vibrometry has been recently applied to noncontact monitoring of cardiac activity, both in terms of cardiac rate and heart rate variability, by measuring the velocity of the skin surface of the chest wall and the neck (optical vibrocardiography). The data were compared with phonocardiography, and the findings were correlated with the heart sounds related to the closure of the mitral valve and the following closure of the aortic and pulmonary valves with characteristic deflections identifiable on the vibrocardiography traces.[25,26]

COMBINATION WITH OTHER IMAGING METHODS

■ ELECTROCARDIOGRAPHY AND PHONOCARDIOGRAPHY

In clinical practice or during a teaching session, one sound channel without an electrocardiogram (ECG) is a fast and easy way to record and store sound signals. However, a simultaneous ECG recording is advisable for accurate timing and documentation of the cardiac cycle.

Assessment of the left ventricular systolic function has been applied to derive the systolic time intervals. The method combines analogic phonocardiography with ECG and external recordings of the carotid pulse. More precise noninvasive assessments of the left ventricular systolic function are performed with acoustic cardiography—a simultaneous ECG and heart sound recording with digital analysis.[15-18]

Pulse Doppler echocardiography is the most common method for predicting optimal atrioventricular synchrony in patients with a complete atrioventricular block and an implanted DDD pacemaker. The possibility of using phonocardiography instead of echocardiography has been demonstrated to be a valid and simple method for this purpose.[27]

■ CARDIAC CATHETERIZATION AND PHONOCARDIOGRAPHY

During radiofrequency ablation, the acoustic energy created by microbubble formation can be detected without echocardiography using digital phonocardiography.[28]

■ ECHOCARDIOGRAPHY AND PHONOCARDIOGRAPHY

Simultaneous timing of heart sounds is used with echocardiography (eg, by assessing the ventricular function). Noise and filtering may limit the precision of phonocardiography.[29]

■ MAGNETIC RESONANCE IMAGING AND PHONOCARDIOGRAPHY

A novel device, the magnetic resonance stethoscope, consists of an acoustic sensor, a signal processing unit, and a coupler to the magnetic resonance imaging system. The system is safe, there is no risk of high-voltage induction or patient burns, it is immune to electromagnetic interference, and it is suitable for all magnetic fields.[30]

THE FUTURE OF PHONOCARDIOGRAPHY

During the past years, improvements in personal computers have made it possible to design new low-cost, high-quality phonocardiographic devices. Spectral phonocardiography enhances

auscultation and is a valid and valuable tool in clinical practice. It can be used to teach an inexperienced listener the art of auscultation. The computerized signal processing method enables automatic analysis of audible heart events and thereby offers a new diagnostic aid in clinical decision making. Digital phonocardiography provides the technology to accurately record and store cardiac auscultatory findings, thus enabling store-and-forward teleconsultation and improved documentation in electronic medical records. The digital processing of heart sounds allows the combination of phonocardiography with other imaging modalities.

REFERENCES

1. McKusick VA, Webb GN, O'Neal Humphries J, et al. On cardiovascular sound: further observations by means of spectral phonocardiography. *Circulation.* 1955;11:849-870.
2. Tavel ME. Cardiac auscultation: a glorious past—and it does have a future! *Circulation.* 2006;113:1255-1259.
3. Woywodt A, Herrmann A, Kielstein JT, Haller H, Haubitz M, Purnhagen H. A novel multimedia tool to improve bedside teaching of cardiac auscultation. *Postgrad Med J.* 2004;80:355-357.
4. Lukkarinen S, Noponen AL. Heart auscultation: audio samples and phonocardiograms. *Evidence-Based Medicine Guidelines* [online]. Available at: http://www.ebm-guidelines.com/. Accessed July 28, 2010.
5. Tavel ME, Katz H. Usefulness of a new sound spectral averaging technique to distinguish an innocent systolic murmur from that of aortic stenosis. *Am J Cardiol.* 2005;95:902-904.
6. Voss A, Mix A, Hubner T. Diagnosing aortic valve stenosis by parameter extraction of heart sound signals. *Ann Biomed Eng.* 2005;33:1167-1174.
7. El-Segaier M, Lilja O, Lukkarinen S, et al. Computer-based detection and analysis of heart sound and murmur. *Ann Biomed Eng.* 2005;33:937-942.
8. Bhatikar SR, Degroff C, Mahajan RL. A classifier based on the artificial network approach for cardiologic auscultation in pediatrics. *Artif Intell Med.* 2005;33:251-260.
9. Noponen AL, Lukkarinen S, Angerla A, et al. Phono-spectrographic analysis of heart murmur in children. *BMC Pediatr.* 2007;7:23.
10. Leatham A. *Auscultation of the Heart and Phonocardiography.* London, United Kingdom: J & A Churchill; 1970.
11. Wang P, Lim CS, Chauhan S, et al. Phonocardiographic signal analysis method using a modified hidden Markov model. *Ann Biomed Eng.* 2007;35:367-374.
12. DeGroff CG, Bhatikar S, Hertzberg J, Shandas R, Valdes-Cruz L, Mahajan RL. Artificial neural network-based method of screening heart murmurs in children. *Circulation.* 2001;103:2711-2716.
13. Van Oort A, Hopman J, De Boo T, et al. The vibratory innocent heart murmur in schoolchildren: a case-control Doppler echocardiographic study. *Pediatric Cardiol.* 1994;15:275-281.
14. Thompson WR, Hayek CS, Tuchinda C, et al. Automated cardiac auscultation for detection of pathologic heart murmurs. *Pediatr Cardiol.* 2001;22:373-379.
15. Marcus GM, Gerber IL, McKeown BH, et al. Association between phonocardiographic third and fourth heart sounds and objective measures of left ventricular function. *JAMA.* 2005;293:2238-2244.
16. Shapiro M, Moyers B, Marcus GM, et al. Diagnostic characteristics of combining phonocardiographic third heart sound and systolic time intervals for the prediction of left ventricular dysfunction. *J Card Fail.* 2007;13:18-24.
17. Efstratiadis S, Michaels AD. Computerized acoustic cardiographic electromechanical activation time correlates with invasive and echocardiographic parameters of left ventricular contractility. *J Card Fail.* 2008;14:577-582.
18. Erne P. Beyond auscultation—acoustic cardiography in the diagnosis and assessment of cardiac disease. *Swiss Med Wkly.* 2008;138:439-452.
19. Tuchinda C, Thompson WR. Cardiac auscultatory recording database: delivering heart sounds through the Internet. *Proc AMIA Symp.* 2001:716-720.
20. Finley JP, Warren AE, Sharratt GP, et al. Assessing children's heart sounds a distance with digital recordings. *Pediatrics.* 2006;118:2322-2325.

21. Mahnke CB, Mulreany MP, Inafuku J, et al. Utility of store-and-forward pediatric telecardiology evaluation in distinguishing normal from pathologic pediatric heart sounds. *Clin Pediatr (Phila)*. 2008;47:919-925.

22. Kovacs F, Kersner N, Kadar K, et al. Computer method for perinatal screening of cardiac murmur using fetal phonocardiography. *Comput Biol Med*. 2009;39:1130-1136.

23. Mittra, AK, Choudhari NK. Time-frequency analysis of foetal heart sound signal for the prediction of prenatal anomalies. *J Med Eng Technol*. 2009;33:296-302.

24. Chourasia VS, Mittra AK. Selection of mother wavelet and denoising algorithm for analysis of foetal phonocardiographic signals. *J Med Eng Technol*. 2009;33:442-448.

25. De Melis M, Morbiducci U, Scalise L. Identification of cardiac events by optical vibrocardiography: comparison with phonocardiography. *Conf Proc IEEE Eng Med Biol Soc*. 2007;2007:2956-2959.

26. Scalise L, Morbiducci U. Non-contact cardiac monitoring from carotid artery using optical vibrocardiography. *Med Eng Phys*. 2008;30:490-497.

27. Miki Y, Ishikawa T, Matsushita K, et al. Novel method of predicting the optimal atrioventricular delay in patients with complete AV block, normal left ventricular function and an implanted DDD pacemaker. *Circ J*. 2009;73:654-657.

28. Kotini P, Mohler S, Ellenbogen KA, et al. Detection of microbubble formation during radiofrequency ablation using phonocardiography. *Europace*. 2006;8:333-335.

29. Aase SA, Torp H, Støylen A. Aortic valve closure: relation to tissue velocities by Doppler and speckle tracking in normal subjects. *Eur J Echocardiogr*. 2008;9:555-559.

30. Frauenrath T, Hezel F, Heinrichs U, et al. Feasibility of cardiac gating free of interference with electro-magnetic fields at 1.5 Tesla, 3.0 Tesla and 7.0 Tesla using an MR-stethoscope. *Invest Radiol*. 2009;44:539-547.

CHAPTER 3

MYOCARDIAL PERFUSION SINGLE PHOTON EMISSION COMPUTED TOMOGRAPHY AND POSITRON EMISSION TOMOGRAPHY

Marcus Carlsson and Juhani Knuuti

INTRODUCTION / 50

PATHOPHYSIOLOGY / 50

SPECT TECHNIQUE / 51
Gated SPECT and Electrocardiogram Triggering / 51
New Detector Technology for SPECT / 54
Attenuation and Its Correction / 54

PET TECHNIQUE / 55
Acquisition / 55
Attenuation and Other Corrections / 55

THE STRESS TEST / 55
Exercise Stress Test / 55
Pharmacologic Stress Test / 55
Medication and Caffeine Before Myocardial Perfusion
    Imaging / 56

RADIOPHARMACEUTICALS / 57
SPECT Tracers / 57
PET Tracers / 57

IMAGING PROTOCOLS / 57
SPECT Protocols / 57
PET Protocols and Data Analysis / 58

HYBRID IMAGING WITH CT / 58

**INDICATIONS FOR MYOCARDIAL PERFUSION SPECT
    AND PET / 60**
Primary Diagnosis of Ischemic Heart Disease / 60
Patients With "Low Risk" Acute Chest Pain / 61
Evaluation of the Physiologic Significance of a Coronary
    Stenosis / 61
Assessment of Ischemia in Patients With Prior
    Revascularization / 62
Risk Assessment Before Major Surgery / 62
Viability Testing / 62

**DIAGNOSTIC ACCURACY, OUTCOME, AND RISK
    ASSESSMENT / 63**

What Determines Whether a Perfusion Imaging Test is
    Useful? / 63
Amount of Ischemic Myocardium / 63
Studies Showing Usefulness of Myocardial Perfusion Imaging in
    Different Clinical Scenarios / 64

PITFALLS / 65
Overreporting / 65
Inadequate Stress Test / 65
Left Bundle Branch Block / 65
Triple-Vessel Disease / 66
High Gastrointestinal Tracer Activity / 66

COMPARISONS WITH OTHER IMAGING MODALITIES / 66
Ischemia Detection / 66
Viability Assessment / 67
Left Ventricular Function / 67

INTRODUCTION

Myocardial perfusion single photon emission computed tomography (SPECT) is a nuclear medicine imaging technique that uses a radioactive perfusion tracer to detect ischemia. Myocardial SPECT can detect, localize, and quantify the degree of ischemic myocardium. The result of a myocardial perfusion SPECT is related to the prognostic outcome of cardiac events (ie, myocardial infarction and death). Therefore, myocardial perfusion SPECT is used to guide treatment in patients with stable angina and after acute coronary syndrome. Myocardial perfusion SPECT is a mature technique, one of the most commonly used cardiac imaging techniques, and part of the international guidelines for treatment of patients with ischemic heart disease.[1-3] There are international guidelines on how to perform,[4] how to report,[5] and when to use[6] myocardial perfusion SPECT. Myocardial positron emission tomography (PET) is a newer nuclear medicine imaging technique that has rapidly become routine in cancer patients. The use in cardiology is also increasing because PET has inherent advantages compared to SPECT (eg, better image resolution and the possibility for absolute quantification of blood flow). However, the limited availability of the technique and especially of the PET perfusion tracers and higher costs are influencing the choice of method, and SPECT has kept its role as the main workhorse for cardiac patients.

PATHOPHYSIOLOGY

Myocardial ischemia is defined as a mismatch between the demand and supply of oxygen to the myocytes, and this is mainly dependent on an adequate myocardial perfusion in various physiologic conditions. The inotropic and chronotropic states determine the myocardial demand, and during physical exercise, the heart rate increases and the force of the myocardium increases to raise the stroke volume and the left ventricular systolic pressure. At normal conditions, the arterioles can dilate during exercise, and perfusion can thus increase from a resting value of 1 mL/min/g to 3 mL/min/g. The maximal vasodilatation of the coronary arteries is even larger; over 5 mL/min/g has been measured, for example, during reactive hyperemia[7] or pharmacologic vaso-dilatation. Coronary artery disease (or ischemic heart disease) affects myocardial perfusion by coronary artery stenoses that increase the resistance of the larger coronary arteries, and thus, the flow is limited. The heart will compensate for this increased resistance by dilatation of the arterioles at rest, thereby preventing a flow decrease. However, this means that part of the flow vasodilator reserve that is supposed to be used at stress is already being used at rest. This explains why patients who have stress-induced ischemia commonly have normal perfusion at rest.

SPECT TECHNIQUE

Myocardial perfusion is depicted at rest and exercise using an intravenous injection of a radioactive perfusion tracer in a peripheral vein. The most commonly used perfusion tracers are technetium 99m (^{99m}Tc)–labeled tetrofosmin (Myoview; GE Healthcare, Little Chalfont, United Kingdom) or sestamibi (Cardiolite; Bristol-Myers Squibb, New York, NY). The formerly most used tracer, thallium, is an elementary compound with similar physiologic properties as potassium and provides a good linear relationship between blood flow and tracer uptake into the myocardium. The radiation dose is higher using thallium, and the image quality is not as good as that obtained with technetium-labeled tracers. The uptake of the perfusion tracer is related to the perfusion of the tissue, which means that only 3% of the injected radioactive material is distributed to the heart. Photons emitted from the radioactive decay (ie, gamma rays) are registered with a gamma camera. The resulting images are coded according to a gray or color scale from no perfusion (black) to maximum perfusion (white in the gray scale or bright colors in most of the color scales). A normal image is shown in Figure 3–1, and a yellow to white color denotes the highest tracer activity in the heart. Images are often displayed in a two-dimensional summary image of the heart called *polar plot* or "*bull's eye*" (Fig. 3–2). A normal finding is an even bright color in all parts of the heart during exercise. When one part of the myocardium shows decreased tracer uptake during stress, a perfusion defect, the images are compared against the

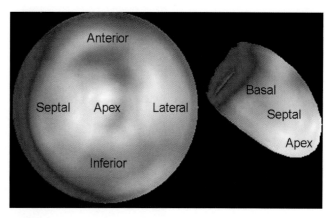

FIGURE 3–2. The perfusion images are routinely presented in a two-dimensional (2D) or three-dimensional (3D) parametric image (polar plot or bull's-eye image). In the 2D image, the entire left ventricle is represented in a circle, where the apex is located in the center and the base of the ventricle is located in the periphery. By convention, the anterior wall is placed upward, the inferior wall downward, the septal wall to the left, and the lateral wall to the right. The muscular perfused part of the septum is shorter than the lateral wall because of the membranous septum, and therefore, there is a peripheral rim of low perfusion tracer uptake to the left in the 2D image. To the right is shown a 3D parametric image of the left ventricle. This image can be freely rotated on the workstation

images obtained at rest. A perfusion defect that is larger at exercise than at rest is interpreted as ischemia (Fig. 3–3A,B). A perfusion defect that does not change between exercise and rest is considered to represent infarcted myocardium but can also be linked with other causes such as hibernating myocardium (Fig. 3–4).

Uptake of the perfusion tracer to the tissues is related to the perfusion also in extracardiac tissues (eg, skeletal muscle and the gastrointestinal tract). This means that an injection at rest will have higher uptake to the gastrointestinal tract compared with an injection at physical exercise because of the higher blood flow to the gastrointestinal tract at rest. During exercise with high sympathetic activity, blood flow is lowered in the gastrointestinal tract and elevated in skeletal muscles. This will affect the image acquisition because the liver and intestines are close to the heart and the extracardiac tracer uptake in the image field of view can be much higher than the uptake of the heart. High extracardiac tracer uptake close to the heart, as a rule of thumb within the width of the heart wall, may necessitate renewed image acquisition. Therefore, before image acquisition, it is recommended to wait for more than 30 minutes after resting injection or injection during pharmacologic stress. In the waiting period, patients are recommended to take a walk in the corridors and eat or drink something to increase the gastrointestinal motility so that the tracer uptake moves away from the heart. After an exercise stress test, images can be acquired 15 minutes after injection.

■ GATED SPECT AND ELECTROCARDIOGRAM TRIGGERING

Electrocardiogram (ECG) triggering or "gating" is routinely used during the gamma camera acquisition, and the acquisition is called *gated SPECT*. The recorded data are placed into 8 to 16 bins or gates depending on the time after the R wave of the ECG. Gated

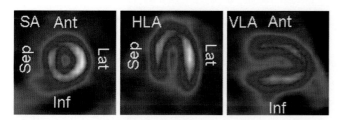

FIGURE 3–1. A normal myocardial perfusion SPECT with an evenly distributed perfusion. The three projections used for visualizing perfusion on myocardial SPECT are shown. The short axis (SA) images are by convention positioned with the inferior (Inf) wall downward, the septum (Sep) to the left, the anterior (Ant) wall upward, and the lateral (Lat) wall to the right. The horizontal long axis (HLA) images are presented with the apex upward, the septum to the left, and the lateral wall to the right. The vertical long axis (VLA) images are presented with the apex toward the right, the anterior wall upward, and the inferior wall downward. Isotope uptake is color coded from black (zero uptake) to yellow-white (100% of maximum uptake within the heart).

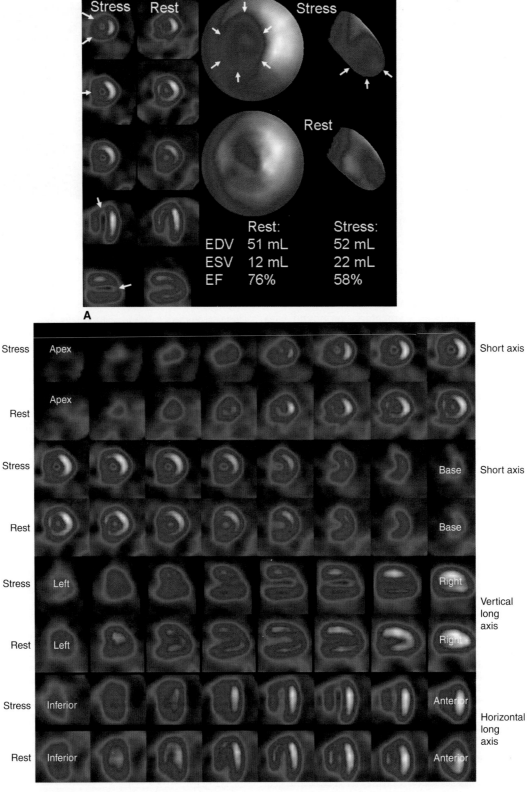

FIGURE 3–3. A. A 66-year-old woman with abdominal pain and no medication or previous history of ischemic heart disease. The exercise test induces abdominal pain and an equivocal ST-segment reaction; therefore, a perfusion single photon emission computed tomography (SPECT) is performed. A mild perfusion decrease in the anteroseptal region is seen at rest, and a severe perfusion defect in the anteroseptal region and apex is seen at stress. Hence, stress-induced ischemia is seen in the left anterior descending (LAD) territory, probably a proximal stenosis after a first diagonal. The reduced activity at rest could be due to breast attenuation. However, at gated SPECT, a mild regional dysfunction is seen in this area, and therefore, resting ischemia or a previous infarction is more likely. The patient was put on medication and referred for coronary angiography because the perfusion defect is large (almost 25% of the left ventricle) and severe because it causes transient ischemic dilatation and postischemic stunning (see Fig. 3–3C). A severe stenosis of the LAD was found and treated with percutaneous coronary intervention. EDV, end-diastolic volume; EF, ejection fraction; ESV, end-systolic volume. **B.** All perfusion images of the 66-year-old patient displayed in short axis, vertical long axis, and horizontal long axis views. By convention, stress images are placed above rest images.

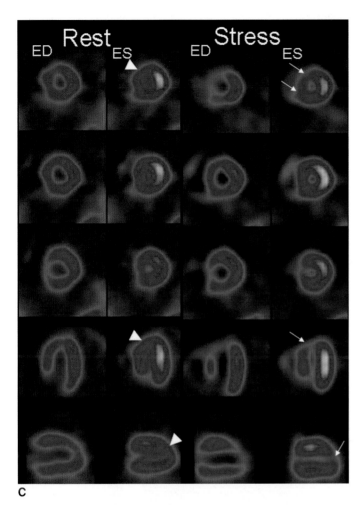

C

FIGURE 3–3. C. Gated SPECT at stress and rest. The frames at end-diastole (ED) and end-systole (ES) are shown. Automatic contour detection yields the end-diastolic and end-systolic volumes, and the ejection fraction can be derived from these volumes. Global function can be visually determined by looking at the endocardial contours at ED and ES. Regional function can be assessed by the increase in counts from ED to ES. Normal regional function is seen as an increase in counts from ED to ES as in the rest images of this patient except in a small area in the apex (arrowheads). At stress, a lack of count increase can be seen in the apex and anteroapical regions (arrows), which implies a decreased regional function in this area.

SPECT enables studies of global and regional ventricular function. Endocardial contours are automatically generated and provide the left ventricular volumes over the cardiac cycle. By calculation of the end-diastolic volume and end-systolic volume, the ejection fraction can be derived (Fig. 3–3C). Left ventricular function is visualized by displaying the images in a cine loop. The information from gated SPECT has been shown to have incremental prognostic value compared with assessment of perfusion only.[8] PET images are often ECG gated in the same manner to obtain functional information.

A perfusion defect that is unchanged between rest and stress can be due to infarction but also due to attenuation artifact, and gated SPECT can be used to differentiate these two (Moving Image 3–1). A myocardial infarct is characterized by reduction in perfusion tracer uptake and decreased regional function (Moving Image 3–2). If normal regional function is seen at gated SPECT in the area of reduced uptake, it is read as an attenuation

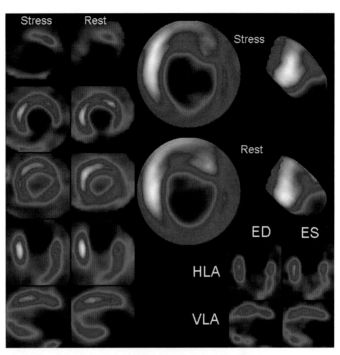

FIGURE 3–4. A 75-year-old man with a previous myocardial infarction and shortness of breath. A large perfusion defect is seen at stress in the apex, inferior wall, and parts of the lateral wall. The perfusion defect is unchanged at rest. The left ventricular volumes are severely increased (end-diastolic volume = 430 mL; end-systolic volume = 350 mL), and the global function is severely depressed (ejection fraction = 17%). Gated single photon emission computed tomography images at end-diastole (ED) and end-systole (ES) in the horizontal long axis (HLA) and vertical long axis (VLA) projections are shown at bottom right. There are no signs of inducible ischemia. The infarcted territory is in more than one vessel. The vessels could be a distal LAD with a large wrap around to the inferior wall, alternatively a dominant right coronary artery supplying the inferior wall and apex. The basal lateral perfusion defect, which is not adjacent with the inferior and apical infarct is probably caused by infarction in the circumflex territory.

artifact, and not as an infarct. Decreased ejection fraction and increased left ventricular volumes without any perfusion defects are seen in cases of cardiomyopathy (Fig. 3–5).

The summed images from gated SPECT are used for assessment of perfusion, and therefore no extra scanning is needed; perfusion and function images are obtained simultaneously. Gated SPECT uses information from many heart beats, and if the heart rhythm is not stable (eg, sinus arrhythmia, premature beats, or atrial fibrillation), gated SPECT cannot be performed. One should bear in mind that the perfusion images display the perfusion as it was at the time of injection. The gated SPECT functional images, however, show function at the time of acquisition. This explains why a perfusion defect representing ischemia can be seen with preserved function at gated SPECT. During the time from injection to scanning, function can be restored. A stress perfusion defect with decreased function compared with the resting images is indicative of postischemic myocardial stunning (Moving Image 3–3). Lower ejection fraction and larger volumes after stress compared with rest are signs of severe ischemia. The increased ventricular volumes caused by postischemic stunning can also be seen on the summed perfusion images as transient ischemic dilatation (TID). TID manifests as a larger blood pool at stress compared with rest; in the images, this is manifested as more of the dark lumen at stress compared with rest (see Fig. 3–3A,B).

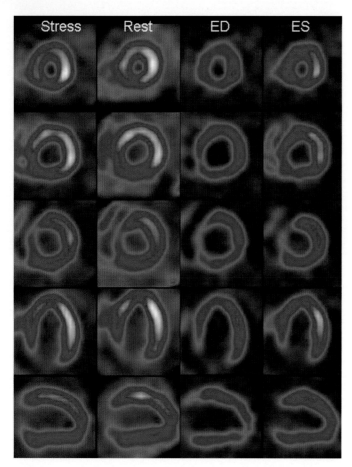

FIGURE 3–5. Gated single photon emission computed tomography (SPECT) of a 44-year-old male intravenous drug addict with a previous episode of sepsis. After antibiotic treatment, a decreased ejection fraction (EF) remains. Myocardial SPECT is performed to assess whether ischemic heart disease is the explanation for the heart failure. No perfusion defects are seen at stress or rest. At gated SPECT, increased left ventricular volumes (end-diastolic volume = 244 mL; end-systolic volume = 167 mL) and decreased EF (31%) were found. The findings of no stress-induced ischemia, no perfusion defects, increased ventricular volumes, and decreased EF are signs of nonischemic cardiomyopathy. ED, end-diastole; ES, end-systole.

■ NEW DETECTOR TECHNOLOGY FOR SPECT

Recent developments have introduced ultrafast cardiac SPECT cameras with acquisition times down to a few minutes and increased spatial resolution.[9,10] This development also provides the possibility to lower the injected radioactive dose to the patient, resulting in effective doses of only a few millisieverts. This has been made possible by new detector technology composed of cadmium-zinc telluride crystals with higher sensitivity, digital detectors instead of photomultiplier tubes, and improved collimator techniques that enable the acquisition of the entire three-dimensional volume continuously without moving the detectors in the conventional half-circle around the patient. The reconstruction algorithms for myocardial perfusion SPECT have also been refined, shortening the acquisition times by 30%. The cost of the new detector technology is roughly double the price for a conventional dedicated cardiac SPECT Anger gamma camera.

■ ATTENUATION AND ITS CORRECTION

Radiation from different parts of the myocardium travels different distances through tissue with varying densities on the way to the gamma camera detector. If there is tissue of high density between the myocardium and the detector, some photons may not reach the detector. This is called attenuation of the signal and may mimic a perfusion defect.[11] Because the body has the same constitution at both stress and rest images, the attenuation will be the same and a similar decrease in counts will be seen at stress and rest. Attenuation causes a decrease in the specificity of the test. Gated SPECT, additional imaging in the prone position, or transmission attenuation correction[11] can be used to overcome this problem (Fig. 3–6). Attenuation correction can be performed by acquiring additional information about the body composition and attenuation properties and then mathematically calculating what the signal would be in the case of no attenuation. Traditionally, transmission information (as opposed to the emission perfusion information from the patient) from radioactive rods orbiting the patient and detected by the gamma camera on the opposite side of

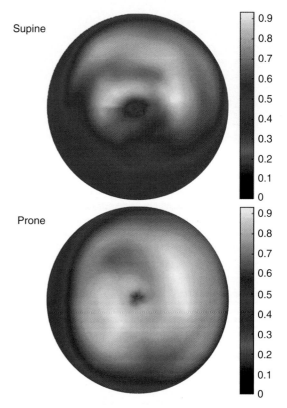

FIGURE 3–6. Supine and prone imaging in a man with chest pain at exercise and an equivocal stress test. Isotope is injected during peak stress, and SPECT images are acquired 15 minutes later in both the supine and prone positions. The supine perfusion image show a moderate reduction in the inferior wall, but the prone image shows an even isotope distribution, indicating attenuation of the radioactive signal. This simple form of attenuation correction can be used without any additional technical devices. Gated SPECT showed normal left ventricular volumes and ejection fraction. See Moving Image 3-1 for the gated SPECT images of this patient. Because of the normal perfusion and function, no resting injection is needed. This approach shortens the examination and lowers the radioactive exposure to the patient. In many nuclear cardiology services, between 25% and 50% of patients' stress images suffice for exclusion of stress-induced ischemia.

the patient has been used. Today, hybrid systems with computed tomography (CT) are available, and the CT information can be used for attenuation correction.[12] The transmitted x-rays give a map of the attenuation of the body. Indeed, attenuation is the basis for all x-ray–based technology, and Hounsfield units in CT are a measure of attenuation. CT can be used to create an attenuation map of the patient, which can correct for attenuation of the photons by the tissues of the body. The information from a low-dose CT scan is superior to that obtained from radioactive rods and is acquired more rapidly.

A simple and inexpensive method to help in identifying attenuation effects without these technical options is to repeat the image acquisition in the prone position. A defect that is present in one position but moves or disappears in the other image acquisition is not caused by an infarct[13,14] (see Fig. 3–6). Prone imaging has therefore been called the "poor man's attenuation correction."

PET TECHNIQUE

PET has technical advantages over SPECT; the spatial resolution is higher, the acquisition is faster, the motion artifacts are less of a problem, attenuation correction is routine, and absolute quantification of perfusion is possible.[15] There are several methodologic differences between SPECT and PET. PET scanners have a different geometry and a different detection principle. Multiple correction algorithms are routinely applied to yield images of absolutely quantitative tracer distribution of the target.

■ ACQUISITION

PET scanning aims to produce a three-dimensional image volume, which is an accurate map of the distribution of tracer in the body. To enable quantification, a series of such volumes is normally generated over time to describe the time-activity curves and investigate the kinetics of tracer uptake in different tissues and blood. The isotopes used in PET emit positrons, which are the antimatter of electrons. The positron is annihilated when colliding with an electron, whereupon two photons are emitted (annihilation radiation) and can be detected by the PET camera. The half-lives of the radioactive PET isotopes are much shorter than those of technetium or thallium used in SPECT (eg, 76 seconds for rubidium 82 [^{82}Rb] and 10 minutes for nitrogen-13 ammonia [^{13}NH$_3$]). In addition, compared with radionuclides emitting single gamma-ray photons, the emission of pairs of 511-keV photons gives PET imaging higher detection efficiency, better uniformity of spatial resolution, and easier correction for attenuation. Gated images for assessment of regional and global function are acquired in the same manner as with SPECT (see previous section on SPECT).

■ ATTENUATION AND OTHER CORRECTIONS

In PET, the photon attenuation correction is routinely used in a robust manner. To exploit the potential of PET to provide quantitative data, a number of other corrections need to be carried out. The geometry of a PET system introduces variation in the detection sensitivity. Normalization corrects this by measuring the count rate for each line of response using a radioactive source. The response time of a detector system is finite. Dead time is the period when a detector is unable to record a new event, and this needs to be corrected also. In addition, to achieve quantitative results, scattered events, random coincidences, and partial volume effects in small targets need to be corrected; these correction methods use mathematical modeling. Furthermore, motion correction is needed when a moving target such as the heart is imaged. Luckily, most of these corrections are performed by the scanners automatically. Partial volume correction for cardiac studies is commonly done after data modeling, and for motion correction, ECG and/or respiratory gating is available.

THE STRESS TEST

■ EXERCISE STRESS TEST

An exercise stress test is recommended as the method of choice when performing myocardial perfusion SPECT, and the perfusion tracer is injected during maximum cardiac exertion. To avoid injecting the perfusion tracer at submaximum exertion and thereby risking a false-negative test, injection should be done when the heart rate is above 85% of the age-predicted maximum. This can be calculated by the following formula: (220 − age) × 0.85. After injection, the patient should continue exercise for 1 minute to make certain that the perfusion tracer has entered the cells and left the blood pool. The workload can be lowered somewhat to enable the patient to continue exercise for 1 whole minute. Contraindications for an exercise stress test and criteria for termination of the test before reaching the age-predicted heart rate are the same as for a standard exercise stress test according to the international recommendations.[16] Contraindications include any acute or ongoing severe cardiopulmonary disease, such as acute coronary syndrome, aortic dissection, cardiac failure or complex arrhythmias with hemodynamic instability, pulmonary embolism, severe hypertension (blood pressure >200/110 mm Hg), and severe aortic stenosis. Absolute indications for early termination of the exercise test include significant decrease in blood pressure, severe angina, sustained ventricular tachycardia, pathologic ST-segment elevation (>1 mm in leads with no Q waves other than V$_1$ or aVR), increasing nervous system symptoms, or signs of poor perfusion. If there are technical difficulties affecting the ability to record ECG and blood pressure, the test should be terminated, and the problems should be fixed before continuing. Relative contraindications include marked ST-segment depression (>3 mm), arrhythmias such as triplets of premature ventricular contractions or supraventricular tachycardia, development of left bundle branch block, and severe hypertension (>250/130 mm Hg).

■ PHARMACOLOGIC STRESS TEST

Pharmacologic stress with adenosine, dipyridamole, regadenoson, or dobutamine can be used to cause coronary vasodilatation in patients who cannot perform a maximum exercise stress test, including patients with orthopedic problems and patients who cannot reach adequate heart rate because of β-blockers or a concomitant disease such as chronic obstructive pulmonary disease or kidney failure. A vasodilator drug is also used in patients with left bundle branch block or a pacemaker with ventricular stimulation because of potential false-positive perfusion images when using the exercise stress test (see "Pitfalls" later). Pharmacologic stress is used most commonly with PET imaging. Direct vasodilatation is caused by adenosine, dipyridamole, and regadenoson. Dobutamine is a sympathomimetic drug with positive inotropic and chronotropic properties that causes a secondary vasodilatation. Pharmacologic stress testing is safe under correct monitoring and patient supervision. ECG, blood pressure, and patient status should be assessed and supervised by a physician, and cessation of the drug and use of antidotes may be necessary.

Adenosine

Adenosine is the most commonly used pharmacologic stress agent and acts as a direct vasodilator on the coronary vessels by binding to the A2A receptor on the arterioles. Adenosine is given as a continuous infusion in a peripheral vein for 5 to 6 minutes. The half-life of adenosine is very short (<10 seconds), and therefore, no antidote is needed. After cessation of the infusion, the effect stops. Adenosine is given at a dose of 140 μg/kg/min, but the dose can be lowered if adverse effects occur. Common adverse effects to adenosine are flushing, headache, chest discomfort, and dyspnea. These adverse effects are unspecific and not related to ischemia; therefore, patients are informed of their benign nature, and most patients can tolerate them. Criteria for early termination of adenosine infusion are persistent high-grade atrioventricular (AV) block or sinoatrial block, severe hypotension, bronchoconstriction, and severe angina. Adenosine causes AV block in high doses, and especially in older patients, transient AV block is seen. Lowering the adenosine dose is often sufficient to avoid high-grade AV block. Blood pressure drops in many patients because of the vasodilatation, but there is rarely a need to stop the infusion. A profound decrease of blood pressure is related to a worse patient status and ischemia, and in some patients, adenosine infusion has to be terminated. Healthy subjects given adenosine do not experience a drop in blood pressure but do experience an increase in the heart rate and stroke volume to maintain the blood pressure. Bronchoconstriction is a rare but potentially severe adverse effect of adenosine and is the reason for the contraindication of adenosine in patients with active asthma or severe chronic obstructive pulmonary disease. In patients with mild chronic obstructive pulmonary disease, premedication with inhalation of β_2 stimulants can be used. Auscultation of the lungs during adenosine infusion can be used to detect bronchoconstriction. Of note is that the dyspnea experienced by most patients is not related to bronchoconstriction. Dyspnea is believed to be caused by stimulation of the peripheral oxygen receptors in the carotid sinus. The safety of adenosine has been assessed in a large study of over 9000 patients; 0.1% of patients experienced bronchoconstrictions, although patients with asthma and severe chronic obstructive pulmonary disease were excluded from receiving adenosine. Two patients experienced severe complications with pulmonary edema and myocardial infarction, respectively. The combination of the adenosine infusion with physical exercise on a bicycle ergometer or treadmill decreases adverse effects. The increase in sympathetic activity during exercise increases blood pressure and decreases the risk of AV block and possibly

bronchoconstriction. Furthermore, the blood supply to the gastrointestinal tract decreases and hence tracer uptake in that region, which is advantageous for the subsequent SPECT acquisition. In patients with left bundle branch block and pacemakers with ventricular stimulation, adenosine infusion should not be combined with physical exercise (see later section "Pitfalls").

Dipyridamole

Dipyridamole acts via the endogenous adenosine of the body by inhibiting the reuptake of adenosine and thereby raising the concentration around the receptor. Because of its long half-life, an antidote is needed, and theophylline is most commonly used. Adverse effects to dipyridamole are similar to those of adenosine.

Regadenoson

Regadenoson is a specific A2A receptor agonist recently made available with similar diagnostic results as adenosine.[17] The effect of regadenoson is sustained, with a half-life of 2 to 3 minutes. Therefore, an antidote such as theophylline is often used. Because of its specific A2A receptor characteristics, regadenoson can be used in chronic obstructive pulmonary disease and asthma patients. Regadenoson was approved in the United States in 2008.

Dobutamine

Dobutamine is a sympathomimetic drug with positive inotropic and chronotropic properties that causes secondary vasodilatation. The infusion rate is increased in steps, starting at 5 or 10 μg/kg/min and increasing every third minute to 20, 30, and 40 μg/kg/min. Blood pressure and ECG are monitored continuously, and criteria for termination of infusion and contraindications are the same as for an exercise stress test. Injection of the radioactive tracer is performed at 85% of the age-predicted heart rate, which often occurs only after adding atropine starting at a dose of 0.25 mg. It is important that β-blockers are discontinued before the test in order to reach the age-predicted heart rate. Common adverse effects of dobutamine are headache, nausea, anxiety, and atypical chest pain. Angina and ventricular arrhythmias need to be monitored, and paroxysmal atrial fibrillation can be triggered by dobutamine. If the termination criteria are followed, severe complications such as myocardial infarction and death are extremely rare. When discontinuing the infusion, the effect of dobutamine lasts longer compared with adenosine, and sometimes an intravenous injection of a β_2-blocker is needed. There are additional contraindications for the use of atropine (eg, narrow-angle glaucoma).

■ MEDICATION AND CAFFEINE BEFORE MYOCARDIAL PERFUSION IMAGING

Oral nitrates should be avoided before stress because of their anti-ischemic effect. If an exercise test or dobutamine infusion is used, β-blockers and heart rate–lowering calcium blockers should be discontinued 48 hours before the injection. A common indication for vasodilator perfusion imaging is inappropriate heart rate response in patients who cannot or who have forgotten to discontinue their medication. The amount of ischemia will be less if anti-ischemic medication is maintained even with vasodilator stress tests,[4] however, with β-blockers, not to the extent that it affects the sensitivity and specificity.[18] Caffeine needs to be discontinued before adenosine, dipyridamole, and regadenoson because of a competitive blockage of the adenosine receptor. Abstinence from caffeine is recommended for preferably 24 hours.

RADIOPHARMACEUTICALS

The characteristics of an ideal perfusion tracer would be uptake to the myocardium in direct proportion to blood flow; high extraction from blood to the myocardium during the first passage; medium half-life to enable time for acquisition but not so long that the radiation dose becomes high; radiation properties that suit the acquisition with regard to energy emission, resolution, and attenuation; and of course, a stable, cheap, and ready supply of the tracer. Unfortunately, there are no tracers today that meet all of these criteria, but three SPECT tracers fulfill several and are therefore used clinically. For PET imaging, three tracers are being used. The radiopharmaceuticals used are injected as a bolus injection in a peripheral vein.

■ SPECT TRACERS

Thallium 201

In the case of thallium, the perfusion tracer and the radioactive substance are one and the same. Thallium 201 (^{201}Tl) can be found in the same group as potassium in the periodic table and is distributed in the body as potassium in proportion to blood flow with a high extraction from the blood. The half-life is rather long, the radiation dose to the patient is high (~18 mSv), and the characteristics for SPECT acquisition are not ideal. After an injection during stress, imaging must be started within 10 minutes because of the so-called redistribution of thallium. Thallium does not stay fixed in the cell after uptake but reenters the blood stream and is continuously redistributed to the body. Therefore, a perfusion defect will disappear at rest because of uptake from thallium in the blood. This means that the same injected dose can be used for both stress and rest images, and the redistribution images at rest are performed 3 to 4 hours after injection. Thallium can also be used for viability testing in the case of a fixed perfusion defect. A late redistribution image the following day is used, and in the case of an infarct, the perfusion defect is still present. A fixed perfusion defect that disappears is an indication of viable myocardium.

^{99m}Tc-Labeled Tetrofosmin or Sestamibi

^{99m}Tc is a radioactive substance and must be linked to a perfusion tracer (eg, tetrofosmin or sestamibi). ^{99m}Tc has good characteristics for SPECT acquisitions and a medium to long half-life of 6 hours. Both perfusion tracers have lower extraction compared with thallium but thereafter remain stable in the cells binding to the mitochondria. This means that injection does not have to be adjacent to the SPECT camera, and the patient can be transported to the acquisition without haste. It also means that a separate resting injection must be performed if the stress image is abnormal. Tetrofosmin and sestamibi have a rather high gastrointestinal uptake, which may cause problems with image acquisition at rest or after pharmacologic stress (see "Pitfalls" later).

■ PET TRACERS

All PET perfusion tracers allow for short imaging protocols and repeated studies due to their short half-lives. A PET perfusion study can thus be performed in a few minutes. Currently, three tracers are mainly used with PET.

^{13}NH$_3$ has high first-pass extraction, and uptake is linear over a wide range of myocardial blood flow except at very high flow rates. Imaging with ^{13}NH$_3$ requires either an on-site cyclotron or proximity to a regional positron radiopharmaceutical source center. Images are of high quality and resolution.

Oxygen 15–labeled water (H$_2$^{15}O) is potentially superior to other tracers because it is metabolically inert and freely diffusible across capillary and cell membranes. However, a drawback is that the tracer is not accumulated in myocardium, but reaches equilibrium between tissue compartments. Thus, images of regional myocardial perfusion distribution are not readily produced by standard image visualization, and image processing for blood pool subtraction is needed; however, the image processing is simple process with current software.

^{82}Rb is a potassium analog that has a first-pass extraction of 65%, and its uptake requires active transport via Na/K-ATPase, which is dependent on coronary flow. Also, with ^{82}Rb, the extraction fraction decreases in a nonlinear manner with increasing blood flow, and this effect is more pronounced when compared with ammonia, although still superior when compared with ^{99m}Tc-labeled SPECT compounds. Image resolution and quality are somewhat compromised due to the high energy of positrons emitted during the decay of ^{82}Rb and due to lower count rates as a result of the ultrashort half-life. An advantage of ^{82}Rb over ^{13}NH$_3$ and H$_2$^{15}O is that it is produced by a strontium 82/^{82}Rb generator without the need for a costly cyclotron.[19]

^{18}F-2-deoxy-2-fluoro-D-glucose (^{18}F-FDG) is widely available due to its success as a metabolic imaging tracer in clinical oncology. It has been known for decades that the tracer is of high value to determine myocardial glucose utilization as an indicator of myocardial viability. Increased ^{18}F-FDG uptake can be observed in ischemic tissue, whereas markedly reduced or absent uptake indicates scar formation. ^{18}F-FDG uptake is heterogeneous in normal myocardium in the fasting state, and therefore, oral glucose loading, nicotinic acid derivatives, and infusion of insulin and glucose have been used to enhance myocardial ^{18}F-FDG uptake.[20]

IMAGING PROTOCOLS

■ SPECT PROTOCOLS

Several different SPECT imaging protocols are being used depending on the local demands and circumstances.

^{201}Tl Protocols

Imaging is performed directly after stress and after 3 to 4 hours at rest using the same isotope injection.

^{99m}Tc Protocols

One-day or 2-day protocols can be used. In the 1-day protocol, the first injection can be at rest or stress, and the injected dose is kept as low as possible. After image acquisition, the second dose is injected, which must be at least 2.5 to 3 times as high as the first dose to override the radioactivity already present in the myocardium. The advantages with a 1-day protocol are that the patients do not need to come back another day and the referring physician can get a quicker reply. The disadvantages are that the radiation dose will be somewhat higher and a perfusion defect can be underestimated if the second dose is too low to override the activity of the first dose. To keep the radiation dose as low as possible, stress imaging can be performed first, and if there is no perfusion abnormality, no rest imaging is needed.

Dual-Isotope Protocols

Resting images are performed with ^{201}Tl, and stress images are performed with a ^{99m}Tc tracer. The advantage is the speed of the protocol; because of different energy peaks, both tracers can be injected shortly after each other without interference. The main disadvantage is that the comparison at rest and stress will be with two different tracers, with differences in, for example, attenuation.

■ PET PROTOCOLS AND DATA ANALYSIS

The patient preparation for PET study is practically the same as for SPECT scans. Drinks containing caffeine need to be avoided during the preceding 12 hours because pharmacologic stressors are commonly used in PET imaging.

The comfortable positioning of the patient on the scanner bed is critical to prevent any motion artifacts during and between the scans. It is strongly recommended that hands are supported upright and not within the field of view. The perfusion imaging protocol depends on which tracer is used. With tracers such as ^{82}Rb and H$_2$^{15}O, the stress study can be performed practically without delay after the rest study. With ^{13}NH$_3$, stress testing is delayed for approximately 30 minutes to allow tracer decay. In all studies, a quality control process is needed to ensure optimal alignment of the CT attenuation and PET emission scans, and if necessary, misalignment needs to be corrected. If the system is capable of list mode acquisition, the data can be collected in ECG-gated mode that allows the simultaneous assessment of regional and global left ventricular wall motion from the same scan data. This is particularly practical when ^{82}Rb is used as tracer. Because the stress images are acquired during stress (and not, as in SPECT, up to an hour after stress), the gated images in PET have higher probability to detect ischemia. The total time required for a whole study session depends on the tracer used. With ^{82}Rb and H$_2$^{15}O, the whole session can be finished in 20 to 30 minutes, and with ^{13}NH$_3$, the session can be finished in 60 to 80 minutes. The protocols can be further shortened significantly because only single stress perfusion imaging may be needed, especially when using quantification, and then the protocol with all tracers can be as short as 10 to 15 minutes.

The PET images can be displayed and analyzed using semi-quantitative or visual assessment as with SPECT. The interpretation is also similar, including the gated images analysis. However, for full quantification, the dynamic image sets need to be processed using dedicated software that is able to perform image segmentation and tracer-specific kinetic modeling (Fig. 3–7). This process typically produces a parametric image in which the original radioactivity values are replaced by physiologic parameters such as perfusion in mL/g/min. Alternatively, numerical values with relative distribution within the left ventricle are reported along with standard image views.

HYBRID IMAGING WITH CT

Currently, all commercially available PET scanners are hybrid devices with multidetector CT in the same gantry as PET. Also with SPECT, combination with a CT is becoming popular. In addition, when using CT for attenuation correction (see sections on SPECT and PET technique earlier), many hybrid systems provide the ability to perform a full diagnostic CT coronary angiography, which can be readily combined with the perfusion or viability images from SPECT or PET.

The efficiency of hybrid imaging with PET/CT is very high because PET imaging protocols are short, allowing both CT angiography and perfusion imaging to be performed in a single session clearly below 30 minutes of total scan duration. The radiation dose from PET perfusion studies is very small; for example, the radiation dose from a single PET perfusion study is 0.8 mSv for H$_2$^{15}O and 1 mSv for ^{3}NH$_3$. Recently, techniques that reduce patient dose in CT have been developed, and the doses have been reduced to as low as 1 to 7 mSv. Therefore, although the use of hybrid imaging causes an increased radiation dose for the patient compared with single imaging, currently comprehensive cardiac PET/CT imaging can be performed with a radiation dose of less than 10 mSv.[21] The new detector technology for SPECT described earlier has decreased imaging time and lowered the dose needed for perfusion imaging. Using these technical developments, a hybrid coronary CT and perfusion stress only SPECT image can be obtained with radiation doses as low as 3 mSv.[12]

The rationale of using hybrid imaging is based on the possibility of simultaneous combination of anatomic and functional information. Because imaging procedures are a significant financial burden to the overall cost of health care, it is important to carefully consider and justify the use of all imaging tests. Coronary artery calcium (CAC) according to the Agatston score has been used a marker of plaque burden, and increased scores are associated with higher cardiovascular risk. There is some evidence that CAC may add incremental value to the perfusion information.[22] For example, the presence of extensive CAC despite a normal relative perfusion distribution increased the sensitivity of detecting coronary stenosis without decreasing specificity, presumably by not missing balanced ischemia.[23] CT coronary angiography is valuable for the evaluation of many subgroups of patients with known or suspected coronary artery disease (CAD), but it provides purely morphologic information that has well-known limitations. It has been shown that only approximately half of the lesions classified as significant in CT are linked with abnormal perfusion.[24,25] The vasomotor tone and coronary collateral flow cannot be estimated because the percent diameter stenosis is only a weak descriptor of coronary resistance. However, myocardial perfusion imaging provides a simple and accurate integrated measure of the effect of all the parameters on coronary resistance and tissue perfusion, thereby optimizing selection of patients who may ultimately benefit from revascularization. However, SPECT and PET imaging do not provide morphologic information. The perfusion imaging only provides information about the existence and severity of perfusion abnormalities, but not about the mechanism; for example, patients with diffuse balanced coronary heart disease and patients with microvascular dysfunction leading to globally compromised perfusion cannot be separated by perfusion imaging.

Short axis

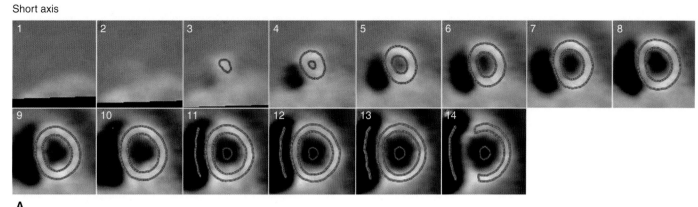

A

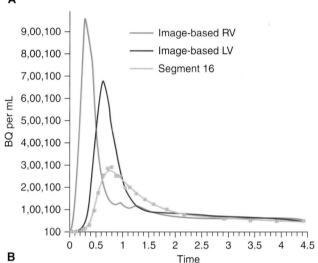

B

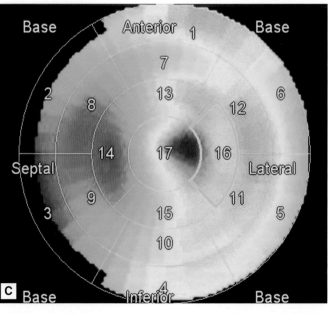

Modelling results			
	F(mL/g/min)	Va	PTF
Global	1.533	0.201	0.631
LAD	1.501	0.201	0.639
LCX	1.764	0.188	0.658
RCA	1.405	0.237	0.683
Seg1	1.701	0.216	0.666
Seg2	1.187	0.308	0.681
Seg3	1.064	0.300	0.688
Seg4	1.680	0.139	0.719
Seg5	1.644	0.169	0.674
Seg6	1.638	0.242	0.637
Seg7	1.517	0.191	0.720
Seg8	1.062	0.289	0.694
Seg9	1.107	0.303	0.691
Seg10	1.625	0.186	0.726
Seg11	1.830	0.168	0.678
Seg12	1.827	0.198	0.679
Seg13	1.598	0.160	0.681
Seg14	1.020	0.321	0.627
Seg15	1.544	0.243	0.642
Seg16	1.861	0.167	0.634
Seg17	1.775	0.142	0.619

D

FIGURE 3–7. An example of analysis of dynamic positron emission tomography perfusion study. The first step is the segmentation of myocardium and definition of myocardial regions of interest (**A**). Thereafter, the time-activity curves of each region are created (**B**) and processed in a mathematical model that produces parametric images or a parametric polar plot (**C**) and a numerical table of results (**D**). F denotes absolute perfusion in mL/min/g in the table. Va indicates the blood volume in the region of interest. PTF denotes the perfusable tissue fraction, which means how much water-perfusable tissue is in the region of interest; a decreased PTF value indicates a low fraction of viable tissue. LAD, left anterior descending artery; LCX, left circumflex artery; LV, left ventricle; RCA, right coronary artery; RV, right ventricle.

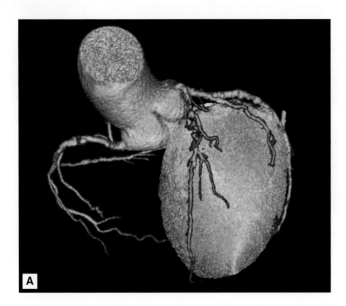
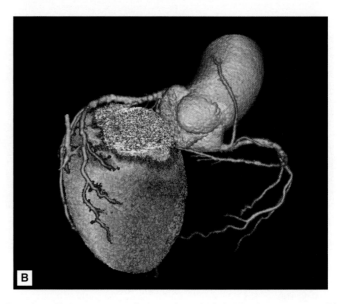

FIGURE 3–8. Hybrid positron emission tomography/computed tomography (CT) image of a patient with coronary artery disease and anterior ischemia. The stress myocardial perfusion is visualized in hybrid CT images using color coding of left ventricular surface. The red and yellow colors denote high perfusion, and green and blue denote reduced perfusion. In this patient, the anterior and septal regions are poorly perfused during stress (**A**, anterior view), and the area supplied by the right coronary artery has very low perfusion (**B**, posterior view).

The analysis of hybrid studies follows the same standard procedures that have been explained earlier. In addition, the analysis of CT angiography includes the standard processes and techniques used in stand-alone situations, such as visual assessment of original transaxial slices, multiplanar reconstructions, and utilization of the quantitative tools available. To make use of the true power of hybrid imaging, the fused images and data should also be used. In fused images, the individual coronary anatomy can be linked with perfusion information (Fig. 3–8).

Hybrid images provide a comprehensive view of the myocardium, the regional myocardial perfusion, and the coronary artery tree, thus eliminating uncertainties in the relationship of perfusion defects and the diseased coronary arteries. This may be particularly helpful in patients with multiple perfusion abnormalities. Combining anatomic information with perfusion also helps to identify and correctly register the subtle irregularities in myocardial perfusion. In patients with suspected CAD, hybrid imaging provided a sensitivity and specificity of 90% and 98%, respectively.[26] Further studies are warranted to ensure the accuracy of hybrid imaging in different clinical populations. Furthermore, the incremental value of hybrid imaging over the stand-alone individual scan needs to be defined, and studies showing the potential effect on treatment, outcome, and cost effectiveness are needed.[12]

INDICATIONS FOR MYOCARDIAL PERFUSION SPECT AND PET

■ PRIMARY DIAGNOSIS OF ISCHEMIC HEART DISEASE

Myocardial perfusion imaging has a key role in the evaluation of patients with symptoms but no history of ischemic heart disease. The patient typically presents with nonacute chest pain or dyspnea of unknown origin (Figs. 3–9 and 3–10). Studies have shown that patients benefitting from myocardial perfusion imaging are

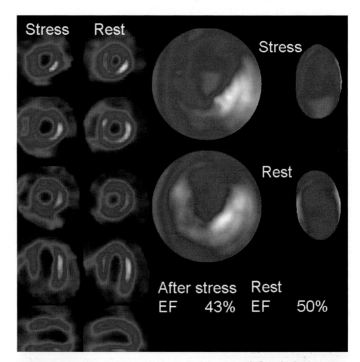

FIGURE 3–9. A 38-year-old man with chest pain at physical exercise. At rest, a mildly decreased perfusion is seen in the anterior wall and apex. At stress, severely decreased perfusion in the same region is seen. At gated single photon emission computed tomography (SPECT), larger volumes and lower ejection fraction (EF) are seen after stress compared with rest, indicating postischemic stunning. Because of severe ischemia, the patient was referred for prompt angiography showing a proximal significant stenosis in the left anterior descending artery, which was treated with percutaneous coronary intervention. The reduced perfusion at rest is most likely caused by resting ischemia because the patient had no history of myocardial infarction. EDV, end-diastolic volume; ESV, end-systolic volume.

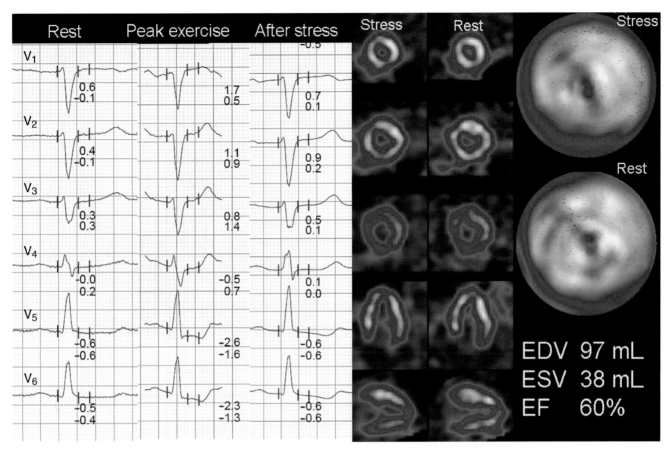

FIGURE 3–10. Equivocal exercise stress test in a 60-year-old woman. Pathologic ST-segment depression but no angina and normal exercise capacity, blood pressure reaction, and heart rate response were found. Because of the uncertain diagnosis, she underwent a myocardial perfusion single photon emission computed tomography (SPECT) study showing normal perfusion at stress and rest and therefore no ischemia. The patient underwent coronary angiography because of acute chest pain; the angiography did not show any pathology. Echocardiography the following day showed moderately decreased ejection fraction that returned to normal the following weeks. A right ventricular biopsy was performed which showed myocyte atrophy and diffuse fibrosis and an MRI did not show any pathology. The diagnosis of Tako-Tsubo cardiomyopathy was made. EDV, end-diastolic volume; EF, ejection fraction; ESV, end-systolic volume.

those with intermediate risk of having ischemic heart disease (eg, an equivocal exercise stress test). Patients with low likelihood (eg, no risk factors and a negative exercise stress test) do not benefit from myocardial perfusion imaging. Patients with high likelihood of ischemic heart disease (eg, risk factors, typical chest pain at physical exertion, and a positive exercise stress test) should not undergo myocardial perfusion imaging but should be treated medically or invasively according to symptoms and risk.

Myocardial perfusion imaging can be the principal diagnostic test if the patient cannot perform an exercise stress test or if ST-segment changes in the resting ECG make the ST-segment response to exercise not interpretable. The former case applies to patients with orthopedic problems that prohibit maximum exercise, and the latter case applies to patients with left bundle branch block or ST-segment depression due to left ventricular hypertrophy. Patients with an equivocal exercise stress test include those who have either significant ST-segment depression or chest pain during exercise but not both. Also, patients who do not reach a sufficient end-exercise heart rate due to rate-limiting medical therapy that cannot be discontinued may undergo a pharmacologic myocardial perfusion imaging study to obtain a diagnosis. Patients with a high CAC score (Agatston >400) with or without chest pain are another group of patients for whom myocardial perfusion SPECT may be appropriate.

■ PATIENTS WITH "LOW RISK" ACUTE CHEST PAIN

Myocardial perfusion imaging can be used to rule out acute coronary syndrome in patients with acute chest pain of unclear origin in whom initial testing with ECG and blood tests was not conclusive. This includes patients with resting images only and injection during or shortly after the episode of acute chest pain (Fig. 3–11), as well as patients with stress and rest imaging admitted for suspected acute coronary syndrome. In this setting, only SPECT data are available.

■ EVALUATION OF THE PHYSIOLOGIC SIGNIFICANCE OF A CORONARY STENOSIS

Stenoses of unclear significance are quite often found at coronary angiography both in patients with stable angina and patients with acute coronary syndrome. Myocardial perfusion imaging can be used to evaluate the flow-limiting effects of the stenosis and to guide therapy. If no or minor ischemia is found, the patient can be treated medically (Fig. 3–12). If a significant amount of the myocardium is jeopardized by ischemia, invasive treatment is indicated. The amount of ischemia at myocardial perfusion imaging correlates with the risk of major adverse cardiac events.

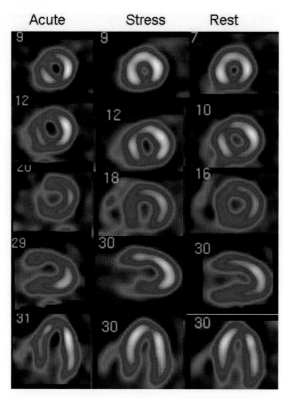

FIGURE 3–11. A case illustrating the use of myocardial perfusion single photon emission computed tomography (SPECT) in unstable and stable angina. A 63-year-old man presented to the emergency department because of acute chest pain but without positive troponins or significant electrocardiogram changes. The perfusion tracer was injected during chest pain, and SPECT showed an anteroseptal perfusion defect (left column) and a depressed ejection fraction (46%). The patient was transferred for emergency coronary angiography and was treated with percutaneous coronary intervention (PCI) for a thrombus in the left anterior descending artery. One year later, the patient had recurrent chest pain at physical activities, and a myocardial stress and rest SPECT study was performed. At stress, a moderately to severely reduced perfusion was seen in a moderately large region in the inferior wall. There was normal perfusion in this region at rest. Hence, the patient had stress-induced ischemia in the right coronary artery (RCA) region. There is a mild reduction in the rest perfusion in the anteroseptal region in this study, but compared with the acute study, the perfusion is better, showing the result of successful PCI treatment. Also, the ejection fraction at gated SPECT is normal (60%). Because of the stress-induced ischemia, the patient was referred to coronary angiography. An occluded RCA was found, which was treated with PCI.

■ ASSESSMENT OF ISCHEMIA IN PATIENTS WITH PRIOR REVASCULARIZATION

Instead of relying on a conventional exercise stress test, a noninvasive imaging study is recommended by guidelines to assess stress-induced ischemia in patients who have undergone revascularization either by percutaneous coronary intervention (PCI) or bypass surgery (Fig. 3–13). The rationale is that because there is already proven CAD, the likelihood of ischemia is higher, and the ST-segment response is often compromised due to previous myocardial infarction in this patient group. Also, myocardial perfusion imaging provides the location and extent of ischemia, which is important in guiding therapy. Another group includes patients who have had an episode of an acute coronary syndrome where coronary angiography has not been performed and where myocardial perfusion imaging is used for risk assessment.

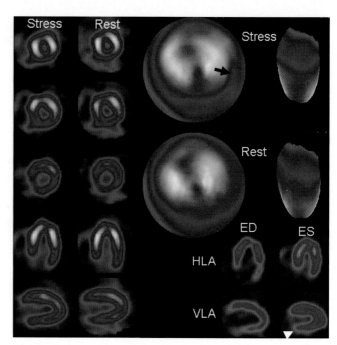

FIGURE 3–12. Myocardial perfusion single photon emission computed tomography (SPECT) in a 52-year-old man who underwent acute percutaneous coronary intervention treatment of an occluded right coronary artery causing an ST-segment elevation myocardial infarction (STEMI). At the angiography, a stenosis was found in the left anterior descending artery (LAD). SPECT was performed for noninvasive evaluation of the patient. There was a minor perfusion defect in the inferolateral wall at rest with slight decrease at stress corresponding to the area of the STEMI. However, in the LAD territory, there was no stress-induced ischemia, and therefore, the patient was treated medically. ED, end-diastole; ES, end-systole; HLA, horizontal long axis; VLA, vertical long axis.

■ RISK ASSESSMENT BEFORE MAJOR SURGERY

Myocardial perfusion imaging can be used to evaluate ischemia in patients with high probability of or known heart disease planned for major surgery. An exercise stress test is often sufficient, but myocardial perfusion imaging can be used in high-risk cases (eg, diabetic and renal failure patients) and especially in cases of vascular surgery.

■ VIABILITY TESTING

Viability testing is important in patients with heart failure to detect the functionally compromised myocardium that is able to recover function by revascularization. With SPECT, an isotope uptake defect seen at rest on myocardial perfusion imaging can be caused by an infarction or decreased perfusion due to a severe stenosis causing resting ischemia. Revascularization is considered useful if a significant part of the dysfunctional myocardium is viable. Late redistribution imaging with thallium can be used, particularly in institutions where other techniques such as PET or magnetic resonance imaging (MRI) are not available (see "Viability Assessment" later). Low-resolution and bad images (too little activity left) at late redistribution hamper the thallium technique, and a reinjection of thallium is often needed. Technetium-labeled tracers can be used for viability testing, and preserved uptake in a myocardial segment implies viable myocytes. Oral nitrate is usually administered before the resting injection when using technetium-labeled tracers for

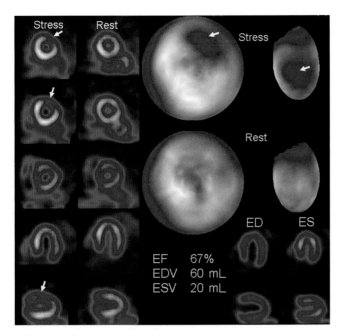

FIGURE 3–13. A 71-year-old woman with previous bypass surgery and several stents placed 4 years earlier presented with recurrent chest pain. Adenosine infusion–induced 1.5-mm ST depression and chest pain, which was relieved by oral nitrates. No perfusion defects were seen at rest, but at stress, there was a moderate decrease in perfusion in a moderately large region in the anterolateral wall. Note the high uptake in the gastrointestinal tract close to the inferior wall. There was no need to repeat the rest acquisition because there was normal perfusion in the adjacent inferior region at stress. Therefore, there could be no stress-induced ischemia in the inferior wall. At coronary angiography, a subtotal occlusion was seen in the venous graft to the first diagonal and marginal branches corresponding to the ischemia; the native vessels were occluded. The grafts to the remaining vessels were open. It was not technically possible to open the venous graft. The size of the ischemia was not so large that a repeat bypass surgery was indicated on a prognostic indication, and the risk of surgery was deemed as too high. Because the patient had angina despite adequate medication, treatment with enhanced extracorporeal counter pulsations (EECP) was tried with good results. ED, end-diastole; EDV, end-diastolic volume; EF, ejection fraction; ES, end-systole; ESV, end-systolic volume.

viability testing to minimize resting ischemia. It is important to note, however, that inducible ischemia itself is an indicator of viability and a resting perfusion defect unchanged during stress in a patient with decreased left ventricular function indicates the need for specific viability testing.

For viability testing with PET, ^{18}F-FDG is used to differentiate between viable and nonviable myocardium in a perfusion defect.[27] ^{18}F-FDG is a glucose analog, and hibernating myocardium maintains metabolic activity; thus, ^{18}F-FDG uptake is enhanced even when perfusion is decreased. The sign of viable hibernating myocardium on PET is typically detected as a decreased perfusion tracer uptake with a maintained ^{18}F-FDG uptake.

DIAGNOSTIC ACCURACY, OUTCOME, AND RISK ASSESSMENT

■ WHAT DETERMINES WHETHER A PERFUSION IMAGING TEST IS USEFUL?

Coronary angiography has been commonly used as reference standard when assessing diagnostic accuracy for noninvasive cardiac imaging tests. However, coronary angiography depicts coronary anatomy, and myocardial perfusion SPECT assesses myocardial perfusion, and the relationship between coronary stenosis and perfusion decrease is not straightforward. Early invasive coronary angiography studies showed that there is no correlation between the reactive hyperemic response and the degree of coronary stenosis.[7] Therefore, one should bear in mind that sensitivity and specificity when using coronary anatomy as the reference method may not be the best markers for the accuracy of a perfusion assessment. Recent studies have demonstrated sensitivity in the range of 85% to 90% and specificity in the range of 80% to 90% for myocardial perfusion SPECT versus coronary angiography.[15,28-33] Older studies showed lower specificity, but the use of attenuation correction, prone imaging, and gated SPECT has resulted in higher specificity, especially in obese and female patients.[13,34] The sensitivity and specificity of PET have been reported as 93% and 92%, respectively.[19]

Research in noninvasive cardiology testing has moved toward evaluating the relationship between the findings of the test and the risk for a major adverse cardiovascular event (MACE)[15] and cost-effectiveness analysis partly because of the problems of diagnostic accuracy mentioned earlier. There is a wealth of scientific evidence on the prognostic value and cost effectiveness of myocardial perfusion SPECT[15,35-38] and, recently, of PET perfusion imaging.[39,40]

■ AMOUNT OF ISCHEMIC MYOCARDIUM

There seems to be a nearly direct relationship between the amount of ischemic myocardium and the risk for a MACE,[41] and when assessing the ischemic myocardium, one needs to take both the extent and the severity of the perfusion defect into account. The myocardium is divided into 17 segments according to the American Heart Association model,[42] and the perfusion is scored for each segment. Zero points are given for no perfusion defect, 1 point is given for mildly reduced perfusion, 2 points are given for moderately reduced perfusion, 3 points are given for severely reduced perfusion, and 4 points are given for absent perfusion. The summed stress score (SSS) is the result of adding the scores for all segments at stress, and the summed rest score (SRS) is the corresponding result at rest. The summed difference score (SDS) is the difference between SSS and SRS. Note that only segments with an SSS can get an SRS; some irregularities in perfusion can be expected at rest in healthy subjects, but at stress, these may disappear. One of the reasons is that the perfusion map is normalized to the maximum perfusion of the heart at stress and rest. At rest, this means that a region with perfusion of 70% of maximum will be the result of a difference between approximately 0.7 and 1.0 mL/min/g or an absolute difference of 0.3 mL/min/g. At stress with a normal maximum perfusion of 3 mL/min/g, the same absolute difference of 0.3 mL/min/g would be 90% of maximum perfusion and would be read as normal. An SSS of 0 to 3 is interpreted as normal.[43,44] With PET, the possibility of quantifying myocardial perfusion in absolute terms is possible and likely provides clinically useful information and makes the technique more accurate, especially in the assessment of severity of disease in patients with multivessel disease[45] (Fig. 3–14). However, more clinical trials are warranted to elucidate the clinical value of quantification of perfusion.

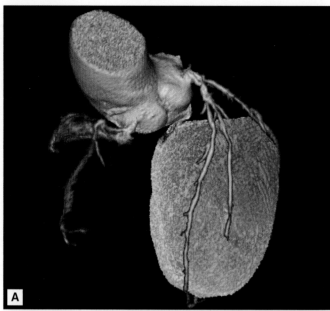

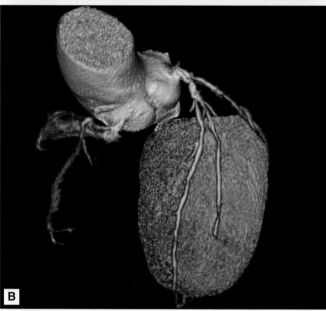

FIGURE 3–14. Hybrid positron emission tomography/computed tomography image of patient with multivessel disease. The images are created similarly as in Fig. 3–8. In this patient, the relative perfusion distribution was normal due to balanced reduction of perfusion in all myocardial regions (**A**). However, quantitative analysis revealed that all regions had very low stress perfusion (**B**)

■ STUDIES SHOWING USEFULNESS OF MYOCARDIAL PERFUSION IMAGING IN DIFFERENT CLINICAL SCENARIOS

Stable Angina

In patients with stable angina, a normal myocardial perfusion imaging study corresponds to an annual risk for a MACE of 0.6% or, in other words, lower risk than the average population.[41] With increasing SSS, the risk increases,[46] and an SSS of 7 to 8 or more representing 10% of the myocardium is associated with an annual risk of MACE of 5%.[47] Studies with myocardial perfusion

imaging have showed that this patient population is a risk group in which medical treatment and risk factor management are associated with higher cardiac death rates compared with treatment with coronary revascularization.[48] However, patients with less extensive ischemia benefit from medical management only compared with coronary revascularization.[49] These results have been reproduced in a substudy of the Clinical Outcomes Utilizing Revascularization and Aggressive Drug Evaluation (COURAGE) trial,[50] where increasing degree of ischemia was associated with increasing rates of MACE and patients with more severe ischemia seemed to experience the greatest benefit from PCI.[15] Several studies in patients with stable angina have shown that using myocardial perfusion SPECT as the initial test before deciding on a coronary angiography saves money compared with an initial coronary angiography especially in patients with intermediate risk of CAD.[51] More frequent coronary revascularizations are performed in patients with initial coronary angiography without a benefit in MACE.[51] These findings have led to the use of myocardial perfusion SPECT and other noninvasive imaging tests as gatekeepers for coronary angiography in patients with intermediate risk for CAD. Patients with low likelihood after initial testing should not undergo myocardial perfusion imaging, and patients with high likelihood can be sent directly to invasive evaluation. Another indication for myocardial perfusion imaging in stable angina is patients who have undergone a coronary angiography in whom stenoses of unclear significance have been found.

Suspected Acute Coronary Syndrome

Myocardial SPECT has two roles in the setting of suspected acute coronary syndrome. It can be used in the emergency department in patients with intermediate risk of acute coronary syndrome with tracer injection during or shortly after chest pain.[6,52-54] The negative predictive value in this patient population is very high (95%-99%), and therefore, patients with a normal scan may be discharged instead of admitted to the hospital. This has been shown to be cost effective.[53,55] In patients who have been admitted to the hospital for suspected acute coronary syndrome with unclear diagnosis after repeated ECG and cardiac biomarkers, a stress test (exercise or pharmacologic) is recommended.[1] Myocardial perfusion SPECT is useful in these patients, especially when abnormalities of the resting ECG hamper ST-segment analysis or when maximum heart rate cannot be reached.

After a Myocardial Infarction

International guidelines include myocardial perfusion imaging as an appropriate test in patients after myocardial infarction for risk assessment if coronary angiography has not been performed or if a coronary stenosis of unclear significance has been found on the primary PCI. However, less data are available in these patient populations on the prognostic value of myocardial perfusion imaging. A systematic review found four observational studies with a total of 2106 patients and concluded that there was independent and incremental prognostic value of myocardial perfusion SPECT after myocardial infarction.[56] More recently, a multinational study showed that early myocardial perfusion SPECT can identify patients who can be discharged early after myocardial infarction.[57]

PITFALLS

■ OVERREPORTING

One of the most common mistakes in myocardial perfusion imaging is overreporting minor defects as ischemia. Small irregularities in the perfusion images are often seen and are not associated with a worse prognosis. Rather, overreporting may lead to unnecessary coronary catheterizations without any benefit to the patient. The parametric maps of perfusion are helpful in locating the ischemia but cannot be the basis for ischemia detection because small areas of irregularities tend to be overestimated on these images. Therefore, the full set of short and long axis images should be evaluated before looking at the parametric images (see Fig. 3–3B). This problem can also be solved by absolute quantification when PET is used (see Fig. 3–14).

■ INADEQUATE STRESS TEST

The perfusion distribution during stress is visualized and compared with rest when assessing ischemia with myocardial perfusion imaging. A stenosis will cause an inability to increase perfusion in the perfusion territory of the corresponding coronary artery during stress, and therefore, adequate stress must be present during injection of the perfusion tracer. In the case of an inadequate stress test, there is the risk of a false-negative test. If an exercise stress test is performed, the limit of at least 85% of predicted maximum heart rate is used. For example, patients on β-blockers often do not reach this level, and in these cases, the perfusion tracer is not injected; instead, a pharmacologic stress test should be performed. In the case of adenosine, dipyridamole, and regadenoson, caffeine abstinence is important before the test because of the competitive inhibition of the binding to the adenosine receptor by caffeine. One recent study used an increased dose of 210 μg/kg/min in patients with recent caffeine intake and showed increased detection of ischemia compared with 140 μg/kg/min and recent caffeine intake.[58] Many patients with chest pain have prescriptions for oral nitrates, and it is important that patients have a 12-hour cessation of long-acting nitrates and at least a 1-hour cessation of short-acting nitrates before the stress injection. Resting injection should likewise be a true rest, and checking the patient's heart rate before injection is an easy way to avoid "false" resting images. Patients exhibiting chest discomfort are often administered short-acting nitrates before resting injection to ensure a true resting perfusion image.

■ LEFT BUNDLE BRANCH BLOCK

Special consideration must be paid to myocardial perfusion SPECT for patients with left bundle branch block (LBBB) on the ECG as well as patients with ventricular stimulation pacemakers causing the ECG to have the appearance of an LBBB. The problem with LBBB in myocardial perfusion SPECT is that many patients seem to have a perfusion defect in the septal half of the heart. The cause of this apparent perfusion deficit is not entirely known and is not seen in all patients with LBBB. What is known empirically is that a stress test where the heart rate increases often causes the perfusion defect to worsen, although no stenosis is found on a subsequent coronary angiography. This is demonstrated in Fig. 3–15 showing a patient with stress-induced LBBB. The stress image shows a perfusion defect in the entire septum but most prominent in the anteroseptal region. At rest, the ECG returns to normal, and the SPECT shows a normal perfusion distribution. Therefore, a pharmacologic vasodilator stress test (eg, adenosine, dipyridamole, or regadenoson) without exercise is used in cases of LBBB to avoid a heart rate increase.

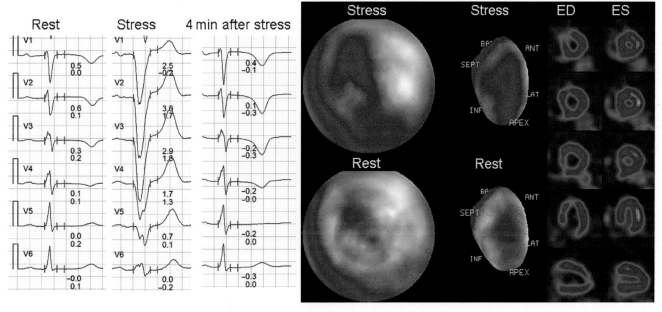

FIGURE 3–15. A former smoker with heredity for ischemic heart disease was admitted to the hospital because of 2 days of recurrent chest pain. Electrocardiogram changes can be seen at rest, but there was no release of troponins. An exercise test was performed because of caffeine intake, and the patient was deemed low risk for acute coronary syndrome. During exercise, a frequency-dependent left bundle branch block (LBBB) developed, and the isotope was inadequately injected despite the LBBB. A perfusion defect was seen in the anteroseptal wall that was not present at rest. This could have been due to the LBBB, and the test was reported as nondiagnostic. Gated single photon emission computed tomography showed normal ejection fraction. A coronary angiography was performed, which showed normal coronary arteries. ANT, anterior; INF, inferior; LAT, lateral; SEPT, septal.

■ TRIPLE-VESSEL DISEASE

Detection of ischemia on standard analysis myocardial perfusion imaging depends on one region having normal perfusion; this region is set to 100%, and the rest of the myocardium is normalized to this normal region. In the case of multivessel disease with physiologically significant stenoses in all coronary vessels, the perfusion will be globally decreased, the region with a 100% signal will be falsely read as normal, and occasionally, so-called balanced *triple-vessel disease* is missed in standard relative perfusion analysis. There are also cases where the perfusion SPECT shows ischemia in one territory but on coronary angiography multivessel disease is found. In these cases, SPECT has detected only the tip of the ischemia iceberg. Therefore, it is important to look for other signs of multivessel coronary disease (eg, the blood pressure reaction and left ventricular volumes and function).[59,60] During exercise stress test, the blood pressure reaction is often pathologic, with a decrease in the blood pressure during the final stages of exercise. A dilatation in the stress perfusion images compared with the rest images (ie, a TID) is also a sign of a pathologic test (Figs. 3–16 and 3–17). This is caused by postischemic stunning where the cardiac contractile function still is depressed after the ischemic event. In these cases, gated SPECT also shows dilated ventricular volumes and decreased ejection fraction after stress compared with rest.

Most of these problems can be avoided by using absolute quantification of myocardial perfusion (see Fig. 3–14).[45] Unfortunately, SPECT does not offer absolute quantification of tissue perfusion, and most clinical routine use of PET imaging is still based on relative analysis of perfusion distribution. Even without quantification, PET has been considered better in complex revascularized patients and obese patients (Fig. 3–18). However, in most patients with bypass surgery, myocardial perfusion SPECT can still be of use (Fig. 3–19).

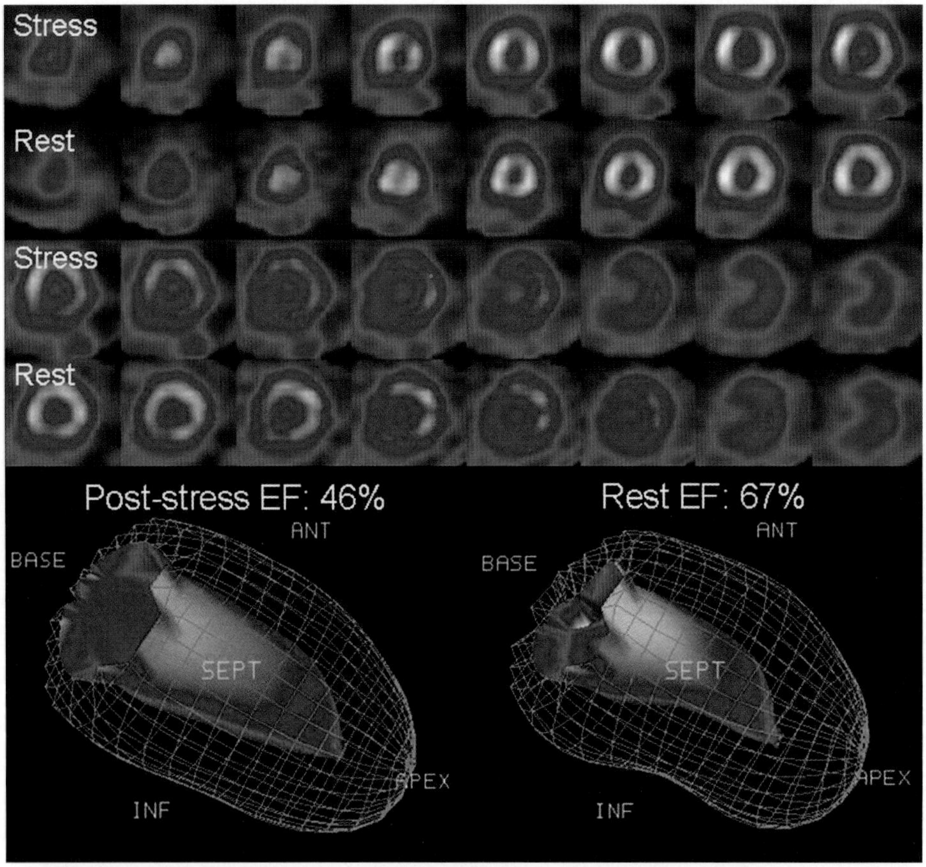

■ HIGH GASTROINTESTINAL TRACER ACTIVITY

Perfusion tracer activity in the gastrointestinal tract adjacent to the heart may cause a false-positive test if present during rest and a false-negative test if present during stress. High uptake is almost always close to the inferior wall and is seldom a problem during exercise. The image acquisition can be repeated in the case of high uptake of perfusion tracer in the regions adjacent to the heart if this leads to problems in interpretation (see Fig. 3–13).

COMPARISONS WITH OTHER IMAGING MODALITIES

There are three roles of myocardial perfusion SPECT and PET that can be compared with other available imaging modalities; these are ischemia detection, assessment of viability/hibernation, and assessment of left ventricular function.

■ ISCHEMIA DETECTION

Myocardial perfusion SPECT is by far the most commonly used cardiac imaging technique to detect ischemia. The use of PET is growing. Other common cardiac imaging techniques used are stress echocardiography and cardiac MRI. Stress echocardiography detects regional function during exercise or dobutamine as an indicator of ischemia. Several studies have shown that stress echocardiography myocardial perfusion SPECT have similar diagnostic and prognostic performance. Stress echocardiography, however is more operator dependent than myocardial perfusion SPECT. Perfusion contrast echocardiography

FIGURE 3–16. An example of balanced triple-vessel disease. Shown is a 42-year-old man with no history of ischemic heart disease for whom the perfusion images show no perfusion defects at stress or rest. However, the left ventricle was dilated at stress compared with rest, so-called *transient ischemic dilatation*. Also, the ejection fraction (EF) decreased after the exercise test compared to rest because of postischemic stunning. These are signs of severe ischemia, and therefore, the test is not normal despite the lack of perfusion defects. Because of global ischemia, the perfusion is decreased homogenously, and no area of normal perfusion and thus no perfusion defects exist. The patient showed triple-vessel disease at coronary angiography and was treated with percutaneous coronary intervention. ANT, anterior; INF, inferior; SEPT, septal.

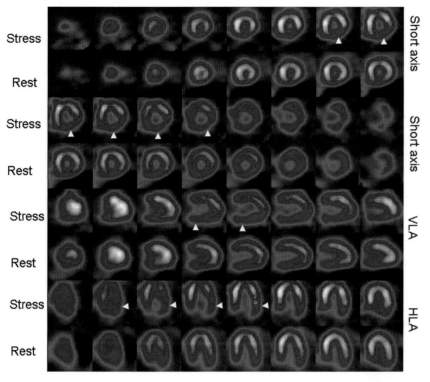

Stress

Rest

Stress

Rest

Stress

Rest

Stress

Rest

Short axis

Short axis

VLA

HLA

FIGURE 3–17. Transient ischemic dilatation. Normal resting perfusion and an inferior perfusion defect (arrowheads) at stress with somewhat unevenly distributed perfusion in the anterior and lateral walls are seen. The dilatation of the ventricle at stress indicates severe ischemia, and therefore, the patient was referred to coronary angiography, which showed triple-vessel disease. HLA, horizontal long axis; VLA, vertical long axis.

has also been recently used for detection of CAD, but its role has not yet been established. Cardiac MRI in patients with suspected CAD is based on either wall motion analysis or first-pass perfusion detection. The accuracy of cardiac MRI is in a similar range as other noninvasive imaging tests in skillful hands. Currently, the availability of MRI scanners for cardiac use is limited. In addition, less evidence about the prognostic value and cost effectiveness of the newer techniques exists.

◼ VIABILITY ASSESSMENT

Multiple imaging techniques have been developed to assess viable and nonviable myocardium by evaluating perfusion, cell membrane integrity, mitochondrial function, glucose metabolism, scar tissue, and contractile reserve. PET, SPECT, and dobutamine stress echocardiography have been extensively evaluated for assessment of viability and prediction of clinical outcome after coronary revascularization. Low-dose dobutamine echocardiography has been successfully used, and an increase in contraction from rest to 5 to 10 μg/kg/min dobutamine is interpreted as viable myocardium. On MRI, late gadolinium enhanced imaging 10 to 20 minutes after contrast injection can be used to visualize the infarct.[61]

In general, nuclear imaging techniques have a high sensitivity for the detection of viability, whereas techniques evaluating contractile reserve have somewhat lower sensitivity but higher specificity. MRI has a high diagnostic accuracy for assessment of the transmural extent of myocardial scar tissue. With this technique, viability

detection is based on indirect estimation of non-scarred myocardium. The fraction of the scar is inversely related to recovery of wall motion after revascularization, but there is no sharp cutoff for accurate prediction of wall motion recovery after revascularization. Because this technique cannot characterize the viable tissue adjacent to scar, low-dose dobutamine infusions have been used with cardiac MRI to improve the accuracy. Thus, the performance of cardiac MRI in detection of viability and predicting recovery of wall motion is similar to other imaging techniques.[62] Of the imaging techniques, ^{18}F-FDG PET is very sensitive; this technique has been used for a long time for viability detection and is still the most documented technique. The evidence is currently mostly based on observational studies or meta-analyses, and there are only two randomized multicenter studies on viability, both of which used PET imaging.[63,64] Patients with a substantial amount of dysfunctional but viable myocardium are likely to benefit from coronary revascularization and may show improvements in regional and global contractile function, symptoms, exercise capacity, and long-term prognosis. In summary, the differences in performance of the various imaging techniques are small, and commonly, the experience and availability determine which technique is used.

◼ LEFT VENTRICULAR FUNCTION

Gated SPECT and gated PET provide automated, mainly user-independent, three-dimensional assessment of left ventricular function. However, the method of choice for left ventricular function is still echocardiography because of its lack of radiation and concomitant assessment of valvular function, which cannot be done by the nuclear imaging methods. Gated SPECT has been extensively validated against other methods, for example MRI.[65]

Moving Image Legends

All moving images are located on the complementary DVD.

MOVING IMAGE 3–1. Gated single photon emission computed tomography (SPECT) images from the patient in Fig. 3–6A. There is normal regional function in the inferior wall supporting the notion of inferior attenuation.

MOVING IMAGE 3–2. Decreased perfusion and regional function in the basal part of the inferior and inferolateral wall with no difference between stress and rest. This is consistent with a myocardial infarction in the right coronary artery territory but no stress-induced ischemia.

MOVING IMAGE 3–3. Decreased perfusion in the apex at rest that increases to a severe and large perfusion defect at stress. The gated single photon emission computed tomography (SPECT) images show a slight reduction in the regional function in the apex at rest. After stress, the left ventricular volumes are dilated, and the global function is depressed. This physiologic phenomenon is called postischemic stunning and is indicative of severe ischemia. A near occlusion was found in the proximal left anterior descending artery on coronary angiography.

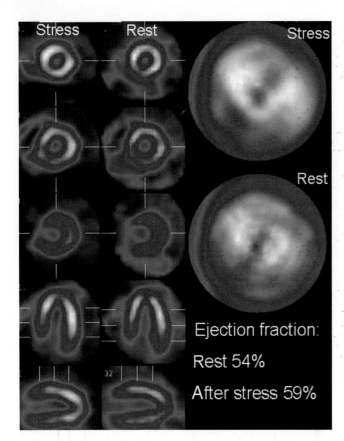

FIGURE 3–18. A 59-year-old man underwent bypass surgery several years earlier and now experiences chest pain. Exercise-induced chest pain and a pathologic ST-segment reaction, but the perfusion images were normal, as were the gated single photon emission computed tomography (SPECT) results. No transient ischemic dilatation was seen. Because of the high probability of ischemia and pathologic exercise test, the patient was referred for a coronary angiography where a significant left anterior descending artery stenosis was found. Symptoms disappeared after percutaneous coronary intervention treatment of the stenosis. This false-negative study exemplifies the lower sensitivity of myocardial perfusion SPECT in patients with previous bypass surgery and the need for the increased diagnostic properties using positron emission tomography in these patients.

REFERENCES

1. Anderson JL, Adams CD, Antman EM, et al. ACC/AHA 2007 guidelines for the management of patients with unstable angina/non-ST-elevation myocardial infarction: a report of the American College of Cardiology/American Heart Association Task Force on Practice Guidelines (Writing Committee to Revise the 2002 Guidelines for the Management of Patients With Unstable Angina/Non-ST-Elevation Myocardial Infarction) developed in collaboration with the American College of Emergency Physicians, the Society for Cardiovascular Angiography and Interventions, and the Society of Thoracic Surgeons endorsed by the American Association of Cardiovascular and Pulmonary Rehabilitation and the Society for Academic Emergency Medicine. *J Am Coll Cardiol.* 2007;50:e1-e157.
2. Gibbons RJ, Abrams J, Chatterjee K, et al. ACC/AHA 2002 guideline update for the management of patients with chronic stable angina—summary article: a report of the American College of Cardiology/American Heart Association Task Force on Practice Guidelines (Committee on the Management of Patients With Chronic Stable Angina). *Circulation.* 2003;107(1):149-158.
3. Van de Werf F, Bax J, Betriu A, et al. Management of acute myocardial infarction in patients presenting with persistent ST-segment elevation: the Task Force on the Management of ST-Segment Elevation Acute Myocardial Infarction of the European Society of Cardiology. *Eur Heart J.* 2008;29:2909-2945.

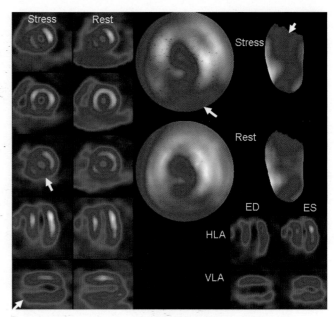

FIGURE 3–19. A 71-year-old man with a previous myocardial infarction 18 years earlier and bypass surgery 12 years ago. The patient developed chest pain during exercise in cold weather, and the exercise stress test was equivocal. Myocardial perfusion single photon emission computed tomography (SPECT) showed a perfusion defect in the apex and anteroapical region at rest. During exercise, a perfusion defect was also seen in the basal inferior region (arrows). Thus, stress-induced ischemia was found in a small region in the native right coronary artery territory, and signs of a myocardial infarction were seen in the distal left anterior descending artery territory. ED, end-diastole; ES, end-systole; HLA, horizontal long axis; VLA, vertical long axis.

4. Hesse B, Tagil K, Cuocolo A, et al. EANM/ESC procedural guidelines for myocardial perfusion imaging in nuclear cardiology. *Eur J Nucl Med Mol Imaging.* 2005;32:855-897.
5. Hendel RC, Wackers FJ, Berman DS, et al. American Society of Nuclear Cardiology consensus statement: reporting of radionuclide myocardial perfusion imaging studies. *J Nucl Cardiol.* 2006;13:e152-e156.
6. Hendel RC, Berman DS, Di Carli MF, et al. ACCF/ASNC/ACR/AHA/ASE/SCCT/SCMR/SNM 2009 appropriate use criteria for cardiac radionuclide imaging: a report of the American College of Cardiology Foundation Appropriate Use Criteria Task Force, the American Society of Nuclear Cardiology, the American College of Radiology, the American Heart Association, the American Society of Echocardiography, the Society of Cardiovascular Computed Tomography, the Society for Cardiovascular Magnetic Resonance, and the Society of Nuclear Medicine: endorsed by the American College of Emergency Physicians. *Circulation.* 2009;119:e561-587.
7. White CW, Wright CB, Doty DB, et al. Does visual interpretation of the coronary arteriogram predict the physiologic importance of a coronary stenosis? *N Engl J Med.* 1984;310:819-824.
8. Sharir T, Germano G, Kavanagh PB, et al. Incremental prognostic value of post-stress left ventricular ejection fraction and volume by gated myocardial perfusion single photon emission computed tomography. *Circulation.* 1999;100:1035-1042.
9. Sharir T, Ben-Haim S, Merzon K, et al. High-speed myocardial perfusion imaging initial clinical comparison with conventional dual detector anger camera imaging. *JACC Cardiovasc Imaging.* 2008;1:156-163.
10. Esteves FP, Raggi P, Folks RD, et al. Novel solid-state-detector dedicated cardiac camera for fast myocardial perfusion imaging: multicenter comparison with standard dual detector cameras. *J Nucl Cardiol.* 2009;16:927-934.
11. Garcia EV. SPECT attenuation correction: an essential tool to realize nuclear cardiology's manifest destiny. *J Nucl Cardiol.* 2007;14:16-24.
12. Kaufmann PA, Di Carli MF. Hybrid SPECT/CT and PET/CT imaging: the next step in noninvasive cardiac imaging. *Semin Nucl Med.* 2009;39(5):341-347.

13. Hayes SW, De Lorenzo A, Hachamovitch R, et al. Prognostic implications of combined prone and supine acquisitions in patients with equivocal or abnormal supine myocardial perfusion SPECT. *J Nucl Med.* 2003;44:1633-1640.

14. Heden B, Persson E, Carlsson M, Pahlm O, Arheden H. Disappearance of myocardial perfusion defects on prone SPECT imaging: comparison with cardiac magnetic resonance imaging in patients without established coronary artery disease. *BMC Med Imaging.* 2009;9:16.

15. Shaw LJ, Narula J. Risk assessment and predictive value of coronary artery disease testing. *J Nucl Med.* 2009;50:1296-1306.

16. Gibbons RJ, Balady GJ, Bricker JT, et al. ACC/AHA 2002 guideline update for exercise testing: summary article: a report of the American College of Cardiology/American Heart Association Task Force on Practice Guidelines (Committee to Update the 1997 Exercise Testing Guidelines). *Circulation.* 2002;106:1883-1892.

17. Mahmarian JJ, Cerqueira MD, Iskandrian AE, et al. Regadenoson induces comparable left ventricular perfusion defects as adenosine: a quantitative analysis from the ADVANCE MPI 2 trial. *JACC Cardiovasc Imaging.* 2009;2:959-968.

18. Yoon AJ, Melduni RM, Duncan SA, Ostfeld RJ, Travin MI. The effect of beta-blockers on the diagnostic accuracy of vasodilator pharmacologic SPECT myocardial perfusion imaging. *J Nucl Cardiol.* 2009;16:358-367.

19. Le Guludec D, Lautamaki R, Knuuti J, Bax JJ, Bengel FM. Present and future of clinical cardiovascular PET imaging in Europe—a position statement by the European Council of Nuclear Cardiology (ECNC). *Eur J Nucl Med Mol Imaging.* 2008;35:1709-1724.

20. Knuuti J, Schelbert HR, Bax JJ. The need for standardisation of cardiac FDG PET imaging in the evaluation of myocardial viability in patients with chronic ischaemic left ventricular dysfunction. *Eur J Nucl Med Mol Imaging.* 2002;29:1257-1266.

21. Kajander S, Ukkonen H, Sipila H, Teras M, Knuuti J. Low radiation dose imaging of myocardial perfusion and coronary angiography with a hybrid PET/CT scanner. *Clin Physiol Funct Imaging.* 2009;29:81-88.

22. Schenker MP, Dorbala S, Hong EC, et al. Interrelation of coronary calcification, myocardial ischemia, and outcomes in patients with intermediate likelihood of coronary artery disease: a combined positron emission tomography/computed tomography study. *Circulation.* 2008;117:1693-1700.

23. Schepis T, Gaemperli O, Koepfli P, et al. Added value of coronary artery calcium score as an adjunct to gated SPECT for the evaluation of coronary artery disease in an intermediate-risk population. *J Nucl Med.* 2007;48:1424-1430.

24. Di Carli MF, Hachamovitch R. New technology for noninvasive evaluation of coronary artery disease. *Circulation.* 2007;115:1464-1480.

25. Meijboom WB, Meijs MF, Schuijf JD, et al. Diagnostic accuracy of 64-slice computed tomography coronary angiography: a prospective, multicenter, multivendor study. *J Am Coll Cardiol.* 2008;52:2135-2144.

26. Namdar M, Hany TF, Koepfli P, et al. Integrated PET/CT for the assessment of coronary artery disease: a feasibility study. *J Nucl Med.* 2005;46:930-935.

27. Sawada SG. Positron emission tomography for assessment of viability. *Curr Opin Cardiol.* 2006;21:464-468.

28. Berman DS, Kang X, Nishina H, et al. Diagnostic accuracy of gated Tc-99m sestamibi stress myocardial perfusion SPECT with combined supine and prone acquisitions to detect coronary artery disease in obese and nonobese patients. *J Nucl Cardiol.* 2006;13:191-201.

29. Dondi M, Fagioli G, Salgarello M, Zoboli S, Nanni C, Cidda C. Myocardial SPECT: what do we gain from attenuation correction (and when)? *Q J Nucl Med Mol Imaging.* 2004;48:181-187.

30. Duvall WL, Croft LB, Corriel JS, et al. SPECT myocardial perfusion imaging in morbidly obese patients: image quality, hemodynamic response to pharmacologic stress, and diagnostic and prognostic value. *J Nucl Cardiol.* 2006;13:202-209.

31. Fricke E, Fricke H, Weise R, et al. Attenuation correction of myocardial SPECT perfusion images with low-dose CT: evaluation of the method by comparison with perfusion PET. *J Nucl Med.* 2005;46:736-744.

32. Masood Y, Liu YH, Depuey G, et al. Clinical validation of SPECT attenuation correction using x-ray computed tomography-derived attenuation maps: multicenter clinical trial with angiographic correlation. *J Nucl Cardiol.* 2005;12:676-686.

33. Mieres JH, Shaw LJ, Arai A, et al. Role of noninvasive testing in the clinical evaluation of women with suspected coronary artery disease: consensus statement from the Cardiac Imaging Committee, Council on Clinical Cardiology, and the Cardiovascular Imaging and Intervention Committee, Council on Cardiovascular Radiology and Intervention, American Heart Association. *Circulation.* 2005;111:682-696.

34. Nishina H, Slomka PJ, Abidov A, et al. Combined supine and prone quantitative myocardial perfusion SPECT: method development and clinical validation in patients with no known coronary artery disease. *J Nucl Med.* 2006;47:51-58.

35. Underwood SR, Anagnostopoulos C, Cerqueira M, et al. Myocardial perfusion scintigraphy: the evidence. *Eur J Nucl Med Mol Imaging.* 2004;31:261-291.

36. Hachamovitch R, Berman DS, Kiat H, Cohen I, Friedman JD, Shaw LJ. Value of stress myocardial perfusion single photon emission computed tomography in patients with normal resting electrocardiograms: an evaluation of incremental prognostic value and cost-effectiveness. *Circulation.* 2002;105:823-829.

37. Abidov A, Hachamovitch R, Hayes SW, et al. Are shades of gray prognostically useful in reporting myocardial perfusion single-photon emission computed tomography? *Circ Cardiovasc Imaging.* 2009;2:290-298.

38. Des Prez RD, Shaw LJ, Gillespie RL, et al. Cost-effectiveness of myocardial perfusion imaging: a summary of the currently available literature. *J Nucl Cardiol.* 2005;12:750-759.

39. Jacklin PB, Barrington SF, Roxburgh JC, et al. Cost-effectiveness of preoperative positron emission tomography in ischemic heart disease. *Ann Thorac Surg.* 2002;73:1403-1409; discussion 1410.

40. Merhige ME, Breen WJ, Shelton V, Houston T, D'Arcy BJ, Perna AF. Impact of myocardial perfusion imaging with PET and (82)Rb on downstream invasive procedure utilization, costs, and outcomes in coronary disease management. *J Nucl Med.* 2007;48:1069-1076.

41. Shaw LJ, Iskandrian AE. Prognostic value of gated myocardial perfusion SPECT. *J Nucl Cardiol.* 2004;11:171-185.

42. Cerqueira MD, Weissman NJ, Dilsizian V, et al. Standardized myocardial segmentation and nomenclature for tomographic imaging of the heart: a statement for healthcare professionals from the Cardiac Imaging Committee of the Council on Clinical Cardiology of the American Heart Association. *Circulation.* 2002;105:539-542.

43. Berman DS, Kang X, Van Train KF, et al. Comparative prognostic value of automatic quantitative analysis versus semiquantitative visual analysis of exercise myocardial perfusion single-photon emission computed tomography. *J Am Coll Cardiol.* 1998;32:1987-1995.

44. Sharir T, Berman DS, Waechter PB, et al. Quantitative analysis of regional motion and thickening by gated myocardial perfusion SPECT: normal heterogeneity and criteria for abnormality. *J Nucl Med.* 2001;42:1630-1638.

45. Knuuti J, Kajander S, Maki M, Ukkonen H. Quantification of myocardial blood flow will reform the detection of CAD. *J Nucl Cardiol.* 2009;16:497-506.

46. Hachamovitch R, Berman DS, Shaw LJ, et al. Incremental prognostic value of myocardial perfusion single photon emission computed tomography for the prediction of cardiac death: differential stratification for risk of cardiac death and myocardial infarction. *Circulation.* 1998;97:535-543.

47. Shaw LJ, Hendel RC, Cerquiera M, et al. Ethnic differences in the prognostic value of stress technetium-99m tetrofosmin gated single-photon emission computed tomography myocardial perfusion imaging. *J Am Coll Cardiol.* 2005;45:1494-1504.

48. Hachamovitch R, Hayes SW, Friedman JD, Cohen I, Berman DS. Comparison of the short-term survival benefit associated with revascularization compared with medical therapy in patients with no prior coronary artery disease undergoing stress myocardial perfusion single photon emission computed tomography. *Circulation.* 2003;107:2900-2907.

49. O'Keefe JH Jr, Bateman TM, Ligon RW, et al. Outcome of medical versus invasive treatment strategies for non-high-risk ischemic heart disease. *J Nucl Cardiol.* 1998;5:28-33.

50. Shaw LJ, Berman DS, Maron DJ, et al. Optimal medical therapy with or without percutaneous coronary intervention to reduce ischemic burden: results from the Clinical Outcomes Utilizing Revascularization and Aggressive Drug Evaluation (COURAGE) trial nuclear substudy. *Circulation.* 2008;117:1283-1291.

51. Shaw LJ, Hachamovitch R, Berman DS, et al. The economic consequences of available diagnostic and prognostic strategies for the evaluation of stable angina patients: an observational assessment of the value of precatheterization ischemia. Economics of Noninvasive Diagnosis (END) Multicenter Study Group. *J Am Coll Cardiol.* 1999;33:661-669.

52. Radensky PW, Hilton TC, Fulmer H, McLaughlin BA, Stowers SA. Potential cost effectiveness of initial myocardial perfusion imaging for assessment of emergency department patients with chest pain. *Am J Cardiol*. 1997;79:595-599.

53. Stowers SA, Eisenstein EL, Th Wackers FJ, et al. An economic analysis of an aggressive diagnostic strategy with single photon emission computed tomography myocardial perfusion imaging and early exercise stress testing in emergency department patients who present with chest pain but nondiagnostic electrocardiograms: results from a randomized trial. *Ann Emerg Med*. 2000;35:17-25.

54. Udelson JE, Beshansky JR, Ballin DS, et al. Myocardial perfusion imaging for evaluation and triage of patients with suspected acute cardiac ischemia: a randomized controlled trial. *JAMA*. 2002;288:2693-2700.

55. Forberg JL, Hilmersson CE, Carlsson M, et al. Negative predictive value and potential cost savings of acute nuclear myocardial perfusion imaging in low risk patients with suspected acute coronary syndrome: a prospective single blinded study. *BMC Emerg Med*. 2009;9:12.

56. Mowatt G, Brazzelli M, Gemmell H, Hillis GS, Metcalfe M, Vale L. Systematic review of the prognostic effectiveness of SPECT myocardial perfusion scintigraphy in patients with suspected or known coronary artery disease and following myocardial infarction. *Nucl Med Commun*. 2005;26:217-229.

57. Mahmarian JJ, Shaw LJ, Filipchuk NG, et al. A multinational study to establish the value of early adenosine technetium-99m sestamibi myocardial perfusion imaging in identifying a low-risk group for early hospital discharge after acute myocardial infarction. *J Am Coll Cardiol*. 2006;48:2448-2457.

58. Reyes E, Loong CY, Harbinson M, Donovan J, Anagnostopoulos C, Underwood SR. High-dose adenosine overcomes the attenuation of myocardial perfusion reserve caused by caffeine. *J Am Coll Cardiol*. 2008;52:2008-2016.

59. Lima RS, Watson DD, Goode AR, et al. Incremental value of combined perfusion and function over perfusion alone by gated SPECT myocardial perfusion imaging for detection of severe three-vessel coronary artery disease. *J Am Coll Cardiol*. 2003;42:64-70.

60. Berman DS, Kang X, Slomka PJ, et al. Underestimation of extent of ischemia by gated SPECT myocardial perfusion imaging in patients with left main coronary artery disease. *J Nucl Cardiol*. 2007;14:521-528.

61. Carlsson M, Arheden H, Higgins CB, Saeed M. Magnetic resonance imaging as a potential gold standard for infarct quantification. *J Electrocardiol*. 2008;41:614-620.

62. Allman KC, Shaw LJ, Hachamovitch R, Udelson JE. Myocardial viability testing and impact of revascularization on prognosis in patients with coronary artery disease and left ventricular dysfunction: a meta-analysis. *J Am Coll Cardiol*. 2002;39:1151-1158.

63. Beanlands RS, Ruddy TD, deKemp RA, et al. Positron emission tomography and recovery following revascularization (PARR-1): the importance of scar and the development of a prediction rule for the degree of recovery of left ventricular function. *J Am Coll Cardiol*. 2002;40:1735-1743.

64. Beanlands RS, Nichol G, Huszti E, et al. F-18-fluorodeoxyglucose positron emission tomography imaging-assisted management of patients with severe left ventricular dysfunction and suspected coronary disease: a randomized, controlled trial (PARR-2). *J Am Coll Cardiol*. 2007; 50:2002-2012.

65. Persson E, Carlsson M, Palmer J, Pahlm O, Arheden H. Evaluation of left ventricular volumes and ejection fraction by automated gated myocardial SPECT versus cardiovascular magnetic resonance. *Clin Physiol Funct Imaging*. 2005;25:135-141.

CHAPTER 4
CORONARY ANGIOGRAPHY

Kjell C. Nikus

DESCRIPTION OF CORONARY ANGIOGRAPHY / 71
Technique / 71

INDICATIONS AND CONTRAINDICATIONS / 71

COMPLICATIONS / 72

CORONARY ANATOMY AND VARIATIONS / 72

ANGIOGRAPHIC CORONARY ARTERY DISEASE / 75

CORONARY ARTERY ANOMALIES / 75
Bridging / 75
Fistulae / 76

COLLATERAL CIRCULATION / 76

ANGIOGRAPHIC ASSESSMENT OF CORONARY FLOW / 76
Angiographic Assessment of Myocardial Blood Flow / 76

ANGIOGRAPHIC FACTORS DETERMINING ECG CHANGES IN ACUTE CORONARY SYNDROMES / 77
Anterior STEMI / 77
Inferior STEMI / 77
Lateral STEMI / 77
Non–ST-Segment Elevation Acute Coronary Syndromes / 77

ANCILLARY METHODS TO STUDY ATHEROSCLEROTIC LESIONS / 77
Intravascular Ultrasound / 78
Novel Invasive Imaging Modalities / 78
Invasive Evaluation of the Physiologic Significance of Stenotic Lesions / 78

MULITMODULAR IMAGING IN CONJUNCTION WITH CORONARY ANGIOGRAPHY / 78

CONCLUSION / 78

DESCRIPTION OF CORONARY ANGIOGRAPHY

Invasive coronary angiography (CA) remains the standard for identifying coronary artery narrowings related to coronary artery disease (CAD). Selective CA, which was first performed by F. Mason Sones in 1959, enables correlation of different clinical syndromes and electrocardiography (ECG) findings with coronary artery anatomy. The method provides the most reliable information for determining appropriate therapy in patients with CAD. CA has become a routine procedure performed on an ambulatory basis in many centers. Technical and logistic improvements have improved patient safety.

The physical requirements for invasive CA performed in a catheterization laboratory include a radiographic system, equipment for physiologic data monitoring and acquisition instrumentation, and equipment for emergency patient care. High-resolution x-ray imaging is required for optimal visualization of the coronary tree, including arterial side branches. Traditional film-based cineangiography has in large part been replaced by digital technology. The digital technique enables immediate online review, quantitative computer analysis, image manipulation capabilities, and increased storage capabilities. During the last few years, direct digital imaging with flat panel technique has become the standard in many catheterization laboratories.

■ TECHNIQUE

Angiography is performed under local anesthesia with small-diameter catheters introduced through a transarterial sheath. The outer diameter of the catheter is specified using French units, where one French unit (F) = 0.33 mm. Normally, 4- or 5-F catheters are used for diagnostic purposes. In the majority of cases, either the femoral or the radial route is used. Through the catheters, which are introduced over a guide wire, iodinated contrast media is injected selectively into the left and right coronary arteries. A few angiographic projections (varying degrees of left, right, cranial, and caudal angulation) are used to enable visualization of the whole coronary tree without superimposition of multiple vessels.

INDICATIONS AND CONTRAINDICATIONS

CA is used to establish or rule out the presence of coronary stenoses, define therapeutic options, and determine prognosis. CA is also used as a research tool for follow-up after invasive procedures or pharmacologic therapy. The American College of Cardiology/American Heart Association (ACC/AHA) Task Force and the European Society of Cardiology established the indications for CA.[1,2] Patients with suspected CAD who have severe stable symptoms and those with certain high-risk features for an adverse outcome should have CA. High-risk criteria include low ejection fraction and poor exercise capacity on an exercise test.

In patients with non–ST-segment elevation acute coronary syndromes (unstable angina and myocardial infarction) with high-risk features (eg, ongoing ischemia, heart failure), CA is recommended during the hospitalization.[3,4] In patients with acute ST-segment elevation myocardial infarction (STEMI), guidelines recommend CA in the acute phase for most patients.[5,6] Primary percutaneous intervention (PCI) is usually performed in the same procedure, immediately after the diagnostic CA, in these patients.

There are no absolute contraindications for CA. Relative contraindications include febrile untreated infection, severe anemia, severe electrolyte imbalance, active bleeding, acute renal failure, and ongoing stroke. Risk factors for significant complications after CA include advanced age, morbid obesity, bleeding diathesis, recent stroke, and dissection or severe atheromatosis of the thoracic aorta.

COMPLICATIONS

With modern technical equipment, major complications are uncommon (<1%) in diagnostic procedures.[7] Vascular complications related to the arterial puncture site are the most frequent complications. Mortality risk is 0.1% or less. Allergic contrast reactions, worsening kidney function, and cerebrovascular accidents are rare complications. Ventricular fibrillation may be provoked by contrast injection into a small side branch, typically the conal branch of the right coronary artery (RCA). Iatrogenic coronary artery dissection is a potential life-threatening complication, which usually is handled by either emergent coronary artery stenting or bypass surgery.

CORONARY ANATOMY AND VARIATIONS

The Coronary Artery Surgery Study (CASS) investigators established the nomenclature that is most often used for coronary artery description.[8] Minor modifications to the criteria were provided by the Bypass Angioplasty Revascularization Investigators (BARI).[9] The coronary artery circulation is composed of two principal arteries, the left coronary artery (LCA) and the RCA, arising from the aorta. The two principal coronary arteries and their larger branches are arranged on the surface of the heart (extramural vessels) and give rise to branches that penetrate the myocardium (intramural vessels). The major epicardial vessels and their second- and third-order branches can be visualized by CA. The network of smaller intramyocardial branches generally is not seen. Not infrequently, the extramural vessels may be covered in part by myocardium and surrounded by cardiac muscle (termed *myocardial bridging*; see later section "Bridging"). Variations in the branching pattern are extremely common in the human heart. According to the BARI classification, the RCA is predominant in approximately 85% of individuals, providing the posterior descending (PD; ie, posterior interventricular) branch and at least one posterolateral (PL) branch (Figs. 4–1 to 4–3).[9] In 7% to 8% of individuals, the coronary circulation is left-dominant; the PL, the PD, and the atrioventricular (AV) nodal branches are all supplied by the terminal portion of the left circumflex coronary artery (LCx; Figs. 4–4 and 4–5). In another 7% to 8% of hearts, there is a codominant or balanced system, in which the RCA gives rise to the PD branch and the LCx gives rise to all the PL branches and, in some individuals, also to a parallel PD branch that supplies part of the interventricular septum (Figs. 4–6 and 4–7).

The proximal or main segment of the LCA is known as the left main (LM) coronary artery (see Fig. 4–3). The left anterior descending (LAD) coronary artery is a direct continuation of the main trunk; it runs along the anterior interventricular groove (see Fig. 4–5). It may terminate before the left ventricular (LV) apex or at the apex (see Fig. 4–3). In most cases, the LAD "wraps" around the apex into the posterior interventricular groove (see Fig. 4–5). One or more left diagonal (LD) branches arise from the LAD, subtending the anterolateral part of the LV (Fig. 4–8). The LAD also gives rise to approximately 10 septal branches (Fig. 4–9; see also Fig. 4–8). One of the proximal

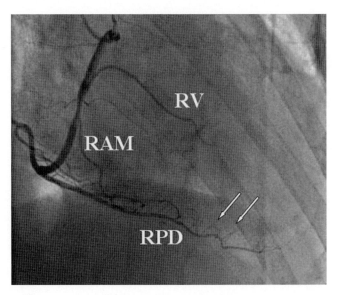

FIGURE 4–1. Right anterior oblique projection of the right coronary artery in right dominant circulation. The large posterior descending (PD) branch subtends the inferior part of the heart giving off small inferoseptal branches (white arrows). In this case, the PD branch reaches the left ventricular apex. A borderline significant stenosis is located at the take-off of the right ventricular (RV) and right acute marginal (RAM) branches. Total occlusion of the artery at this point would result in right ventricular transmural ischemia with ST-segment elevation in the right-sided electrocardiogram leads (V_3R-V_5R) and less often in lead V_1. RPD, right posterior descending branch.

septal branches is usually larger than the others and supplies the region of the bundle of His and bundle branches of the conduction system (see Fig. 4–9). The LCx arises from the LM and gives off branches to the upper lateral LV wall and the left

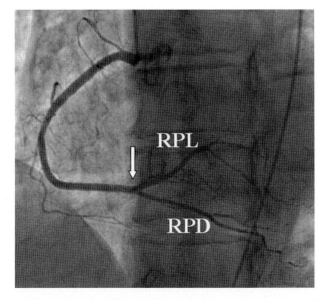

FIGURE 4–2. Left anterior oblique projection of the right coronary artery (RCA) in right dominant circulation. At the crux cordis (white arrow), the point where the atrioventricular and interventricular grooves converge, the artery bifurcates into the posterior descending (PD) and posterolateral (PL) branches. The PD branch runs along the interventricular groove, whereas the PL branches spread out over the infero (postero) lateral aspect of the heart. RPD, right posterior descending branch; RPL, right posterolateral branch.

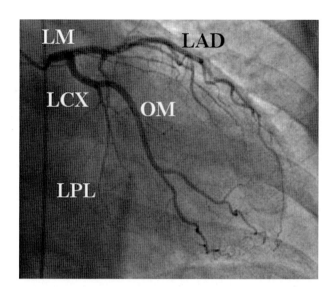

FIGURE 4–3. Right anterior oblique caudal projection showing the left coronary artery in right dominant circulation. The left main coronary artery (LM) bifurcates into the two main left-sided epicardial coronary arteries, the left anterior descending (LAD) artery and the left circumflex (LCx) artery. The LAD extends to the left ventricular (LV) apex but does not reach the inferior part of the heart because the patient has a big posterior descending branch of the right coronary artery (RCA). Occlusion of the LAD in this patient would not result in ST-segment elevations in the inferior leads II, III, and aVF. The LCx divides into a large obtuse marginal (OM) branch subtending the anterolateral part of the LV and small posterolateral (PL) branches. The infero (postero) lateral part of the LV is subtended by the RCA. In this patient, occlusion of the proximal part of the LCx would result in a lateral ST-segment elevation myocardial infarction because of the anatomy (small PL branches, large OM branch). The electrocardiography findings would be practically identical if the occlusion were in the OM branch. LPL, left posterolateral branch.

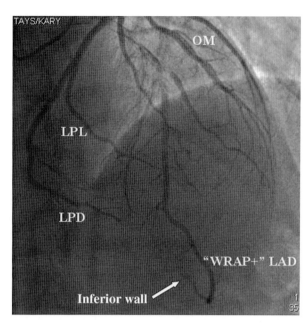

FIGURE 4–5. In left dominant circulation (left anterior oblique cranial projection), the left anterior descending (LAD) artery runs along the anterior interventricular groove, reaches the apex, and wraps around the apex into the inferior interventricular groove. A distal occlusion of this artery would result in inferior ST-segment elevation myocardial infarction: ST-segment elevation in leads II, III, and aVF and reciprocal ST-segment depression in leads aVL and I. The left circumflex artery is also big, giving off obtuse marginal (OM) and left posterolateral (LPL) branches and a left posterior descending (LPD) branch.

atrium (see Fig. 4–3). In approximately two-thirds of cases, the LCx terminates between the lateral margin of the LV and the posterior interventricular sulcus (Fig. 4–10). The left obtuse marginal (OM) branches arise at a right or an acute angle from the LCx and descends vertically toward the apex of the heart

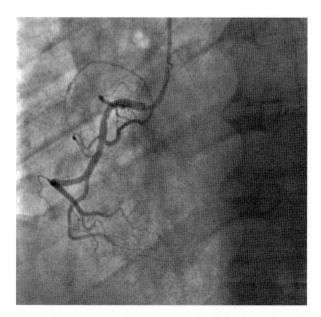

FIGURE 4–4. In left dominant circulation (left anterior oblique projection), the right coronary artery is small, giving off right ventricular (RV) and right acute marginal branches, which supply the RV almost exclusively. Occlusion of this type of arteries results in ST-segment elevation in the right precordial leads V₁ and V₂ (sometimes V₃) and reciprocal ST-segment depression in lead V₆. The electrocardiography findings may be misinterpreted as anterior ST-segment elevation myocardial infarction caused by left anterior descending artery occlusion. Due to the absence of contralateral ischemia (no cancellation of injury vectors), the ST elevations may be quite impressive despite the limited area of ischemia.

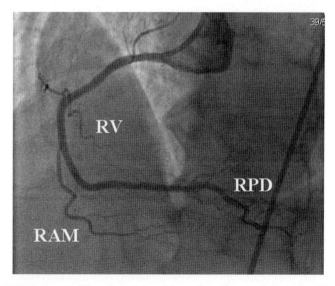

FIGURE 4–6. In balanced circulation (left anterior oblique projection), the right coronary artery periphery consists of a large right posterior descending (RPD) branch, but no posterolateral (PL) branches are present. Right ventricular (RV) and right acute marginal (RAM) branches are indicated.

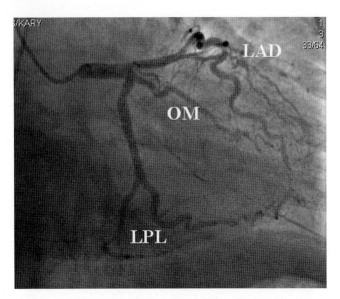

FIGURE 4–7. In balanced circulation (right anterior oblique caudal projection), the left posterolateral (LPL) periphery of the left circumflex (LCx) artery is big. A high obtuse marginal (OM) branch is also present in this patient. LAD, left anterior descending artery.

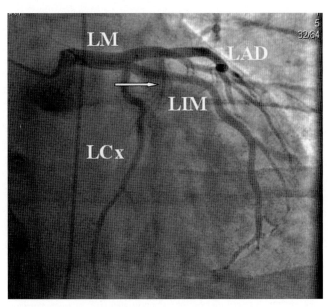

FIGURE 4–9. Left coronary artery in caudal projection. The left coronary artery trifurcates into the left anterior descending (LAD) artery, the left circumflex (LCx) artery, and the left intermediate (LIM) artery. In patients with a large intermediate branch, the LCx typically has no or only minor obtuse marginal branches. The large first septal branch is indicated (arrow). LM, left main artery.

(see Fig. 4–3). In approximately one-third of individuals, the LM trifurcates; the intermediate (IM) branch (ramus intermedius) comes off between the LAD and the LCx (see Fig. 4–9). The direct origin of the LAD and the LCx by separate ostia from the aorta without an LM coronary artery is a rare occurrence.

The RCA usually gives rise to a large branch along the acute margin (RAM branch) of the heart (see Fig. 4–1). In most individuals (right dominance), the RCA gives off the PL and PD branches at the crux cordis (see Fig. 4–2). The AV nodal branch

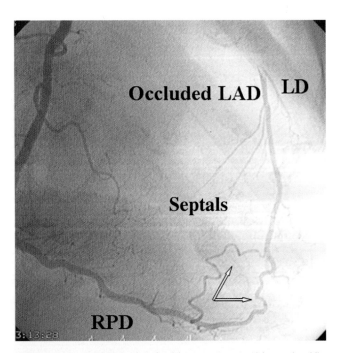

FIGURE 4–8. Contrast injection into the right coronary artery (right anterior oblique projection) shows well developed (Rentrop grade 3) collateral channels (arrows) from the right posterior descending (RPD) branch to the chronically occluded left anterior descending (LAD) artery. A small left diagonal (LD) branch and some septal branches of the LAD also fill retrogradely.

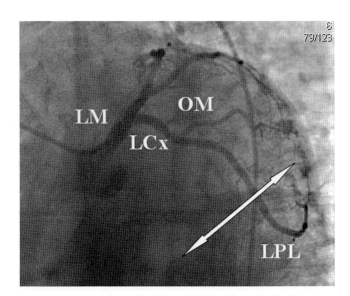

FIGURE 4–10. Left anterior oblique caudal ("spider") projection of the left coronary artery. The level of occlusion in the left circumflex (LCx) artery is critical for determining whether the electrocardiogram (ECG) will show ST-segment elevation myocardial infarction (STEMI) or non–ST-segment elevation myocardial infarction. In proximal occlusion, before the obtuse marginal (OM) branch, STEMI will be present. If the occlusion is distal to the obtuse margin of the heart (two-headed arrow) (distal to the OM branch), the ECG shows ST-segment depression or is without significant ST-segment changes in the 12-lead ECG. LM, left main artery; LPL, left posterolateral branch.

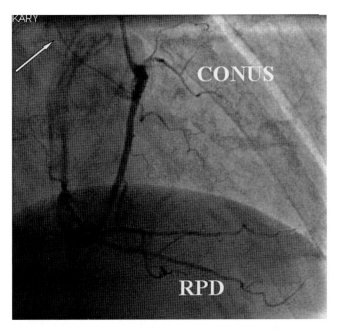

FIGURE 4–11. The conus branch more often takes off as the first side branch of the right coronary artery than via a separate ostium of the aorta. It subtends the right side of the interventricular septum and the right ventricular outflow tract. Patients with large conus branches do not show ST-segment elevation in lead V_1 in anterior ST-segment elevation myocardial infarction caused by left anterior descending artery occlusion (protection of the right side of the septum by the side branch). The small side branch to the sinus node is indicated by an arrow. RPD, right posterior descending branch.

arises from the PL branch. The most proximal side branch, the conus branch, subtends the right part of the interventricular septum to a varying extent (Fig. 4–11). In approximately 50% of individuals, the conus branch takes off directly from the aorta, either through a separate ostium (two-thirds of individuals) or through a common ostium with the RCA (one-third of individuals). The branch to the sinus node arises from the proximal RCA in the majority of individuals (see Fig. 4–11). In approximately 45% of human hearts, the sinus node is supplied by a branch arising within the first few millimeters of the course of the LCx.

ANGIOGRAPHIC CORONARY ARTERY DISEASE

CAD is defined as more than 50% angiographic diameter stenosis in one or more of the epicardial coronary arteries. Based on disease severity, obstructive CAD is classified as single-, double-, or triple-vessel disease. Stenoses less than 50% are considered as non–symptom generating, except in cases with dynamic obstruction. It has been suggested that acute coronary syndromes predominantly occur at the site of coronary stenoses with less than 50% diameter reduction,[10] presumably related to thin-cap fibroatheromas. This finding has been questioned in more recent studies.[11] Scoring systems have been developed to more specifically characterize the coronary vasculature with respect to the number of lesions and their functional impact, location, and complexity.[12,13] Recently, the SYNTAX score was developed as an angiographic grading tool.[14]

CORONARY ARTERY ANOMALIES

Coronary artery anomalies occur in 1% to 5% of individuals and represent those angiographic findings in which the origin, course, or termination of the arteries is infrequently encountered.[15,16] Coronary anomalies may or may not cause myocardial ischemia. High take-off above the junction of the sinus and from the tubular part of the aorta and multiple coronary ostia usually represent no major clinical problems but may pose a challenge for the interventionalist to perform selective CA.

Some coronary artery anomalies are very difficult to visualize at angiography, and even if they are visualized, their course may be delineated inaccurately. Hence, multimodular imaging should be considered in cases with signs of myocardial ischemia or unexplained syncope in young individuals, where no other etiologies are evident.

Anomalous origin of the LCA from the pulmonary artery (ALCAPA) is one of the most serious congenital coronary artery anomalies. Approximately 90% of untreated infants die in the first year of life, and only a few patients survive to adulthood.[17] CA usually helps confirm the diagnosis of ALCAPA and demonstrates collateral circulation between the RCA and LCA and a coronary "steal" phenomenon into the pulmonary artery. Anomalous origin of the RCA from the pulmonary artery (ARCAPA) is a very rare congenital abnormality.

Anomalous origin of a coronary artery from the opposite (or noncoronary) sinus (ACOS) taking an interarterial (ie, between the aorta and the pulmonary artery) course carries a high risk for sudden cardiac death. The RCA arises from the left sinus of Valsalva as a separate vessel or as a branch of a single coronary artery in 0.03% to 0.17% of patients who undergo angiography.[18] The most common course of an anomalous RCA arising from the left sinus of Valsalva is interarterial; this variant can be associated with sudden cardiac death in up to 30% of patients. The LCA arises from the right sinus of Valsalva as a separate vessel or as a branch of a single coronary artery in 0.09% to 0.11% of patients who undergo angiography.[19] An interarterial course may be seen in up to 75% of patients with this anomaly, who are at high risk for sudden cardiac death due to the acute angle of the ostium, the stretch of the intramural segment, and the compression between the commissure of the right and left coronary cusps.

Duplication of the LAD artery in otherwise normal hearts has been reported to occur in 0.13% to 1% of the general population.[20] Duplication of the LAD artery consists of a short LAD artery, which courses and terminates in the anterior interventricular sulcus without reaching the apex, and a long LAD artery, which originates from either the LAD artery proper or the LCA and then enters the distal anterior interventricular sulcus and courses to the apex. In patients having bypass surgery, the cardiac surgeon needs to be informed about this anomaly to be able to place the arteriotomy optimally.

■ BRIDGING

Myocardial bridging is caused by a band of myocardial muscle overlying a segment of a coronary artery. It is most commonly localized in the middle segment of the LAD artery. There is some discrepancy between the prevalence of myocardial bridging at angiography (0.5%-2.5%) and the prevalence at pathologic analysis (15%-85%).[21] The cause for this discrepancy is presumed to be the fact that myocardial bridging often occurs without overt symptoms, so that patients are rarely referred for CA. In some cases, however, myocardial bridging is responsible for angina pectoris, myocardial infarction, life-threatening arrhythmias, or even death. The standard of reference for diagnosing myocardial bridges is CA, at which a typical "milking" effect and a "step down–step up" phenomenon induced by systolic compression of the tunneled segment may be seen. In multidetector computed tomography, myocardial bridging is present in approximately one-third of cases. By this method, the intramyocardial location of the involved coronary arterial segment is easily recognized. Myocardial bridging does not cause ischemia in the vast majority of individuals.

■ FISTULAE

Coronary artery fistula is a condition in which a communication exists between one or two coronary arteries and either a cardiac chamber, the coronary sinus, the superior vena cava, or the pulmonary artery. This condition is seen in approximately 0.1% to 0.2% of all patients who undergo selective CA.[22] It more commonly involves the RCA (60% of cases) than the LCA (40%). In coronary artery fistula, the involved coronary artery is dilated because of increased blood flow and is often tortuous to an extent determined by the shunt volume. The most common site of drainage is the right ventricle (45% of cases), followed by the right atrium (25%) and the pulmonary artery (15%).[23] The fistula drains into the left atrium or left ventricle in less than 10% of cases. When the shunt leads into a right-sided cardiac chamber, the hemodynamics resemble those of an extracardiac left-to-right shunt; when the connection is to a left-sided cardiac chamber, the hemodynamics mimic those of aortic insufficiency. Myocardial perfusion may be diminished for that portion of the myocardium supplied by the abnormally connecting coronary artery. This situation represents a hemodynamic steal phenomenon and may lead to myocardial ischemia.

COLLATERAL CIRCULATION

After total or near-total occlusion of a coronary artery, perfusion of ischemic myocardium occurs through collaterals, which are vascular channels that interconnect epicardial coronary arteries. Previously occluded vessel branches are usually manifested as truncated stumps on angiography. The part of the vessel distal to the occlusion is frequently filled late in the contrast injection by antegrade ("bridging") collaterals or collaterals that originate from the same or an adjacent vessel. In fresh total occlusions, typically represented by STEMI, no collateral flow may be evident from CA. Functioning collaterals maintain myocardial viability but are not as effective as the native vessel for oxygen distribution. Some grade of effort angina is typical for patients with occluded coronary arteries and collateral

flow. The Rentrop classification is used for defining the grade of established coronary filling.[24] Briefly, grade 0 represents no collateral opacification, grade 1 represents filling of side branches, and grade 2 represents partial and grade 3 complete filling of the main branch by collateral vessels (see Fig. 4–8).

ANGIOGRAPHIC ASSESSMENT OF CORONARY FLOW

In 1985, the Thrombolysis in Myocardial Infarction (TIMI) investigators introduced a simple, quantitative grading of coronary flow to assess the efficiency of coronary reperfusion therapy.[25] This grading system has been widely accepted as a standard in the angiographic grading of coronary blood flow both in clinical trials and as a useful tool in routine clinical work. TIMI flow grade 0 represents no antegrade flow beyond the vessel obstruction. TIMI flow grade 1 represents perfusion of contrast material distal to the occlusion, but the entire coronary bed distal to the occlusion is not opacified. TIMI flow grade 2 represents slower rate of entry of contrast material into the distal vessel when compared with other areas of the coronary tree. TIMI flow grade 3 represents normal contrast filling. TIMI flow grade 3 has been associated with improved outcome in acute STEMI, but normal blood flow in the epicardial vessels does not necessarily equate to normal myocardial blood flow.

To overcome limitations of the original TIMI flow grading system, a quantitative measure, the TIMI frame count, was introduced.[26] In this method, the number of cine frames required for contrast material to reach standard distal coronary landmarks of a coronary artery is counted. In addition, the length of the corresponding artery is taken into consideration by introducing vessel-corrected TIMI frame counts. Corrected TIMI frame count ≤27 frames was defined as normal epicardial perfusion. TIMI frame counting is an objective and quantitative index of epicardial blood flow and is an independent predictor of in-hospital mortality after acute myocardial infarction. The method is simple and reproducible but, like the TIMI flow grade, is not a specific measure of myocardial blood flow.

■ ANGIOGRAPHIC ASSESSMENT OF MYOCARDIAL BLOOD FLOW

Optimal reperfusion therapy has been defined in several studies as achievement of normalization of both epicardial coronary perfusion and myocardial perfusion. The so-called *no-reflow phenomenon*, an open epicardial artery without flow into the myocardium, predicts adverse clinical events and left ventricular remodeling. Two different angiographic methods have been described for assessment of myocardial perfusion on the angiogram. One is myocardial blush grade,[27] an index based on the intensity of contrast opacity of the infarcted area, and the other is TIMI myocardial perfusion grading,[28] which focuses on the velocity of contrast opacity clearance. Both methods have proven useful for the assessment of microvascular flow and prediction of clinical outcomes after myocardial infarction. It has been proposed that the duration of blush reflects the perfusion level of myocardium.

However, visual assessment of these methods is categorical, subjective, and operator dependent, and quantitative angiographic indexes of myocardial perfusion are under development.[29]

ANGIOGRAPHIC FACTORS DETERMINING ECG CHANGES IN ACUTE CORONARY SYNDROMES

In the preangiography era, autopsy was used as the gold standard for ECG correlations with anatomy. It was not until the early 1970s, that the field of ECG in ischemic heart disease began to flourish, concomitantly with the advent of CA, echocardiography, and nuclear medicine.[30] In the absence of confounding factors, like left bundle branch block (LBBB), the ECG contains clinically important information about the culprit artery, size of artery, and site of occlusion in the acute occlusive stage of an acute myocardial infarction. This is true especially for the hyperacute occlusive stage ("preinfarction syndrome"), represented in the ECG by ST-segment elevation without new Q waves, or signs of myocardial reperfusion (inverted T waves).[31] This represents the "golden hour" for reperfusion treatment. Many investigators have correlated ECG findings in acute STEMI with CA and found wide variation in sensitivity and specificity. A number of anatomic factors, easily appreciated from CA, affect the predictive power of the ECG in these situations.

Knowledge of morphologic ECG interpretation enables individual decision making in the acute phase of STEMI. Decisions about type of reperfusion therapy and where to send the patient (local hospital vs tertiary care center) can be based on the ECG findings and the clinical history of the patient.[32] The diagnostic information in the ECG should also be used in the catheterization laboratory by the invasive cardiologist. Especially in multivessel disease, where the infarct-related artery has opened, the ECG pinpoints the culprit lesion, which needs to be treated. In cases with cardiogenic shock, when ECG data for culprit artery identification are used optimally, a guiding catheter may be inserted immediately into the culprit artery, saving critical minutes to open the occluded artery.

■ ANTERIOR STEMI

In anterior STEMI, when the maximal ST-segment elevation is in leads V_2 to V_4, the culprit artery is almost exclusively the LAD. In a minority of cases, the LM coronary artery, the LD, the LCx, or the RCA may be the culprit artery. In anterior STEMI, both the level of LAD occlusion and the size of the artery modify the ECG pattern. When the occlusion is proximal to the first LD branch, the anterolateral segment of the LV will be involved in the ischemic process, and ST-segment elevation will be present in lead aVL. Typically, reciprocal ST-segment depression is seen in lead III. However, if the LAD is large, wrapping around the LV apex, ischemia of two anatomically opposite regions, the anterolateral and the inferior, results in a cancellation of injury vectors, with resultant attenuation of the ST-segment elevations. If the occlusion is distal to the first diagonal branch, the size of the artery will determine the ECG pattern. In small LADs, the ST segments in the extremity leads will be isoelectric (anteroseptal

ischemia), whereas in large LADs, there will be ST-segment elevation in the inferior leads II, III, and aVF, with reciprocal ST-segment depression in lead aVL (see Fig. 4–5). In some cases with anterior STEMI with proximal occlusion of the LAD, there is no ST-segment elevation in lead aVL. Instead, the ECG shows ST-segment elevation in lead aVR and ST-segment depression in lead V_6.[33]

■ INFERIOR STEMI

In patients with ST-segment elevation maximally in the inferior leads II, III, and aVF, the culprit artery is either the RCA or the LCx. Many different algorithms have been developed to determine the infarct-related artery.[34] These algorithms are mainly based on the fact that in RCA occlusions, the ischemic area is located more inferiorly and to the right, whereas in LCX occlusion, the injury vector points more into the posterior and lateral directions. In Figs. 4–1, 4–4, 4–5, and 4–10, anatomic aspects that determine the ECG patterns are presented. Involvement of the right ventricle induces ST-segment elevation in the right-sided precordial leads (V_3R-V_5R) and, in some cases, also in lead V_1 (- V_2 - V_3).

■ LATERAL STEMI

When the maximal ST-segment elevation is in leads I, aVL, V_5, or V_6, the LCx is usually the culprit artery (see Fig. 4–3). In addition, a few cases with distal LAD occlusions may present with this pattern due to apicolateral ischemia.

■ NON–ST-SEGMENT ELEVATION ACUTE CORONARY SYNDROMES

Information about coronary anatomy from the ECG is more limited in cases with non–ST-segment elevation acute coronary syndromes. However, there are situations where the CA findings can be predicted with high certainty. If the ECG shows widespread ST-segment depression, maximally in leads V_4 and V_5 with inverted T waves in these leads, and concomitant ST-segment elevation in lead aVR (circumferential subendocardial ischemia), there is a high probability of left main and/or severe three-vessel CAD.[35] This represents a high-risk subgroup with a high in-hospital event rate. CA on an emergency basis is recommended. ST-segment depression maximally in the right-sided chest leads (irrespective of the direction of the T wave) represents a mirror-image STEMI, where the ischemia is on the posterior wall of the LV. Additional leads V_7 to V_9 typically show ST elevations. The coronary artery occlusion is typically distal to the first obtuse marginal branch of a small LCx (see Fig. 4–10).

ANCILLARY METHODS TO STUDY ATHEROSCLEROTIC LESIONS

CA quantifies luminal obstruction. The degree of stenosis is usually reported by comparing diseased segments of the coronary tree with nearby segments without evident stenosis. However, CA is limited in its ability to quantitate the extent of distribution of atherosclerosis. The vessel lumen filled with contrast media is well appreciated by CA, but the method gives practically no information about the characteristics of the vessel wall. In cases with evenly distributed atherosclerotic plaques, the CA finding may even be interpreted as normal or near-normal. Advances in the understanding of the pathophysiology of atherosclerotic plaque demonstrate that in certain stages of plaque progression, the plaque is vulnerable to rupture. Vulnerable plaques may go undetected by CA. One clear advantage with CA is the possibility to continue the diagnostic workup with other invasive methods with the patient still in the catheterization laboratory. Both anatomy and physiology of the coronary arteries can be easily studied with these ancillary methods.

■ INTRAVASCULAR ULTRASOUND

Intravascular ultrasound (IVUS) visualizes the arterial wall in a format analogous to a histologic cross-section. IVUS provides detailed information about the quality and extent of atherosclerotic lesions in the vessel wall. IVUS is well suited as an ancillary method to CA to be performed simultaneously. The IVUS catheter is introduced into the coronary artery through a guiding catheter over a thin wire. Longitudinal or three-dimensional display of the coronary artery wall for tissue characterization is best performed with an automatic pullback device. Soft plaques can be differentiated from fibrotic lesions, and calcification within the vessel wall causes echo dropout behind the calcification. Thrombi and dissections are visible on IVUS. For diagnostic purposes, IVUS is indicated in borderline significant or angiographically suboptimally visualized lesions, such as tortuous coronary anatomy. IVUS studies have demonstrated that coronary atherosclerosis is more diffuse than appreciated by the use of CA.[36] One drawback with IVUS is the lack of solid data for its value in guiding therapeutic decisions.

■ NOVEL INVASIVE IMAGING MODALITIES

Even higher resolutions of plaques are provided by optical coherence tomography, a catheter-based imaging modality introduced during the last few years.[37,38] The method enables measurement of the thickness of the fibrous cap, which is considered critical for the risk of plaque disruption with sudden thrombotic vessel occlusion. Integrated backscatter analysis ("virtual histology") converts radiofrequency backscatter signals provided by ultrasound into color-coded regions to characterize different types of atherosclerotic plaques.[38] The real value of these promising new methods to guide therapy needs to be proven.

■ INVASIVE EVALUATION OF THE PHYSIOLOGIC SIGNIFICANCE OF STENOTIC LESIONS

The presence of myocardial ischemia is an important risk factor for an adverse clinical outcome. Revascularization of stenotic coronary lesions that induce ischemia can improve a patient's functional status and outcome. For stenotic lesions that do not induce ischemia, however, the benefit of revascularization is less clear, and medical therapy alone is likely to be equally effective.[39] Especially in patients with multivessel CAD, determining which

lesions cause ischemia and warrant stenting can be difficult. CA, the standard technique for guiding PCI in patients with multivessel CAD, may underestimate or overestimate a lesion's functional severity. Fractional flow reserve (FFR) is an index of the physiologic significance of a coronary stenosis and is defined as the ratio of maximal blood flow in a stenotic artery to normal maximal flow.[40] It can be easily measured during CA by calculating the ratio of distal coronary pressure measured with a coronary pressure guidewire to aortic pressure measured simultaneously with the guiding catheter. FFR in a normal coronary artery equals 1.0. An FFR value of 0.80 or less identifies ischemia-causing coronary stenoses with an accuracy of more than 90%.[41] The information provided by FFR is similar to that obtained with myocardial perfusion studies, but it is more specific and has a better spatial resolution because every artery or segment is analyzed separately and masking of one ischemic area by another, more severely ischemic zone is avoided. Deferring PCI in nonischemic stenotic lesions as assessed by FFR is associated with an annual rate of death or myocardial infarction of approximately 1% in patients with single-vessel CAD, which is lower than the rate after routine stenting.[39] However, deferring PCI in lesions with an FFR of less than 0.75 to 0.80 may result in worse outcomes than those obtained with revascularization.[42] It was recently shown that routine measurement of FFR in patients with multivessel CAD who are undergoing PCI with drug-eluting stents significantly reduces the rate of the composite end point of death, nonfatal myocardial infarction, and repeat revascularization at 1 year.[40]

MULITMODULAR IMAGING IN CONJUNCTION WITH CORONARY ANGIOGRAPHY

It is not unusual to find normal or near-normal coronary arteries in patients with a clinical picture of acute coronary syndrome. *Takotsubo cardiomyopathy*, first described in Japan in 1991,[43] is a cardiac syndrome characterized by ECG features mimicking acute STEMI, transient LV dysfunction, and minimal release of biomarkers of myocardial injury.[44] LV ventriculography performed in conjunction with CA shows a typical pattern of apical dyskinesis and basal hyperkinesis.

Another clinical entity encountered in the era of invasive STEMI treatment is *acute pulmonary embolism*. Patients with acute chest discomfort and ST-segment elevations in the right precordial leads and angiographically normal coronary arteries typically show hyperkinetic contractions on LV ventriculogram. Bedside echocardiography can easily be performed after the invasive evaluation, followed by pulmonary angiography for definite diagnosis. In massive pulmonary embolism, catheter-directed thrombectomy can be performed with the patient in the catheterization laboratory through a transvenous catheter.[45]

CONCLUSION

CA is the standard for identifying coronary artery narrowing related to CAD. New diagnostic methods like cardiac computed tomography allow noninvasive anatomic assessment of the coronary tree and offer alternatives especially for patients with low or intermediate probability for coronary artery stenoses. Available tests, including CA, all have advantages and drawbacks. The choice of imaging method should be tailored to each person based on the clinical judgment of patient risk, clinical history, and local expertise. CA will remain the method of choice in situations with high probability for an invasive therapeutic procedure, especially in acute coronary syndromes.

REFERENCES

1. Scanlon PJ, Faxon DP, Audet AM, et al. ACC/AHA guidelines for coronary angiography: executive summary and recommendations. A report of the American College of Cardiology/American Heart Association Task Force on Practice Guidelines (Committee on Coronary Angiography) developed in collaboration with the Society for Cardiac Angiography and Interventions. *Circulation.* 1999;99:2345-2357.

2. Fox K, Garcia MA, Ardissino D, et al. Guidelines on the management of stable angina pectoris: executive summary: the Task Force on the Management of Stable Angina Pectoris of the European Society of Cardiology. *Eur Heart J.* 2006;27:1341-1381.

3. Braunwald E, Antman EM, Beasley JW, et al. ACC/AHA guideline update for the management of patients with unstable angina and non-ST-segment elevation myocardial infarction–2002: summary article: a report of the American College of Cardiology/American Heart Association Task Force on Practice Guidelines (Committee on the Management of Patients With Unstable Angina). *Circulation.* 2002;106:1893-1900.

4. Bertrand ME, Simoons ML, Fox KA, et al. Management of acute coronary syndromes in patients presenting without persistent ST-segment elevation. *Eur Heart J.* 2002;23:1809-1840.

5. Antman EM, Hand M, Armstrong PW, et al. 2007 focused update of the ACC/AHA 2004 guidelines for the management of patients with ST-elevation myocardial infarction: a report of the American College of Cardiology/American Heart Association Task Force on Practice Guidelines: developed in collaboration with the Canadian Cardiovascular Society endorsed by the American Academy of Family Physicians: 2007 Writing Group to Review New Evidence and Update the ACC/AHA 2004 Guidelines for the Management of Patients with ST-Elevation Myocardial Infarction, writing on behalf of the 2004 writing committee. *Circulation.* 2008;117:296-329.

6. Van de Werf F, Ardissino D, Betriu A, et al. Management of acute myocardial infarction in patients presenting with ST-segment elevation. The Task Force on the Management of Acute Myocardial Infarction of the European Society of Cardiology. *Eur Heart J.* 2003;24:28-66.

7. Reddy BK, Brewster PS, Walsh T, et al. Randomized comparison of rapid ambulation using radial, 4 French femoral access, or femoral access with AngioSeal closure. *Catheter Cardiovasc Interv.* 2004;62:143-149.

8. Principal Investigators of CASS and Their Associates. National Heart, Lung and Blood Institute Coronary Artery Surgery Study (CASS). *Circulation.* 1981;63(Suppl 1):I1-I81.

9. The BARI Protocol. Protocol for the Bypass Angioplasty Revascularization Investigation. *Circulation.* 1991;84(Suppl V):V-1–V-27.

10. Ambrose JA, Tannenbaum MA, Alexopoulos D, et al. Angiographic progression of coronary artery disease and the development of myocardial infarction. *J Am Coll Cardiol.* 1988;12:56-62.

11. Manoharan G, Ntalianis A, Muller O, et al. Severity of coronary arterial stenoses responsible for acute coronary syndromes. *Am J Cardiol.* 2009;103:1183-1188.

12. Leaman DM, Brower RW, Meester GT, et al. Coronary artery atherosclerosis: severity of the disease, severity of angina pectoris and compromised left ventricular function. *Circulation.* 1981;63:285-299.

13. Ryan TJ, Faxon DP, Gunnar RM, et al. Guidelines for percutaneous transluminal coronary angioplasty. A report of the American College of Cardiology/American Heart Association Task Force on Assessment of Diagnostic and Therapeutic Cardiovascular Procedures (Subcommittee on Percutaneous Transluminal Coronary Angioplasty). *Circulation.* 1988;78:486-502.

14. Sianos G, Morel MA, Kappetein AP, et al. The SYNTAX score: an angiographic tool grading the complexity of coronary artery disease. *EuroIntervention.* 2005;1:219-227.

15. von Kodolitsch Y, Franzen O, Lund GK, et al. Coronary artery anomalies part II: recent insights from clinical investigations. *Z Kardiol.* 2005; 94:1-13.

16. Kim SY, Seo JB, Do KH, et al. Coronary artery anomalies: classification and ECG-gated multi-detector row CT findings with angiographic correlation. *Radiographics.* 2006;26:317-333.

17. Wesselhoeft H, Fawcett JS, Johnson AL. Anomalous origin of the left coronary artery from the pulmonary trunk. Its clinical spectrum, pathology, and pathophysiology, based on a review of 140 cases with seven further cases. *Circulation.* 1968;38:403-425.

18. Yamanaka O, Hobbs RE. Coronary artery anomalies in 126,595 patients undergoing coronary arteriography. *Cathet Cardiovasc Diagn.* 1990;21:28-40.

19. Chaitman BR, Lesperance J, Saltiel J, et al. Clinical, angiographic, and hemodynamic findings in patients with anomalous origin of the coronary arteries. *Circulation.* 1976;53:122-131.

20. Sajja LR, Farooqi A, Shaik MS, et al. Dual left anterior descending coronary artery: surgical revascularization in 4 patients. *Tex Heart Inst J.* 2000;27:292-296.

21. Amoroso G, Battolla L, Gemignani C, et al. Myocardial bridging on left anterior descending coronary artery evaluated by multidetector computed tomography. *Int J Cardiol.* 2004;95:335-337.

22. Said SA, el Gamal MI, van der Werf T. Coronary arteriovenous fistulas: collective review and management of six new cases—changing etiology, presentation, and treatment strategy. *Clin Cardiol.* 1997;20:748-752.

23. McNamara JJ, Gross RE. Congenital coronary artery fistula. *Surgery.* 1969;65:59-69.

24. Rentrop KP, Cohen M, Blanke H, et al. Changes in collateral channel filling immediately after controlled coronary artery occlusion by an angioplasty balloon in human subjects. *J Am Coll Cardiol.* 1985;5: 587-592.

25. The TIMI Study Group. The Thrombolysis in Myocardial Infarction (TIMI) trial: phase I findings. *N Engl J Med.* 1985;312:932-936.

26. Gibson CM, Murphy SA, Rizzo MJ, et al. Relationship between TIMI frame count and clinical outcomes after thrombolytic administration. Thrombolysis in Myocardial Infarction (TIMI) Study Group. *Circulation.* 1999;99:1945-1950.

27. van't Hof AW, Liem A, Suryapranata H, et al. Angiographic assessment of myocardial reperfusion in patients treated with primary angioplasty for acute myocardial infarction: myocardial blush grade. Zwolle Myocardial Infarction Study Group. *Circulation.* 1998;97:2302-2306.

28. Gibson CM, Cannon CP, Murphy SA, et al. Relationship of TIMI myocardial perfusion grade to mortality after administration of thrombolytic drugs. *Circulation.* 2000;101:125-130.

29. Ding S, Pu J, Qiao ZQ, et al. TIMI myocardial perfusion frame count: a new method to assess myocardial perfusion and its predictive value for short-term prognosis. *Catheter Cardiovasc Interv.* 2010;75:722-732.

30. Sclarovsky S. *Electrocardiography of Acute Myocardial Ischaemic Syndromes.* London, United Kingdom: Martin Dunitz Ltd; 1999.

31. Eskola MJ, Holmvang L, Nikus KC, et al. The electrocardiogram window of opportunity to treat vs. the different evolving stages of ST-elevation myocardial infarction: correlation with therapeutic approach, coronary anatomy, and outcome in the DANAMI-2 trial. *Eur Heart J.* 2007;28: 2985-2991.

32. Nikus KC, Eskola MJ, Niemela KO, et al. Modern morphologic electrocardiographic interpretation—a valuable tool for rapid clinical decision making in acute ischemic coronary syndromes. *J Electrocardiol.* 2005;38:4-6.

33. Eskola MJ, Nikus KC, Holmvang L, et al. Value of the 12-lead electrocardiogram to define the level of obstruction in acute anterior wall myocardial infarction: correlation to coronary angiography and clinical outcome in the DANAMI-2 trial. *Int J Cardiol.* 2009;131:378-383.

34. Fiol M, Cygankiewicz I, Carrillo A, et al. Value of electrocardiographic algorithm based on "ups and downs" of ST in assessment of a culprit artery in evolving inferior wall acute myocardial infarction. *Am J Cardiol.* 2004;94:709-714.

35. Nikus KC, Eskola MJ, Virtanen VK, et al. ST-depression with negative T waves in leads V4-V5—a marker of severe coronary artery disease in non-ST elevation acute coronary syndrome: a prospective study of angina

at rest, with troponin, clinical, electrocardiographic, and angiographic correlation. *Ann Noninvasive Electrocardiol.* 2004;9:207-214.

36. Mintz GS, Painter JA, Pichard AD, et al. Atherosclerosis in angiographically "normal" coronary artery reference segments: an intravascular ultrasound study with clinical correlations. *J Am Coll Cardiol.* 1995;25: 1479-1485.

37. Prati F, Regar E, Mintz GS, et al. Expert review document on methodology, terminology, and clinical applications of optical coherence tomography: physical principles, methodology of image acquisition, and clinical application for assessment of coronary arteries and atherosclerosis. *Eur Heart J.* 2010;31:401-415.

38. Garcia-Garcia HM, Gonzalo N, Regar E, et al. Virtual histology and optical coherence tomography: from research to a broad clinical application. *Heart.* 2009;95:1362-1374.

39. Pijls NH, van Schaardenburgh P, Manoharan G, et al. Percutaneous coronary intervention of functionally nonsignificant stenosis: 5-year follow-up of the DEFER study. *J Am Coll Cardiol.* 2007;49:2105-2111.

40. Tonino PA, De Bruyne B, Pijls NH, et al. Fractional flow reserve versus angiography for guiding percutaneous coronary intervention. *N Engl J Med.* 2009;360:213-224.

41. Pijls NH, Van Gelder B, Van der Voort P, et al. Fractional flow reserve. A useful index to evaluate the influence of an epicardial coronary stenosis on myocardial blood flow. *Circulation.* 1995;92:3183-3193.

42. Legalery P, Schiele F, Seronde MF, et al. One-year outcome of patients submitted to routine fractional flow reserve assessment to determine the need for angioplasty. *Eur Heart J.* 2005;26:2623-2629.

43. Dote K, Sato H, Tateishi H, et al. Myocardial stunning due to simultaneous multivessel coronary spasms: a review of 5 cases. *J Cardiol.* 1991;21: 203-214.

44. Pernicova I, Garg S, Bourantas C, et al. Takotsubo cardiomyopathy: a review of the literature. *Angiology.* 2010;61:166-173.

45. Kuo WT, Gould MK, Louie JD, et al. Catheter-directed therapy for the treatment of massive pulmonary embolism: systematic review and meta-analysis of modern techniques. *J Vasc Interv Radiol.* 2009;20:1431-1440.

CHAPTER 5
CARDIAC COMPUTED TOMOGRAPHY

Monvadi B. Srichai and João A. C. Lima

GENERAL INFORMATION ON CARDIAC COMPUTED TOMOGRAPHY / 81
Introduction / 81
Specific Technical Aspects / 81
Specific Clinical Considerations / 85

STANDARD APPLICATIONS FOR CARDIAC COMPUTED TOMOGRAPHY / 86
Coronary Artery Evaluation / 86
Pulmonary Vein Evaluation / 87
Congenital Heart Disease / 89
Pericardial Disease / 89
Cardiac Masses / 91

EVOLVING APPLICATIONS FOR CARDIAC COMPUTED TOMOGRAPHY / 94
Myocardial Evaluation / 94
Valvular Heart Disease / 96

MULTIMODAL APPLICATIONS / 97
Coronary Artery Disease / 97
Congenital Cardiovascular Disease / 97
Secondary Assessment for Cardiac Structure and Function / 98

MULTIMODAL CASE EXAMPLES / 98
Case 1 / 98
Case 2 / 98

GENERAL INFORMATION ON CARDIAC COMPUTED TOMOGRAPHY

■ INTRODUCTION

Cardiac computed tomography (CT) has become one of the fast growing areas of cardiovascular imaging since the advent of multidetector scanners in 1998. Early cross-sectional CT imaging of the heart was performed using electron beam CT. Continued advancements in multidetector CT (MDCT) scanners as well as their widespread availability, however, have further increased the utility of cardiac MDCT for evaluation of a variety of cardiovascular diseases.

CT uses rapidly rotating x-ray sources and detectors to create an image. The x-ray sources and detectors are mounted opposite one another on a ring, and the rotating unit is called the gantry. The patient is placed inside the ring, and radiation that is not absorbed by the patient passes into multiple detectors, and,

through a process known as filtered back projection, a cross-sectional image is generated (Fig. 5–1). Images are acquired in an axial (transverse) plane in thin sections to yield isotropic voxels, matching that of in-plane spatial resolution. CT angiography (CTA) of the cardiovascular system refers to CT scanning that is performed during the injection of an iodinated contrast agent. Although much information can be obtained from a non-contrast CT, optimal evaluation of cardiac structures, including vascular anatomy, usually requires CTA.

Important aspects of cardiac CT imaging include:

1. High temporal resolution with electrocardiogram (ECG) synchronization of data acquisition to minimize cardiac motion artifacts
2. High spatial resolution with isotropic voxels to allow for oblique reconstructions without loss of resolution
3. Contrast resolution
4. Radiation dose

Image quality optimization mainly consists of elimination of artifacts related to cardiac motion, respiratory motion, and partial volume effects. Different aspects of CT imaging, including collimation, pitch, breath-hold period, field of view, reconstruction interval, rate and volume of intravenous contrast administration, reconstruction algorithm, and radiation dose, affect overall image quality. Unfortunately, no single set of optimal scan parameters currently suffices for all cardiac CT applications on all CT systems. Instead, CT techniques often reflect a combination of personal or institutional preferences coupled with individual manufacturer capabilities and tailored, to a large extent, to the individual patient's specific clinical needs.

■ SPECIFIC TECHNICAL ASPECTS

Scanner Design

The gantry design of all MDCT scanners is similar with only minor variations. Single-source systems consist of a single set of x-ray source and detectors, and dual-source systems have two sets of x-ray sources and detectors mounted on the gantry. Detector geometry and postprocessing algorithms are system specific and somewhat dependent on the number of detectors used in the gantry design and number of slices generated, currently anywhere from 4 to 320 slices. Special three-dimensional (3D) back-projection algorithms are used to correct for artifacts that arise from the cone-beam geometry that results from the oblique x-ray projections of thin collimated slices generated from the gantry.[1] Thin-slice collimations (0.5-0.625 mm) with reconstructed slice thickness of 0.4 to 0.7 mm allow for near isotropic voxels, which are important for oblique reconstructions. Gantry speed rotations of 280 to 420 ms/360° allow for high temporal resolution in the range of 140 to 210 ms. Further improvements in temporal resolution are obtained with the use of dual-source technology and multisegment postprocessing algorithms, which are important for functional assessment of the heart as well as for improving image quality in patients with fast heart rates.

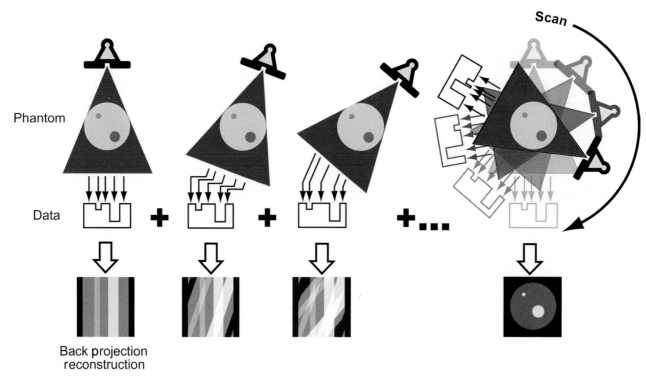

FIGURE 5–1. Generation of a computed tomography image using filtered back projection.

ECG Referencing

Normal motion of the heart is a source of significant motion artifact on conventional CT imaging. Because cardiac motion varies throughout the cardiac cycle, often in a predictable manner, synchronization of data acquisition to the heart cycle allows for combination of data acquired from consecutive gantry rotations in volumetric data sets with minimal blurring artifact related to cardiac motion.

The ECG signal is commonly used for synchronization. The time between two consecutive heartbeats is defined by the R-R interval (the interval between consecutive R waves of the ECG; 1000 ms for a heart rate of 60 beats per minute). Depending on the acquisition mode, the R-R interval of the ECG signal is used to either *prospectively* trigger data acquisition or to *retrospectively* determine the timing of reconstruction of the image data sets.

With prospective triggering, data acquisition is timed to the ECG R peak after a preselected delay within the following cardiac cycle at a given table position. After table movement, data are again sampled based on the next available R trigger (Fig. 5–2). With retrospective ECG gating, a conventional spiral data set is acquired with simultaneous tracing and recording of the patient's ECG. Following data acquisition, image data and ECG data are merged to allow for ECG-related image reconstruction after scanning (Fig. 5–3). In contrast to other CT spiral acquisitions, cardiac algorithms usually require a substantially reduced pitch factor (0.2-0.3) in order to allow image reconstruction at any time point of the cardiac cycle. A comparison of these two acquisition techniques is shown in Table 5–1.

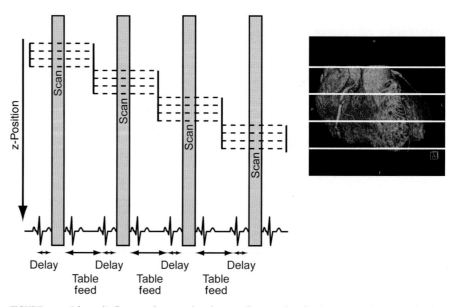

FIGURE 5–2. Schematic diagram of prospective electrocardiogram triggering for computed tomography data acquisition and reconstruction.

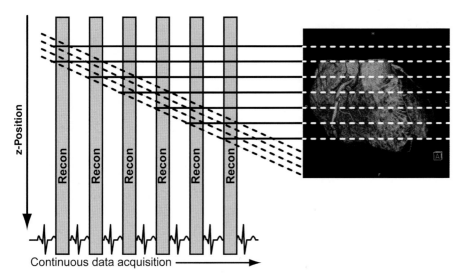

FIGURE 5-3. Schematic diagram of retrospective electrocardiogram triggering for computed tomography data acquisition and reconstruction.

cardiac cycles (two to four heartbeats) in order to fill a data segment more rapidly (Fig. 5–4). However, with multisector reconstructions, image quality may be degraded due to blurring artifacts related to differences in the position of cardiac structures from cycle to cycle even within the same phase of the cycle. In this regard, multisegment reconstruction is most useful when coupled to gantry rotation and the patient's heart rate using a computerized algorithm.[2,3] Dual-source CT scanners achieve improved temporal resolution (75-83 ms depending on scanner) with simultaneous scanning using two sets of sources and detectors, and similar to single-source scanners, multisector reconstruction algorithms can further improve the temporal resolution.

Temporal Resolution

Temporal resolution is the amount of time needed to acquire the necessary x-ray data in order to reconstruct an image.[2] In cardiac MDCT, an image can be generated using half-scan reconstruction algorithms, and hence, temporal resolution for a particular scanner corresponds to the time needed for the gantry to rotate half of a full 360° rotation, or 175 ms with a 350 ms/360° rotation speed. Further improvements in temporal resolution can be achieved with multisector reconstruction algorithms, which are based on merging data of adjacent

Spatial Resolution

Spatial resolution is mainly dependent on detector width, slice collimations, and data sampling. Coronary arteries are small, ranging from 1 to 5.5 mm in diameter.[4] Nitroglycerin given just prior to scanning is often used to dilate the coronary arteries.[5,6] With current generation MDCT scanners, there have been great improvements in spatial resolution, particularly in the z-axis resolution, leading to near isotropic voxels with spatial resolution up to 0.4 × 0.4 × 0.4 mm.[7] These advances have greatly enhanced visualization of small structures such as the coronary arteries

TABLE 5-1. Basic Advantages and Disadvantages of Data Acquisition Schemes

	Prospective Triggering	Retrospective Gating
Advantages	Pulsed radiation Low radiation exposure	Spiral acquisition Volumetric data set Full coverage of cardiac cycle Variable data reconstruction High reproducibility Allows for dose modulation
Disadvantages	Sequential (not volumetric) data acquisition Predefined timing necessary Partial R-R interval covered Irregular heartbeats may cause mis-registration	Continuous radiation High radiation exposure

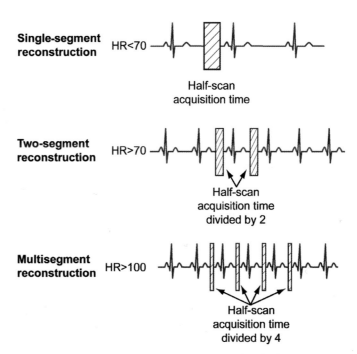

FIGURE 5-4. Schematic diagram of single-segment and multisegment computed tomography data reconstruction. HR, heart rate.

but still remain inferior to conventional coronary angiography, which has a spatial resolution of 0.2×0.2 mm.[8]

Contrast Administration

Several considerations are important to be aware of with contrast use in cardiac imaging. First, because image quality is greatly dependent on regularity of the heart rhythm, nonionic contrast is used to prevent perturbations in the heart rate during image acquisition.[9] Second, patients with cardiac disease may have low cardiac outputs, and as such, the timing of contrast arrival into the regions of interest can be variable. Hence, it is important to accurately track contrast delivery times individually for each patient. Third, because imaging time is so short in cardiac imaging, contrast osmolarity also becomes an important factor. In particular, when using third-generation scanners with very short imaging times, maximal opacification with greater osmolarity is advantageous. Finally, the physiologic impact of receiving contrast media must be taken into consideration because this can also affect the timing of contrast arrival.

Two types of contrast timing methods have been employed in current MDCT scanning systems. The first involves determining the circulation time by giving a small-volume test bolus (10-20 cc) of contrast and observing the time of its arrival in the heart, also known as a timing run. The second involves imaging a specific region of interest (eg, ascending aorta), and once the contrast density attenuation reaches a prespecified point, image acquisition starts, also known as bolus tracking. Again, exact values are dependent on scanner type, contrast type, amount and delivery method, scan delay time, and individual preference.

Post Processing

Because cardiac MDCT data are acquired with near-isotropic resolution, oblique multiplanar and thin maximum intensity projection reconstructions, including curved reformations, are used, in addition to standard axial two-dimensional (2D) evaluation, for evaluation of the cardiac structures. These oblique reconstructions are particularly important for visualization of the coronary vessels throughout their course in both a longitudinal and axial plane to the vessel of interest for the assessment of atherosclerotic plaque and luminal stenosis (Fig. 5–5). In addition to 2D evaluations, volume- and shaded surface-rendered 3D reconstructions with advanced visualization algorithms allow for the extraction of specific overlying structures such as bones, lung tissue and vessels, and soft tissue structures to focus on cardiac anatomy. These volume-rendered 3D images (Fig. 5–6) are invaluable for understanding complex cardiac anatomy (eg, anomalous coronary arteries) and in surgical planning. Shaded surface displays are commonly used for visualization of internal structures from a specified point simulating an endoscopic or angioscopic view (Fig. 5–7) and can provide important information on the internal relationship of structures, which may be important for guiding procedures (eg, pulmonary vein isolation).

Retrospective ECG gating allows for the reconstruction of volumetric image data sets during multiple phases of the cardiac cycle. Although currently temporal resolution is still limited (75 ms at best), qualitative evaluation of wall motion and

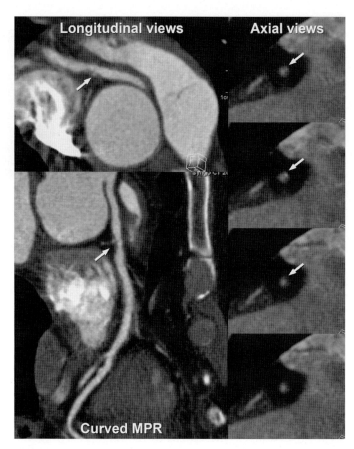

FIGURE 5–5. Computed tomography images using multiplanar straight and curved reconstructions demonstrating moderate mixed calcified and noncalcified plaque (arrow) in the right coronary artery demonstrated on both longitudinal and axial views of the vessel of interest. MPR, multiplanar reconstruction.

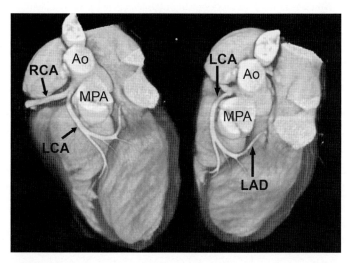

FIGURE 5–6. Computed tomography images demonstrating 3D, volume-rendered reconstructions that demonstrate anomalous origin of the left coronary system from the proximal right coronary artery (RCA). Ao, aorta; LAD, left anterior descending; LCA, left coronary artery; MPA, main pulmonary artery.

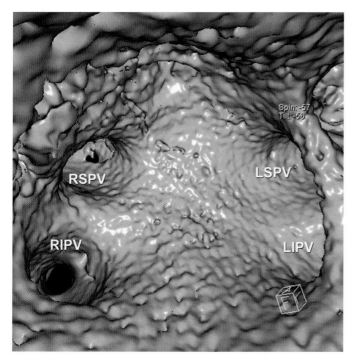

FIGURE 5–7. Computed tomography image demonstrates shaded surface–rendered reconstruction of the interior of the left atrium and draining pulmonary veins. LIPV, left inferior pulmonary vein; LSPV, left superior pulmonary vein; RIPV, right inferior pulmonary vein; RSPV, right superior pulmonary vein.

valve function can be made. Additionally, precise quantitative calculation of ventricular volumes and ejection fraction can be obtained from the data sets.[10-13]

Radiation Considerations

Radiation dose exposure is largely dependent on the acquisition protocol used. Typical effective radiation doses for coronary CTA are 5 to 12 mSv, although doses as high as 36 mSv have been reported with some protocols. In comparison, the typical radiation dose for chest CT is 5 to 7 mSv and that of a chest x-ray is <0.1 mSv. Several methods can be used to reduce overall radiation dose. These include minimizing scan length, reducing tube voltage (eg, 100 kVp instead of 120 kVp), using ECG dose modulation schemes in which tube current is lowered during acquisition of nondesired phases, reducing amperage (mA), limiting scan field of view, using step and shoot scanning (eg, prospective gating techniques), and increasing the table speed or pitch.[14] The ability to use one or multiple dose-reduction schemes is dependent on multiple factors including patient body habitus, patient heart rate, and CT scanner capabilities.

■ SPECIFIC CLINICAL CONSIDERATIONS

MDCT represents an important diagnostic imaging modality in the evaluation of patients for cardiac disease. Although MDCT has the ability to provide spectacular 3D information for a variety of diseases, specific technical and clinical aspects must be considered for each individual patient.

Motion Artifacts

Cardiac motion is a significant source of motion artifact for conventional CT imaging. Fast gantry speed CT scanners with resultant high temporal resolution and ECG-gated acquisitions, either prospective or retrospective, are used in cardiac CT imaging to improve image quality by minimizing cardiac motion artifact. Given the limited temporal resolution offered by current MDCT technologies, image quality can also be improved through optimization of the patient's heart rate. Reconstruction is commonly performed during mid to late diastole, when there is minimal cardiac motion. Diastolic time is approximately two-thirds of the cardiac cycle; however, with increasing heart rate, the proportion of the cardiac cycle spent in diastole decreases.[1,15] β-Blockers are often used to both lower the heart rate and promote regularity of the heart rhythm or decrease arrhythmias. Depending on the optimal diastolic time interval desired, oral or intravenous β-blockers have been shown to be safe when administered to patients prior to CT scanning.[15-17] In patients unable to tolerate β-blockers (eg, severe asthmatics), calcium channel blockers may provide a similar benefit.

Respiratory motion is another potential source of motion artifact that can degrade image quality on CT imaging. The use of multidetector scanners with wide coverage and minimizing scan length are methods that can decrease overall scan acquisition time and hence the amount of time required for the patient to breath-hold. Thus, for coronary imaging, scan acquisition coverage is limited to the heart. By contrast, for evaluation of a patient with bypass grafts, coverage needs to be increased to include any aortocoronary bypass grafts. This necessitates increased scan acquisition time and hence increased breath-hold time. It is important to instruct the patient prior to image acquisition on the importance of breath-holding during scan acquisition. For patients unable to breath-hold the requisite amount of time needed for scan acquisition, methods to reduce scan acquisition time or use of alternative imaging techniques should be considered.

Contrast Administration

Many cardiac CT imaging applications require the concomitant administration of intravenous iodinated contrast to improve visualization and distinction of the cardiac structures. For cardiac CT imaging, regularity of the heart rate and rhythm throughout image acquisition is important in order to optimize image quality, and potential changes in heart rate and rhythm may occur with administration of intravenous contrast. Care should be taken to screen patients with potential contraindications to contrast use, including a history of prior reaction to iodinated contrast and/or known renal insufficiency.

Image Quality

Image quality is important for diagnosis. Spatial resolution, temporal resolution, and contrast resolution are all important aspects for image quality related to CT scanners and protocol design. However, several patient-specific parameters, including body habitus, heart rate and rhythm, respiratory status, and cardiac structure being imaged, are also important aspects for

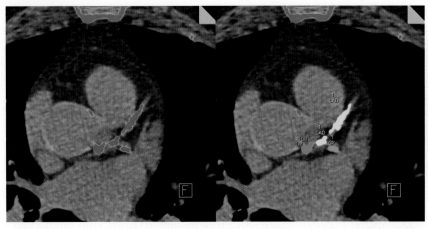

Artery	No. of lesions (1)	Volume [mm³] (3)	Equiv. mass [mg/cm³ CaHA] (4)	Score (2)
LM	1	353.9	103.01	441.9
LAD	1	464.8	109.03	593.4
CX	1	600.4	156.36	770.2
RCA	**0**	**0.0**	**0.00**	**0.0**
Total	3	1419.1	368.40	1805.5

Threshold = 130 HU (96.6 mg/cm³ CaHA)

(1) Lesion is volume based
(2) Equivalent Agatston score
(3) Isotropic interpolated volume
(4) Calibration factor: 0.743

FIGURE 5–8. Coronary calcium scoring. CX, circumflex; LAD, left anterior descending; LM, left main; RCA, right coronary artery.

diagnostic image quality. Patients with high body mass index often require a high tube current in order to produce diagnostic quality images with low image noise. Depending on the CT scanner, different methods may be used to achieve diagnostic image quality while minimizing overall radiation dose. As mentioned earlier, heart rate can be optimized for cardiac CT imaging by the administration of β-blockers to increase diastolic time. Patients with irregular heart rhythms may also benefit from β-blocker administration to regularize the heart rate (eg, suppress premature contractions). However, these drugs may be of no benefit in a patient with irregularly irregular rhythm, as in atrial fibrillation. Finally, it is important to note that although higher specifications and restrictions on these patient-specific parameters may be necessary for imaging small mobile structures such as the coronary arteries, these restrictions may not be so stringent when imaging other larger cardiac structures such as the pulmonary veins or pericardium.

STANDARD APPLICATIONS FOR CARDIAC COMPUTED TOMOGRAPHY

■ CORONARY ARTERY EVALUATION

Goals in the assessment of coronary artery disease include identification of coronary plaques and flow-limiting coronary stenoses, measurement of atherosclerotic burden, and characterization of plaque components.[18] Identification and quantification of calcified plaques can be performed using a noncontrast CT study. Further information on atherosclerotic burden, presence of noncalcified or mixed plaques, and assessment for stenoses requires a contrast CT study.

Noncontrast CT for Calcium Scoring

Atherosclerotic coronary calcifications are often found in patients with long-standing coronary atherosclerosis. Elevated levels of coronary calcification have been shown to correspond to increased risk of myocardial events.[19-22] Current clinical indications for quantification of coronary calcium are in patients with atypical chest pain, as well as asymptomatic patients with

traditional cardiovascular risk factors.[23] Noncontrast CT is currently the only method available to accurately quantify the coronary calcium plaque burden. Coronary artery calcium is assessed through the measurement of the number of pixels in the CT image with a density ≥130 Hounsfield units (HU) to calculate a total calcium score,[24] a calcium volumetric score,[25] or an absolute calcium mass[26] (Fig. 5–8). Each method has shown similar reproducibility,[27-29] and most software processing programs can easily provide all three scores simultaneously. A high coronary calcium score is a sensitive but nonspecific marker for obstructive coronary artery disease (CAD), and changes in the calcium score have not been shown to correspond to changes in cardiovascular event risk.[23]

Contrast Coronary CTA

Coronary Artery Disease Noncalcified atherosclerotic plaques in the coronary arteries can be visualized using contrast-enhanced CT. The high spatial resolution and soft tissue delineation can provide information about the content of atherosclerotic plaques and coronary artery wall,[30] including distinction between low-density lipid-rich (47 ± 9 HU) versus higher density fibrous (104 ± 28 HU) plaques.[31,32] Several studies have demonstrated the high sensitivity (72%-99%) and specificity (86%-97%) and particularly the high negative predictive value (97%-100%) of MDCT when compared against the gold standards of x-ray coronary angiography and intravascular ultrasound for the detection of significant CAD.[33-39] More importantly, with increasing number of detectors and faster gantry speeds leading to an improvement in image resolution, there has been a significant increase in the number of evaluable segments compared with early-generation scanners. The presence of coarse calcifications with related blooming and streak artifact, however, still remains problematic in regard to accurate interpretation of degree of luminal narrowing.

Coronary Anomalies Anomalies of the coronary arteries affect approximately 1% of the population, with 87% of these individuals having anomalies of the origin and distribution and 13% having coronary artery fistulae.[40,41] The true incidence of ectopic origin of the coronary arteries from the aorta in the population is unknown but estimated to be between 0.17% and 0.6%. Cardiac catheterization has traditionally been the preferred imaging modality for characterization of coronary artery anomalies. However, given the complex 3D nature of these anomalies, not infrequently, conventional angiography incompletely delineates the anatomic origin and course of the coronary artery. CTA of the coronary arteries has therefore become one of the accepted standards for complete evaluation of coronary artery anomalies. With the high spatial resolution, volumetric acquisition, and orientation in any plane, CT can accurately depict the origin and course of coronary artery anomalies with high sensitivity, although specificity is reduced in patients with high heart rates due to the limited temporal resolution even with cardiac gating.[42,43]

Assessment of Stent Patency With the growth of nonsurgical revascularization techniques, there has been an enormous increase in the number of patients with CAD who receive coronary artery stents.[44,45] Hence, early identification of in-stent restenosis is important in the management of these patients. MDCT has shown variable success for evaluation of in-stent restenosis with steady improvements noted when using newer 64-slice systems offering improvement in spatial resolution, particularly when using dedicated reconstruction kernels.[45-53] However, there is still high variability of stent lumen visibility depending on the stent type, size, orientation, and surrounding tissue (Fig. 5–9). Sharp reconstruction kernels, in addition to the routine medium kernels, may provide improvement in visible lumen diameter as well as more realistic intraluminal attenuation values.[44,45]

Assessment of Bypass Grafts Surgical revascularization of CAD is accomplished by coronary artery bypass grafting in which a graft (arterial or venous) is used to bypass an occluded or stenosed coronary artery. Compared with the native coronary arteries, reversed saphenous vein and internal mammary artery grafts are easier to visualize due to the reduced overall motion, larger lumen, and less convoluted course. Familiarity with the common types of grafts used and placement can aid in both planning and interpretation of images (Fig. 5–10). Venous

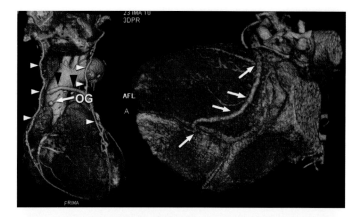

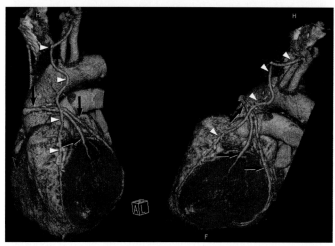

FIGURE 5–10. Volume-rendered computed tomography images demonstrating different bypass graft types including free saphenous vein grafts (black arrowheads), in situ internal mammary artery grafts (white arrowheads), sequential bypass grafts (white arrows), and "Y" or "T" grafts (black arrows). OG, occluded graft.

conduits are generally wider and longer than their arterial counterparts but have reduced long-term patency.

With the MDCT technique, special considerations must be taken into account during data acquisition. Because most patients have an in situ mammary artery graft, image acquisition must cover the entire thorax in order to visualize the proximal anastomosis and origin of the internal mammary arteries. Given the larger volume of coverage, adjustments in contrast dose and scan delay timing after contrast administration should be made to ensure adequate contrast enhancement of the bypass grafts and native coronary artery vessels during image acquisition. MDCT has been shown to have high sensitivity (97%-100%) and specificity (98%) for diagnosing graft occlusion, although somewhat lower sensitivity (75%-82%) and specificity (88%-92%) for detecting significant stenoses.[54,55]

■ PULMONARY VEIN EVALUATION

There has been an increase in the number of interventional procedures performed for the treatment of atrial arrhythmias. In particular, atrial fibrillation, which affects approximately 2 million people in the United States,[56] can now be treated using an

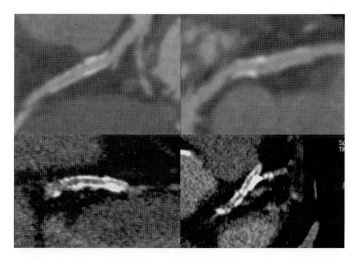

FIGURE 5–9. Oblique multiplanar reconstructed computed tomography images demonstrating patent (top row) and occluded stents (bottom row).

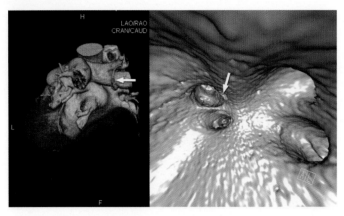

FIGURE 5–11. Volume-rendered computed tomography (left) and corresponding shaded surface reconstruction (right) of the interior of the left atrium demonstrating pulmonary venous anatomy with additional draining vein on the right.

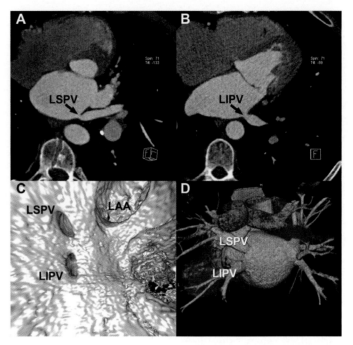

FIGURE 5–13. Multiplanar reformatted computed tomography images demonstrating significant stenosis of the left superior (**A**) and left inferior (**B**) pulmonary vein ostia. Three-dimensional shaded surface endoluminal view (**C**) and volume-rendered (**D**) images demonstrate the anatomy. LAA, left atrial appendage; LIPV, left inferior pulmonary vein; LSPV, left superior pulmonary vein.

ablation technique, often pulmonary vein isolation. Imaging evaluation of the left atrial anatomy and pulmonary venous anatomy can aid the eletrophysiologist in preprocedural planning and can be used to asses for postprocedural complications. Three-dimensional visualization of the left atrium and pulmonary venous anatomy is often used to guide the electrophysiologist in navigating the left atrial cavity during catheter ablation.

The location, size, and number of pulmonary veins need to be defined. Ostial branches, which are venous branches noted within 5 mm of the atriopulmonary venous junction, are also important to note. Commonly, there are four pulmonary veins with separate ostia into the left atrium. Knowledge of aberrant pulmonary veins (Fig. 5–11) such as accessory or conjoined veins and incidental left atrial diverticula can help guide procedures to ensure isolation of the electrical potentials arising from all the pulmonary veins and avoid potential complications from attempts to enter atrial diverticula. Diagnosis of the presence of left atrial thrombus, especially prevalent in the left atrial appendage, is important to prevent iatrogenic systemic embolism (Fig. 5–12).

Postprocedural complications of radiofrequency ablation include endocardial scarring (Fig. 5–13), pulmonary vein dissection, and perforation.[57] Small pleural or pericardial effusions, small atrial septal defects, and pulmonary venous stenosis are also potential complications. Serious complications include stroke, hemopericardium, hemothorax, pulmonary vein thrombosis, and hemodynamically significant pulmonary vein stenosis, which can result in pulmonary veno-occlusive disease including focal pulmonary edema.[58] Pulmonary vein stenosis may develop up to 8 months after the procedure. Current ablation techniques, however, have greatly diminished the complication rate of pulmonary venous stenosis.

Imaging of the left atrial and pulmonary venous anatomy can be performed with CT or magnetic resonance imaging (MRI). CTA imaging can be performed as a gated or nongated study and should encompass the area from the aortic arch through the apex of the heart during a single breath-hold.[59] Postprocessing of the image data sets, including 2D multiplanar reconstructions of the pulmonary venous ostia and atrial appendage, and 3D volume-rendered and shaded surface displays demonstrate the complex anatomy. Depending on the software vendor,

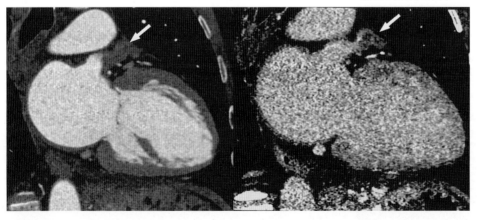

FIGURE 5–12. Early (left) and delayed (right) first-pass perfusion computed tomography image in two-chamber view of the heart demonstrating persistent filling defect in the left atrial appendage representing thrombus (arrow).

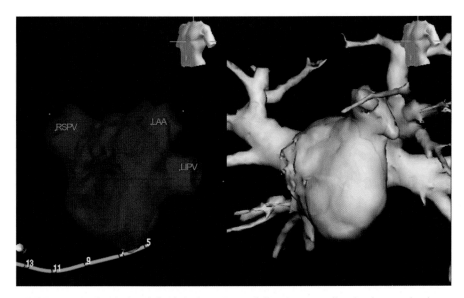

FIGURE 5–14. Synchronization of electrical voltage 3D map (left) and corresponding 3D volume-rendered computed tomography image (right) of the left atrium used for guiding electrophysiology intervention. LAA, left atrial appendage; LIPV, left inferior pulmonary vein; RSPV, right superior pulmonary vein.

Because congenital heart disease often involves abnormalities in both the right and left heart chambers, the timing of data acquisition is set such that there is optimal contrast enhancement seen in both sides of the heart. In cases with intracardiac shunting, imaging can be performed early (within 5 seconds of contrast administration) and late (approximately 30 seconds after contrast administration) in order to determine the degree and direction of shunting.[62] Images can be evaluated using multiplanar reconstructions, maximum intensity projections and 3D volume rendered image sets. Data can also be reconstructed in multiple phases through the cardiac cycle for calculation of cardiac volumes and function.

volumetric CT data sets acquired through the left atrium can be synchronized and fused with electrical mapping systems in the electrophysiology laboratory (Fig. 5–14).

■ CONGENITAL HEART DISEASE

Over the past five decades, the number of adults with congenital heart disease has grown due to the advances in cardiac surgery, intensive care, and noninvasive diagnosis.[60] Approximately 85% of infants with cardiovascular anomalies can be expected to survive into adulthood, and with further advancements in surgical techniques, this number may continue to grow.[61] Although surgical correction of an anomaly may reestablish a relatively normal pattern of blood flow, these adult survivors still remain at significant risk for developing complications from their operative procedures or from lingering effects of the original anomaly. Hence, these patients need to be followed closely regardless of their stage of treatment. As such, comprehensive imaging evaluation of the cardiovascular anatomy, flow, and function is important in the management of these patients. Cardiac MDCT with its fast acquisition times and capacity to obtain volumetric 3D information with high spatial resolution has often been used in the anatomic evaluation of congenital heart disease (Fig. 5–15). Advantages of CT compared with other imaging modalities such as cardiac MRI include short examination, fewer requirements for sedation, simultaneous evaluation of airways and lung parenchyma, and high spatial resolution. Disadvantages include radiation exposure, use of iodinated contrast, and lack of hemodynamic information.

CT imaging protocol is dependent on the structure of interest and information needed. For patients with abnormalities in the vascular system, image acquisition is usually started a few centimeters above the aortic arch and continued to the diaphragm.

■ PERICARDIAL DISEASE

Diseases of the pericardium encompass a spectrum of disorders including congenital malformations and infection-related, infarction-related, metabolic, autoimmune, traumatic, neoplastic, and idiopathic disorders. Depending on the disease process, clinical manifestations of pericardial involvement can vary. Suspected pericardial

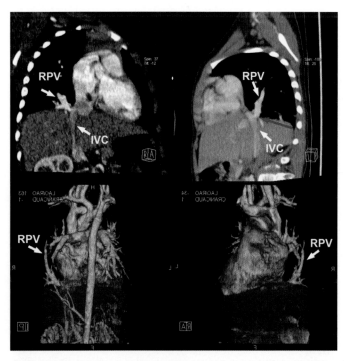

FIGURE 5–15. Multiplanar reformatted (top row) and three-dimensional volume-rendered (bottom row) computed tomography images demonstrating partial anomalous pulmonary venous return of the right-sided pulmonary veins (RPV) into the subdiaphragmatic inferior vena cava (IVC) with some narrowing noted at the ostium (red arrow).

disease is usually initially evaluated with echocardiography. However, CT imaging can also provide additional valuable information.

CT imaging has been widely accepted for the evaluation of structural changes in the pericardium. The best quality images in the evaluation of pericardial disease are obtained with the use of cardiac gating and fast imaging to minimize motion blurring, although more prominent pericardial disease findings may be evident even on conventional studies performed for other indications. On CT, the pericardium is usually well delineated from the adjacent low-attenuation fat. Anatomic features of pericardial disease such as pericardial thickening, pericardial calcification, and pericardial effusion or masses are easily detected and evaluated with CT. Limited tissue characterization of pericardial fluid/masses can make it difficult to differentiate thickened pericardium from an exudative pericardial effusion with high protein content. Functional and hemodynamic information is also limited with CT. However, CT is the most sensitive technique for detection of pericardial calcification.

Pericardial Effusion

The CT appearance of pericardial effusion is often not very specific for a particular etiology, and further evaluation is usually necessary to help narrow the range of differential possibilities. CT attenuation measurements can provide initial characterization of pericardial fluid. On CT, simple effusions have attenuation similar to that of water. In contrast, more proteinaceous fluid (exudates or inspissated fluid collections) will have attenuation greater than water on CT.[63] CT characteristics of malignant effusions may be similar to hemorrhagic effusions, depending on blood content, and are often associated with an irregularly thickened pericardium or pericardial nodularity. In addition, because of the wide field of view, associated abnormalities of the mediastinum and lungs may also be detected during the examination.[64]

Acute Pericarditis

Acute pericarditis may or may not be accompanied by pericardial effusion and some degree of myocarditis depending on etiology. Clinical symptoms and serologic markers of inflammation can often support the diagnosis. CT imaging can be used to aid in the diagnosis, especially when other tests prove inconclusive. Structural changes of the pericardium such as thickening, inflammation, pericardial effusion, and associated myocarditis or other concomitant heart disease and mediastinal pathology can be demonstrated.

Constrictive Pericarditis

Chronic inflammation of the pericardium can lead to constrictive pericarditis, which is characterized by impaired ventricular filling. The process may extend to involve the underlying myocardium, resulting in reduced ventricular function. The etiology of constrictive pericardial disease has often been attributed to antecedent acute pericarditis due to infectious, inflammatory, or idiopathic causes. However, other etiologies such as neoplastic diseases, postradiation therapy, postcardiac surgery, and

remote nonpenetrating or penetrating cardiac trauma have been frequently seen. Accurate diagnosis and differentiation from restrictive cardiomyopathy are important because curative treatment for constrictive pericarditis is possible with surgical pericardiectomy. Initial diagnostic workup usually includes 2D, Doppler, and tissue Doppler echocardiography with analysis of respiratory changes associated or not with changes of preload. However, equivocal findings may be present in up to one-third of patients with possible pericardial constriction, and further testing is usually required.

Direct visualization of the pericardium can be performed with CT for measurement of pericardial thickness. However, the finding of a thickened pericardium is not necessarily confirmatory of constrictive pericarditis. In addition, up to 20% of patients with constrictive pericarditis may present with normal-thickness pericardium on current imaging methods.[65] CT can also demonstrate characteristic anatomic features for constrictive pericarditis including a conical or tubular diastolic ventricular shape, an associated pericardial effusion, pericardial calcification (Fig. 5–16), and secondary sequelae including dilated atria, hepatic veins, and pulmonary veins, which can further support the diagnosis of constrictive pericarditis.

Pericardial Masses

The differential diagnosis of pericardial masses includes pericardial cyst, hematoma, neoplasm, loculated effusions, or pseudoaneurysms. Although often detected initially with echocardiography, evaluation with CT can be helpful in diagnosis and treatment. CT characteristics such as tissue attenuation,

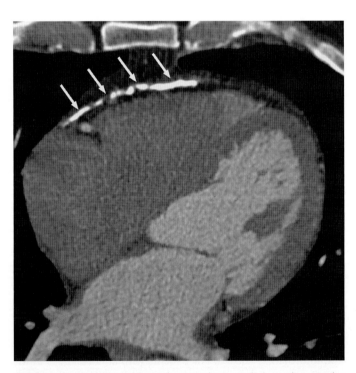

FIGURE 5–16. Multiplanar reformatted computed tomography image demonstrating pericardial calcifications (arrows) that can be seen in constrictive pericarditis.

degree of contrast enhancement, and presence or absence of blood flow into the mass can help differentiate among pericardial masses. In addition, the size, anatomic extent, associated lesions, vascularity, and effects on cardiac function of the masses can be clarified. Furthermore, CT can guide other diagnostic testing, such as biopsy, and facilitate treatment and follow-up.

Congenital Pericardial Lesions

Congenital defects of the pericardium comprise partial left, right, or diaphragmatic or total absence of the pericardium. Most patients are asymptomatic, although approximately 30% may have additional congenital abnormalities. Complete absence of the pericardium poses a risk of homolateral cardiac displacement and amplified heart mobility and an increased risk of traumatic aortic type A dissection. Partial left-sided defects can be complicated by cardiac strangulation caused by herniation of the left atrial appendage, atrium, or left ventricle through the defect. Although the diagnosis can be suggested by chest x-ray and echocardiography, definitive diagnosis and complete evaluation of the pericardium can be performed with CT.

■ CARDIAC MASSES

Cardiac masses may be divided into benign or malignant lesions. Benign cardiac tumors include cardiac neoplasms, pseudotumors such as thrombi, and normal structures that resemble masses. Malignant cardiac tumors include both primary and secondary malignancies that can affect the heart. Echocardiography is often the initial diagnostic test to evaluate cardiac masses but often provides limited information on tissue characterization and extent of extracardiac involvement or presence of metastatic disease. Therefore, cross-sectional imaging with CT can provide additional information including the precise location of cardiac tumors (eg, paracardiac, mural, or intracavitary), the extent of disease, the presence of associated effusions, and the presence of metastases[66] (Fig. 5–17). Additionally, CT imaging findings including tissue characterization may suggest the tumor type, which can be important in treatment planning (Table 5–2).

Depending on the size and location of the cardiac mass, CT image acquisition is tailored to obtain the necessary information. Noncontrast CT imaging can provide limited information regarding the nature of cardiac masses, but contrast CT imaging with cardiac gating can better assess the precise location, size, and extent of cardiac masses.

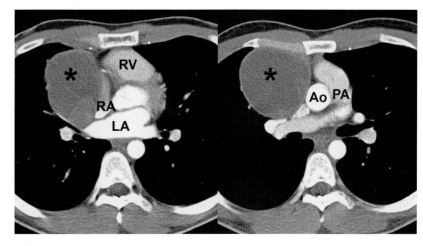

FIGURE 5–17. Axial computed tomography image demonstrating a large paracardiac mass (asterisk) with associated compression of the right atrium (RA). Further workup of the mass revealed a thymoma arising from the anterior mediastinum. Ao, aorta; LA, left atrium; PA, pulmonary artery; RV, right ventricle.

TABLE 5–2. CT Characteristic Features of Cardiac Masses

Mass	CT Characteristics	Distribution and Features
Thrombus	Hypodense	Atrial appendage, left ventricular aneurysms
Myxoma	Heterogeneous hypodense	Attachment to interatrial septum; commonly in left atrium
Papillary fibroelastoma	Hypodense	Solitary, mobile, pedunculated
Lipoma	Hypodense	Encapsulated mass with smooth contour
Fibroma	Hypodense with areas of calcification	Large, solitary, intramyocardial
Rhabdomyoma	Hypodense	Multicentric masses, intramural or intracavitary
Teratoma	Heterogeneous often with calcification in the form of teeth	Multicentric
Hemangioma	Heterogeneous with interdispersed calcification	Commonly in epicardial layer of myocardium
Angiosarcoma	Hypodense nodular lesions	Commonly affect right atrium; frequent extension
Rhabdomyosarcoma	Hypodense	Pericardial infiltration rare
Lymphoma	Hypodense or isodense	Multiple circumscribed polypoid masses or ill-defined infiltrative lesion

CT, computed tomography.

Benign Cardiac Neoplasms

Benign cardiac masses include myxoma, papillary fibroelastomas, lipoma, and rhabdomyoma. Benign tumors tend to affect the left-sided chambers of the heart. Although these lesions are histologically benign, they can act malignantly via secondary effects on the heart and vasculature. Therefore, successful treatment depends on the early detection and characterization of these masses.

Myxoma Myxomas on CT often demonstrate a distinct, intracavitary sphere, typically with calcification, heterogeneous hypoattenuation consistent with its gelatinous nature,[67-69] and neovascularization.[70] They commonly demonstrate a narrow base of attachment (somewhat pedunculated), and attachment to the interatrial septum virtually cements the diagnosis.[76,71] Functional consequences of large myxomas can be seen in cine cardiac CT in which the tumor mass may prolapse into the ventricles or cause obstruction of the atrioventricular valves.

Papillary Fibroelastoma Papillary fibroelastomas are avascular papillomas lined with endothelium. Depending on the size, location, and mobility, these masses may not be well seen on CT, especially if cardiac gating is not used. However, on CT they often appear as small (<2 cm in diameter), solitary, mobile, pedunculated, hypodense,[72] homogeneous valvular, or endocardial masses that flutter or prolapse with cardiac motion.[69]

Lipoma Lipomas typically occur in adults, although they can also be seen in children. They generally occur as solitary masses that can arise from the epicardial surface spreading into the pericardial space[73] or from the interatrial septum or endocardial surface as a broad base from which they can grow into any of the cardiac chambers.[74] Lipomas are seen as encapsulated masses demonstrating the hypodense[75] attenuation of fat on CT. There is often lack of contrast enhancement, but use of contrast can increase their conspicuity. In addition, a smooth contour and capsule can further distinguish benign lipomas from the irregular, multilobar liposarcomas.[69]

Although not a tumor, lipomatous hypertrophy of the interatrial septum can be confused with the truly neoplastic lipoma. Lipomatous hypertrophy results from an increase in cell number, or hyperplasia, seen in obese, elderly individuals as an unencapsulated fatty infiltration, defined formally as any deposit of fat in the atrial septum at the level of the fossa ovalis that exceeds 2 cm in transverse diameter.[76] In addition to characteristic sparing of the fossa ovalis seen on echocardiography, this tissue may appear wedge shaped or as diffuse septal thickening on CT.

Fibroma On CT, fibromas commonly appear as a large solitary, calcified mass within the ventricular myocardium. This is in contrast to other intramyocardial tumors including rhabdomyomas, which are often multicentric, and rhabdomyosarcomas, which are frequently cystic or necrotic.[77] On CT, fibromas are commonly hypodense due to the dense, fibrous tissue with bright areas of calcification.[78,79]

Rhabdomyoma Cardiac rhabdomyomas account for the majority of cardiac tumors seen in infants.[71,77] Unlike other cardiac tumors, rhabdomyomas frequently regress over time and thus are treated conservatively. However, complications can result from an obstructive syndrome or from severe arrhythmias.[80] On imaging studies, rhabdomyomas can be seen in both right and left ventricular myocardium and interventricular septum. They may be intracavitary or intramural and are often multiple rather than single. On CT, rhabdomyomas appear hypodense to myocardium after contrast administration.

Teratomas Cardiac teratomas generally occur in infants and children as a predominantly right-sided pericardial mass.[81] Although considered benign, these tumors are often accompanied by pericardial effusions, which may progress to cardiac tamponade with subsequent respiratory distress and cyanosis.[81,82] However, surgical resection is often curative.[83] CT imaging of teratomas demonstrates a heterogenous, multicystic appearance with calcification, often in the form of teeth, and can confirm the diagnosis of teratoma over other tumors.[71,77]

Hemangiomas Cardiac hemangiomas are rare, benign, vascular tumors of the heart. They usually occur in the epicardial layer but can involve all the cardiac chambers. Symptoms are usually the result of tumor compression of surrounding structures or embolization.[84] On noncontrast CT, cardiac hemangiomas have a heterogeneous density with occasional interspersed calcification.[69] In addition, they enhance intensely with contrast, which may be inhomogeneous due to interspersed calcification and fibrous septa within the mass.[85]

Malignant Cardiac Neoplasms

Malignant cardiac masses include metastatic neoplasms, primary cardiac sarcomas, and primary cardiac lymphoma. Although no single finding is specific, malignant cardiac tumors commonly affect the right-sided chambers of the heart, demonstrate inhomogeneity of tumor tissue, appear infiltrative, and are associated with pericardial or pleural effusion.[86]

Metastatic Disease Most metastases to the heart occur from lung or breast cancer, but they can also occur from melanoma, lymphoma, and leukemia.[87-89] Involvement of cardiac structures primarily occurs through the lymphatic pathway, although hematogenous, contiguous, or transvenous extension does occur.[90] Cardiac involvement is commonly seen as a late manifestation of primary tumor extension,[91] but characteristic vascular involvement signs may help facilitate diagnosis. Pulmonary vein extension may signal bronchogenic carcinoma, inferior vena caval extension can be seen with renal cell and hepatocellular carcinoma, and superior vena caval extension may indicate supracardiac tumors such as thymic carcinomas.[92] CT imaging of metastases can demonstrate nodular masses or pericardial thickening often with contrast enhancement due to vascularity of the lesions.[93,94] Other common features of malignancy include right-sided involvement, ventricular infiltration, and hemorrhagic pericardial effusion.[95]

Sarcoma Cardiac sarcomas are extremely rare tumors occurring in less than 0.2% of the population but represent the most common primary malignant cardiac tumor seen in adults.[96] These tumors may originate in the epicardium or pericardium, involve the myocardium and cardiac valves, and cause nonspecific signs and symptoms that make clinical diagnosis difficult. There are several subtypes of sarcomas including angiosarcoma, osteosarcoma, fibrosarcoma, malignant fibrous histiocytoma, leiomyosarcoma, myxosarcoma, synovial sarcoma, neurofibrosarcoma, lymphosarcoma, reticulum cell sarcoma, and undifferentiated sarcoma.

Angiosarcoma is a tumor of endothelial cells and represents the most prevalent subtype. These tumors most commonly affect the right atrium; are highly vascular lesions with hemorrhagic, necrotic foci; and frequently invade the pericardium with associated hemorrhagic effusion that can lead to cardiac tamponade.[97] On CT, angiosarcomas appear as hypodense irregular or nodular lesions, often arising from the right atrial free wall with heterogeneous enhancement, or in the case of pericardial infiltration, they may appear as pericardial effusion or thickening.[98]

Rhabdomyosarcomas are striated muscle tumors that represent the most common cardiac malignancy in infants and children.[99] These tumors may arise anywhere within the heart, involving any cardiac chamber or valve,[100] although pericardial infiltration is rare.[71] On CT, these tumors demonstrate low attenuation with a smooth or irregular contour that enhances with contrast.[101] Extracardiac extension into the pulmonary arteries, aorta, or valvular structures can be demonstrated with CT.[100]

Fibrosarcomas consist primarily of malignant fibroblasts and comprise 5% of all primary cardiac tumors.[102,103] They commonly affect the left atrium, and valvular involvement is found in as many as 50%. On CT, fibrosarcomas appear as a low-attenuation, often obliterative mass. Fibrosarcomas may infiltrate the pericardium by direct invasion[104] or tumor deposition nodules,[105] or they may primarily involve the pericardium, appearing similar to malignant mesothelioma.[96]

Osteosarcomas in the heart consist of malignant bone-producing tumor cells.[96] Primary osteosarcomas commonly arise in the left atrium usually accompanied by signs and symptoms of congestive heart failure.[106] CT may show dense calcifications within a low-attenuation, left-sided mass.[107] However, early lesions may have minimal calcification and can be mistaken for dystrophic calcifications. Other distinguishing features include a broad base of attachment and an aggressive growth pattern with extension into the pulmonary veins or atrial septum or infiltrative growth along the epicardium.[108-110]

Leiomyosarcoma is a malignant tumor with smooth muscle differentiation. It may arise from the subendocardium of the cardiac chambers but more commonly arises from smooth muscle of the pulmonary veins and arteries and then spreads into the heart.[96] CT imaging demonstrates lobulated, irregular, low-attenuation masses.[111]

Liposarcoma is a malignant mesenchymal tumor that consists of lipoblasts. These tumors are extremely rare.[96] They tend to arise in the atria but have been reported to occur in any cardiac chamber, the pericardium, and cardiac valves.[112,113] Unlike benign lipomas, liposarcomas have little or no macroscopic fat.[69] CT imaging demonstrates a large, multilobular, heterogeneous mass with areas of necrosis and hemorrhage.[100]

Lymphomas Primary cardiac lymphoma includes lymphoma that is mostly confined to the heart or pericardium,[96] as opposed to the more common cardiac spread of non-Hodgkin lymphoma.[114] These lymphomas are commonly aggressive B-cell lymphomas.[71,115] Although there is increased prevalence in immunocompromised patients, these lymphomas are also seen in immunocompetent patients.[115] Cardiac lymphoma may appear as either multiple circumscribed polypoid masses[116] or an ill-defined infiltrative lesion.[117,118] Cardiac lymphomas are less likely than sarcomas to have necrosis.[96] They commonly arise in the right side of the heart but may involve any chamber. Pericardial effusions are common and may be the only finding at the time of imaging. On CT, lymphomas appear hypodense or isodense relative to myocardium and demonstrate heterogeneous contrast enhancement.[115,118]

Pseudotumors

Normal Cardiac Structures Due to the complex nature of the cardiac anatomy and the unique individual variations seen, normal cardiac structures can often be mistaken for cardiac tumors. In particular, fetal remnants (eg, Eustachian valve, Chiari network) or normal variants (eg, prominent trabeculations, false tendons) may give the impression of a cardiac tumor. Given the 3D nature of cross-sectional imaging with CT, differentiation of normal cardiac structures from cardiac tumors can be made. In addition, the distinction between cardiac neoplasms versus other cardiac masses can also be made.

Thrombi Intracavitary cardiac thrombi probably represent the most common masses seen in cardiac imaging. In patients with atrial arrhythmias or other predisposing factor for atrial blood flow stasis (eg, mitral stenosis), they can frequently be seen along the posterolateral wall of the left atrium or within the left atrial appendage.[119] In patients with cardiomyopathy, ventricular thrombi can form in areas of slow blood flow such as ventricular aneurysm or regions with dysfunctional myocardium. On CT, thrombi generally exhibit homogeneous hypodense attenuation after contrast administration.[120] Care should be taken to distinguish slow flow with incomplete opacification, which may be seen on first-pass imaging, from true thrombi, which in general will remain hypodense on delayed imaging after contrast administration. (see Fig 5–12)

Vegetation Intracardiac masses related to infective endocarditis are usually diagnosed with echocardiography in the appropriate clinical setting. However, in cases where the diagnosis is uncertain, CT imaging can aid in excluding a cardiac tumor. In general, vegetations exhibit CT imaging characteristics similar to thrombi. Because vegetations are often nonvascular, they generally do not enhance with contrast administration. Although distinction from cardiac tumor is possible, tissue differentiation between thrombi and vegetations is generally not possible with CT, and accurate diagnosis relies on incorporating the patient's accompanying clinical features and the effect on cardiac structures (eg, location and/or evidence of destruction) (Fig. 5–18).

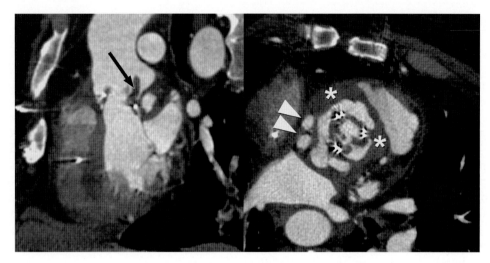

FIGURE 5–18. Multiplanar reformatted computed tomography images demonstrating a bioprosthetic valve in the aortic position with thickened leaflets, large vegetation (black arrow), thickening of the aortic annulus (asterisks), and disruption suggestive of aortic root abscess (white arrowheads).

EVOLVING APPLICATIONS FOR CARDIAC COMPUTED TOMOGRAPHY

■ MYOCARDIAL EVALUATION

Myocardial structural assessment, including evaluation for viability and prognosis based on the presence of inflammation, scar, and diffuse fibrosis, is usually performed by MRI and/or nuclear cardiac imaging techniques. MDCT does not currently provide sufficient spatial or contrast-to-noise information to allow for quantification of such processes. However, often cardiac CT is the method of choice in the assessment of left ventricular (LV) structure and function because of patient care logistics, convenience, or contraindications to alternative imaging modalities.

Chamber Size and Functions

Multiple studies have documented the diagnostic value of cardiac CT to evaluate LV size and global and regional LV function.[121-124] The use of retrospective ECG gating allows for collection of imaging data for reconstruction throughout the cardiac cycle, which can then be used for evaluation of wall motion and function. In routine clinical practice, functional analysis is most commonly performed to evaluate the left ventricle and aortic valve. Precise evaluation of LV function is important for diagnosis, therapy, and follow-up of patients with cardiovascular diseases.

Endocardial excursion and the extent and timing of systolic myocardial wall thickening are used for LV functional assessment of cardiac CT images. Wall motion may be reported as normal, hypokinetic, akinetic, dyskinetic, or aneurysmal. Quantitative functional evaluation relies on methods to segment the ventricular cavity. Definition of the intraventricular cavity is dependent on the software vendor used. Commonly, either a Hounsfield threshold cutoff value or endocardial contouring of the intraventricular cavity is performed to distinguish

the cavity from myocardium. Ejection fraction, stroke volume, and cardiac output can then be derived from the calculated ventricular volumes. In general, when compared with cardiac magnetic resonance (CMR), cardiac CT demonstrates excellent agreement for assessment of LV ejection fraction and regional wall motion.[122,123]

It is important to note that newer, more recent low-dose coronary CTA (CCTA) protocols often use prospective triggering methods with collection of imaging data only during diastole at a substantially lower radiation exposure. These CCTA techniques preclude quantitative and qualitative functional analyses due to lack of additional phases through systole.

Myocardial Viability

The ability to distinguish dysfunctional but viable myocardium from nonviable tissue after acute or chronic ischemia has important implications for the therapeutic management of patients with CAD.[125,126] Image-based characterization of myocardial scar morphology can identify those patients with hibernating myocardium who may achieve functional systolic recovery with revascularization.[127] The assessment of myocardial viability and infarct morphology with delayed contrast-enhanced MRI has been well validated over the past several years and is considered the noninvasive imaging gold standard for detection of myocardial fibrosis.

The recent advent of MDCT technology has expanded its potential for a more comprehensive evaluation of cardiovascular diseases. Although hypoattenuation in the noncontrast scan (due to fatty degeneration of the infarcted area) or during the contrast-enhanced coronary angiography scan has been shown to demonstrate areas of previous myocardial infarction, it is largely underestimated by MDCT.[128,129] Delayed MDCT myocardial imaging can accurately identify and characterize morphologic features of acute and healed myocardial infarction, including infarct size, transmurality, and the presence of microvascular

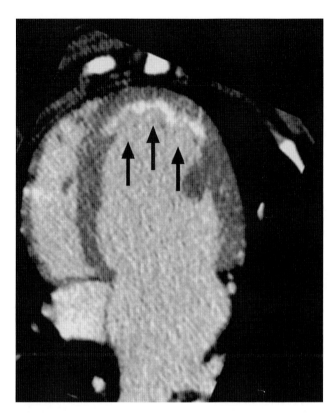

FIGURE 5–19. Multiplanar reformatted computed tomography image taken approximately 5 minutes after contrast administration demonstrating subendocardial contrast enhancement (arrows) involving the apical segments of the left ventricle.

obstruction and collagenous scar.[130,131] Infarcted myocardial tissue by MDCT is characterized by well-delineated hyperenhanced regions (Fig. 5–19), whereas regions of microvascular obstruction by MDCT are characterized by hypoenhancement on imaging early after myocardial infarction.[130,131] The mechanism of myocardial hyperenhancement and hypoenhancement in acutely injured myocardial territories after iodinated contrast administration is similar to that proposed for delayed gadolinium-enhanced MRI.[125] Under conditions of normal myocyte function, sarcolemmal membranes serve to exclude iodine from the intracellular space. After myocyte necrosis, however, membrane dysfunction ensues, and iodine molecules are able to penetrate the cell. Because 75% of the total myocardial volume is intracellular, large increases in the volume of distribution are achieved, which results in marked hyperenhancement relative to the noninjured myocytes. The mechanism of hyperenhancement of healed myocardial infarction or collagenous scar is thought to be related to an accumulation of contrast media in the interstitial space between collagen fibers and thus an increased volume of distribution compared with that of tightly packed myocytes. The low signal intensity of microvascular obstruction regions despite restoration of normal flow through the infarct-related artery is explained by the death and subsequent cellular debris blockage of intramyocardial capillaries at the core of the damaged region. These obstructed capillaries do not allow contrast material to flow into the damaged bed, which results in a region of low

signal intensity compared with normal myocardium. In minutes to hours, contrast material is able to penetrate this "no reflow" region, and the necrotic myocytes that reside in that myocardial territory then become hyperenhanced as iodine is internalized by the cell. In weeks, the microvascular obstruction area is replaced by collagenous scar tissue, and the former dark areas now become bright. Because the transmurality of delayed enhancement predicts functional recovery after revascularization,[127] the better spatial resolution of MDCT, as compared with CMR, may influence the accuracy of viability assessment, but thus far, no study has tested this hypothesis.

Myocardial Ischemia

The use of CT imaging for evaluation of myocardial perfusion has been documented in the past by investigators using electron beam CT.[132] However, it was not until the development of 64-slice CT systems that the combination of coronary angiography with stress-induced myocardial perfusion assessment could be reliably performed.[133,134] Currently, the greatest limitation to CT coronary angiography is the presence of severely calcified coronary segments, stents, or other artifacts that limit luminal visualization. Patients with calcified arteries tend to be older and/or have advanced CAD. Their studies are challenging from a diagnostic viewpoint because vulnerable plaques and stenotic lesions may be hidden underneath large amounts of calcium accumulated in the outer portions of atherosclerotic plaques encompassing one or more segments. Although progress in multidetector technology has improved our ability to study such patients, greater coverage and improved temporal resolution are unlikely to eliminate the problem, which is in large part intrinsic to the pathogenesis of atherosclerosis—namely, plaques grow outwardly first and tend to accumulate calcium as part of the healing process, therefore creating a natural shield to x-ray penetration. This is a particular limitation to the CT evaluation of older persons, patients with advanced CAD, and patients with prior coronary artery bypass graft surgery or multiple stent implantations, as well as patients with diseases such as chronic renal failure that accelerate plaque calcification. Furthermore, coronary anatomic information is much more valuable when combined with a functional test, because decisions regarding treatment are based on the detection of myocardial ischemia.[135] The poor correlation between anatomic modalities such as invasive coronary angiography[136,137] and MDCT[138] with stress perfusion tests underscores the fact that one cannot substitute for the other.

Myocardial perfusion measurements by MDCT are derived from the upslope differences in contrast enhancement between the ischemic and remote areas (Fig. 5–20). Current-generation, 64-detector scanners still have limited coverage of the heart, resulting in the base of the heart being scanned earlier in time than the apex, making comparisons in signal intensities between the two areas problematic. In this regard, the introduction of wide-coverage MDCT technology that would allow the entire heart to be imaged in one gantry rotation (Fig. 5–21) combined with the capability of programming such gated image acquisitions to occur only during specific portions of a given

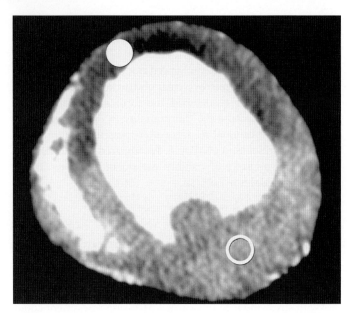

FIGURE 5–20. Multiplanar reformatted computed tomography image during first-pass myocardial perfusion demonstrating localized region of low attenuation anteriorly (white dot) when compared with corresponding inferior wall, which demonstrates relatively normal perfusion (white circle).

cardiac cycle has created a brand new horizon of possibilities to reduce radiation exposure enough to enable the performance of combined angiography and myocardial perfusion assessment during stress, which associated with the angiographic and delayed enhanced images should provide a comprehensive cardiac assessment. Also, with more coverage, scan times will likely decrease, potentially reducing the amount of contrast material per scan. Such techniques would be ideal for the assessment of patients with chest pain who also have calcified coronaries, as well as for the follow-up of patients with advanced heart disease after coronary artery bypass surgery or multiple stent implantations. Using iodine molecules as a tracer, current research has demonstrated that by measuring the concentration in time of the tracer in the myocardium, MDCT can determine absolute blood flow in different regions of the myocardium.[133] Recent

attention to patients with chest pain but no obstructive epicardial CAD (syndrome X) has demonstrated that in a substantial proportion of these individuals, microvascular processes can be identified by perfusion reserve measurements in association with traditional CAD risk factors such as hypercholesterolemia, hypertension, and smoking, as well as with diabetes.[139] The possibility of quantifying epicardial coronary plaque while also assessing microvascular disease during maximal vasodilatation enables coronary MDCTA to characterize macrovascular atherosclerosis as well as microvascular dysfunction secondary to atherosclerosis or other disease processes. The capability of quantifying myocardial blood flow by contrast-enhanced MDCT could represent a "quantum leap" in our ability to assess and characterize the entire process of cardiac atherosclerosis.

◼ VALVULAR HEART DISEASE

Valvular heart disease is an important part of cardiology. Often detected by physical examination, imaging studies can help clarify the affected valve, define the valvular anatomy, and assess the degree of valve dysfunction and its effect on cardiac chamber morphology and function. The cardiac valves are normally very thin, pliable, mobile structures. Hence, imaging techniques to assess valve disease need to have high spatial and temporal resolution. Traditionally, transthoracic echocardiography with its acceptable spatial resolution and high temporal resolution with near real-time imaging is the imaging modality of choice in the assessment of valve disease. Quantification of valvular stenosis and valve area, valvular regurgitation, and effective orifice area and an assessment of ventricular function can be easily performed. Transesophageal echocardiography can further define valvular anatomy and dysfunction in patients with infective endocarditis or in patients with poor acoustic windows. Although cardiac CT can provide high spatial resolution of valvular anatomy, moderate temporal resolution limits assessment of valvular flow and function.

Native Valves

Information on valve morphology, leaflet abnormalities, and valve motion is possible with CT (Fig. 5–22) but remains inferior to

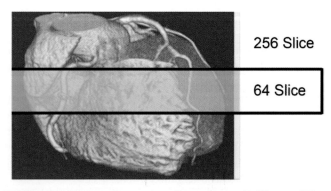

FIGURE 5–21. Diagrammatic comparison of heart coverage with different multidetector computed tomography systems.

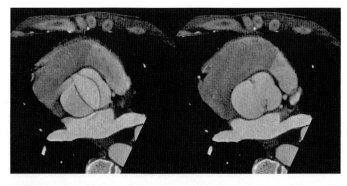

FIGURE 5–22. Multiplanar reformatted computed tomography image during systole (left) and diastole (right) demonstrating bicuspid aortic valve.

echocardiographic techniques.[140,141] However, information from CT can be helpful in inconclusive cases. Valvular characteristics such as leaflet morphology (thickening, calcifications, and poor leaflet coaptation), congenital lesions, and abnormalities of the valvular and subvalvular apparatus can be demonstrated on CT.[142] Severity of the stenosis can be assessed by planimetry of the orifice area during valve opening,[143-145] and the severity of regurgitant lesions can be assessed by measuring the effective regurgitant orifice area by planimetry during valve closure.[142] In addition, measurement of aortic valve Agatston calcium score has been shown to correlate with severity of aortic valve gradient by echocardiography.[146,147] Indirect characteristics such as dilation of chambers or vascular structures (eg, dilated left ventricle and/or dilated aortic root in aortic regurgitation) and increased ventricular wall thickness (eg, right ventricular hypertrophy in pulmonic stenosis) provide further information on the severity of the secondary hemodynamic impairment.

Prosthetic Valves

Prosthetic heart valves and annuloplasty rings are implanted every year around the world and have become extremely useful devices in cardiac disease (Fig. 5–23). Prosthetic valves can be divided into two main classes: mechanical prostheses and biologic or tissue valves. Mechanical valves are classified into three major groups: caged-ball, tilting-disc, and bileaflet valves. Today, the most widely used mechanical valve is the bileaflet valve, although older caged-ball valves are still seen in patients for follow-up. Tissue valves include heterografts, homografts, and autografts. CT has not been extensively studied for the evaluation of prosthetic valve dysfunction. As with echocardiography, artifacts related to the metal used in the implants may limit accurate evaluation for prosthetic valve function. However, cardiac CT assessment of prosthetic valves, particularly mechanical

valves, may provide additional information to that provided by echocardiography, leading to a more complete assessment of valvular function and hemodynamics.[148]

Infective Endocarditis

Infective endocarditis involves the endocardial surface, most commonly affecting the heart valves, but also mural endocardium. Characteristic vegetations are comprised of platelets, fibrin, inflammatory cells, and microorganisms. In general, vegetations exhibit CT imaging characteristics similar to thrombi and generally do not enhance with contrast administration. Abnormalities in valve structure, including the presence of prosthetic valves, are often predisposing factors for the development of endocarditis. In addition to the presence of vegetations, CT imaging can aid in the identification of perivalvular extension, myocardial or perivalvular abscess formation, fistula formation, and pseudoaneurysms, particularly along the intervalvular fibrosa (see Fig. 5–18). In particular, prosthetic valve endocarditis can be difficult to evaluate with echocardiography due to acoustic shadowing related to the prosthesis, and in those situations, CT imaging has the ability to provide important additional information.[142]

MULTIMODAL APPLICATIONS

■ CORONARY ARTERY DISEASE

A comprehensive assessment of CAD should include information on coronary artery anatomy and functional information regarding the hemodynamic relevance of lesions in order to guide revascularization procedures. At present, there is much debate regarding the optimal management of patients with stable CAD, and several guidelines recommend evidence of functional ischemia prior to revascularization of stenoses.[149-151] Although there has been some experience with the use of MDCT for the evaluation of myocardial perfusion for assessment of functional significance of coronary artery lesions, at present, current MDCT systems still have limited coverage of the heart and prohibitive radiation doses to use for this indication. As such, standard noninvasive evaluation of hemodynamic significance of coronary lesions can be performed by stress nuclear perfusion, stress echocardiography, or stress CMR techniques. Information on segmental perfusion or wall motion response to either a physiologic or pharmacologic stressor can then be used to evaluate functional consequences of coronary artery lesions found on MDCT.

■ CONGENITAL CARDIOVASCULAR DISEASE

Echocardiography and invasive left and right cardiac catheterization are the primary cardiac imaging modalities used to evaluate congenital cardiovascular disease. However, echocardiography is limited by the small field of view, limited acoustic windows, and operator dependence. Cardiac angiography is limited by overlapping of adjacent vascular structures, difficulty in demonstrating the systemic and pulmonary vascular systems simultaneously, invasive nature of the procedure with risk for

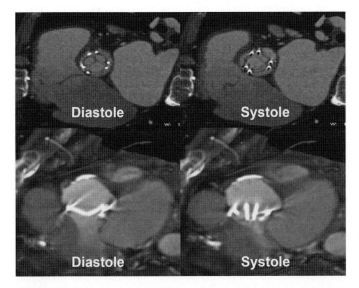

FIGURE 5–23. Multiplanar reformatted computed tomography images demonstrating a bioprosthetic valve (top) and a bileaflet tilting-disc mechanical valve (bottom).

complications, relatively high risk of ionizing radiation, and use of iodinated contrast material.

CT has been used in the anatomic and structural evaluation of congenital cardiovascular disease. With the wide field of view, information on intracardiac and extracardiac morphology, including systemic and pulmonary vascular anomalies, can be readily evaluated. Technologic developments in CT with high temporal and spatial resolution have further allowed for evaluation using multiplanar reformations, which are essential because each vascular structure has its own axis, and the cardiac heart axes are also unique to each individual. Furthermore, acquisition of multiphasic information on CT allows for assessment of cardiac chamber size and function, which is particularly useful for quantitative evaluation of structures not easily evaluated with echocardiography such as the right ventricle, or evaluations that may not be possible with CMR due to the presence of ferromagnetic implants such as closure devices or pacemakers. At present, MDCT evaluation is primarily limited to evaluation of anatomic structural disease, and further assessment of hemodynamic significance of anatomic lesions (eg, shunt quantification) requires additional data from either echocardiography, CMR, or invasive cardiac catheterization in a multimodal imaging approach depending on the patient's underlying disease.

■ SECONDARY ASSESSMENT FOR CARDIAC STRUCTURE AND FUNCTION

Echocardiography is the primary imaging modality of choice for the evaluation of cardiac structure and function. It is a cost-effective technique, widely available, portable, does not expose the patient to ionizing radiation, and provides the necessary information for management of patients with cardiac disease. However, there are several limitations with echocardiography, including operator dependence, narrow field of view, limited cardiac views dependent on limited acoustic windows, and often poor acoustic windows in patients with emphysema or large body habitus. In addition, acoustic shadowing due to high attenuators such as calcifications or metallic implants (eg, valve replacement) can further limit visualization of intracardiac structures. As a result, the complex geometry and orientation of certain cardiac structures may be difficult to fully evaluate with echocardiography.

CMR imaging has often been used as an alternative noninvasive imaging modality for evaluation of cardiac structure and function. Similar to echocardiography, CMR does not expose the patient to ionizing radiation and allows complete evaluation of cardiac and vascular structures in any field of view with a wider field of view when compared with echocardiography and can provide anatomic, functional, and hemodynamic information. In addition to anatomic structure, CMR can provide more information on tissue characterization (eg, myocardial scar or intracardiac mass) than other available techniques, which is important in patient management. CMR is evolving into the reference standard for quantification of global and regional right and left ventricular volumes and function, evaluation of valvular anatomy, and assessment of cardiovascular mass. However, the limited availability, contraindications in certain

patients (eg, pacemakers), and artifacts in patients with certain metallic implants (eg, atrial septal defect closure devices) limit its widespread use.

Cardiac CTA is most commonly used for anatomic evaluation of CAD and congenital heart disease. Although it is not the primary imaging modality for assessment of cardiac structure and function, it can be used as a supplement to echocardiography and CMR imaging. In certain cases, cardiac CTA can provide useful information on right and left ventricular size and function, evaluation of valvular disease, and assessment of intracardiac mass, particularly when there are limitations or contraindications to other available techniques, as discussed earlier. An important limitation with cardiac CTA is the need for ionizing radiation. In addition, for assessment of cardiac function, imaging must be performed throughout the cardiac cycle, leading to a substantial radiation dose penalty compared with other cardiac CT techniques that limit radiation dose to certain periods of the cardiac cycle. Therefore, CTA in this setting should be performed only in selected patients in whom the necessary information is not obtainable with other imaging techniques such as CMR.

MULTIMODAL CASE EXAMPLES

■ CASE 1

A 70-year-old woman with hypertension presents for evaluation of occasional chest pain not related to exertion. Current medication was amlodipine. The patient was normotensive with a blood pressure of 127/82 mm Hg and heart rate of 70 bpm. Total cholesterol was 190 mg/dL, with high-density lipoprotein of 55 mg/dL and low-density lipoprotein of 130 mg/dL. Framingham risk score was calculated to be 5%. The patient was referred for exercise nuclear stress test. She exercised for 10 minutes on the Bruce protocol with no complaints during stress and no ischemic changes on ECG. Single photon emission CT imaging performed at rest and stress demonstrated small area of mild ischemia in the basal inferior wall (Fig. 5–24). However, attenuation artifact in this same area limited the specificity of these findings. The patient was referred for coronary CTA, which demonstrated long segments of severe stenoses involving the proximal and mid right coronary artery, which was confirmed on x-ray angiography (Fig. 5–25). The patient was treated with aggressive medical management without revascularization.

■ CASE 2

A 55-year-old man with lone atrial fibrillation presents for evaluation of left atrial and pulmonary vein anatomy prior to pulmonary vein isolation procedure. Transesophageal echocardiography performed for evaluation of left atrial thrombus revealed an abnormal cystic structure noted in the interatrial septum (Fig. 5–26) without significant enhancement after injection of agitated saline. Cardiac CT imaging performed for further definition of left atrial anatomy revealed evidence of atrial septal aneurysm with unusual configuration, which corresponded to the cystic abnormality visualized on the echocardiogram (Fig. 5–27).

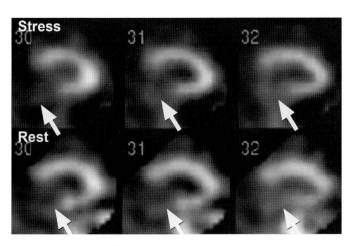

FIGURE 5–24. Stress and rest technetium 99m–sestamibi single photon emission computed tomography images demonstrating perfusion defect involving the basal inferior wall (arrows) on stress images that partially fills in on rest images suggestive of mixed myocardial infarct with peri-infarct ischemia.

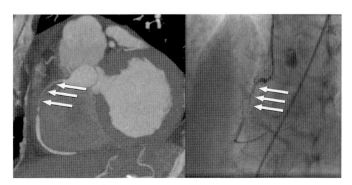

FIGURE 5–25. Multiplanar reformatted coronary computed tomography angiography (left) and corresponding x-ray coronary angiography (right) images demonstrating occluded right coronary artery with bridging collaterals (arrows).

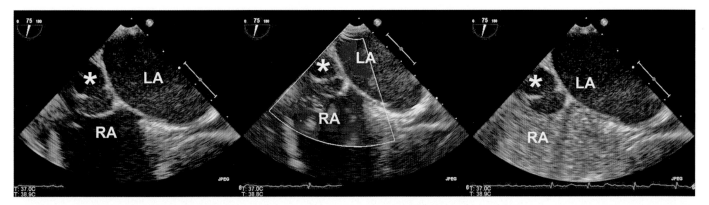

FIGURE 5–26. Transesophageal echocardiography images with transducer rotated to 75° in two dimensions (left), color Doppler (middle), and after administration of agitated saline (right) demonstrating cystic-appearing structure (asterisk) in the interatrial septum. LA, left atrium; RA, right atrium.

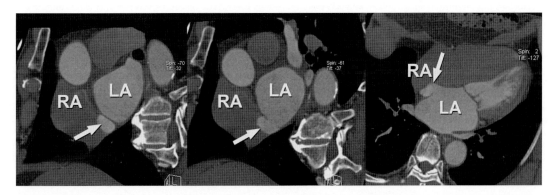

FIGURE 5–27. Multiplanar reformatted computed tomography images in short axial (left and middle) and long axis (right) views of the heart demonstrating large interatrial septal aneurysm (arrows) with unusual cystic appearance (left) depending on orientation of slice plane. LA, left atrium; RA, right atrium.

ACKNOWLEDGMENTS

We gratefully acknowledge Martha Helmers for her hard work in preparing the final figures for this chapter.

REFERENCES

1. Wintersperger BJ, Nikolaou K. Basics of cardiac MDCT: techniques and contrast application. *Eur Radiol.* 2005;15(Suppl 2):B2-B9.
2. Flohr T, Ohnesorge B. Heart rate adaptive optimization of spatial and temporal resolution for electrocardiogram-gated multislice spiral CT of the heart. *J Comput Assist Tomogr.* 2001;25:907-923.
3. Schroeder S, Kopp AF, Baumbach A, et al. Noninvasive detection and evaluation of atherosclerotic coronary plaques with multislice computed tomography. *J Am Coll Cardiol.* 2001;37:1430-1435.
4. de Feyter PJ, Nieman K. New coronary imaging techniques: what to expect? *Heart.* 2002;87:195-197.
5. Kopp AF, Schroeder S, Kuettner A, et al. Non-invasive coronary angiography with high resolution multidetector-row computed tomography. Results in 102 patients. *Eur Heart J.* 2002;23:1714-1725.
6. Gerber TC, Kuzo RS, Karstaedt N, et al. Current results and new developments of coronary angiography with use of contrast-enhanced computed tomography of the heart. *Mayo Clin Proc.* 2002;77:55-71.
7. Nikolaou K, Flohr T, Knez A, et al. Advances in cardiac CT imaging: 64-slice scanner. *Int J Cardiovasc Imaging.* 2004;20:535-540.
8. Pannu HK, Flohr TG, Corl FM, Fishman EK. Current concepts in multidetector row CT evaluation of the coronary arteries: principles, techniques, and anatomy. *Radiographics.* 2003;23(Spec No):S111-S125.
9. Hill JA. Nonionic contrast use in cardiac angiography. *Invest Radiol.* 1993;28 (Suppl 5):S48-S53; discussion S54.
10. Gilard M, Pennec PY, Cornily JC, et al. Multi-slice computer tomography of left ventricular function with automated analysis software in comparison with conventional ventriculography. *Eur J Radiol.* 2006;59:270-275.
11. Dirksen MS, Bax JJ, de Roos A, et al. Usefulness of dynamic multislice computed tomography of left ventricular function in unstable angina pectoris and comparison with echocardiography. *Am J Cardiol.* 2002;90:1157-1160.
12. Mahnken AH, Spuentrup E, Niethammer M, et al. Quantitative and qualitative assessment of left ventricular volume with ECG-gated multislice spiral CT: value of different image reconstruction algorithms in comparison to MRI. *Acta Radiol.* 2003;44:604-611.
13. Juergens KU, Grude M, Maintz D, et al. Multi-detector row CT of left ventricular function with dedicated analysis software versus MR imaging: initial experience. *Radiology.* 2004;230:403-410.
14. Budoff MJ. Maximizing dose reductions with cardiac CT. *Int J Card Imaging.* 2009; 25(Suppl 2):279-287.
15. Boudoulas H, Rittgers SE, Lewis RP, Leier CV, Weissler AM. Changes in diastolic time with various pharmacologic agents: implication for myocardial perfusion. *Circulation.* 1979;60:164-169.
16. Boudoulas H, Lewis RP, Rittgers SE, Leier CV, Vasko JS. Increased diastolic time: a possible important factor in the benefical effect of propranolol in patients with coronary artery disease. *J Cardiovasc Pharmacol.* 1979;1:503-513.
17. Shim SS, Kim Y, Lim SM. Improvement of image quality with beta-blocker premedication on ECG-gated 16-MDCT coronary angiography. *AJR Am J Roentgenol.* 2005;184:649-654.
18. Fayad ZA, Fuster V. Clinical imaging of the high-risk or vulnerable atherosclerotic plaque. *Circ Res.* 2001;89:305-316.
19. O'Malley PG, Greenberg BA, Taylor AJ. Cost-effectiveness of using electron beam computed tomography to identify patients at risk for clinical coronary artery disease. *Am Heart J.* 2004;148:106-113.
20. Rumberger JA, Behrenbeck T, Breen JF, Sheedy PF 2nd. Coronary calcification by electron beam computed tomography and obstructive coronary artery disease: a model for costs and effectiveness of diagnosis as compared with conventional cardiac testing methods. *J Am Coll Cardiol.* 1999;33:453-462.
21. Raggi P, Callister TQ, Cooil B, Russo DJ, Lippolis NJ, Patterson RE. Evaluation of chest pain in patients with low to intermediate pretest probability of coronary artery disease by electron beam computed tomography. *Am J Cardiol.* 2000;85:283-288.
22. Clouse ME. How useful is computed tomography for screening for coronary artery disease? Noninvasive screening for coronary artery disease with computed tomography is useful. *Circulation.* 2006;113:125-146; discussion 125-146.
23. O'Rourke RA, Brundage BH, Froelicher VF, et al. American College of Cardiology/American Heart Association Expert Consensus document on electron-beam computed tomography for the diagnosis and prognosis of coronary artery disease. *Circulation.* 2000;102:126-140.
24. Agatston AS, Janowitz WR, Hildner FJ, Zusmer NR, Viamonte M Jr, Detrano R. Quantification of coronary artery calcium using ultrafast computed tomography. *J Am Coll Cardiol.* 1990;15:827-832.
25. Callister TQ, Cooil B, Raya SP, Lippolis NJ, Russo DJ, Raggi P. Coronary artery disease: improved reproducibility of calcium scoring with an electron-beam CT volumetric method. *Radiology.* 1998;208:807-814.
26. Hong C, Becker CR, Schoepf UJ, Ohnesorge B, Bruening R, Reiser MF. Coronary artery calcium: absolute quantification in nonenhanced and contrast-enhanced multi-detector row CT studies. *Radiology.* 2002;223:474-480.
27. Hong C, Bae KT, Pilgram TK. Coronary artery calcium: accuracy and reproducibility of measurements with multi-detector row CT—assessment of effects of different thresholds and quantification methods. *Radiology.* 2003;227:795-801.
28. Becker CR, Kleffel T, Crispin A, et al. Coronary artery calcium measurement: agreement of multirow detector and electron beam CT. *AJR Am J Roentgenol.* 2001;176:1295-1298.
29. Horiguchi J, Yamamoto H, Akiyama Y, Marukawa K, Hirai N, Ito K. Coronary artery calcium scoring using 16-MDCT and a retrospective ECG-gating reconstruction algorithm. *AJR Am J Roentgenol.* 2004;183:103-108.
30. Becker CR, Ohnesorge BM, Schoepf UJ, Reiser MF. Current development of cardiac imaging with multidetector-row CT. *Eur J Radiol.* 2000;36:97-103.
31. Becker CR, Nikolaou K, Muders M, et al. Ex vivo coronary atherosclerotic plaque characterization with multi-detector-row CT. *Eur Radiol.* 2003;13:2094-2098.
32. Nikolaou K, Becker CR, Muders M, et al. Multidetector-row computed tomography and magnetic resonance imaging of atherosclerotic lesions in human ex vivo coronary arteries. *Atherosclerosis.* 2004;174:243-252.
33. Pugliese F, Mollet NR, Runza G, et al. Diagnostic accuracy of non-invasive 64-slice CT coronary angiography in patients with stable angina pectoris. *Eur Radiol.* 2006;16:575-582.
34. Mollet NR, Cademartiri F, van Mieghem CA, et al. High-resolution spiral computed tomography coronary angiography in patients referred for diagnostic conventional coronary angiography. *Circulation.* 2005;112:2318-2323.
35. Nieman K, Oudkerk M, Rensing BJ, et al. Coronary angiography with multi-slice computed tomography. *Lancet.* 2001;357:599-603.
36. Ropers D, Baum U, Pohle K, et al. Detection of coronary artery stenoses with thin-slice multi-detector row spiral computed tomography and multiplanar reconstruction. *Circulation.* 2003;107:664-666.
37. Schroeder S, Kopp AF, Baumbach A, et al. Noninvasive detection of coronary lesions by multislice computed tomography: results of the New Age pilot trial. *Catheter Cardiovasc Interv.* 2001;53:352-358.
38. Kuettner A, Trabold T, Schroeder S, et al. Noninvasive detection of coronary lesions using 16-detector multislice spiral computed tomography technology: initial clinical results. *J Am Coll Cardiol.* 2004;44:1230-1237.
39. Leber AW, Knez A, von Ziegler F, et al. Quantification of obstructive and nonobstructive coronary lesions by 64-slice computed tomography: a comparative study with quantitative coronary angiography and intravascular ultrasound. *J Am Coll Cardiol.* 2005;46:147-154.
40. Baltaxe HA, Wixson D. The incidence of congenital anomalies of the coronary arteries in the adult population. *Radiology.* 1977;122:47-52.
41. Yamanaka O, Hobbs RE. Coronary artery anomalies in 126,595 patients undergoing coronary arteriography. *Cathet Cardiovasc Diagn.* 1990;21:28-40.
42. Manghat NE, Morgan-Hughes GJ, Marshall AJ, Roobottom CA. Multidetector row computed tomography: imaging congenital coronary artery anomalies in adults. *Heart.* 2005;91:1515-1522.
43. White CS, Laskey WK, Stafford JL, NessAiver M. Coronary MRA: use in assessing anomalies of coronary artery origin. *J Comput Assist Tomogr.* 1999;23:203-207.
44. Maintz D, Seifarth H, Raupach R, et al. 64-slice multidetector coronary CT angiography: in vitro evaluation of 68 different stents. *Eur Radiol.* 2006;16:818-826.

45. Seifarth H, Raupach R, Schaller S, et al. Assessment of coronary artery stents using 16-slice MDCT angiography: evaluation of a dedicated reconstruction kernel and a noise reduction filter. *Eur Radiol.* 2005;15:721-726.

46. Maintz D, Grude M, Fallenberg EM, Heindel W, Fischbach R. Assessment of coronary arterial stents by multislice-CT angiography. *Acta Radiol.* 2003;44:597-603.

47. Kruger S, Mahnken AH, Sinha AM, et al. Multislice spiral computed tomography for the detection of coronary stent restenosis and patency. *Int J Cardiol.* 2003;89:167-172.

48. Ligabue G, Rossi R, Ratti C, Favali M, Modena MG, Romagnoli R. Noninvasive evaluation of coronary artery stents patency after PTCA: role of multislice computed tomography. *Radiol Med (Torino).* 2004;108: 128-137.

49. Mahnken AH, Buecker A, Wildberger JE, et al. Coronary artery stents in multislice computed tomography: in vitro artifact evaluation. *Invest Radiol.* 2004;39:27-33.

50. Maintz D, Seifarth H, Flohr T, et al. Improved coronary artery stent visualization and in-stent stenosis detection using 16-slice computed-tomography and dedicated image reconstruction technique. *Invest Radiol.* 2003;38:790-795.

51. Schuijf JD, Bax JJ, Jukema JW, et al. Feasibility of assessment of coronary stent patency using 16-slice computed tomography. *Am J Cardiol.* 2004;94:427-430.

52. Hong C, Chrysant GS, Woodard PK, Bae KT. Coronary artery stent patency assessed with in-stent contrast enhancement measured at multi-detector row CT angiography: initial experience. *Radiology.* 2004;233:286-291.

53. Gilard M, Cornily JC, Rioufol G, et al. Noninvasive assessment of left main coronary stent patency with 16-slice computed tomography. *Am J Cardiol.* 2005;95:110-112.

54. Anders K, Baum U, Schmid M, et al. Coronary artery bypass graft (CABG) patency: assessment with high-resolution submillimeter 16-slice multidetector-row computed tomography (MDCT) versus coronary angiography. *Eur J Radiol.* 2006;57:336-344.

55. Marano R, Storto ML, Maddestra N, Bonomo L. Non-invasive assessment of coronary artery bypass graft with retrospectively ECG-gated four-row multi-detector spiral computed tomography. *Eur Radiol.* 2004;14: 1353-1362.

56. Go AS, Hylek EM, Phillips KA, et al. Prevalence of diagnosed atrial fibrillation in adults: national implications for rhythm management and stroke prevention: the AnTicoagulation and Risk Factors in Atrial Fibrillation (ATRIA) Study. *JAMA.* 2001;285:2370-2375.

57. Lacomis JM, Wigginton W, Fuhrman C, Schwartzman D, Armfield DR, Pealer KM. Multi-detector row CT of the left atrium and pulmonary veins before radio-frequency catheter ablation for atrial fibrillation. *Radiographics.* 2003;23(Spec No):S35-S48; discussion S48-S50.

58. Ghaye B, Szapiro D, Dacher JN, et al. Percutaneous ablation for atrial fibrillation: the role of cross-sectional imaging. *Radiographics.* 2003;23(Spec No):S19-S33; discussion S48-S50.

59. Pilleul F, Merchant N. MRI of the pulmonary veins: comparison between 3D MR angiography and T1-weighted spin echo. *J Comput Assist Tomogr.* 2000;24:683-687.

60. Warnes CA, Liberthson R, Danielson GK, et al. Task force 1: the changing profile of congenital heart disease in adult life. *J Am Coll Cardiol.* 2001;37:1170-1175.

61. Moller JH. Alexander S. Nadas Lecture. Fifty years of pediatric cardiology and challenges for the future. *Circulation.* 1994;89:2479-2483.

62. Funabashi N, Asano M, Sekine T, Nakayama T, Komuro I. Direction, location, and size of shunt flow in congenital heart disease evaluated by ECG-gated multislice computed tomography. *Int J Cardiol.* 2006;112:399-404.

63. Tomoda H, Hoshiai M, Furuya H, et al. Evaluation of pericardial effusion with computed tomography. *Am Heart J.* 1980;99:701-706.

64. Wang ZJ, Reddy GP, Gotway MB, Yeh BM, Hetts SW, Higgins CB. CT and MR imaging of pericardial disease. *Radiographics.* 2003;23(Spec No):S167-S180.

65. Talreja DR, Edwards WD, Danielson GK, et al. Constrictive pericarditis in 26 patients with histologically normal pericardial thickness. *Circulation.* 2003;108:1852-1857.

66. Link KM, Lesko NM. MR evaluation of cardiac/juxtacardiac masses. *Top Magn Reson Imaging.* 1995;7:232-245.

67. Tsuchiya F, Kohno A, Saitoh R, Shigeta A. CT findings of atrial myxoma. *Radiology.* 1984;151:139-143.

68. Masui T, Takahashi M, Miura K, Naito M, Tawarahara K. Cardiac myxoma: identification of intratumoral hemorrhage and calcification on MR images. *AJR Am J Roentgenol.* 1995;164:850-852.

69. Grebenc ML, Rosado de Christenson ML, Burke AP, Green CE, Galvin JR. Primary cardiac and pericardial neoplasms: radiologic-pathologic correlation. *Radiographics.* 2000;20:1073-1103.

70. Kim YK, Yong HS, Kang EY, Woo OH. Left atrial myxoma with neovascularization: detected on cardiac computed tomography angiography. *Int J Cardiovasc Imaging.* 2009;25(Suppl 1):95-98.

71. Shapiro LM. Cardiac tumours: diagnosis and management. *Heart.* 2001;85:218-222.

72. Alkadhi H, Leschka S, Hurlimann D, Jenni R, Genoni M, Wildermuth S. Fibroelastoma of the aortic valve. Evaluation with echocardiography and 64-slice CT. *Herz.* 2005;30:438.

73. King SJ, Smallhorn JF, Burrows PE. Epicardial lipoma: imaging findings. *AJR Am J Roentgenol.* 1993;160:261-262.

74. Grande AM, Minzioni G, Pederzolli C, et al. Cardiac lipomas. Description of 3 cases. *J Cardiovasc Surg (Torino).* 1998;39:813-815.

75. Conces DJ Jr, Vix VA, Tarver RD. Diagnosis of a myocardial lipoma by using CT. *AJR Am J Roentgenol.* 1989;153:725 726.

76. Araoz PA, Mulvagh SL, Tazelaar HD, Julsrud PR, Breen JF. CT and MR imaging of benign primary cardiac neoplasms with echocardiographic correlation. *Radiographics.* 2000;20:1303-1319.

77. Beghetti M, Gow RM, Haney I, Mawson J, Williams WG, Freedom RM. Pediatric primary benign cardiac tumors: a 15-year review. *Am Heart J.* 1997;134:1107-1114.

78. Brown JJ, Barakos JA, Higgins CB. Magnetic resonance imaging of cardiac and paracardiac masses. *J Thorac Imaging.* 1989;4:58-64.

79. Valente M, Cocco P, Thiene G, et al. Cardiac fibroma and heart transplantation. *J Thorac Cardiovasc Surg.* 1993;106:1208-1212.

80. Muhler EG, Turniski-Harder V, Engelhardt W, von Bernuth G. Cardiac involvement in tuberous sclerosis. *Br Heart J.* 1994;72:584-590.

81. Seguin JR, Coulon P, Huret C, Grolleau-Roux R, Chaptal PA. Intrapericardial teratoma in infancy: a rare disease. *J Cardiovasc Surg (Torino).* 1986;27: 509-511.

82. Beghetti M, Prieditis M, Rebeyka IM, Mawson J. Images in cardiovascular medicine. Intrapericardial teratoma. *Circulation.* 1998;97:1523-1524.

83. Tollens T, Casselman F, Devlieger H, et al. Fetal cardiac tamponade due to an intrapericardial teratoma. *Ann Thorac Surg.* 1998;66:559-560.

84. Lo LJ, Nucho RC, Allen JW, Rohde RL, Lau FY. Left atrial cardiac hemangioma associated with shortness of breath and palpitations. *Ann Thorac Surg.* 2002;73:979-981.

85. Oshima H, Hara M, Kono T, Shibamoto Y, Mishima A, Akita S. Cardiac hemangioma of the left atrial appendage: CT and MR findings. *J Thorac Imaging.* 2003;18:204-206.

86. Hoffmann U, Globits S, Schima W, et al. Usefulness of magnetic resonance imaging of cardiac and paracardiac masses. *Am J Cardiol.* 2003;92:890-895.

87. Abraham KP, Reddy V, Gattuso P. Neoplasms metastatic to the heart: review of 3314 consecutive autopsies. *Am J Cardiovasc Pathol.* 1990;3: 195-198.

88. Klatt EC, Heitz DR. Cardiac metastases. *Cancer.* 1990;65:1456-1459.

89. Lam KY, Dickens P, Chan AC. Tumors of the heart. A 20-year experience with a review of 12,485 consecutive autopsies. *Arch Pathol Lab Med.* 1993;117:1027-1031.

90. Schoen FJ, Berger BM, Guerina NG. Cardiac effects of noncardiac neoplasms. *Cardiol Clin.* 1984;2:657-670.

91. Roberts WC. Primary and secondary neoplasms of the heart. *Am J Cardiol.* 1997;80:671-682.

92. Restrepo CS, Largoza A, Lemos DF, et al. CT and MR imaging findings of malignant cardiac tumors. *Curr Probl Diagn Radiol.* 2005;34:1-11.

93. Barakos JA, Brown JJ, Higgins CB. MR imaging of secondary cardiac and paracardiac lesions. *AJR Am J Roentgenol.* 1989;153:47-50.

94. Funari M, Fujita N, Peck WW, Higgins CB. Cardiac tumors: assessment with Gd-DTPA enhanced MR imaging. *J Comput Assist Tomogr.* 1991;15:953-958.

95. Schvartzman PR, White RD. Imaging of cardiac and paracardiac masses. *J Thorac Imaging.* 2000;15:265-273.

96. Burke A, Virmani R. *Atlas of Tumor Pathology: 3rd Series, Fascicle 16.* Washington, DC: Armed Forces Institute of Pathology; 1996:98.

97. Janigan DT, Husain A, Robinson NA. Cardiac angiosarcomas. A review and a case report. *Cancer.* 1986;57:852-859.

98. Rettmar K, Stierle U, Sheikhzadeh A, Diederich KW. Primary angiosarcoma of the heart. Report of a case and review of the literature. *Jpn Heart J.* 1993;34:667-683.

99. Hwa J, Ward C, Nunn G, Cooper S, Lau KC, Sholler G. Primary intraventricular cardiac tumors in children: contemporary diagnostic and management options. *Pediatr Cardiol.* 1994;15:233-237.

100. Araoz PA, Eklund HE, Welch TJ, Breen JF. CT and MR imaging of primary cardiac malignancies. *Radiographics.* 1999;19:1421-1434.

101. Jack CM, Cleland J, Geddes JS. Left atrial rhabdomyosarcoma and the use of digital gated computed tomography in its diagnosis. *Br Heart J.* 1986;55:305-307.

102. Gilkeson RC, Chiles C. MR evaluation of cardiac and pericardial malignancy. *Magn Reson Imaging Clin N Am.* 2003;11:173-186, viii.

103. McAllister HA Jr, Hall RJ, Cooley DA. Tumors of the heart and pericardium. *Curr Probl Cardiol.* 1999;24:57-116.

104. Itoh A, Okubo S, Nakanishi N, et al. Recurrent epicardial fibrosarcoma which arose 12 years after the first resection. *Eur Heart J.* 1991;12:270-272.

105. Shih WJ, McCullough S, Smith M. Diagnostic imagings for primary cardiac fibrosarcoma. *Int J Cardiol.* 1993;39:157-161.

106. Burke AP, Virmani R. Osteosarcomas of the heart. *Am J Surg Pathol.* 1991;15:289-295.

107. Chaloupka JC, Fishman EK, Siegelman SS. Use of CT in the evaluation of primary cardiac tumors. *Cardiovasc Intervent Radiol.* 1986;9:132-135.

108. Yashar J, Witoszka M, Savage DD, et al. Primary osteogenic sarcoma of the heart. *Ann Thorac Surg.* 1979;28:594-600.

109. Schneiderman H, Fordham EW, Goren CC, McCall AR, Rosenberg MS, Rozek S. Primary cardiac osteosarcoma: multidisciplinary aspects applicable to extraskeletal osteosarcoma generally. *CA Cancer J Clin.* 1984;34:110-117.

110. Reynolds JS Jr, Gregoratos G, Gordon MJ, Bloor CM. Primary osteosarcoma of the heart. *Am Heart J.* 1985;109:598-600.

111. Takamizawa S, Sugimoto K, Tanaka H, Sakai O, Arai T, Saitoh A. A case of primary leiomyosarcoma of the heart. *Intern Med.* 1992;31:265-268.

112. Paraf F, Bruneval P, Balaton A, et al. Primary liposarcoma of the heart. *Am J Cardiovasc Pathol.* 1990;3:175-180.

113. Murtra M, Mestres CA, Igual A, et al. Primary liposarcoma of the right ventricle and pulmonary artery: surgical excision and replacement of the pulmonic valve by a Bjork-Shiley tilting disc valve. *Thorac Cardiovasc Surg.* 1983;31:172-174.

114. Roberts WC, Glancy DL, DeVita VT Jr. Heart in malignant lymphoma (Hodgkin's disease, lymphosarcoma, reticulum cell sarcoma and mycosis fungoides). A study of 196 autopsy cases. *Am J Cardiol.* 1968;22:85-107.

115. Ceresoli GL, Ferreri AJ, Bucci E, Ripa C, Ponzoni M, Villa E. Primary cardiac lymphoma in immunocompetent patients: diagnostic and therapeutic management. *Cancer.* 1997;80:1497-1506.

116. Versluis PJ, Lamers RJ, van Belle AF. Primary malignant lymphoma of the heart: CT and MRI features. *Rofo.* 1995;162:533-534.

117. Tada H, Asazuma K, Ohya E, et al. Images in cardiovascular medicine. Primary cardiac B-cell lymphoma. *Circulation.* 1998;97:220-221.

118. Dorsay TA, Ho VB, Rovira MJ, Armstrong MA, Brissette MD. Primary cardiac lymphoma: CT and MR findings. *J Comput Assist Tomogr.* 1993;17:978-981.

119. Freedberg RS, Kronzon I, Rumancik WM, Liebeskind D. The contribution of magnetic resonance imaging to the evaluation of intracardiac tumors diagnosed by echocardiography. *Circulation.* 1988;77:96-103.

120. Restrepo CS, Largoza A, Lemos DF, et al. CT and MR imaging findings of benign cardiac tumors. *Curr Probl Diagn Radiol.* 2005;34:12-21.

121. Juergens KU, Grude M, Fallenberg EM, et al. Using ECG-gated multidetector CT to evaluate global left ventricular myocardial function in patients with coronary artery disease. *AJR Am J Roentgenol.* 2002;179:1545-1550.

122. Juergens KU, Seifarth H, Maintz D, et al. MDCT determination of volume and function of the left ventricle: are short-axis image reformations necessary? *AJR Am J Roentgenol.* 2006;186:S371-S378.

123. Mahnken AH, Koos R, Katoh M, et al. Sixteen-slice spiral CT versus MR imaging for the assessment of left ventricular function in acute myocardial infarction. *Eur Radiol.* 2005;15:714-720.

124. van der Vleuten PA, Willems TP, Gotte MJ, et al. Quantification of global left ventricular function: comparison of multidetector computed tomography and magnetic resonance imaging. A meta-analysis and review of the current literature. *Acta Radiol.* 2006;47:1049-1057.

125. Wu KC, Lima JA. Noninvasive imaging of myocardial viability: current techniques and future developments. *Circ Res.* 2003;93:1146-1158.

126. Pagley PR, Beller GA, Watson DD, Gimple LW, Ragosta M. Improved outcome after coronary bypass surgery in patients with ischemic cardiomyopathy and residual myocardial viability. *Circulation.* 1997;96:793-800.

127. Kim RJ, Wu E, Rafael A, et al. The use of contrast-enhanced magnetic resonance imaging to identify reversible myocardial dysfunction. *N Engl J Med.* 2000;343:1445-1453.

128. Sanz J, Weeks D, Nikolaou K, et al. Detection of healed myocardial infarction with multidetector-row computed tomography and comparison with cardiac magnetic resonance delayed hyperenhancement. *Am J Cardiol.* 2006;98:149-155.

129. Mahnken AH, Koos R, Katoh M, et al. Assessment of myocardial viability in reperfused acute myocardial infarction using 16-slice computed tomography in comparison to magnetic resonance imaging. *J Am Coll Cardiol.* 2005;45:2042-2047.

130. Lardo AC, Cordeiro MA, Silva C, et al. Contrast-enhanced multidetector computed tomography viability imaging after myocardial infarction: characterization of myocyte death, microvascular obstruction, and chronic scar. *Circulation.* 2006;113:394-404.

131. Gerber BL, Belge B, Legros GJ, et al. Characterization of acute and chronic myocardial infarcts by multidetector computed tomography: comparison with contrast-enhanced magnetic resonance. *Circulation.* 2006;113:823-833.

132. Lerman LO, Siripornpitak S, Maffei NL, Sheedy PF 2nd, Ritman EL. Measurement of in vivo myocardial microcirculatory function with electron beam CT. *J Comput Assist Tomogr.* 1999;23:390-398.

133. George RT, Jerosch-Herold M, Silva C, et al. Quantification of myocardial perfusion using dynamic 64-detector computed tomography. *Invest Radiol.* 2007;42:815-822.

134. George RT, Resar J, Silva C, et al. Combined computed tomography coronary angiography and perfusion imaging accurately detects the physiologic significance of coronary stenoses in patients with chest pain. In: *AHA Scientific Sessions 2006.* Dallas, TX: American Heart Association; 2006.

135. Smith SC Jr, Feldman TE, Hirshfeld JW Jr, et al. ACC/AHA/SCAI 2005 guideline update for percutaneous coronary intervention: a report of the American College of Cardiology/American Heart Association Task Force on Practice Guidelines (ACC/AHA/SCAI Writing Committee to Update 2001 Guidelines for Percutaneous Coronary Intervention). *Circulation.* 2006;113:e166-e286.

136. Rodes-Cabau J, Candell-Riera J, Angel J, et al. Relation of myocardial perfusion defects and nonsignificant coronary lesions by angiography with insights from intravascular ultrasound and coronary pressure measurements. *Am J Cardiol.* 2005;96:1621-1626.

137. Ragosta M, Bishop AH, Lipson LC, et al. Comparison between angiography and fractional flow reserve versus single-photon emission computed tomographic myocardial perfusion imaging for determining lesion significance in patients with multivessel coronary disease. *Am J Cardiol.* 2007;99:896-902.

138. Schuijf JD, Wijns W, Jukema JW, et al. Relationship between noninvasive coronary angiography with multi-slice computed tomography and myocardial perfusion imaging. *J Am Coll Cardiol.* 2006;48:2508-2514.

139. Buchthal SD, den Hollander JA, Merz CN, et al. Abnormal myocardial phosphorus-31 nuclear magnetic resonance spectroscopy in women with chest pain but normal coronary angiograms. *N Engl J Med.* 2000;342:829-835.

140. Shanewise JS, Cheung AT, Aronson S, et al. ASE/SCA guidelines for performing a comprehensive intraoperative multiplane transesophageal echocardiography examination: recommendations of the American Society of Echocardiography Council for Intraoperative Echocardiography and the Society of Cardiovascular Anesthesiologists Task Force for Certification in Perioperative Transesophageal Echocardiography. *J Am Soc Echocardiogr.* 1999;12:884-900.

141. Baumert B, Plass A, Bettex D, et al. Dynamic cine mode imaging of the normal aortic valve using 16-channel multidetector row computed tomography. *Invest Radiol.* 2005;40:637-647.

142. Manghat NE, Rachapalli V, Van Lingen R, Veitch AM, Roobottom CA, Morgan-Hughes GJ. Imaging the heart valves using ECG-gated 64-detector row cardiac CT. *Br J Radiol.* 2008;81:275-290.

143. Debl K, Djavidani B, Seitz J, et al. Planimetry of aortic valve area in aortic stenosis by magnetic resonance imaging. *Invest Radiol.* 2005;40:631-636.

144. John AS, Dill T, Brandt RR, et al. Magnetic resonance to assess the aortic valve area in aortic stenosis: how does it compare to current diagnostic standards? *J Am Coll Cardiol.* 2003;42:519-526.

145. LaBounty TM, Sundaram B, Agarwal P, Armstrong WA, Kazerooni EA, Yamada E. Aortic valve area on 64-MDCT correlates with transesophageal echocardiography in aortic stenosis. *AJR Am J Roentgenol.* 2008;191:1652-1658.

146. Morgan-Hughes GJ, Roobottom CA. Aortic valve calcification on computed tomography predicts the severity of aortic stenosis. *Clin Radiol.* 2004;59:208; author reply 208-209.

147. Cowell SJ, Newby DE, Burton J, et al. Aortic valve calcification on computed tomography predicts the severity of aortic stenosis. *Clin Radiol.* 2003;58:712-716.

148. LaBounty TM, Agarwal PP, Chughtai A, Kazerooni EA, Wizauer E, Bach DS. Hemodynamic and functional assessment of mechanical aortic valves using combined echocardiography and multidetector computed tomography. *J Cardiovasc Comput Tomogr.* 2009;3:161-167.

149. Smith SC Jr, Feldman TE, Hirshfeld JW Jr, et al. ACC/AHA/SCAI 2005 guideline update for percutaneous coronary intervention: a report of the American College of Cardiology/American Heart Association Task Force on Practice Guidelines (ACC/AHA/SCAI Writing Committee to Update the 2001 Guidelines for Percutaneous Coronary Intervention). *J Am Coll Cardiol.* 2006;47:e1-e121.

150. Fox K, Garcia MA, Ardissino D, et al. Guidelines on the management of stable angina pectoris: executive summary: the Task Force on the Management of Stable Angina Pectoris of the European Society of Cardiology. *Eur Heart J.* 2006;27:1341-1381.

151. Gibbons RJ, Abrams J, Chatterjee K, et al. ACC/AHA 2002 guideline update for the management of patients with chronic stable angina—summary article: a report of the American College of Cardiology/American Heart Association Task Force on practice guidelines (Committee on the Management of Patients With Chronic Stable Angina). *J Am Coll Cardiol.* 2003;41:159-168.

CHAPTER 6

CARDIAC MAGNETIC RESONANCE IMAGING IN ISCHEMIC HEART DISEASE

Erik Hedström, Martin Ugander, and Håkan Arheden

PATHOPHYSIOLOGY AND THE ISCHEMIC CASCADE / 104
   Acute Coronary Syndrome / 104
   Chronic Ischemia / 107

CARDIOVASCULAR MAGNETIC RESONANCE IMAGING / 109
   CMR Contrast Agents / 109
   Myocardium at Risk / 110
   Viability and Infarct Imaging / 112
   Myocardial Perfusion MRI / 119
   Noninvasive Coronary Angiography / 121

SUMMARY / 122

This chapter will focus on acute and chronic ischemic heart disease (IHD); the underlying pathophysiology; and the assessment of myocardial function, perfusion, infarct size, and myocardium at risk, all by cardiovascular magnetic resonance (CMR).

PATHOPHYSIOLOGY AND THE ISCHEMIC CASCADE

Understanding of CMR imaging in both acute and chronic IHD necessitates understanding of the sequence of pathophysiologic events that occur during ischemia. IHD is a dominating cause of death in Western countries and an emerging problem in developing countries. The development of IHD is related to both hereditary factors and lifestyle factors including smoking, diet, and lack of exercise. This section provides an overview of pathophysiology of ischemia with a focus on the mechanisms relevant to the etiology, diagnosis, and treatment of acute myocardial ischemia, stress-induced ischemia, myocardial stunning, hibernation, and infarction. These mechanisms are discussed in relation to the ischemic cascade, findings of myocardial perfusion and function at rest and stress, and the assessment of myocardial viability and the need for coronary revascularization.

The temporal sequence of events referred to as the ischemic cascade[1] is illustrated in Fig. 6–1. Ischemia can be described as an imbalance between myocardial oxygen supply and demand. Ischemia can thus be conceptualized in two different ways. Reduced supply in the resting condition is exemplified by myocardial ischemia in the setting of plaque rupture, thrombus formation, and acute coronary occlusion. By comparison, a person may have adequate myocardial perfusion at rest despite having a stenosis in a coronary artery. Upon physical exertion, demand is increased, and myocardial ischemia may ensue despite unchanged supply, or rather, inability to increase supply in order to meet increased demand. In terms of treatment, a situation where myocardial oxygen supply is insufficient in relation to demand (ischemia) can be alleviated by increasing supply (ie, increased perfusion following surgical or percutaneous revascularization), but also by reducing demand (ie, β-blocker therapy). If possible, both the supply and the demand sides of the ischemic imbalance can be therapeutically targeted.

■ ACUTE CORONARY SYNDROME

Acute coronary syndrome[2] (ACS) refers to clinical symptoms related to acute myocardial ischemia, sometimes called *unstable coronary artery disease.* If myocardium is affected by severe enough ischemia for a sufficient duration of time, the ultimate consequence is irreversible cell death. This is represented by infarction, seen at the top extreme of the ischemic cascade (see Fig. 6–1). During the healing process, the dead myocytes are replaced by connective tissue, forming a fibrotic scar, and myocardial contraction in the affected region cannot be restored. Furthermore, patients undergoing myocardial infarction are often subject to repeated infarction and, dependent on infarct size and location, negative left ventricular remodeling with possible dilatation and heart failure. For restoration of blood supply in ACS, either medical thrombolysis or percutaneous coronary intervention (PCI) may be used. However, the restoration of epicardial flow by PCI is not necessarily associated with restored myocardial microvascular flow, and thus, other means for restoring microvascular flow may be needed.

Major determinants of final infarct size include determinants of the severity of ischemia, which depends on the degree of collateralization, preconditioning, size of the myocardium at risk, duration of ischemia, and metabolic demand during ischemia including core body temperature. The most common cause of myocardial infarction is rupture of an atherosclerotic plaque with formation of a thrombus leading to occlusion of a coronary artery.[3] The rupture of a plaque results in exposure of collagen, lipids, smooth muscle cells, and tissue factors to the blood, leading to activation of platelets and the coagulation system.[4-6] Glycoprotein (GP) IIb/IIIa receptors on the surface of the platelets enable aggregation of platelets through cross-bridges of fibrinogen, and several vasoactive and procoagulative mediators are released. Treatment resulting in inhibition of these receptors is therefore of interest. A GPIIb/IIIa inhibitor is often used as adjuvant therapy in PCI because it may prevent obstruction of microvascular vessels, thus increasing microvascular blood flow after the restoration of epicardial flow.[7] The same agent has previously been proven to attenuate circulating inflammatory markers,[8] which are likely to take part in formation of the scar.

In ACS, the occlusion of a coronary artery results in a sudden imbalance in myocardial supply and demand. However, a more gradual development of occlusive atherosclerotic disease, as seen in many patients, may lead to recruitment of functional collateral vessels. These functional collaterals provide perfusion to myocardium that otherwise would be at risk of infarction during

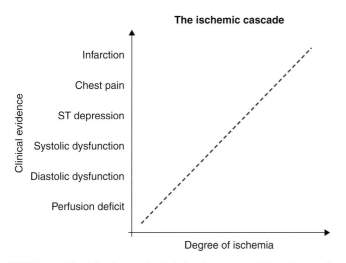

FIGURE 6–1. The ischemic cascade. As ischemia progresses, information on the severity is most sensitive when using imaging modalities that depict ischemia followed by imaging modalities that depict function. Electrocardiographic changes are usually a late-stage sign of ischemia preceding chest pain.

coronary occlusion and thus alleviate the ischemic burden on the myocardium supplied by the affected coronary artery during acute occlusion.[9] In addition, the myocardium may be protected by preconditioning caused by repeated episodes of ischemia due to spontaneous closing and opening of the occluded artery during ischemia. Both collateral flow and preconditioning attenuate the ischemic injury and reduce final infarct size. Notably, the presence of native collaterals differs between species,[10] which is one explanation for the diverse results from studies of the impact of duration of ischemia on final infarct size in different animal models.

Myocardium at Risk

Apart from collateralization and preconditioning, a major determinant of final infarct size is the size of the myocardium subjected to ischemia. This is called myocardium at risk and depends on where in the coronary arterial bed the occlusion occurs. Myocardium at risk represents the maximum amount of myocardium that might be infarcted as a result of the ischemia.

A myocardial salvage index can be calculated to estimate how much of the jeopardized myocardium (myocardium at risk) has been salvaged due to reperfusion therapy. This is calculated as follows: (myocardium at risk – final infarct size)/myocardium at risk.

Regarding salvage of jeopardized myocardium (ie, myocardium at risk), animal data have shown that the duration of ischemia needed to cause 50% of the myocardium to develop into infarction is approximately 40 minutes in pig and rat and 3 hours in dog. For humans, the corresponding time to reach 50% infarction is just under 5 hours (Fig. 6–2).[11] Thus, when studying the efficiency of treatment with regard to infarct evolution, conclusions drawn from animal studies may not be directly translatable to humans, at least not with regard to time scale. This is especially important to consider when planning phase III studies, where animal research is commonly used as a basis for justifying the expected effects of a treatment in humans.

Infarct Evolution

Reimer et al[12] showed in 1977 that a myocardial infarct evolves gradually during ischemia as a "wave front" that originates at the endocardium and spreads toward the epicardium as a function of time. Final infarct size is thus also related to the duration of ischemia, defined as the time from onset of occlusion to restoration of perfusion of the ischemic myocardium. The time course of infarct evolution has been well described for several species.[10,13-20] In man, however, estimation of the time course of infarct evolution during occlusion of a coronary artery has been adapted from studies with physiologically diverse inclusion criteria that have been compensated for by the inclusion of large numbers of patients. The Gruppo Italiano per lo Studio della Streptochinasi nell'Infarto Miocardico 1 study (GISSI-1)[21] and Second International Study of Infarct Survival (ISIS-2)[22] showed that fibrinolytic therapy within 1 hour from the onset of symptoms results in a more than 50% reduction in mortality. Results from previous studies also indicate that treatment within 6 hours from onset of symptoms results in a mortality reduction twice that of treatment 6 to 12 hours after onset of pain.[23] Overall, this shows that, similarly to the results from animal models, early reperfusion is of great value in patients. Recently, the infarct evolution in man was directly studied in a group of patients with strict inclusion criteria that closely mimicked an experimental setting.[11] Two representative cases for early and late reperfusion in man are shown in Fig. 6–3, relating the final infarct size determined by late gadolinium enhancement CMR imaging to the myocardium at risk determined by myocardial perfusion single photon emission computed tomography (SPECT) imaging. Results from this study demonstrate that infarct evolution in man is considerably slower than in pigs, rats, or dogs[11] (Fig. 6–4).

The aerobic metabolism in ischemic myocardium ceases within 10 seconds of acute coronary occlusion. This initially manifests itself as impaired myocardial relaxation, otherwise known as diastolic dysfunction. Relaxation is the energy-dependent phase of the contractile cycle in the cardiac myocyte, and it is limited by the supply of energy from adenosine triphosphate (ATP). ATP is necessary during relaxation in order to pump Ca^{2+} from the cytosol back into the sarcoplasmatic reticulum through ATP-dependent Ca^{2+} channels.[24] Hence, following reduction in the supply of ATP, relaxation is the first process to be influenced. Within minutes, as ischemia persists, reduced amounts of creatine phosphate[25] and the free energy hydrolysis of ATP[26] both contribute to the continued reduction in the amount of ATP. Thus, the accumulated ATP debt further impacts on the ATP-dependent transport of Ca^{2+}, and contraction is impaired. Systolic dysfunction is the result of this compromised contraction in addition to compromised relaxation. In acute occlusion, anaerobic metabolism is quickly inhibited as a result of accumulation of metabolites.[27] In combination with accumulation of metabolites, the myocyte cell membrane eventually ruptures, thereby defining the necrosis that is the hallmark of infarction. Rupture of cell membrane leads to inability to exclude small molecules, which is an excellent marker for cell death.[28]

Myocardial infarction is first seen in the endocardial layers of the myocardium. The endocardium is most sensitive to ischemia

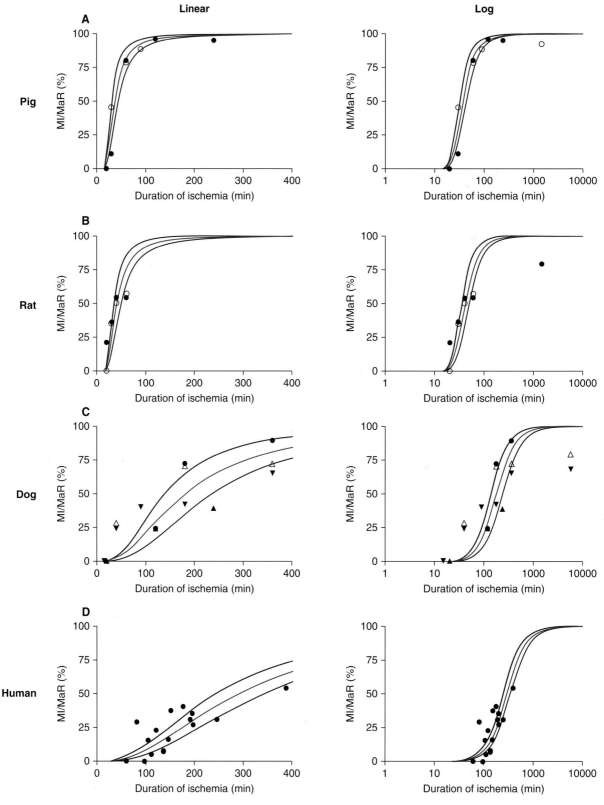

FIGURE 6–2. Myocardial infarct size in relation to myocardium at risk with respect to duration of ischemia in different species. A linear and logarithmic time scale is presented in the left and right panels, respectively. **A.** Data from previous studies in pigs (black circle = Fujiwara et al[14]; white circle = Näslund et al[13]). **B.** Data from previous studies in rats (black circle = Hale and Kloner[19]; white circle = Arheden et al[15]). **C.** Data from previous studies in dogs (white triangle = Reimer and Jennings[16]; black circle = Kloner et al[17]; upward black triangle = Fujiwara et al[14]; downward black triangle = Reimer et al[18]). **D.** Human data (Hedström et al[11]). The brown and blue lines represent the 95% confidence intervals. MaR, myocardium at risk; MI, myocardial infarction. Reproduced from Hedström E, Engblom H, Frogner F, et al. Infarct evolution in man studied in patients with first-time coronary occlusion in comparison to different species: implications for assessment of myocardial salvage. *J Cardiovasc Magn Reson*. 2009;11:38.

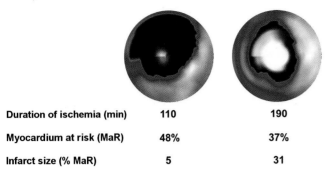

Duration of ischemia (min)	110	190
Myocardium at risk (MaR)	48%	37%
Infarct size (% MaR)	5	31

FIGURE 6–3. Fusion of polar plots from myocardial perfusion single photon emission computed tomography (MPS) acquired acutely and late gadolinium-enhanced (LGE) cardiac magnetic resonance (CMR) images acquired 1 week after acute myocardial infarction (MI) in two patients subjected to ischemia for 110 and 190 minutes, respectively. The MPS polar plots indicate myocardium at risk (MaR; black) in the otherwise well-perfused myocardium (yellow). The center of the polar plot represents the left ventricular apex, and the periphery represents the basal parts of the left ventricle. Final MI size by LGE CMR is shown in white, where brightness indicates MI transmurality from 0% (black) to 100% (white). Reproduced from Hedström E, Engblom H, Frogner F, et al. Infarct evolution in man studied in patients with first-time coronary occlusion in comparison to different species: implications for assessment of myocardial salvage. *J Cardiovasc Magn Reson.* 2009;11:38.

because myocardial depolarization and contraction originate in the endocardium and spread toward the epicardium. In contrast, repolarization and relaxation a short time later originate in the epicardium and spread toward the endocardium. The endocardium thereby has a shorter time span for myocardial perfusion during diastole compared with the epicardium. Furthermore, the largest-caliber coronary arteries lie on the epicardial surface of the myocardium, and the most fine-caliber arterioles are localized in the endocardium. The endocardium is preferentially subjected to the highest pressures of systolic ejection due to the ensuing pressure gradient from endocardium to epicardium. Taken together, the endocardium is the region of the myocardium that is most susceptible to the imbalances of supply and

demand in ischemia and is the first to succumb to infarction. Whereas the endocardial lateral borders of infarction are established early, the transmural extent of infarction extends in a wave-front manner throughout the myocardial wall. The time course of this wave front relates to the duration of ischemia.[12,16] The endocardial lateral borders of the final infarct are therefore roughly equivalent to the lateral borders of myocardium at risk. Importantly, this is not the case at earlier stages of occlusion or when infarction has been aborted.[29]

■ CHRONIC ISCHEMIA

In the setting of chronic IHD due to slow accumulation of atherosclerotic plaque over years, a more subtle progression through the ischemic cascade may occur compared with the setting of acute coronary occlusion. Patients may present in several different physiologic states of myocardial dysfunction that have not yet led to infarction or scar in the myocardium.

The term *nonviable myocardium* will here be used to describe myocardium that has been irreversibly damaged by infarction. The terms *viability* and *viable myocardium* have been used extensively in the literature to selectively describe reversibly dysfunctional myocardium while excluding normally functioning myocardium, which also is alive.[30] However, the term *viable* will be used to describe all myocardium—normal and dysfunctional—that is not irreversibly damaged.[31] Consequently, the term *dysfunctional but viable myocardium* will instead be used to selectively describe myocardium with intact cell membranes and that is in a state of potentially reversible dysfunction. Dysfunction in this setting refers to reduced systolic function.

The first event in the ischemic cascade may often be observed as compromised perfusion. Reduced perfusion may be caused by progressive stenosis due to the development of atherosclerotic plaque.[32] Diastolic dysfunction is usually thought to precede systolic function. The notion that diastolic dysfunction can exist in isolation, however, is a subject of debate.[33,34] Because a reduced amount of ATP impairs relaxation and causes diastolic

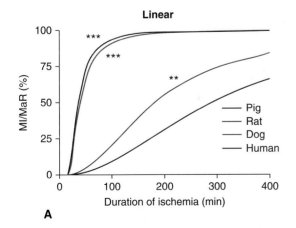

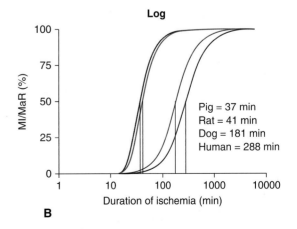

FIGURE 6–4. Infarct progression for different species. Comparison of the infarct progression slope (**A**) and the time to reach 50% myocardial infarction (MI) of the myocardium at risk (MaR) (**B**) for the different species. There was a significantly slower infarct evolution in man compared with pigs, rats, and dogs. Consequently, the time to reach 50% MI of the MaR was longer for humans compared with pigs, rats, and dogs. *** = $P < .001$; ** = $P < .01$. Reproduced from Hedström E, Engblom H, Frogner F, et al. Infarct evolution in man studied in patients with first-time coronary occlusion in comparison to different species: implications for assessment of myocardial salvage. *J Cardiovasc Magn Reson.* 2009;11:38.

dysfunction, although it has not been studied, it is reasonable to assume that increasing the deficit of ATP will affect contraction as well. Studies using sensitive measures of systolic function, such as tissue Doppler imaging by echocardiography, have identified previously undetectable reduced systolic function in patients who exhibit diastolic dysfunction.[33,35] Furthermore, it has also been proposed that diastolic filling is facilitated by the kinetic energy of the blood that enters from the pulmonary veins during ventricular systole.[36,37] This would imply that diastolic dysfunction could be augmented by reduced function during systole.

Following the reduction of myocardial function, further ATP debt affects the ATP-dependent Na^+/K^+ pump in the cell membrane.[38] Disturbances in depolarization and repolarization and, ultimately, failure to sustain the membrane potential can be observed as changes in the electrocardiogram (ECG). The accumulation of metabolites eventually leads to the development *of chest pain,* possibly due to the accumulation of adenosine.[39] Finally, if ischemia persists long enough, the result is irreversible cell rupture and infarction.

In summary, the ischemic cascade (see Fig. 6–1) describes a sequence of physiologic observations that are involved in the development of dysfunctional but viable myocardium. However, subtypes of dysfunctional but viable myocardium can readily be identified based on unique combinations of physiologic characteristics and their appropriate treatment. Notably, accurate classification by necessity includes assessment of perfusion, function, and viability. By definition, it is not possible to accurately classify dysfunctional but viable myocardium from a pathophysiologic perspective if any one of these three physiologic characteristics is left out of an assessment. Dysfunctional but viable myocardium can be categorized into subtypes based on important differences with regard to presence or absence of compromised perfusion, function, cellular integrity, and need for revascularization. The characteristics of different categories of ischemically compromised myocardium are summarized in Table 6–1.

Stress-Induced Ischemia

Stress-induced ischemia is characterized by viable myocardium that has normal perfusion and function at rest, but where perfusion and function are compromised at stress. Stress leads to an increased oxygen demand that typically can be achieved by, for example, physical exertion, increased sympathetic discharge leading to increased heart rate, increased blood pressure, and increased wall tension.[40] Stress can also be induced pharmacologically. Patients exhibiting stress-induced ischemia will benefit from revascularization, particularly those with a large extent of stress-induced ischemia.[41]

One should be aware that this definition of stress-induced ischemia represents a simplified definition that is presented for purposes of comparison. It should be acknowledged that situations may occur where the duration of stress-induced ischemia is short enough to only induce a reduction in perfusion, but not sufficient enough to induce a reduction in contractile function. Likewise, situations may occur where the duration or severity of ischemia due to stress may be sufficient to induce a prolonged but ultimately reversible reduction in function. The occurrence of prolonged resting dysfunction following the reversal of ischemia is called *stunned myocardium.*

Stunned Myocardium

Stunned myocardium is characterized by a prolonged post-ischemic reduction in function in the presence of normal perfusion and the absence of infarction.[42] The classic definition of stunning stems from observations of a prolonged but reversible reduction in systolic function following successful restoration of perfusion in the setting of experimental occlusion and reperfusion[43] and, later, acute occlusion and reperfusion in the clinical setting of ST-segment elevation myocardial infarction.[44,45] In these settings, rest and stress perfusion will both have been restored to normal, and the observed reduction in function will spontaneously resolve with time. Therefore, it is not necessary to revascularize stunned myocardium according to this classical definition.

The cellular mechanisms governing stunning have not been completely elucidated. Dominant views include the influence of oxidant stress from reactive oxygen species, as well as disturbances in calcium homeostasis.[46,47] There are, however, situations where stunning occurs as a result of stress-induced ischemia, and thus, these patients would require revascularization. Such scenarios can be referred to as *repetitive stunning.*

Repetitive Stunning

Reduced function at rest is an important part of the definition of dysfunctional but viable myocardium, including stunning. As discussed earlier, stress-induced ischemia of sufficient severity and duration may

TABLE 6–1. Physiologic Characteristics Used to Define Different Categories of Ischemically Compromised Myocardium

	Function		Perfusion			
	Rest	Stress	Rest	Stress	Cell Death	Need for Revasc.
Normal	Norm	Norm	Norm	Norm	No	No
Stress-induced ischemia	Norm	↓	Norm	↓	No	Yes
Stunning	↓	↓	Norm	Norm	No	No
Repetitive stunning	↓	↓	Norm	↓	No[a]	Yes
Hibernation	↓	↓	↓	↓	No[a]	Yes
Infarction	↓	↓	↓	↓	Yes	No

[a] Repetitive stunning or hibernation may induce cellular morphologic changes, which are characterized by both adaptive and degenerative features,[59] but not widespread necrosis as is seen in myocardial infarction.

Norm, normal; Revasc., revascularization.

induce a reduction in function that persists until the next ischemic episode despite the return of normal resting perfusion between ischemic episodes. This has been observed in both experimental animals[48] and patients with chest pain upon exertion.[49] These patients have stress-induced ischemia, and if they are not revascularized, the risk of stunning is present whenever these patients are subjected to sufficient stress. Furthermore, such repetitive stunning cumulatively induces a greater reduction in postischemic resting function than one episode alone.[50,51] In summary, myocardium exhibiting repetitive stunning is repeatedly stunned by stress-induced ischemia and should therefore be revascularized.

Hibernating Myocardium

Hibernating myocardium[52] is defined as "a state of persistently impaired myocardial and left ventricular function at rest due to reduced coronary blood flow that can be partially or completely restored to normal if the myocardial oxygen supply/demand relationship is favorably altered, either by improving blood flow and/or by reducing demand."[53] Thus, hibernating myocardium is characterized by a chronic reduction in resting function as an adaptation to reduced resting perfusion in the absence of infarction. Clinical studies have shown that myocardium with reduced function and perfusion at rest may regain function following improvement in resting perfusion by revascularization.[54-58]

The ultrastructural and histologic morphology of hibernating myocardium has been studied using transmural needle biopsies taken at the time of open heart surgery. In summary, the features include signs of atrophy, most notably in the contractile myofibrils, and signs of degeneration and possibly dedifferentiation, most notably in the interstitial space.[59] The severity of interstitial fibrosis has been shown to increase with increased duration of the symptomatic ischemia.[60] Also, the amount of myocytes with excess glycogen is exponentially related to the time required for functional recovery following revascularization.[61] Importantly though, noninvasive assessment of changes in perfusion and metabolism cannot currently distinguish between myocardium of mild or severe histologic degeneration.[62]

Controversy exists regarding whether hibernating myocardium with reduction in both resting function and perfusion readily exists or whether the more common mechanism for resting dysfunction is repeated episodes of stress-induced ischemia due to a reduced coronary flow reserve leading to stunning in myocardium with otherwise normal resting perfusion.[59]

An experimental model of hibernation in swine sustained for 1 month has shown normal resting perfusion in one third of the volume of dysfunctional but viable myocardium.[63] However, studies of patients with chronic IHD have shown normal resting perfusion in approximately 90% of regions of the left ventricle identified as having dysfunctional but viable myocardium.[64,65] These clinical data support the notion that dysfunctional but viable myocardium is predominantly comprised of repetitive stunning. By comparison, a review of 26 studies comprising 372 patients undergoing quantitative assessment of resting myocardial blood flow in dysfunctional but viable myocardium showed that 49% of the patients were found to have significantly

reduced resting perfusion in dysfunctional but viable myocardium compared with normal myocardium.[59] Furthermore, others have identified hibernating myocardium in >20% of the left ventricle in as many as 30% to 40% of patients with IHD and a left ventricular ejection fraction ≤30%.[66,67] It is possible that these differences in findings regarding the prevalence of hibernating myocardium reflect differences in patient selection criteria in these reports.

The notion that dysfunctional but viable myocardium with reduced resting perfusion does exist is supported by findings of serially assessed improvement in resting perfusion and function following revascularization.[54-58] These data favor the concept that hibernating myocardium with some degree of reduced resting perfusion is a considerable component of dysfunctional but viable myocardium.

Of importance for the clinician, reduced perfusion at stress is prevalent regardless of whether the dysfunctional but viable myocardium is due to repetitive stunning or hibernation. Both situations merit revascularization. Reduced resting perfusion appears to be less prevalent in dysfunctional but viable myocardium but can nonetheless exist. Furthermore, it is likely that both hibernation and repetitive stunning may coexist in the same patient and even the same region of myocardium.[68] This implies a downregulation in function as an adaptation to reduced resting perfusion, but also an exacerbation of the compromise in function and perfusion at stress. Hence, the exact differentiation between hibernation and repetitive stunning may be of limited clinical importance. The identification of dysfunctional but viable myocardium in need of revascularization, regardless of subtype, is of paramount importance.[69]

CARDIOVASCULAR MAGNETIC RESONANCE IMAGING

■ CMR CONTRAST AGENTS

Paramagnetic Contrast Agents

Despite the excellent soft tissue contrast shown by CMR, some situations may benefit from increased tissue contrast. The paramagnetic CMR contrast agents predominantly affect the image contrast by shortening the longitudinal relaxation time, T1, which is measured in milliseconds. The effects induced by magnetic resonance (MR) contrast agents are typically discussed in terms of 1/T1, called R1, the relaxation rate (ms^{-1}), which is increased in the presence of paramagnetic contrast agents.[70,71] Importantly, the contrast agent itself is not visualized by CMR. Rather, CMR visualizes the relaxation-altering effect that the paramagnetic agent exerts on the hydrogen protons in its immediate vicinity. This effect depends on the number of protons available to affect, the distance to these protons, and the rotational tumbling frequency of the water-particle complex[72] and is related to the contrast agent concentration and its relaxivity (ie, how "good" the contrast agent is at affecting the protons) (Fig. 6–5). The relaxivity in vitro for the agents most often used today is approximately 4 s^{-1} mM^{-1} at 20 MHz and 37°C. The contrast agent concentration in a certain tissue depends on the

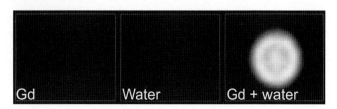

FIGURE 6–5. Three viability images of syringes filled with gadolinium (Gd), water, and Gd added to water. The syringe with Gd alone is dark in the image because no protons are available to affect. Also, the syringe with water alone becomes dark in the viability images. When Gd is added, the protons are affected, and the image becomes bright. This is also the case with edema and infarction where Gd affects the protons in the compartment.

pharmacokinetics of the contrast agent and tissue architecture. In vitro, the contrast agent concentration is considered to be linearly related to relaxivity. In vivo, however, this is limited by additional relaxation effects.[73] The signal intensity in the image is therefore not necessarily linearly related to the relaxation rate. Contrast agent concentration in a tissue, however, is proportional to the change in R1 (ΔR1), defined as the difference between R1 before and after contrast administration. Thus, R1 and ΔR1 can be quantified by using a Look-Locker sequence[74] or modified Look-Locker sequence for pixel mapping of R1.[75] A Look-Locker sequence uses an inversion pulse followed by multiple small flip angle excitation pulses. Thereby the longitudinal relaxation rate of the tissue can be estimated. This may be used in order to determine contrast agent concentrations in different regions within the myocardium, such as infarcted and normal myocardium.

The most common paramagnetic agent used today is gadolinium (Gd), which has seven unpaired electrons and thus high relaxivity.[72] Because Gd is toxic, it is chelated to a ligand, such as diethylene triamine pentaacetic acid (DTPA), 1,4,7,10-tetraazacyclododecane-1,4,7,10-tetraacetic acid (DOTA), or DTPA bismethyl amide (DTPA-BMA), in order to reduce toxicity.[76] Gd bound to ligands such as those mentioned distributes in the extracellular space[77] in the same way as inulin[78] and acts mainly on R1.

Nephrogenic Systemic Fibrosis

Recently, some Gd-based contrast agents have been suggested to be related to a rare but severe disease called nephrogenic systemic fibrosis (NSF).[79] The disease is typically characterized by fibrosis of the skin and connective tissues. It is recommended that estimated glomerular filtration rate (eGFR) be assessed in patients above age 60 and patients with hypertension, diabetes, or hepatorenal disease. In cases of eGFR <30 mL/min, it is recommended that the examination using Gd-based contrast agents be cancelled. For patients with eGFR <60 mL/min, it is recommended that the dose be reduced to 0.1 mmol/kg. Patients with hepatorenal syndrome and patients with reduced renal function who have had or are awaiting liver transplantation should be considered at risk of NSF if eGFR is <60 mL/min. It is proposed that the value of the examination should be considered and that contrast agent may be administered, even in

patients with low eGFR. Finally, there are macrocyclic contrast agents that have not been associated with NSF, and one might argue that these agents should be used preferentially. The numbers of proven cases of NSF are low in total, and the incidence may be decreased further by using adequate dose and choice of agent to be administered and using postexamination dialysis in certain cases.[80,81]

Intravascular MR Contrast Agents

Intravascular MR contrast agents have been thought to overcome some of the limitations of extravascular contrast agents (eg, in angiography where the contrast stays in the vessel without extravasation). These agents have been tested for coronary artery MR imaging (MRI),[82,83] infarct imaging,[84-86] and determination of microvascular obstruction.[87] The most promising applications are for angiography, but their clinical potential has not yet been fully explored.

■ MYOCARDIUM AT RISK

T2-Weighted MRI

Both clinical and experimental studies of treatment for acute myocardial infarction are facilitated by accurate measurement of myocardial infarct size expressed as percentage of the myocardium at risk.[88,89] The number of patients needed for a certain power is significantly lower when infarct size is normalized to myocardium at risk. The reference standard in clinical research for quantifying myocardium at risk is myocardial perfusion SPECT (MPS) (see Chapter 3). Quantifying myocardium at risk by MPS, however, requires that a radioactive tracer is injected prior to opening the occluded coronary artery. The tracers technetium 99m (^{99m}Tc) -sestamibi and ^{99m}Tc-tetrofosmin both distribute in the myocardium in proportion to blood flow[90] and are taken up by the viable myocytes, probably by a potential-driven transport of the lipophilic cation[91] and binding to the mitochondria. Very little change in myocardial distribution is seen over time. The tracer does not redistribute and has a half-life of 6 hours. Imaging can typically be performed up to 4 hours after injection.[92] Importantly, because the myocardial uptake is fast and redistribution is minimal, image acquisition will represent the perfusion of the myocardium at the time of tracer injection. Thus, if the tracer is injected during occlusion, image acquisition undertaken following reperfusion will still represent the perfusion of the myocardium as it was during occlusion.[93,94] However, there are issues with using MPS to quantify myocardium at risk, such as the logistics of radiotracer availability, need for administration before opening of the occluded coronary artery, and possible interference with post-PCI care when acquiring images. Considering these limitations with MPS imaging, other clinical methods to quantify myocardium at risk are warranted.

T2-weighted CMR has been demonstrated to show myocardium at risk in experimental studies[95-97] (Fig. 6–6). Similar findings in human studies have suggested that T2-weighted imaging may be related to myocardium at risk.[98-101] Recently, T2-weighted short tau inversion recovery (STIR) CMR imaging was directly validated in humans using MPS imaging as reference method

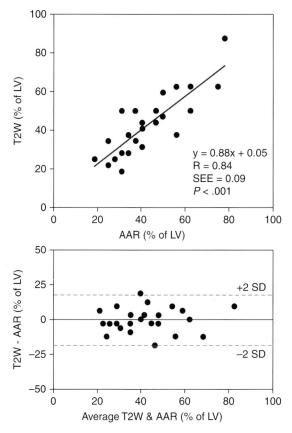

FIGURE 6–6. Agreement between areas at risk (AAR) determined by microspheres and T2-weighted (T2W) magnetic resonance imaging in an experimental model of myocardial infarction. LV, left ventricle; SD, standard deviation; SEE, standard error of estimate. Reproduced with permission from Aletras AH, Tilak GS, Natanzon A, et al. Retrospective determination of the area at risk for reperfused acute myocardial infarction with T2-weighted cardiac magnetic resonance imaging: histopathological and displacement encoding with stimulated echoes (DENSE) functional validations. *Circulation.* 2006;113:1865-1870.

and demonstrated that myocardium at risk can be quantified in humans at 1 day and at 1 week after the acute event.[102] T2-STIR MRI is thus a promising tool for measuring myocardium at risk simultaneously with final infarct size 1 week after the acute event (Fig. 6–7).

The brightness in T2 images is believed to be mainly related to increased free-water content caused by edema, which prolongs T2 relaxation.[103] This prolongation has been suggested to be related to the duration of ischemia.[104] The increase in T2 following acute ischemia is relatively small. Thus, images may only show subtle signal intensity changes. As a result, surface coil intensity correction and through-plane motion need to be compensated for. Recent enhancements include black-blood T2-STIR,[102,105] single-shot, bright-blood, T2-prepared steady-state free precession (SSFP) during free breathing,[99] and hybrid T2 bright-blood turbo spin echo (TSE) SSFP techniques with high signal-to-noise ratio and contrast-to-noise ratio[97] and single breath-hold T2 mapping.[106] The bright-blood sequences may help solve the issue of difficulties differentiating slow-flowing blood from edema of the myocardial wall, whereas T2 mapping provides the ability for absolute quantification of tissue T2.

Contrast-Enhanced SSFP MRI

In a recent study, quantification of myocardium at risk with contrast-enhanced SSFP MRI was demonstrated and validated using MPS imaging as reference method[107] (Fig. 6–8).

Endocardial Extent of Infarction

It has been argued that the endocardial extent of infarction can be used as a surrogate measure of myocardium at risk.[108,109]

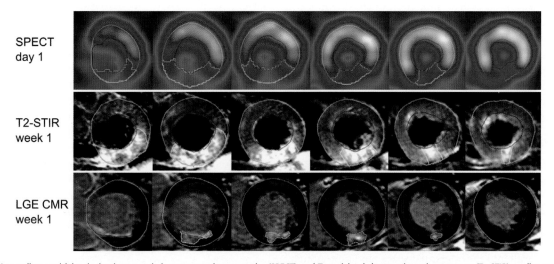

FIGURE 6–7. Myocardium at risk by single photon emission computed tomography (SPECT) and T2-weighted short tau inversion recovery (T2-STIR) cardiac magnetic resonance (CMR) and final infarct size by late gadolinium-enhanced (LGE) CMR in one typical patient. Short axis slices at the same ventricular level of SPECT on day 1, T2-STIR at week 1, and LGE CMR at week 1 in a patient with reperfused right coronary occlusion resulting in an inferior infarct. The epicardium is traced in green, the endocardium is traced in red, and the affected region is traced in yellow. Note the similarity in size of the perfusion defect during coronary occlusion by SPECT and by T2-STIR CMR 1 week later, which demonstrates that T2-STIR at week 1 can be used to quantify myocardium at risk. Reprinted from Carlsson M, Ubachs JF, Hedstrom E, Heiberg E, Jovinge S, Arheden H. Myocardium at risk after acute infarction in humans on cardiac magnetic resonance: quantitative assessment during follow-up and validation with single-photon emission computed tomography. *JACC Cardiovasc Imaging.* 2009;2:569-576. Copyright 2009, with permission from Elsevier.

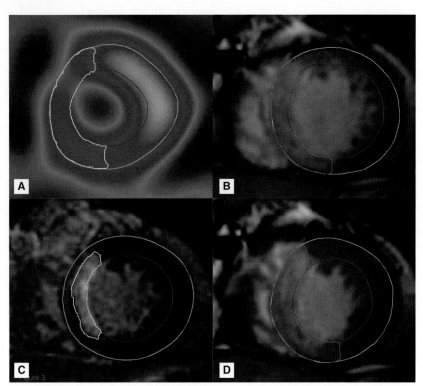

FIGURE 6–8. Corresponding left ventricular short axis views from a patient with anterior ST-segment elevation myocardial infarction. Myocardium at risk determined by (**A**) myocardial perfusion single photon emission computed tomography, (**B**) gadolinium-enhanced steady-state free precession (SSFP) at end-diastole, (**C**) infarct size images with late gadolinium enhancement, and (**D**) gadolinium-enhanced SSFP at end-systole. Reproduced from Sorensson P, Heiberg E, Saleh N, et al. Assessment of myocardium at risk with contrast enhanced steady-state free precession cine cardiovascular magnetic resonance compared to single-photon emission computed tomography. *J Cardiovasc Magn Reson.* 2010;12:25.

However, there are clinical situations with early reperfusion and a high degree of salvage or aborted infarction when the endocardial extent of infarction cannot be measured or is inaccurate.[29] Thus, in these situations, salvage should not be calculated based on the endocardial extent of infarction because it is not a reliable quantitative measure of myocardium at risk (Fig. 6–9).

■ VIABILITY AND INFARCT IMAGING

Late Gd Enhancement MRI

In vivo and ex vivo experiments have demonstrated that infarct size can be accurately assessed using late Gd-enhanced (LGE) CMR (Figs. 6–10 and 6–11).[110-112] Depiction of myocardial infarction relies on the pharmacokinetics and biodistribution of Gd chelate (ie, Gd-DTPA, Gd-DOTA, or Gd-DTPA-BMA). Importantly, the Gd chelates are small enough to readily pass across the vessel wall into the interstitial space but large enough that they will not pass across the cell wall. Thus, these Gd chelates are referred to as extracellular contrast agents. Healthy cells have intact cell membranes and exclude the tracers. Thus, extracellular MR contrast media distributes in proportion to the extracellular space.[77] Animal experiments using echoplanar MR with isotope validation indicate that the extracellular space

is approximately 20% in normal myocardium, 30% in myocardium at risk or salvaged myocardium, and 90% in necrosis where cells with ruptured sarcolemmas can no longer exclude the contrast agent[15] (Fig. 6–12).

The concept of using paramagnetic agents for enhancement of image contrast was illustrated already by Bloch in 1946.[70] The use of Gd-DTPA as a nonspecific contrast agent for CMR was discussed in 1984 by Weinmann et al,[71] and the basics for using segmented inversion-recovery gradient-recalled echo imaging was described in 1990 by Edelman et al[113] for enhanced image contrast originally for liver imaging. This was further developed by Simonetti et al[114] who introduced the technique for imaging of myocardial infarction. Image contrast between the infarcted region and normal myocardium was further accentuated by both using an extracellular contrast agent and adjusting the image acquisition so that the inversion time (TI) was set to null the signal from normal myocardium. To reduce motion artifacts, the acquisition is synchronized to diastasis during the latter part of diastole in order to minimize the effect of cardiac movement on image quality. General motion artifacts are also reduced by adding gradient-moment refocusing. The normal myocardium shows up as black in a magnitude-based inversion-recovery image, because the TI is set to null the signal from normal myocardium. Because normal myocardium has a distribution volume of approximately 20%,[77] the infarcted region with a distribution volume of approximately 90% will show as bright due to the increased relaxation rate related to the relatively higher contrast agent concentration in this region (Fig. 6–13). It should be noted that the contrast agents most often used distribute passively into the extracellular space and do not accumulate in or bind to the injured myocardium.[115] Furthermore, in cases of acute occlusion, the ischemic region may still appear bright despite absence of contrast agent[116] (Fig. 6–14). This is related to the use of magnitude images where a region lacking contrast agent will display an image intensity that is similar for reperfused infarction and nonreperfused ischemia. However, this ischemic region does not necessarily represent infarction because if this ischemic region is reperfused in a timely manner, a high degree of salvage can be expected. This potential pitfall may be avoided when imaging with a phase-sensitive inversion-recovery sequence, as described below.

Extracellular MR Contrast Dynamics

The enhancement of an infarcted region by LGE CMR is initially (during approximately the first 5 minutes after injection) related primarily to blood flow.[117] After approximately 10 minutes, a pseudo–steady-state is reached (Fig. 6–15), and contrast agent concentration throughout the body declines with renal

Myocardium at risk

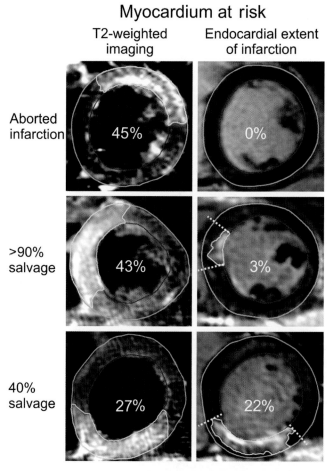

FIGURE 6–9. Myocardium at risk by T2-weighted imaging and endocardial extent of infarction. Short axis slices at the same ventricular level of T2-weighted imaging and late gadolinium-enhanced (LGE) cardiac magnetic resonance (CMR) for endocardial extent of infarction in three patients after reperfusion of an acute coronary occlusion. The endocardial borders are traced in red, the epicardial borders are traced in green, and the affected region is traced in yellow (myocardium at risk [MaR] for T2-weighted imaging and infarction for LGE CMR). The borders of the endocardial extent of infarction are indicated by dashed lines. Within each image, the total MaR is given as a percentage of left ventricular wall. The upper panel shows a patient with an aborted infarction, the middle panel shows a patient with >90% myocardial salvage, and the lower panel shows a patient with 40% myocardial salvage. Note the difference in size of the MaR by T2-weighted imaging and endocardial extent of infarction for the patient with an aborted infarction and the patient with >90% myocardial salvage. Reproduced from Ubachs JF, Engblom H, Erlinge D, et al. Cardiovascular magnetic resonance of the myocardium at risk in acute reperfused myocardial infarction: comparison of T2-weighted imaging versus the circumferential endocardial extent of late gadolinium enhancement with transmural projection. *J Cardiovasc Magn Reson.* 2010;12:18.

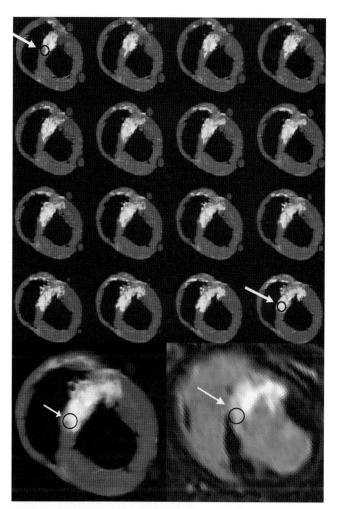

FIGURE 6–10. Comparison between ex vivo and in vivo viability images. **Top four rows:** T1-weighted short axis ex vivo cardiac magnetic resonance (CMR) images (repetition time/echo time, 20 ms/3.2 ms; flip angle, 70°; number of signal averages, two; isotropic resolution, 0.5 mm) in an image stack of 16 consecutive thin 0.5-mm thick ex vivo sections. Sections are arranged from base to apex starting at upper left and advancing left to right, then top to bottom. The arrow with circle shows a region that is not completely infarcted in the top row and almost completely infarcted in the bottom row. **Bottom left:** Image shows average of 16 thin ex vivo sections corresponding to one 8-mm thick section. **Bottom right:** In vivo inversion-recovery CMR image (repetition time/echo time/inversion time, 3.8 ms/1.1 ms/230-290 ms; flip angle, 15°; resolution, 1.56 x 1.56 mm) shows good agreement with averaged ex vivo image. Note partial volume effect seen as the relatively intermediate signal intensity on bottom right image where arrow with circle shows same region as for the corresponding ex vivo images. Reproduced from Heiberg E, Ugander M, Engblom H, et al. Automated quantification of myocardial infarction from MR images by accounting for partial volume effects: animal, phantom, and human study. *Radiology.* 2008;246:581-588.

clearance and is fully cleared after approximately 24 hours in a person with normal renal function. At this pseudo–steady-state, extracellular MR contrast agents are distributed in body tissues according to their fractional tissue distribution volume (the fraction of the tissue volume in which the contrast agent can distribute).[77] In the case of extracellular contrast agents, the fractional distribution volume corresponds to the extracellular space available in the compartment. For instance, normal myocardium has approximately 20% extracellular space (Fig. 6–16), whereas the blood pool has approximately 50% extracellular space (1-hematocrit). Acutely infarcted myocardium has undergone sarcolemmal rupture, and thus, the formerly intracellular space is exposed to and has become contiguous with the extracellular space, totaling approximately 90%.[77] Moreover, the tissue subjected to ischemia and reperfusion is swollen due to edema for hours to days.

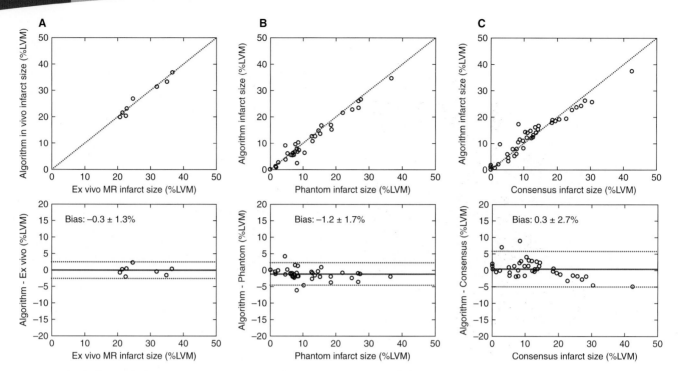

FIGURE 6–11. Graphs show results for performance of automatic algorithm for calculation of myocardial infarct size where partial volume is taken into account (see Fig. 6–10). **Top:** Results comparing algorithm with reference infarct size. Dotted line is line of identity. **Bottom:** Difference calculated by subtracting result with algorithm from reference infarct volume. **A.** Animal data. **B.** Computer phantom data. **C.** Patient data. Consensus infarct size denotes the mean of manual measurements from three observers. LVM, left ventricular mass; MR, magnetic resonance. Reproduced from Heiberg E, Ugander M, Engblom H, et al. Automated quantification of myocardial infarction from MR images by accounting for partial volume effects: animal, phantom, and human study. *Radiology.* 2008;246:581-588.

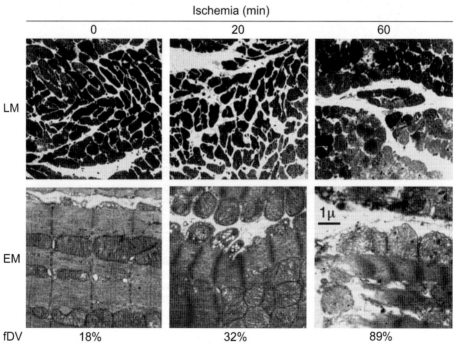

FIGURE 6–12. Light microscopic (LM, top; magnification, 380×) and electron microscopic (EM, bottom; magnification, 32,500×) sections of hearts subjected to regional moderate (20-minute) and severe (60-minute) ischemia and then reperfusion. The LM sections obtained from normal and injured regions are stained with 1% toluidine blue dye. The normal myocardium (0-minute ischemia, top left) is compact and consists of darkly stained myocytes and intact microvasculature; at EM (bottom left), it shows abundant contractile bands, mitochondria of normal size, and intact sarcolemma. At LM, after 20 minutes of ischemia (top middle), most cells appear to be normal. Some cells, however, are lightly stained, which is consistent with intracellular edema, and appear as scattered small islands of grouped cells. In some areas, the myocardium is less compact, with increased distance between the myocyte bundles, which is suggestive of increased extracellular volume. At EM, after 20 minutes of ischemia (bottom middle), most of the cells are viable. A few cells show irreversible injury. At LM, after 60 minutes of ischemia (top right), the majority of cells are lightly stained and swollen. The space between the myocyte bundles is increased compared with that in the normal myocardium. At EM, after 60 minutes of ischemia (bottom right), irreversible injury in all cells is evident, as reflected in the presence of amorphous matrix densities in the mitochondria and discontinuous sarcolemma. fDV, fractional distribution volume. Reproduced with permission from Arheden H, Saeed M, Higgins CB, et al. Reperfused rat myocardium subjected to various durations of ischemia: estimation of the distribution volume of contrast material with echo-planar MR imaging. *Radiology.* 2000;215:520-528.

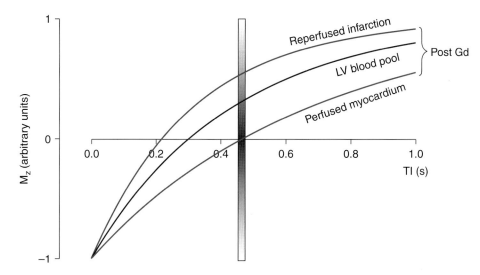

FIGURE 6–13. Longitudinal magnetization recovery curves in the situation when contrast agent has access to the injured myocardium. The reperfused infarct is enhanced in the magnetic resonance (MR) image, due to a larger tissue distribution volume for contrast agent in this region. Optimal inversion time (TI) is chosen as the time when the signal from viable myocardium is nulled. This time point is indicated by the intensity bar, which also indicates the MR image contrast, where black in the MR image corresponds to an M_z of 0, whereas bright regions in the MR image correspond to an M_z closer to −1 or 1. Gd, gadolinium; LV, left ventricle; M_z, magnetic moment in the z direction. Reproduced with permission from Hedström E, Arheden H, Eriksson R, Johansson L, Ahlstrom H, Bjerner T. Importance of perfusion in myocardial viability studies using delayed contrast-enhanced magnetic resonance imaging. *J Magn Reson Imaging.* 2006;24:77-83.

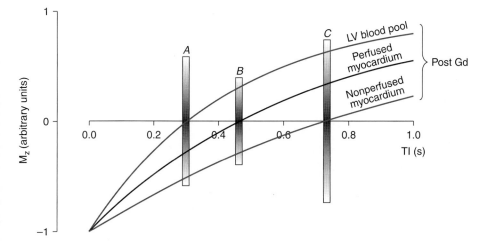

FIGURE 6–14. Longitudinal magnetization recovery curves after administration of an extracellular gadolinium (Gd)-based contrast agent, in the situation when contrast agent does not have access to the injured myocardium (nonperfused). Infarcted or not, in the absence of contrast agent, this region would still be hyperintense if the signal from perfused myocardium were nulled (see Fig. 6–19B). The higher signal intensity in nonperfused myocardium is related to the modulus reconstruction of the magnetic resonance image and is due to absence of contrast agent in this region. The signal intensity bars A, B, and C indicate nulling of the signal from blood, perfused myocardium, and nonperfused myocardium, respectively, and correspond to Fig. 6–19. Curves are derived from measured relaxation rate (R1) values applying a Look-Locker sequence 21 minutes after contrast agent administration but are presented as real data for clarity. LV, left ventricle; M_z, magnetic moment in z direction; TI, inversion time. Reproduced with permission from Hedström E, Arheden H, Eriksson R, Johansson L, Ahlstrom H, Bjerner T. Importance of perfusion in myocardial viability studies using delayed contrast-enhanced magnetic resonance imaging. *J Magn Reson Imaging.* 2006;24:77-83.

First-Pass Dynamics

The first pass of MR contrast agent is usually used to acquire short axis images for assessment of myocardial perfusion at rest and stress to determine presence of stress-induced ischemia (see later section "Myocardial Perfusion MRI").

An MR contrast agent that has been injected into a peripheral vein, usually the brachial vein, enters the right atrium from the superior vena cava, continues sequentially to the right ventricle and the lungs, and then appears in the left atrium, left ventricle, aorta, the coronary arteries, and the myocardium. If structures like thrombi or tumors are present anywhere in the great vessels or cardiac chambers, these exclude the MR contrast during the first pass and therefore appear dark. If they stay dark after the myocardium has enhanced, they are likely thrombi or other structures with low vascularization. If they enhance intermediately, they may be sparsely vascularized tumors like lipomas or fibromas. If they enhance to the same extent as myocardium or more, they may represent highly vascularized tumors such as sarcomas. First-pass images acquired in the four-chamber view may therefore be used to diagnose these conditions.

Extravasation of an extracellular MR contrast medium during the first pass through the capillary bed is high, up to 40%, which challenges imaging of vessels and direct quantification of myocardial perfusion (see earlier section "Intravascular MR Contrast Agents").

Early Images and Microvascular Obstruction

A dark core of microvascular obstruction may be seen in larger infarcts at first-pass perfusion, early Gd enhancement (EGE), and LGE MR imaging[118] (Fig. 6–17). This core is visualized with a much slower initial rise of enhancement and is typically located at the subendocardial level. This hypoenhanced core usually persists for several minutes but starts to decrease in size after approximately 5 minutes. The optimal time to detect and quantify microvascular obstruction is therefore suggested to be approximately 2 to 4 minutes after contrast injection.[119] The term microvascular obstruction comes from the severe

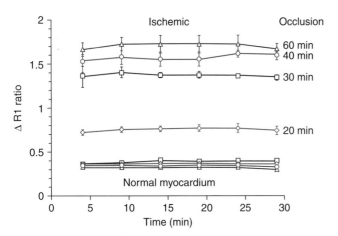

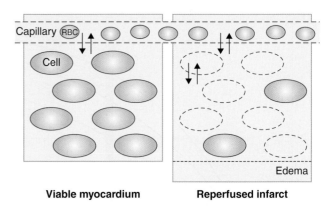

FIGURE 6–15. Change in relaxation rate (ΔR1) ratios are illustrated as a function of time after injection of 0.2 mmol/kg gadodiamide in hearts subjected to 20, 30, 40, and 60 minutes of coronary arterial occlusion followed by 1 hour of reperfusion. Note that the ΔR1 ratios in normal and injured myocardium are constant for 30 minutes after the injection; this suggests that the ΔR1 ratios represent the partition coefficient. The ΔR1 ratios increased with the duration of occlusion. Reproduced with permission from Arheden H, Saeed M, Higgins CB, et al. Reperfused rat myocardium subjected to various durations of ischemia: estimation of the distribution volume of contrast material with echo-planar MR imaging. *Radiology.* 2000;215:520-528.

FIGURE 6–16. Schematic drawing of contrast agent distribution. The contrast agent distributes passively in the extracellular space, indicated in yellow. In reperfused infarction (right), the tissue distribution volume is increased compared with viable myocardium. This is mainly due to loss of cellular membrane integrity and to some extent related to edema. RBC, red blood cell. Adapted with permission from Arheden H, Saeed M, Higgins CB, et al. Measurement of the distribution volume of gadopentetate dimeglumine at echo-planar MR imaging to quantify myocardial infarction: comparison with 99mTc-DTPA autoradiography in rats. *Radiology.* 1999;211:698-708.

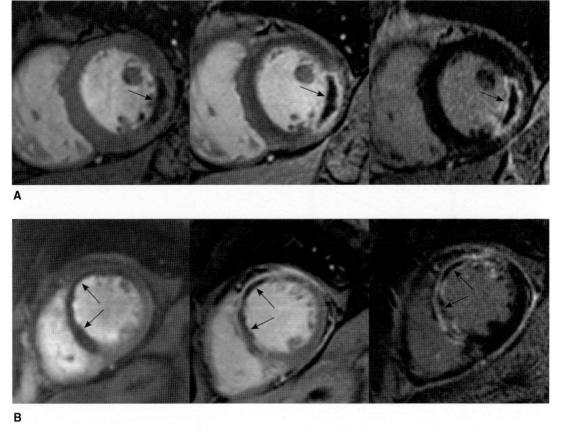

FIGURE 6–17. A. Cardiac magnetic resonance (CMR) images from a patient with acute lateral myocardial infarction. Arrows point to microvascular obstruction (MO; areas of hypoenhancement) on first-pass perfusion (left), early gadolinium enhancement (EGE; middle), and late gadolinium enhancement (LGE; right). **B.** CMR images from a patient with acute anterior myocardial infarction. Arrows point to MO on (areas of hypoenhancement) first-pass perfusion (left), EGE (middle), and LGE (right). Reproduced from Mather AN, Lockie T, Nagel E, et al. Appearance of microvascular obstruction on high resolution first-pass perfusion, early and late gadolinium enhancement CMR in patients with acute myocardial infarction. *J Cardiovasc Magn Reson.* 2009;11:33.

capillary damage due to microemboli obstructing the micro-vasculature, endothelial damage, and myocardial inflammation. Administration of a GPIIb/IIIa inhibitor seems to increase blood flow on the microvascular level,[7] and microvascular obstruction is seen to a lesser extent in patients receiving this treatment early after pain onset.

A CMR report should include information on the amount of microvascular obstruction because this determines outcome, predicts event-free survival,[120] and is more common in larger infarcts.[121] The region of microvascular obstruction is resorbed and heals to thin scar over time.[122]

Late Gd Enhancement

LGE CMR images are acquired for visualization and quantification of myocardial necrosis, microvascular obstruction, healed myocardial infarction (scar), and other types of fibrosis due to cardiomyopathies or myocarditis.

LGE CMR has emerged as a powerful tool for accurate and high-resolution assessment of myocardial viability.[123] Validation studies have demonstrated the ability of LGE CMR to differentiate between viable and nonviable myocardium independent of wall motion, reperfusion status, or infarct age.[110,124,125] Studies in humans have shown infarct transmurality to be predictive of recovery of regional function following acute infarction,[126,127] elective revascularization,[128-132] and β-blocker therapy.[133] Infarct size by LGE CMR is prognostically significant independent of measures of systolic function.[134] It has been shown that myocardial infarction by LGE CMR exceeding approximately one quarter of the left ventricle in the acute setting will predict negative remodeling (increased end-diastolic volume and reduced ejection fraction) over time.[135]

LGE CMR images are typically acquired 10 to 30 minutes after Gd-based contrast agent administration.[136] The size of measured infarct on LGE CMR images does not change if images are acquired between 10 and 30 minutes after contrast agent injection (see "Extracellular MR Contrast Dynamics" earlier).[136] Myocardial infarct size overestimation has been suggested when imaging is performed too early after Gd administration (<10 minutes), and therefore, this should be taken into consideration.

LGE CMR performed within the first 24 hours after an acute infarction may result in overestimation of infarct size in experimental[137,138] and human[135,139-142] studies. This might be ascribed to edema within the core of the infarction but may also be attributed to edema of the peri-infarction zone. The core of the infarction is known to shrink over the first 24 hours. Infarct size continues to decline over the first year[142] (Fig. 6–18). The time line for when infarct size is no longer overestimated has not been fully evaluated, and the pathophysiologic background of enhancement and its overestimation of myocardial infarction size during the first week after infarction are not completely understood. Notably, LGE CMR accurately depicts infarct size in the setting of chronic fibrotic scar.[110] Because LGE may be used both for acute and chronic infarction, a T2-weighted sequence sensitive for edema may be added to differentiate one from the other.[98]

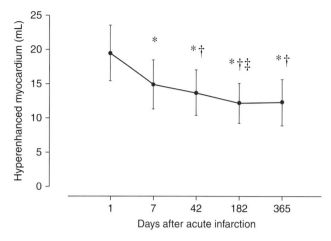

FIGURE 6–18. Hyperenhancement caused by acute infarction decreases over time with the most pronounced decrease during the first week. Vertical bars indicate standard error of the mean. $*P = .05$ versus day 1; $†P = .05$ versus day 7; $‡P = .05$ versus day 42. Published with permission from Engblom H, Hedstrom E, Heiberg E, Wagner GS, Pahlm O, Arheden H. Rapid initial reduction of hyperenhanced myocardium after reperfused first myocardial infarction suggests recovery of the peri-infarction zone: one-year follow-up by MRI. *Circ Cardiovasc Imaging.* 2009;2:47-55.

Importance of Finding the Optimal Inversion Time

Usually, infarct size by LGE CMR is considered adequate for clinical applications if imaging is undertaken using the optimal TI for nulling the signal from normal myocardium. The optimal value of TI for nulling the signal from normal myocardium depends on the scanner manufacturer and sequence timing parameters, as well as contrast agent dose, time after contrast agent administration, and renal clearance. To facilitate finding the optimal TI for nulling signal from normal myocardium, a Look-Locker sequence may be applied[74] (Fig. 6–19). In this sequence, the images are acquired as described earlier for determination of relaxation rate, and each image acquired is associated with the time after the inversion pulse. Thus, one can choose the TI when the signal from the normal myocardium is nulled in the image. To facilitate finding the optimal TI using a Look-Locker sequence, one needs to acquire representative images while choosing imaging parameters similar to those that are to be used for the subsequent viability sequence.

Phase-Sensitive LGE

The inversion-recovery sequence adapted by Simonetti et al[114] was further developed by Kellman et al.[143-145] They introduced a reconstructed image considering not only the magnitude, but also the phase of the magnetization during recovery. The phase-sensitive inversion-recovery (PSIR) sequence is therefore not so dependent on selecting the optimal TI for nulling the signal from normal myocardium (Fig. 6–20). The normal myocardium is presented as black in the image, and contrast/brightness can be adjusted for enhancing the image contrast further. The phase-sensitive reconstructed image is typically the image that is most useful for diagnosis. In cases with artifactual nulling of the signal from structures other than normal myocardium in the phase-sensitive reconstructed image, however,

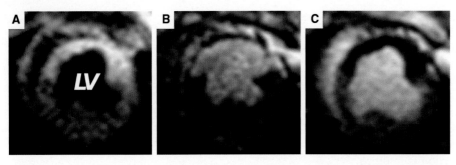

FIGURE 6–19. A short-axis image of the left ventricle acquired 21 minutes after contrast agent administration using a Look-Locker sequence consisting of 70 images, in a setting of coronary artery occlusion in pig. Three different inversion times have been chosen when the signal was nulled from blood (**A**), perfused myocardium (**B**), and non-perfused myocardium (**C**). The correct inversion time to choose for viability studies would be the one depicted in B. Compare Fig. 6–14 for longitudinal relaxation curves. Reproduced with permission from Hedström E, Arheden H, Eriksson R, Johansson L, Ahlstrom H, Bjerner T. Importance of perfusion in myocardial viability studies using delayed contrast-enhanced magnetic resonance imaging. *J Magn Reson Imaging*. 2006;24:77-83.

the standard magnitude image acquired simultaneously may be used for diagnosis. In such cases, this image is still dependent on the optimal TI for nulling the signal from normal myocardium. Therefore, the aim should be to select an appropriate TI to facilitate diagnosis, even when using a PSIR sequence.

In patients with arrhythmias, the standard magnitude or PSIR images may be difficult to interpret due to different timings of acquisition in the cardiac cycle resulting in motion artifacts. In the case of arrhythmias, it is also of value to image every other heart beat to allow recovery of the signal before the next inversion pulse.

In these situations, a single-shot SSFP sequence may also be applied.[146] This yields higher image contrast due to decreased blurriness and less motion artifacts (Fig. 6–21). Moreover, this sequence can be acquired during free breathing with respiratory gating or with a very short breath-hold (1 second) and may

therefore also be applied in patients who are not able to hold their breath for the duration of a typical breath-hold sequence (15 to 25 seconds).[147] The downside of the single-shot SSFP sequence is a decreased sensitivity to detect small areas of fibrosis/infarct.

Relation of LGE CMR to Other Methods for Viability Assessment

An important challenge in the identification of dysfunctional but viable myocardium is the determination of myocardial viability, particularly in the setting of chronic IHD. Several noninvasive imaging techniques offer this possibility, and they include thallium-201 and [99mTc] tracers used for MPS, 18-fluorodeoxyglucose (18-FDG) positron emission tomography (PET), dobutamine stress echocardiography, dobutamine stress CMR, and LGE CMR.

A comprehensive review of non-CMR techniques for viability assessment was undertaken for 105 studies of just over 3000 patients. In these studies, regional functional improvement following revascularization occurred in 53% of the evaluated segments that were identified as dysfunctional but viable prior to intervention. The overall mean weighted sensitivity and specificity of the techniques was 84% and 69%, respectively, for identification of regional functional improvement after revascularization.[148] Furthermore, pooled data have highlighted the prognostic importance of viability testing by showing that patients with significant viability who were revascularized showed a greater than 50% reduction in cardiac event rate compared with both patients who were treated medically and patients without viability who were treated either medically or with revascularization.[149]

Human LGE CMR studies have demonstrated excellent repeatability[137] and good agreement compared with 18-FDG PET,[129,150,151] MPS,[152-154] and myocardial contrast echocardiography.[155] The assessment of infarct size by MPS, however, can both overestimate[153] and underestimate[152] infarct size by LGE CMR. Importantly, one study showed that 47% of subendocardial infarcts identified by LGE CMR were missed by MPS[152]; this is likely attributable to the limited resolution in MPS. In addition, LGE CMR can be used to definitively assess viability in patients with suspected attenuation artifacts by MPS.[156] The spatial resolution in LGE CMR is much greater than in MPS and can resolve small periprocedural infarctions not detected by other techniques.[157,158]

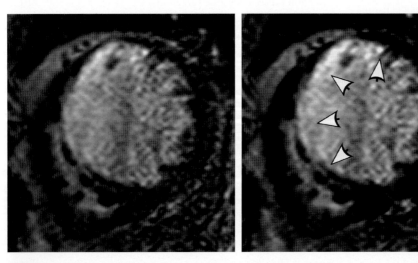

FIGURE 6–20. The standard magnitude image (left) and the reconstructed phase-sensitive image (right) in a patient with anterior and septal infarction. The inversion time is not correctly chosen to null the signal from normal myocardium. Despite this, the reconstructed image shows excellent image contrast with a homogeneous dark myocardial wall with bright infarction (arrowheads).

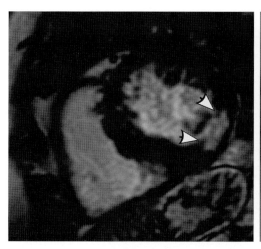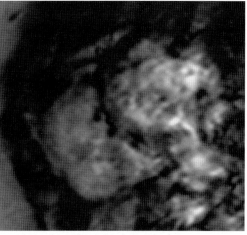

FIGURE 6–21. A T1-weighted single-shot steady-state free precession sequence applied in a patient with arrhythmia (left). The signal from normal myocardium is well nulled, and the bright inferior infarction is easily delineated (arrowheads). For comparison regarding motion artifacts, a standard sequence is shown (right).

Low-dose dobutamine stress CMR imaging involves an infusion of a low dose of dobutamine in order to assess whether or not an improvement can be seen in regional contractile function, as a measure of dysfunctional but viable myocardium. Improvement in regional function assessed by low-dose dobutamine stress CMR has shown close agreement with viability by PET[159] and a sensitivity of 89% and specificity of 94% for predicting improvement in function following revascularization.[160] Moreover, assessment using grid tagging[161] and dobutamine has shown a similarly high sensitivity of 89% and specificity of 93% for predicting functional improvement after revascularization.[162]

Studies comparing low-dose dobutamine stress and LGE CMR have shown conflicting results. Two studies have shown similar or better results with LGE CMR compared with low-dose dobutamine when it comes to predicting functional recovery following revascularization.[163,164] However, other studies have shown that contractile reserve with dobutamine is superior to LGE CMR for predicting functional recovery[165] and may add information particularly regarding the potential for functional recovery of segments with intermediate infarct transmurality.[166] Thus, the relative contributions of contractile reserve and viability by LGE CMR to functional recovery and prognostic benefit following revascularization are worthy of further study.[167]

In summary, LGE CMR has developed as the reference standard for assessment of transmurality and extent of infarction. It offers the advantages of increased spatial resolution over alternative techniques. In particular, LGE CMR is an imaging technique whereby nonviable infarction is imaged directly through an increased tissue distribution volume of contrast agent in nonviable tissue, as opposed to relying on the absence of signal or analysis of regional function as with nuclear and echocardiographic techniques, respectively.

■ MYOCARDIAL PERFUSION MRI

The importance of assessing stress-induced ischemia in the detection of coronary artery disease is paramount. The data on stress perfusion testing are extensive in the setting of MPS, which is the clinically most prevalent imaging modality for myocardial ischemia stress testing. Numerous studies using MPS have shown that the risk of cardiac events increases with the extent and severity of stress perfusion defects assessed by MPS.[41] Furthermore, the number of lives saved due to treatment with revascularization compared with medical treatment increases with the amount of ischemic myocardium identified by MPS.[168]

Pooled analysis of 79 studies (8964 patients) using MPS to detect coronary artery disease by invasive angiography showed a weighted mean sensitivity of 86% and specificity of 74%.[31] Of patients with normal MPS studies, only those with a high suspicion for coronary artery disease are referred for invasive coronary angiography. Therefore, the relatively low specificity for MPS may reflect such a referral bias. The percentage of normal MPS studies in a population with a low likelihood of coronary artery disease is called the *normalcy rate*. Thus, normalcy is a better descriptor of the performance of a test in a population without disease. The normalcy rate for MPS in 10 studies (543 patients) was 89%.[31]

For CMR, stress by external work has limitations because it is awkward to attempt physical exertion when lying supine in an MR scanner. Importantly, this inevitably leads to motion artifacts from both breathing and bulk motion. Thus, image interpretation becomes difficult, and sensitivity and specificity of the examination during external work are low.

Pharmacologic stress can be undertaken using either a vasodilator agent, such as adenosine or dipyridamole, for assessment of perfusion or a β-agonist, such as dobutamine with or without the addition of atropine, for assessment of regional contractile function. In CMR, these agents are used in the same fashion as they are used in MPS and stress echocardiography.

Stress Perfusion With Adenosine or Dipyridamole

CMR has an emerging role in the assessment of perfusion. Quantitative analysis of first-pass contrast kinetics has been used to identify stenosis by invasive coronary angiography and has been shown to correspond to perfusion by PET[169] and perfusion by microspheres.[170] Stress perfusion CMR is hampered by a lack of standardization with regard to the most optimal sequence parameters for image acquisition. There is continued development in the field, with the ultimate goal of achieving a method that can provide quantitative pixel maps of the absolute blood flow in the myocardium in units of mL/min/g tissue, analogous to PET.[171,172] In the absence of that level of methodologic maturity, CMR perfusion assessment is performed by visual analysis,

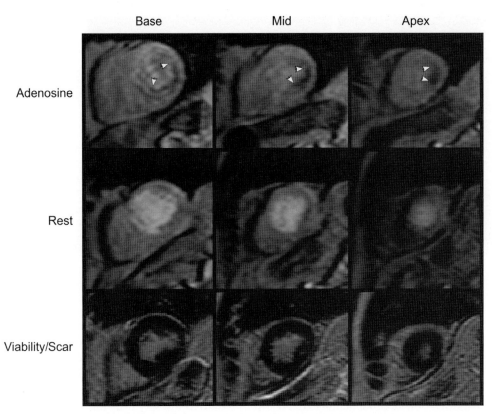

FIGURE 6–22. Myocardial perfusion magnetic resonance imaging (MRI) in a patient with significant stenosis in the left circumflex coronary artery (LCx) at the basal, midventricular, and apical level. Upper row shows first-pass perfusion at adenosine stress, middle row shows corresponding images at rest, and lower row shows corresponding late gadolinium-enhanced (LGE) MRIs. A region in the lateral wall is dark at all levels during adenosine stress (arrowheads). This perfusion defect is less prominent at rest. LGE MRIs show smaller regions of LGE. The difference between perfusion defect at stress and LGE is the region with stress-induced ischemia.

which yields sensitivity in excess of 90% and specificity of approximately 70%.

Adenosine and dipyridamole have almost identical effects. Adenosine acts directly on vascular smooth muscle, causing nearly maximal vasodilatation, whereas dipyridamole prevents breakdown of adenosine that is produced naturally in tissue. The basic principle of vasodilator stress perfusion CMR is that the vasodilator causes an up to five-fold increase in blood flow to healthy myocardium, whereas myocardium subtended by a stenotic artery will have an impeded ability to upregulate blood flow and thus exhibits a relatively delayed arrival of the first pass of an intravenously administered bolus of a contrast agent. This delayed arrival is visualized as a hypointense region corresponding to the distribution of a coronary artery (Fig. 6–22).

A multicenter multivendor trial comparing MPS and CMR stress perfusion found that CMR outperformed MPS with regard to overall diagnostic accuracy.[169] However, that study had several limitations in design. Most notably, gated MPS was not used in the MPS analysis, despite it being known that gated MPS adds significantly to the diagnostic accuracy of MPS.[173-175] Despite the challenges with CMR stress perfusion imaging, prognostic studies have begun to be published that show similar results to MPS. Importantly, a positive CMR stress perfusion examination performed on patients being evaluated for unclear chest pain

in the emergency department is independently associated with poor prognosis.[176] By comparison, a normal CMR stress perfusion study is associated with a greater than 99% probability of 3-year event-free survival.[176-179] In addition, the presence of a reversible perfusion defect by CMR is prognostically poor in a way that is complementary to the prognostic value of LGE CMR for identifying myocardial infarction.[180]

Adenosine infusion is safe.[181] During the stress study, patients should be monitored regarding heart rate and rhythm, blood pressure, and symptoms. Adenosine/dipyridamole should not be used in patients with poor pulmonary function or atrioventricular block IIa or higher due to the risk of adenosine-induced complete atrioventricular block.

Stress Function With High-Dose Dobutamine

The results from dobutamine stress CMR are reproducible, and high levels of specificity and sensitivity have been shown (~80%-90%).[182] Imaging is undertaken at rest and during increased stress levels. Because dobutamine and atropine are used for increasing contractility, they are primarily useful for assessment of abnormalities of myocardial contraction[177,182,183] (Fig. 6–23).

The administration of dobutamine usually follows a scheme with an increased body weight–adjusted infusion rate over time. High-dose dobutamine increases myocardial oxygen demand,

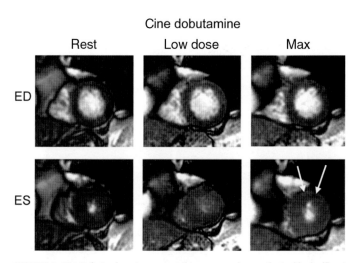

FIGURE 6–23. Dobutamine stress magnetic resonance in a patient with significant in-stent left anterior descending artery stenosis. Arrows point to region with decreased contractility at high dose. ED, end-diastole; ES, end-systole; max, maximum. Reproduced with permission from Paetsch I, Jahnke C, Wahl A, et al. Comparison of dobutamine stress magnetic resonance, adenosine stress magnetic resonance, and adenosine stress magnetic resonance perfusion. *Circulation*. 2004;110:835-842.

and thus, myocardial regions supplied by a stenotic coronary artery typically develop abnormalities in myocardial contractility due to inadequate ability to upregulate the supply of oxygenated blood. The high-dose regimen is needed to increase sensitivity and specificity for visualizing wall motion abnormalities.

Adverse effects are rare[184]; however, patients should be monitored regarding heart rate and rhythm, blood pressure, wall motion abnormalities, and symptoms. Because wall motion abnormalities precede ST-segment changes in the ischemic cascade, and wall motion may be visualized during scanning, a standard single-lead ECG, as available at the scanner, is adequate for rhythm monitoring. However, the dobutamine regimen should not be used in patients with severe hypertension, significant aortic stenosis, unstable angina pectoris, or other debilitating systemic disease.

Images are acquired during rest and increased pharmacologic stress. To image the contractility defects, fast imaging is required. Either SSFP or real-time images are used, often as a short breath-hold sequence of approximately 5 seconds acquiring approximately 30 to 40 images per heartbeat with a spatial resolution of 1.5 × 1.5 mm. When using real-time imaging, the wall motion abnormalities can be visualized during the examination and thus can be used for monitoring the patient.[185] However, the real-time images have lower spatial and temporal resolution than breath-hold images, and thus breath-hold images are preferred. Improved parallel real-time imaging may enhance image quality despite faster acquisition and thus facilitate evaluation of wall motion, while also shortening the scan time.[186] Similar to CMR stress perfusion, a normal CMR high-dose dobutamine stress study is associated with a greater than 99% probability of 3-year event-free survival.[177]

Sensitivity of the examination may be increased by adding tagging prepulses to the acquisition.[187] The tagging prepulses are applied

perpendicular to the imaging plane and appear in the images as dark lines. Thus, local tissue deformation and contractility may be visualized and assessed. Recent developments include other tissue tracking methods such as displacement encoding with stimulated echoes (DENSE),[188] harmonic phase imaging (HARP),[189] and strain-encoded CMR.[190] The dysfunctional region by strain-encoded CMR has been shown to correspond to region of infarction by LGE CMR.[191] Furthermore, phase-contrast strain measurements can be performed for assessment of regional function.[192] However, these acquisitions are currently too time consuming to be used for monitoring the patient during stress imaging.

To evaluate the images for diagnosis, the cine loops of the left ventricle are usually analyzed in 17 segments according to the American Heart Association.[193] Because these segments are based on a standard coronary anatomy, one should be aware that the segments shown may be supplied by other coronary arteries than expected. In particular, there is considerable overlap between the perfusion territories subtended by the left circumflex and right coronary arteries.[194] Collateral vessels also may contribute to variations from typical patterns. Thus, it is not possible to define which coronary artery has a stenosis or occlusion based on wall motion alone. The images in each segment are usually first graded by quality as good, acceptable, or poor. The wall motion is graded as normal, hypokinetic, akinetic, or dyskinetic. The wall motion score is thereafter divided by the number of diagnostic segments. The findings are considered to be diagnostic for ischemia either if wall motion is not increasing during increased stress or if systolic wall thickening is lacking. A reduction in wall motion or wall thickening is also considered to be indicative of ischemia.

■ NONINVASIVE CORONARY ANGIOGRAPHY

CMR can be used to perform noninvasive coronary angiography analogously to computed tomography (CT). A recent comprehensive meta-analysis confirmed that CT with 16-slice detectors or more shows a significantly better sensitivity and specificity for significant stenosis compared with CMR, although only five head-to-head studies exist.[195] One head-to-head study showed that CT had a greater number of evaluable coronary artery segments compared with CMR.[196] Interestingly, CMR was able to provide an accurate diagnosis in two thirds of the cases in which coronary segments were unevaluable by CT due to extensive calcification. CMR coronary angiography has also been shown to be able to quantify an increased coronary artery wall thickness in patients with nonsignificant coronary artery disease compared with controls.[197]

A whole-heart SSFP coronary artery MR angiography was described in 2003 that enables coronary imaging in three dimensions without the use of MR contrast agent[198] (Fig 6–24). This sequence has been used in clinical trials with promising results.[199,200]

Advantages with CMR include the lack of radiation exposure, but drawbacks include longer examination time and lower spatial resolution, in addition to the lower diagnostic accuracy. Evaluation

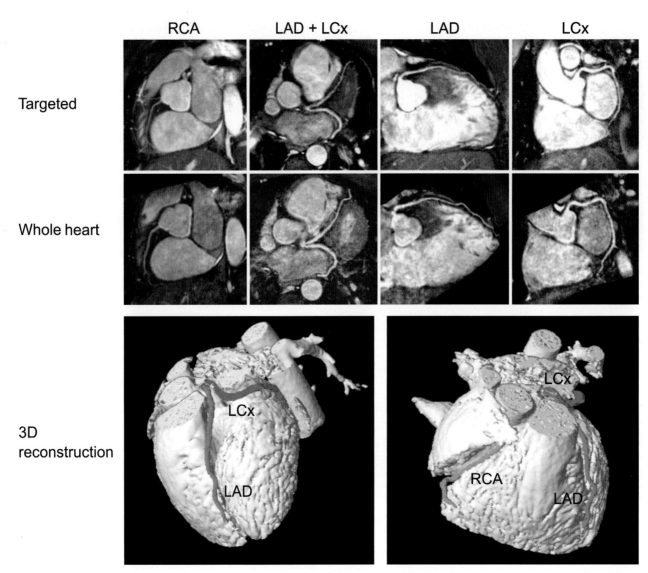

FIGURE 6–24. Coronary arteries of a volunteer that were imaged using a transverse targeted sequence (top row) and reformatted from a whole-heart sequence (middle row). Note that by using the whole-heart sequence, image contrast to the background is improved, especially in the more distal segments of the left anterior descending (LAD) and left circumflex (LCx) arteries. The bottom row shows three-dimensional (3D) reconstructions following computer-assisted image segmentation, which enables the major coronary vessels (right coronary artery [RCA], LAD, and LCx) to be visualized. Reproduced with permission from Weber OM, Martin AJ, Higgins CB. Whole-heart steady-state free precession coronary artery magnetic resonance angiography. *Magn Reson Med.* 2003;50:1223-1228.

of suspected anomalous coronary artery anatomy is possibly the strongest indication for CMR coronary angiography.[201]

SUMMARY

CMR is complementary to and often provides incremental value over other imaging modalities for assessment of IHD. Of specific and proven value is LGE CMR for determination of viability and scar. In combination with stress perfusion imaging and cine imaging for function, CMR is the only modality that can integrate assessment of function, perfusion, and viability in one session, which is necessary for a comprehensive evaluation of viable but dysfunctional myocardium. The recent introduction of assessments for myocardium at risk adds to CMR's versatility.

CMR is usually less observer dependent compared with other competing modalities and does not use radiation, and most applications are noninvasive. CMR is as close to a one-stop shop for ischemic heart disease as a modality can get.

REFERENCES

1. Nesto RW, Kowalchuk GJ. The ischemic cascade: temporal sequence of hemodynamic, electrocardiographic and symptomatic expressions of ischemia. *Am J Cardiol.* 1987;59:23C-30C.
2. Braunwald E, Antman EM, Beasley JW, et al. ACC/AHA guidelines for the management of patients with unstable angina and non-ST-segment elevation myocardial infarction. A report of the American College of Cardiology/American Heart Association Task Force on Practice Guidelines (Committee on the Management of Patients With Unstable Angina). *J Am Coll Cardiol.* 2000;36:970-1062.

3. Libby P, Bonow RO, Mann DL, Zipes DP. *Braunwald's Heart Disease: A Textbook of Cardiovascular Medicine.* Philadelphia, PA: Saunders Elsevier; 2008.

4. Rapaport SI, Rao LV. The tissue factor pathway: how it has become a "prima ballerina." *Thromb Haemost.* 1995;74:7-17.

5. Davies MJ. The composition of coronary-artery plaques. *N Engl J Med.* 1997;336:1312-1314.

6. Fuster V, Stein B, Ambrose JA, Badimon L, Badimon JJ, Chesebro JH. Atherosclerotic plaque rupture and thrombosis. Evolving concepts. *Circulation.* 1990;82:II47-59–II47-59.

7. Neumann FJ, Gawaz M, Dickfeld T, et al. Antiplatelet effect of ticlopidine after coronary stenting. *J Am Coll Cardiol.* 1997;29:1515-1519.

8. Karlsson K, Marklund SL. Heparin-induced release of extracellular superoxide dismutase to human blood plasma. *Biochem J.* 1987;242:55-59.

9. Ramanathan KB, Wilson JL, Ingram LA, Mirvis DM. Effects of immature recruitable collaterals on myocardial blood flow and infarct size after acute coronary occlusion. *J Lab Clin Med.* 1995;125:66-71.

10. Maxwell MP, Hearse DJ, Yellon DM. Species variation in the coronary collateral circulation during regional myocardial ischaemia: a critical determinant of the rate of evolution and extent of myocardial infarction. *Cardiovasc Res.* 1987;21:737-746.

11. Hedström E, Engblom H, Frogner F, et al. Infarct evolution in man studied in patients with first-time coronary occlusion in comparison to different species: implications for assessment of myocardial salvage. *J Cardiovasc Magn Reson.* 2009;11:38.

12. Reimer KA, Lowe JE, Rasmussen MM, Jennings RB. The wavefront phenomenon of ischemic cell death. 1. Myocardial infarct size vs duration of coronary occlusion in dogs. *Circulation.* 1977;56:786-794.

13. Näslund U, Häggmark S, Johansson G, Pennert K, Reiz S, Marklund SL. Effects of reperfusion and superoxide dismutase on myocardial infarct size in a closed chest pig model. *Cardiovasc Res.* 1992;26:170-178.

14. Fujiwara H, Matsuda M, Fujiwara Y, et al. Infarct size and the protection of ischemic myocardium in pig, dog and human. *Jpn Circ J.* 1989;53:1092-1097.

15. Arheden H, Saeed M, Higgins CB, et al. Reperfused rat myocardium subjected to various durations of ischemia: estimation of the distribution volume of contrast material with echo-planar MR imaging. *Radiology.* 2000;215:520-528.

16. Reimer KA, Jennings RB. The "wavefront phenomenon" of myocardial ischemic cell death. II. Transmural progression of necrosis within the framework of ischemic bed size (myocardium at risk) and collateral flow. *Lab Invest.* 1979;40:633-44.

17. Kloner RA, Ellis SG, Lange R, Braunwald E. Studies of experimental coronary artery reperfusion. Effects on infarct size, myocardial function, biochemistry, ultrastructure and microvascular damage. *Circulation.* 1983;68:I8-I15.

18. Reimer KA, Vander Heide RS, Richard VJ. Reperfusion in acute myocardial infarction: effect of timing and modulating factors in experimental models. *Am J Cardiol.* 1993;72:13G-21G.

19. Hale SL, Kloner RA. Effect of early coronary artery reperfusion on infarct development in a model of low collateral flow. *Cardiovasc Res.* 1987;21:668-673.

20. Shen YT, Fallon JT, Iwase M, Vatner SF. Innate protection of baboon myocardium: effects of coronary artery occlusion and reperfusion. *Am J Physiol.* 1996;270:H1812-H1818.

21. Effectiveness of intravenous thrombolytic treatment in acute myocardial infarction. Gruppo Italiano per lo Studio della Streptochinasi nell'Infarto Miocardico (GISSI). *Lancet.* 1986;1:397-402.

22. ISIS-2 (Second International Study of Infarct Survival) Collaborative Group. Randomised trial of intravenous streptokinase, oral aspirin, both, or neither among 17,187 cases of suspected acute myocardial infarction: ISIS-2. *Lancet.* 1988;2:349-360.

23. Boersma E, Simoons ML. Reperfusion strategies in acute myocardial infarction. *Eur Heart J.* 1997;18:1703-1711.

24. Opie LH. *The Heart, Physiology, from Cell to Circulation.* Philadelphia, PA: Lippincott-Raven; 1998.

25. Korge P, Byrd SK, Campbell KB. Functional coupling between sarcoplasmic-reticulum-bound creatine kinase and Ca(2+)-ATPase. *Eur J Biochem.* 1993;213:973-980.

26. Cross HR, Clarke K, Opie LH, Radda GK. Is lactate-induced myocardial ischaemic injury mediated by decreased pH or increased intracellular lactate? *J Mol Cell Cardiol.* 1995;27:1369-1381.

27. Whitman G, Kieval R, Wetstein L, Seeholzer S, McDonald G, Harken A. The relationship between global myocardial ischemia, left ventricular function, myocardial redox state, and high energy phosphate profile. A phosphorous-31 nuclear magnetic resonance study. *J Surg Res.* 1983;35:332-339.

28. Steenbergen C, Hill ML, Jennings RB. Volume regulation and plasma membrane injury in aerobic, anaerobic, and ischemic myocardium in vitro. Effects of osmotic cell swelling on plasma membrane integrity. *Circ Res.* 1985;57:864-875.

29. Ubachs JF, Engblom H, Erlinge D, et al. Cardiovascular magnetic resonance of the myocardium at risk in acute reperfused myocardial infarction: comparison of T2-weighted imaging versus the circumferential endocardial extent of late gadolinium enhancement with transmural projection. *J Cardiovasc Magn Reson.* 2010;12:18.

30. Rizzello V, Poldermans D, Bax JJ. Assessment of myocardial viability in chronic ischemic heart disease: current status. *Q J Nucl Med Mol Imaging.* 2005;49:81-96.

31. Underwood SR, Anagnostopoulos C, Cerqueira M, et al. Myocardial perfusion scintigraphy: the evidence. *Eur J Nucl Med Mol Imaging.* 2004;31:261-291.

32. Naghavi M, Libby P, Falk E, et al. From vulnerable plaque to vulnerable patient: a call for new definitions and risk assessment strategies. Part I. *Circulation.* 2003;108:1664-1672.

33. Yip G, Wang M, Zhang Y, Fung JW, Ho PY, Sanderson JE. Left ventricular long axis function in diastolic heart failure is reduced in both diastole and systole: time for a redefinition? *Heart.* 2002;87:121-125.

34. Shmuylovich L, Kovacs SJ. Load-independent index of diastolic filling: model-based derivation with in vivo validation in control and diastolic dysfunction subjects. *J Appl Physiol.* 2006;101:92-101.

35. Nikitin NP, Witte KK, Clark AL, Cleland JG. Color tissue Doppler-derived long-axis left ventricular function in heart failure with preserved global systolic function. *Am J Cardiol.* 2002;90:1174-1177.

36. Carlsson M, Ugander M, Heiberg E, Arheden H. The quantitative relationship between longitudinal and radial function in left, right, and total heart pumping in humans. *Am J Physiol Heart Circ Physiol.* 2007;293:H636-H644.

37. Carlsson M, Ugander M, Mosen H, Buhre T, Arheden H. Atrioventricular plane displacement is the major contributor to left ventricular pumping in healthy adults, athletes, and patients with dilated cardiomyopathy. *Am J Physiol Heart Circ Physiol.* 2007;292:H1452-H1459.

38. Eisner DA, Smith TW. The Na-K pump and its effectors in cardiac muscle. In: Fozzard HA, ed. *The Heart and Cardiovascular System.* 2nd ed. New York, NY: Raven Press; 1992.

39. Sylven C. Mechanisms of pain in angina pectoris—a critical review of the adenosine hypothesis. *Cardiovasc Drugs Ther.* 1993;7:745-759.

40. Ardehali A, Ports TA. Myocardial oxygen supply and demand. *Chest.* 1990;98:699-705.

41. Hachamovitch R, Berman DS, Shaw LJ, et al. Incremental prognostic value of myocardial perfusion single photon emission computed tomography for the prediction of cardiac death: differential stratification for risk of cardiac death and myocardial infarction. *Circulation.* 1998;97:535-543.

42. Braunwald E, Kloner RA. The stunned myocardium: prolonged, postischemic ventricular dysfunction. *Circulation.* 1982;66:1146-1149.

43. Heyndrickx GR, Millard RW, McRitchie RJ, Maroko PR, Vatner SF. Regional myocardial functional and electrophysiological alterations after brief coronary artery occlusion in conscious dogs. *J Clin Invest.* 1975;56:978-985.

44. Lavallee M, Cox D, Patrick TA, Vatner SF. Salvage of myocardial function by coronary artery reperfusion 1, 2, and 3 hours after occlusion in conscious dogs. *Circ Res.* 1983;53:235-247.

45. Bush LR, Buja LM, Samowitz W, et al. Recovery of left ventricular segmental function after long-term reperfusion following temporary coronary occlusion in conscious dogs. Comparison of 2- and 4-hour occlusions. *Circ Res.* 1983;53:248-263.

46. Bolli R. Mechanism of myocardial "stunning." *Circulation.* 1990;82:723-738.

47. Moens AL, Claeys MJ, Timmermans JP, Vrints CJ. Myocardial ischemia/reperfusion-injury, a clinical view on a complex pathophysiological process. *Int J Cardiol.* 2005;100:179-190.

48. Homans DC, Sublett E, Dai XZ, Bache RJ. Persistence of regional left ventricular dysfunction after exercise-induced myocardial ischemia. *J Clin Invest.* 1986;77:66-73.

49. Ambrosio G, Betocchi S, Pace L, et al. Prolonged impairment of regional contractile function after resolution of exercise-induced angina. Evidence of myocardial stunning in patients with coronary artery disease. *Circulation.* 1996;94:2455-2464.

50. Nicklas JM, Becker LC, Bulkley BH. Effects of repeated brief coronary occlusion on regional left ventricular function and dimension in dogs. *Am J Cardiol.* 1985;56:473-478.

51. Homans DC, Laxson DD, Sublett E, Lindstrom P, Bache RJ. Cumulative deterioration of myocardial function after repeated episodes of exercise-induced ischemia. *Am J Physiol.* 1989;256:H1462-H1471.

52. Braunwald E, Rutherford JD. Reversible ischemic left ventricular dysfunction: evidence for the "hibernating myocardium." *J Am Coll Cardiol.* 1986;8:1467-1470.

53. Rahimtoola SH. The hibernating myocardium. *Am Heart J.* 1989;117:211-221.

54. Nienaber CA, Brunken RC, Sherman CT, et al. Metabolic and functional recovery of ischemic human myocardium after coronary angioplasty. *J Am Coll Cardiol.* 1991;18:966-978.

55. Takeishi Y, Tono-oka I, Kubota I, et al. Functional recovery of hibernating myocardium after coronary bypass surgery: does it coincide with improvement in perfusion? *Am Heart J.* 1991;122:665-670.

56. Maes A, Flameng W, Borgers M, et al. Regional myocardial blood flow, glucose utilization and contractile function before and after revascularization and ultrastructural findings in patients with chronic coronary artery disease. *Eur J Nucl Med.* 1995;22:1299-1305.

57. Altehoefer C, vom Dahl J, Messmer BJ, Hanrath P, Buell U. Fate of the resting perfusion defect as assessed with technetium-99m methoxy-isobutyl-isonitrile single-photon emission computed tomography after successful revascularization in patients with healed myocardial infarction. *Am J Cardiol.* 1996;77:88-92.

58. Paluszkiewicz L, Kwinecki P, Jemielity M, Szyszka A, Dyszkiewicz W, Cieslinski A. Myocardial perfusion correlates with improvement of systolic function of the left ventricle after CABG. Dobutamine echocardiography and Tc-99m-MIBI SPECT study. *Eur J Cardiothorac Surg.* 2002;21:32-35.

59. Heusch G, Schulz R, Rahimtoola SH. Myocardial hibernation: a delicate balance. *Am J Physiol Heart Circ Physiol.* 2005;288:H984-H999.

60. Schwarz ER, Schoendube FA, Kostin S, et al. Prolonged myocardial hibernation exacerbates cardiomyocyte degeneration and impairs recovery of function after revascularization. *J Am Coll Cardiol* 1998;31:1018-1026.

61. Vanoverschelde JL, Depre C, Gerber BL, et al. Time course of functional recovery after coronary artery bypass graft surgery in patients with chronic left ventricular ischemic dysfunction. *Am J Cardiol.* 2000;85:1432-1439.

62. Schwarz ER, Schaper J, vom Dahl J, et al. Myocyte degeneration and cell death in hibernating human myocardium. *J Am Coll Cardiol.* 1996;27:1577-1585.

63. Hughes GC, Landolfo CK, Yin B, et al. Is chronically dysfunctional yet viable myocardium distal to a severe coronary stenosis hypoperfused? *Ann Thorac Surg.* 2001;72:163-168.

64. Marinho NV, Keogh BE, Costa DC, Lammerstma AA, Ell PJ, Camici PG. Pathophysiology of chronic left ventricular dysfunction. New insights from the measurement of absolute myocardial blood flow and glucose utilization. *Circulation.* 1996;93:737-744.

65. Hernandez-Pampaloni M, Bax JJ, Morita K, Dutka DP, Camici PG. Incidence of stunned, hibernating and scarred myocardium in ischaemic cardiomyopathy. *Eur J Nucl Med Mol Imaging.* 2005;32:314-321.

66. Auerbach MA, Schoder H, Hoh C, et al. Prevalence of myocardial viability as detected by positron emission tomography in patients with ischemic cardiomyopathy. *Circulation.* 1999;99:2921-2926.

67. al-Mohammad A, Mahy IR, Norton MY, et al. Prevalence of hibernating myocardium in patients with severely impaired ischaemic left ventricles. *Heart.* 1998;80:559-564.

68. Bonow RO. Identification of viable myocardium. *Circulation.* 1996;94:2674-2680.

69. Allman KC, Shaw LJ, Hachamovitch R, Udelson JE. Myocardial viability testing and impact of revascularization on prognosis in patients with coronary artery disease and left ventricular dysfunction: a meta-analysis. *J Am Coll Cardiol.* 2002;39:1151-1158.

70. Bloch F. Nuclear induction. *Phys Rev.* 1946;70:460-474.

71. Weinmann HJ, Brasch RC, Press WR, Wesbey GE. Characteristics of gadolinium-DTPA complex: a potential NMR contrast agent. *AJR Am J Roentgenol.* 1984;142:619-624.

72. Lauffer RB. Paramagnetic metal complexes as water proton relaxation agents for NMR imaging: theory and design. *Chem Rev.* 1987;87:901-927.

73. Donahue KM, Weisskoff RM, Burstein D. Water diffusion and exchange as they influence contrast enhancement. *J Magn Reson Imaging.* 1997;7:102-110.

74. Look DC, Locker DR. Time saving in measurement of NMR and EPR relaxation times. *Rev Sci Instrum.* 1970;41:250-251.

75. Messroghli DR, Walters K, Plein S, et al. Myocardial T1 mapping: application to patients with acute and chronic myocardial infarction. *Magn Reson Med.* 2007;58:34-40.

76. Kroll H, Korman S, Siegel E, et al. Excretion of yttrium and lanthanum chelates of cyclohexane 1,2-trans diamine tetraacetic acid and diethylenetriamine pentaacetic acid in man. *Nature.* 1957;180:919-920.

77. Arheden H, Saeed M, Higgins CB, et al. Measurement of the distribution volume of gadopentetate dimeglumine at echo-planar MR imaging to quantify myocardial infarction: comparison with 99mTc-DTPA autoradiography in rats. *Radiology.* 1999;211:698-708.

78. Kruhoffer P. Inulin as an indicator for the extracellular space. *Acta Physiol Scand.* 1945;11:16-36.

79. Grobner T, Prischl FC. Gadolinium and nephrogenic systemic fibrosis. *Kidney Int.* 2007;72:260-264.

80. Altun E, Martin DR, Wertman R, Lugo-Somolinos A, Fuller ER 3rd, Semelka RC. Nephrogenic systemic fibrosis: change in incidence following a switch in gadolinium agents and adoption of a gadolinium policy—report from two U.S. universities. *Radiology.* 2009;253:689-696.

81. Martin DR, Krishnamoorthy SK, Kalb B, et al. Decreased incidence of NSF in patients on dialysis after changing gadolinium contrast-enhanced MRI protocols. *J Magn Reson Imaging.* 2010;31:440-446.

82. Stuber M, Botnar RM, Danias PG, et al. Contrast agent-enhanced, free-breathing, three-dimensional coronary magnetic resonance angiography. *J Magn Reson Imaging.* 1999;10:790-799.

83. Sandstede JJ, Pabst T, Wacker C, et al. Breath-hold 3D MR coronary angiography with a new intravascular contrast agent (feruglose)—first clinical experiences. *Magn Reson Imaging.* 2001;19:201-205.

84. Schmiedl U, Moseley ME, Sievers R, et al. Magnetic resonance imaging of myocardial infarction using albumin-(Gd-DTPA), a macromolecular blood-volume contrast agent in a rat model. *Invest Radiol.* 1987;22:713-721.

85. Wendland MF, Saeed M, Geschwind JF, Mann JS, Brasch RC, Higgins CB. Distribution of intracellular, extracellular, and intravascular contrast media for magnetic resonance imaging in hearts subjected to reperfused myocardial infarction. *Acad Radiol.* 1996;3(Suppl 2):S402-S404.

86. Schwitter J, Saeed M, Wendland MF, et al. Influence of severity of myocardial injury on distribution of macromolecules: extravascular versus intravascular gadolinium-based magnetic resonance contrast agents. *J Am Coll Cardiol.* 1997;30:1086-1094.

87. Bremerich J, Wendland MF, Arheden H, et al. Microvascular injury in reperfused infarcted myocardium: noninvasive assessment with contrast-enhanced echoplanar magnetic resonance imaging. *J Am Coll Cardiol.* 1998;32:787-793.

88. Feiring AJ, Johnson MR, Kioschos JM, Kirchner PT, Marcus ML, White CW. The importance of the determination of the myocardial area at risk in the evaluation of the outcome of acute myocardial infarction in patients. *Circulation.* 1987;75:980-987.

89. Jennings RB, Hawkins HK, Lowe JE, Hill ML, Klotman S, Reimer KA. Relation between high energy phosphate and lethal injury in myocardial ischemia in the dog. *Am J Pathol.* 1978;92:187-214.

90. Sinusas AJ, Shi Q, Saltzberg MT, et al. Technetium-99m-tetrofosmin to assess myocardial blood flow: experimental validation in an intact canine model of ischemia. *J Nucl Med.* 1994;35:664-671.

91. Younès A, Songadele JA, Maublant J, Platts E, Pickett R, Veyre A. Mechanism of uptake of technetium-tetrofosmin. II: uptake into isolated adult rat heart mitochondria. *J Nucl Cardiol.* 1995;2:327-333.

92. Sridhara BS, Braat S, Rigo P, Itti R, Cload P, Lahiri A. Comparison of myocardial perfusion imaging with technetium-99m tetrofosmin versus thallium-201 in coronary artery disease. *Am J Cardiol.* 1993;72:1015-1019.

93. Gibbons RJ, Verani MS, Behrenbeck T, et al. Feasibility of tomographic 99mTc-hexakis-2-methoxy-2-methylpropyl-isonitrile imaging for the assessment of myocardial area at risk and the effect of treatment in acute myocardial infarction. *Circulation.* 1989;80:1277-1286.

94. Sinusas AJ, Trautman KA, Bergin JD, et al. Quantification of area at risk during coronary occlusion and degree of myocardial salvage after

reperfusion with technetium-99m methoxyisobutyl isonitrile. *Circulation.* 1990;82:1424-1437.

95. Aletras AH, Tilak GS, Natanzon A, et al. Retrospective determination of the area at risk for reperfused acute myocardial infarction with T2-weighted cardiac magnetic resonance imaging: histopathological and displacement encoding with stimulated echoes (DENSE) functional validations. *Circulation.* 2006;113:1865-1870.

96. Tilak GS, Hsu LY, Hoyt RF Jr, Arai AE, Aletras AH. In vivo T2-weighted magnetic resonance imaging can accurately determine the ischemic area at risk for 2-day-old nonreperfused myocardial infarction. *Invest Radiol.* 2008;43:7-15.

97. Aletras AH, Kellman P, Derbyshire JA, Arai AE. ACUT2E TSE-SSFP: a hybrid method for T2-weighted imaging of edema in the heart. *Magn Reson Med.* 2008;59:229-235.

98. Abdel-Aty H, Zagrosek A, Schulz-Menger J, et al. Delayed enhancement and T2-weighted cardiovascular magnetic resonance imaging differentiate acute from chronic myocardial infarction. *Circulation.* 2004;109:2411-2416.

99. Kellman P, Aletras AH, Mancini C, McVeigh ER, Arai AE. T2-prepared SSFP improves diagnostic confidence in edema imaging in acute myocardial infarction compared to turbo spin echo. *Magn Reson Med.* 2007;57:891-897.

100. Friedrich MG, Abdel-Aty H, Taylor A, Schulz-Menger J, Messroghli D, Dietz R. The salvaged area at risk in reperfused acute myocardial infarction as visualized by cardiovascular magnetic resonance. *J Am Coll Cardiol.* 2008;51:1581-1587.

101. O'Regan DP, Ahmed R, Karunanithy N, et al. Reperfusion hemorrhage following acute myocardial infarction: assessment with T2* mapping and effect on measuring the area at risk. *Radiology.* 2009;250:916-922.

102. Carlsson M, Ubachs JF, Hedstrom E, Heiberg E, Jovinge S, Arheden H. Myocardium at risk after acute infarction in humans on cardiac magnetic resonance: quantitative assessment during follow-up and validation with single-photon emission computed tomography. *JACC Cardiovasc Imaging.* 2009;2:569-576.

103. Frank JA, Feller MA, House WV. Measurement of proton nuclear magnetic resonance longitudinal relaxation times and water content in infarcted canine myocardium and induced pulmonary injury. *Clin Res.* 1976;24:217A-223A.

104. Johnston DL, Brady TJ, Ratner AV, et al. Assessment of myocardial ischemia with proton magnetic resonance: effects of a three hour coronary occlusion with and without reperfusion. *Circulation.* 1985;71:595-601.

105. García-Dorado D, Oliveras J, Gili J, et al. Analysis of myocardial oedema by magnetic resonance imaging early after coronary artery occlusion with or without reperfusion. *Cardiovasc Res.* 1993;27:1462-1469.

106. Giri S, Chung YC, Merchant A, et al. T2 quantification for improved detection of myocardial edema. *J Cardiovasc Magn Reson.* 2009;11:56.

107. Sorensson P, Heiberg E, Saleh N, et al. Assessment of myocardium at risk with contrast enhanced steady-state free precession cine cardiovascular magnetic resonance compared to single-photon emission computed tomography. *J Cardiovasc Magn Reson.* 2010;12:25.

108. Ortiz-Perez JT, Meyers SN, Lee DC, et al. Angiographic estimates of myocardium at risk during acute myocardial infarction: validation study using cardiac magnetic resonance imaging. *Eur Heart J.* 2007;28:1750-1758.

109. Wright J, Adriaenssens T, Dymarkowski S, Desmet W, Bogaert J. Quantification of myocardial area at risk with T2-weighted CMR: comparison with contrast-enhanced CMR and coronary angiography. *JACC Cardiovasc Imaging.* 2009;2:825-831.

110. Kim RJ, Fieno DS, Parrish TB, et al. Relationship of MRI delayed contrast enhancement to irreversible injury, infarct age, and contractile function. *Circulation.* 1999;100:1992-2002.

111. Hsu LY, Natanzon A, Kellman P, Hirsch GA, Aletras AH, Arai AE. Quantitative myocardial infarction on delayed enhancement MRI. Part I: animal validation of an automated feature analysis and combined thresholding infarct sizing algorithm. *J Magn Reson Imaging.* 2006;23:298-308.

112. Heiberg E, Ugander M, Engblom H, et al. Automated quantification of myocardial infarction from MR images by accounting for partial volume effects: animal, phantom, and human study. *Radiology.* 2008;246:581-588.

113. Edelman RR, Wallner B, Singer A, Atkinson DJ, Saini S. Segmented turboFLASH: method for breath-hold MR imaging of the liver with flexible contrast. *Radiology.* 1990;177:515-521.

114. Simonetti OP, Kim RJ, Fieno DS, et al. An improved MR imaging technique for the visualization of myocardial infarction. *Radiology.* 2001;218:215-223.

115. Decking UKM, Pai VM, Wen H, Balaban RS. Does binding of Gd-DTPA to myocardial tissue contribute to late enhancement in a model of acute myocardial infarction? *Magn Reson Med.* 2003;49:168-171.

116. Hedström E, Arheden H, Eriksson R, Johansson L, Ahlstrom H, Bjerner T. Importance of perfusion in myocardial viability studies using delayed contrast-enhanced magnetic resonance imaging. *J Magn Reson Imaging.* 2006;24:77-83.

117. Diesbourg LD, Prato FS, Wisenberg G, et al. Quantification of myocardial blood flow and extracellular volumes using a bolus injection of Gd-DTPA: kinetic modeling in canine ischemic disease. *Magn Reson Med.* 1992;23:239-253.

118. Mather AN, Lockie T, Nagel E, et al. Appearance of microvascular obstruction on high resolution first-pass perfusion, early and late gadolinium enhancement CMR in patients with acute myocardial infarction. *J Cardiovasc Magn Reson.* 2009;11:33.

119. Kramer CM, Barkhausen J, Flamm SD, Kim RJ, Nagel E. Standardized cardiovascular magnetic resonance imaging (CMR) protocols, Society for Cardiovascular Magnetic Resonance: Board of Trustees Task Force on Standardized Protocols. *J Cardiovasc Magn Reson.* 2008;10:35.

120. Wu KC, Zerhouni EA, Judd RM, et al. Prognostic significance of microvascular obstruction by magnetic resonance imaging in patients with acute myocardial infarction. *Circulation.* 1998;97:765-772.

121. Nijveldt R, Beek AM, Hofman MB, et al. Late gadolinium-enhanced cardiovascular magnetic resonance evaluation of infarct size and microvascular obstruction in optimally treated patients after acute myocardial infarction. *J Cardiovasc Magn Reson.* 2007;9:765-770.

122. Bogaert J, Kalantzi M, Rademakers FE, Dymarkowski S, Janssens S. Determinants and impact of microvascular obstruction in successfully reperfused ST-segment elevation myocardial infarction. Assessment by magnetic resonance imaging. *Eur Radiol.* 2007;17:2572-2580.

123. Shan K, Constantine G, Sivananthan M, Flamm SD. Role of cardiac magnetic resonance imaging in the assessment of myocardial viability. *Circulation.* 2004;109:1328-1334.

124. Fieno DS, Kim RJ, Chen EL, Lomasney JW, Klocke FJ, Judd RM. Contrast-enhanced magnetic resonance imaging of myocardium at risk: distinction between reversible and irreversible injury throughout infarct healing. *J Am Coll Cardiol.* 2000;36:1985-1991.

125. Rehwald WG, Fieno DS, Chen EL, Kim RJ, Judd RM. Myocardial magnetic resonance imaging contrast agent concentrations after reversible and irreversible ischemic injury. *Circulation.* 2002;105:224-229.

126. Choi KM, Kim RJ, Gubernikoff G, Vargas JD, Parker M, Judd RM. Transmural extent of acute myocardial infarction predicts long-term improvement in contractile function. *Circulation.* 2001;104:1101-1107.

127. Beek AM, Kuhl HP, Bondarenko O, et al. Delayed contrast-enhanced magnetic resonance imaging for the prediction of regional functional improvement after acute myocardial infarction. *J Am Coll Cardiol.* 2003;42:895-901.

128. Kim RJ, Wu E, Rafael A, et al. The use of contrast-enhanced magnetic resonance imaging to identify reversible myocardial dysfunction. *N Engl J Med.* 2000;343:1445-1453.

129. Knuesel PR, Nanz D, Wyss C, et al. Characterization of dysfunctional myocardium by positron emission tomography and magnetic resonance: relation to functional outcome after revascularization. *Circulation.* 2003;108:1095-1100.

130. Selvanayagam JB, Kardos A, Francis JM, et al. Value of delayed-enhancement cardiovascular magnetic resonance imaging in predicting myocardial viability after surgical revascularization. *Circulation.* 2004;110:1535-1541.

131. Schvartzman PR, Srichai MB, Grimm RA, et al. Nonstress delayed-enhancement magnetic resonance imaging of the myocardium predicts improvement of function after revascularization for chronic ischemic heart disease with left ventricular dysfunction. *Am Heart J.* 2003;146:535-541.

132. Ugander M, Cain PA, Johnsson P, Palmer J, Arheden H. Chronic nontransmural infarction has a delayed recovery of function following revascularization. *BMC Cardiovasc Disord.* 2010;10:4.

133. Bello D, Shah DJ, Farah GM, et al. Gadolinium cardiovascular magnetic resonance predicts reversible myocardial dysfunction and remodeling in patients with heart failure undergoing beta-blocker therapy. *Circulation.* 2003;108:1945-1953.

134. Wu KC, Weiss RG, Thiemann DR, et al. Late gadolinium enhancement by cardiovascular magnetic resonance heralds an adverse prognosis in nonischemic cardiomyopathy. *J Am Coll Cardiol.* 2008;51:2414-2421.

135. Lund GK, Stork A, Muellerleile K, et al. Prediction of left ventricular remodeling and analysis of infarct resorption in patients with reperfused myocardial infarcts by using contrast-enhanced MR imaging. *Radiology.* 2007;245:95-102.

136. Mahrholdt H, Wagner A, Holly TA, et al. Reproducibility of chronic infarct size measurement by contrast-enhanced magnetic resonance imaging. *Circulation.* 2002;106:2322-2327.

137. Saeed M, Lund G, Wendland MF, Bremerich J, Weinmann H, Higgins CB. Magnetic resonance characterization of the peri-infarction zone of reperfused myocardial infarction with necrosis-specific and extracellular nonspecific contrast media. *Circulation.* 2001;103:871-876.

138. Fieno DS, Hillenbrand HB, Rehwald WG, et al. Infarct resorption, compensatory hypertrophy, and differing patterns of ventricular remodeling following myocardial infarctions of varying size. *J Am Coll Cardiol.* 2004;43:2124-2131.

139. Choi CJ, Haji-Momenian S, Dimaria JM, et al. Infarct involution and improved function during healing of acute myocardial infarction: the role of microvascular obstruction. *J Cardiovasc Magn Reson.* 2004;6:917-925.

140. Baks T, van Geuns RJ, Duncker DJ, et al. Prediction of left ventricular function after drug-eluting stent implantation for chronic total coronary occlusions. *J Am Coll Cardiol.* 2006;47:721-725.

141. Ripa RS, Nilsson JC, Wang Y, Sondergaard L, Jorgensen E, Kastrup J. Short- and long-term changes in myocardial function, morphology, edema, and infarct mass after ST-segment elevation myocardial infarction evaluated by serial magnetic resonance imaging. *Am Heart J.* 2007;154:929-936.

142. Engblom H, Hedstrom E, Heiberg E, Wagner GS, Pahlm O, Arheden H. Rapid initial reduction of hyperenhanced myocardium after reperfused first myocardial infarction suggests recovery of the peri-infarction zone: one-year follow-up by MRI. *Circ Cardiovasc Imaging.* 2009;2:47-55.

143. Kellman P, Dyke CK, Aletras AH, McVeigh ER, Arai AE. Artifact suppression in imaging of myocardial infarction using B1-weighted phased-array combined phase-sensitive inversion recovery. *Magn Reson Med.* 2004;51:408-412.

144. Kellman P, Arai AE, McVeigh ER, Aletras AH. Phase-sensitive inversion recovery for detecting myocardial infarction using gadolinium-delayed hyperenhancement. *Magn Reson Med.* 2002;47:372-383.

145. Kellman P, Larson AC, Hsu LY, et al. Motion-corrected free-breathing delayed enhancement imaging of myocardial infarction. *Magn Reson Med.* 2005;53:194-200.

146. Rosendahl L, Ahlander B-M, Björklund P-G, Blomstrand P, Brudin L, Engvall JE. Image quality and myocardial scar size determined with magnetic resonance imaging in patients with permanent atrial fibrillation: a comparison of two imaging protocols. *Clin Physiol Funct Imaging.* 2010;30:122-129.

147. Li W, Li BSY, Polzin JA, Mai VM, Prasad PV, Edelman RR. Myocardial delayed enhancement imaging using inversion recovery single-shot steady-state free precession: initial experience. *J Magn Reson Imaging.* 2004;20:327-330.

148. Bax JJ, Poldermans D, Elhendy A, Boersma E, Rahimtoola SH. Sensitivity, specificity, and predictive accuracies of various noninvasive techniques for detecting hibernating myocardium. *Curr Probl Cardiol.* 2001;26:141-186.

149. Bax JJ, van der Wall EE, Harbinson M. Radionuclide techniques for the assessment of myocardial viability and hibernation. *Heart.* 2004;90(Suppl 5):v26-v33.

150. Klein C, Nekolla SG, Bengel FM, et al. Assessment of myocardial viability with contrast-enhanced magnetic resonance imaging: comparison with positron emission tomography. *Circulation.* 2002;105:162-167.

151. Kuhl HP, Lipke CS, Krombach GA, et al. Assessment of reversible myocardial dysfunction in chronic ischaemic heart disease: comparison of contrast-enhanced cardiovascular magnetic resonance and a combined positron emission tomography-single photon emission computed tomography imaging protocol. *Eur Heart J.* 2006;27:846-853.

152. Wagner A, Mahrholdt H, Holly TA, et al. Contrast-enhanced MRI and routine single photon emission computed tomography (SPECT) perfusion imaging for detection of subendocardial myocardial infarcts: an imaging study. *Lancet.* 2003;361:374-379.

153. Hedstrom E, Palmer J, Ugander M, Arheden H. Myocardial SPECT perfusion defect size compared to infarct size by delayed gadolinium-enhanced magnetic resonance imaging in patients with acute or chronic infarction. *Clin Physiol Funct Imaging.* 2004;24:380-386.

154. Slomka PJ, Fieno D, Thomson L, et al. Automatic detection and size quantification of infarcts by myocardial perfusion SPECT: clinical validation by delayed-enhancement MRI. *J Nucl Med.* 2005;46:728-735.

155. Janardhanan R, Moon JC, Pennell DJ, Senior R. Myocardial contrast echocardiography accurately reflects transmurality of myocardial necrosis and predicts contractile reserve after acute myocardial infarction. *Am Heart J.* 2005;149:355-362.

156. McCrohon JA, Lyne JC, Rahman SL, Lorenz CH, Underwood SR, Pennell DJ. Adjunctive role of cardiovascular magnetic resonance in the assessment of patients with inferior attenuation on myocardial perfusion SPECT. *J Cardiovasc Magn Reson.* 2005;7:377-382.

157. Ricciardi MJ, Wu E, Davidson CJ, et al. Visualization of discrete microinfarction after percutaneous coronary intervention associated with mild creatine kinase-MB elevation. *Circulation.* 2001;103:2780-2783.

158. Steuer J, Bjerner T, Duvernoy O, et al. Visualisation and quantification of peri-operative myocardial infarction after coronary artery bypass surgery with contrast-enhanced magnetic resonance imaging. *Eur Heart J.* 2004;25:1293-1299.

159. Baer FM, Voth E, Schneider CA, Theissen P, Schicha H, Sechtem U. Comparison of low-dose dobutamine-gradient-echo magnetic resonance imaging and positron emission tomography with [18F]fluorodeoxyglucose in patients with chronic coronary artery disease. A functional and morphological approach to the detection of residual myocardial viability. *Circulation.* 1995;91:1006-1015.

160. Baer FM, Theissen P, Schneider CA, et al. Dobutamine magnetic resonance imaging predicts contractile recovery of chronically dysfunctional myocardium after successful revascularization. *J Am Coll Cardiol.* 1998;31:1040-1048.

161. Zerhouni EA. Myocardial tagging by magnetic resonance imaging. *Coron Artery Dis.* 1993;4:334-339.

162. Sayad DE, Willett DL, Hundley WG, Grayburn PA, Peshock RM. Dobutamine magnetic resonance imaging with myocardial tagging quantitatively predicts improvement in regional function after revascularization. *Am J Cardiol.* 1998;82: 1149-1151, A10.

163. Van Hoe L, Vanderheyden M. Ischemic cardiomyopathy: value of different MRI techniques for prediction of functional recovery after revascularization. *AJR Am J Roentgenol.* 2004;182:95-100.

164. Gutberlet M, Frohlich M, Mehl S, et al. Myocardial viability assessment in patients with highly impaired left ventricular function: comparison of delayed enhancement, dobutamine stress MRI, end-diastolic wall thickness, and TI201-SPECT with functional recovery after revascularization. *Eur Radiol.* 2005;15:872-880.

165. Wellnhofer E, Olariu A, Klein C, et al. Magnetic resonance low-dose dobutamine test is superior to SCAR quantification for the prediction of functional recovery. *Circulation.* 2004;109:2172-2174.

166. Kaandorp TA, Bax JJ, Schuijf JD, et al. Head-to-head comparison between contrast-enhanced magnetic resonance imaging and dobutamine magnetic resonance imaging in men with ischemic cardiomyopathy. *Am J Cardiol.* 2004;93:1461-1464.

167. Kim RJ, Manning WJ. Viability assessment by delayed enhancement cardiovascular magnetic resonance: will low-dose dobutamine dull the shine? *Circulation.* 2004;109:2476-2479.

168. Hachamovitch R, Hayes SW, Friedman JD, Cohen I, Berman DS. Comparison of the short-term survival benefit associated with revascularization compared with medical therapy in patients with no prior coronary artery disease undergoing stress myocardial perfusion single photon emission computed tomography. *Circulation.* 2003;107:2900-2907.

169. Schwitter J, Wacker CM, van Rossum AC, et al. MR-IMPACT: comparison of perfusion-cardiac magnetic resonance with single-photon emission computed tomography for the detection of coronary artery disease in a multicentre, multivendor, randomized trial. *Eur Heart J.* 2008;29:480-489.

170. Lee DC, Simonetti OP, Harris KR, et al. Magnetic resonance versus radionuclide pharmacological stress perfusion imaging for flow-limiting stenoses of varying severity. *Circulation.* 2004;110:58-65.

171. Hsu LY, Rhoads KL, Holly JE, Kellman P, Aletras AH, Arai AE. Quantitative myocardial perfusion analysis with a dual-bolus contrast-enhanced first-pass MRI technique in humans. *J Magn Reson Imaging.* 2006;23:315-322.

172. Kellman P, Aletras AH, Hsu LY, McVeigh ER, Arai AE. T2* measurement during first-pass contrast-enhanced cardiac perfusion imaging. *Magn Reson Med.* 2006;56:1132-1134.

173. Lima RS, Watson DD, Goode AR, et al. Incremental value of combined perfusion and function over perfusion alone by gated SPECT myocardial

perfusion imaging for detection of severe three-vessel coronary artery disease. *J Am Coll Cardiol.* 2003;42:64-70.

174. De Winter O, Velghe A, Van de Veire N, et al. Incremental prognostic value of combined perfusion and function assessment during myocardial gated SPECT in patients aged 75 years or older. *J Nucl Cardiol.* 2005;12:662-670.

175. Matsumoto N, Sato Y, Suzuki Y, et al. Incremental prognostic value of cardiac function assessed by ECG-gated myocardial perfusion SPECT for the prediction of future acute coronary syndrome. *Circ J.* 2008;72:2035-2039.

176. Ingkanisorn WP, Kwong RY, Bohme NS, et al. Prognosis of negative adenosine stress magnetic resonance in patients presenting to an emergency department with chest pain. *J Am Coll Cardiol.* 2006;47:1427-1432.

177. Jahnke C, Nagel E, Gebker R, et al. Prognostic value of cardiac magnetic resonance stress tests: adenosine stress perfusion and dobutamine stress wall motion imaging. *Circulation.* 2007;115:1769-1776.

178. Pilz G, Jeske A, Klos M, et al. Prognostic value of normal adenosine-stress cardiac magnetic resonance imaging. *Am J Cardiol.* 2008;101:1408-1412.

179. Lerakis S, McLean DS, Anadiotis AV, et al. Prognostic value of adenosine stress cardiovascular magnetic resonance in patients with low-risk chest pain. *J Cardiovasc Magn Reson.* 2009;11:37.

180. Steel K, Broderick R, Gandla V, et al. Complementary prognostic values of stress myocardial perfusion and late gadolinium enhancement imaging by cardiac magnetic resonance in patients with known or suspected coronary artery disease. *Circulation.* 2009;120:1390-1400.

181. Cerqueira MD, Verani MS, Schwaiger M, Heo J, Iskandrian AS. Safety profile of adenosine stress perfusion imaging: results from the Adenoscan Multicenter Trial Registry. *J Am Coll Cardiol.* 1994;23:384-389.

182. Nagel E, Lehmkuhl HB, Bocksch W, et al. Noninvasive diagnosis of ischemia-induced wall motion abnormalities with the use of high-dose dobutamine stress MRI: comparison with dobutamine stress echocardiography. *Circulation.* 1999;99:763-770.

183. Paetsch I, Jahnke C, Wahl A, et al. Comparison of dobutamine stress magnetic resonance, adenosine stress magnetic resonance, and adenosine stress magnetic resonance perfusion. *Circulation.* 2004;110:835-842.

184. Wahl A, Paetsch I, Gollesch A, et al. Safety and feasibility of high-dose dobutamine-atropine stress cardiovascular magnetic resonance for diagnosis of myocardial ischaemia: experience in 1000 consecutive cases. *Eur Heart J.* 2004;25:1230-1236.

185. Schalla S, Nagel E, Lehmkuhl H, et al. Comparison of magnetic resonance real-time imaging of left ventricular function with conventional magnetic resonance imaging and echocardiography. *Am J Cardiol.* 2001;87:95-99.

186. Kozerke S, Tsao J, Razavi R, Boesiger P. Accelerating cardiac cine 3D imaging using k-t BLAST. *Magn Reson Med.* 2004;52:19-26.

187. Kuijpers D, Ho KYJAM, van Dijkman PRM, Vliegenthart R, Oudkerk M. Dobutamine cardiovascular magnetic resonance for the detection of myocardial ischemia with the use of myocardial tagging. *Circulation.* 2003;107:1592-1597.

188. Aletras AH, Wen H. Mixed echo train acquisition displacement encoding with stimulated echoes: an optimized DENSE method for in vivo functional imaging of the human heart. *Magn Reson Med.* 2001;46:523-534.

189. Osman NF, McVeigh ER, Prince JL. Imaging heart motion using harmonic phase MRI. *IEEE Trans Med Imaging.* 2000;19:186-202.

190. Bergvall E, Cain P, Arheden H, Sparr G. A fast and highly automated approach to myocardial motion analysis using phase contrast magnetic resonance imaging. *J Magn Reson Imaging.* 2006;23:652-661.

191. Garot J, Lima JAC, Gerber BL, et al. Spatially resolved imaging of myocardial function with strain-encoded MR: comparison with delayed contrast-enhanced MR imaging after myocardial infarction. *Radiology.* 2004;233:596-602.

192. Bergvall E, Hedstrom E, Bloch KM, Arheden H, Sparr G. Spline-based cardiac motion tracking using velocity-encoded magnetic resonance imaging. *IEEE Trans Med Imaging.* 2008;27:1045-1053.

193. Cerqueira MD, Weissman NJ, Dilsizian V, et al. Standardized myocardial segmentation and nomenclature for tomographic imaging of the heart: a statement for healthcare professionals from the Cardiac Imaging Committee of the Council on Clinical Cardiology of the American Heart Association. *Circulation.* 2002;105:539-542.

194. Persson E, Palmer J, Pettersson J, et al. Quantification of myocardial hypoperfusion with 99m Tc-sestamibi in patients undergoing prolonged coronary artery balloon occlusion. *Nucl Med Commun.* 2002;23:219-228.

195. Schuetz GM, Zacharopoulou NM, Schlattmann P, Dewey M. Meta-analysis: noninvasive coronary angiography using computed tomography versus magnetic resonance imaging. *Ann Intern Med.* 2010;152:167-177.

196. Ozgun M, Rink M, Hoffmeier A, et al. Intraindividual comparison of 3D coronary MR angiography and coronary CT angiography. *Acad Radiol.* 2007;14:910-916.

197. Kim WY, Stuber M, Bornert P, Kissinger KV, Manning WJ, Botnar RM. Three-dimensional black-blood cardiac magnetic resonance coronary vessel wall imaging detects positive arterial remodeling in patients with nonsignificant coronary artery disease. *Circulation.* 2002;106:296-299.

198. Weber OM, Martin AJ, Higgins CB. Whole-heart steady-state free precession coronary artery magnetic resonance angiography. *Magn Reson Med.* 2003;50:1223-1228.

199. Sakuma H, Ichikawa Y, Suzawa N, et al. Assessment of coronary arteries with total study time of less than 30 minutes by using whole-heart coronary MR angiography. *Radiology.* 2005;237:316-321.

200. Sakuma H, Ichikawa Y, Chino S, Hirano T, Makino K, Takeda K. Detection of coronary artery stenosis with whole-heart coronary magnetic resonance angiography. *J Am Coll Cardiol.* 2006;48:1946-1950.

201. Taylor AM, Thorne SA, Rubens MB, et al. Coronary artery imaging in grown up congenital heart disease: complementary role of magnetic resonance and x-ray coronary angiography. *Circulation.* 2000;101:1670-1678.

CHAPTER 7

ELECTROCARDIOGRAPHY OF ISCHEMIC HEART DISEASE

Henrik Engblom and David G. Strauss

INTRODUCTION / 128

ECG ASPECTS OF MYOCARDIAL ISCHEMIA / 129
Pathophysiology of Myocardial Ischemia due to Decreased Blood Supply / 129
The Ischemic Cascade in Coronary Occlusion / 129
Transmural Ischemia due to Coronary Occlusion: ST-Segment Deviation / 130
Clinical Implications / 131

ECG ASPECTS OF MYOCARDIAL INFARCTION / 131
Pathophysiology of Myocardial Infarction / 131
Infarct-Related ECG Changes / 131
The Pathologic Q Wave / 131
Clinical Implications / 131

QUANTITATIVE ASSESSMENT OF MYOCARDIAL ISCHEMIA AND INFARCTION USING THE 12-LEAD ECG / 132
ECG Analysis of Ischemia Location, Size, and Severity / 132
ECG Acuteness (Time-Course) of Ischemia / 132
ECG Characterization of Infarction / 133

MULTIMODAL IMAGING TO UNCOVER THE PATHOPHYSIOLOGIC BASIS FOR ECG CHANGES RELATED TO MYOCARDIAL ISCHEMIA AND INFARCTION / 135
Myocardial Ischemia by ECG Compared With Myocardial Perfusion SPECT / 135
Infarct Characteristics by ECG Compared With CMR / 135

DISCLAIMER   140

INTRODUCTION

The 12-lead electrocardiogram (ECG) is still the most frequently used diagnostic method in patients with suspected ischemic heart disease (IHD). Practically all patients presenting at the emergency room with chest pain have an ECG recorded to exclude or confirm unstable IHD and ongoing myocardial ischemia. In many regions, ECG is recorded in ambulances on patients with typical or atypical chest pain, dizziness, fainting, irregular heartbeat, and other clinical symptoms or signs. Furthermore, inducible ECG changes found during an exercise or pharmacologic stress test are frequently used to diagnose significant coronary artery stenosis in the situation of stable IHD. The frequent use of ECG as a diagnostic method in suspected IHD worldwide is due to several factors. First, the ECG provides a unique perspective of the condition of the myocardium by exploring its electrical activity, which is not depicted by other imaging modalities of the heart. Second, it is an inexpensive examination that is not associated with any risk for the patient, and it can be performed within a few minutes. Third, the technique is widely available, even in the developing parts of the world. Finally, the medical community has a long experience with the method because it has been around for more than 100 years.

Currently, the standard clinical ECG is displayed in 12 leads, 6 limb leads, and 6 precordial leads. This results in 12 views of the electrical activity of the myocardium. Body surface potential mapping (BSPM) is a method that provides additional views of the body surface potential distribution by performing recordings at multiple sites (24-240 sites) on the body surface. BSPM has evolved from the so-called classical forward and inverse problems of ECG. The former focuses on how the electrical activity from electrical sources present in the heart is propagated to the epicardium (near-field problem) or to the body surface (far-field problem).[1] The latter focuses on how the electrical activity recorded at the body surface can be used to derive details about the electrical activity in the heart (ie, epicardial potentials).[2] Both problems require high spatial resolution information from the body surface, which can be obtained through BSPM. Thus, BSPM has previously been shown to be useful for detecting myocardial infarction.[3-6] BSPM will not be discussed further in this chapter.

Although there are clear advantages to using additional leads in certain circumstances, problems may occur even when using only the 10 electrodes of the standard 12-lead ECG. Multiple electrodes and wires interfere with auscultation, echocardiograms, resuscitation efforts, and chest x-rays. Noise levels due to limb movement detected by multiple leads make interpretation difficult, and the discomfort to patients caused by so many electrodes tends to be high. Additionally, rapid and accurate electrode placement can be difficult in emergency situations. Fewer electrodes placed at more easily accessed locations could facilitate ECG acquisition for both patients and staff. An example of a reduced lead set is the EASI lead system, which uses five torso electrodes, four recording and one ground. The EASI lead system has been shown to emulate the 12-lead ECG reasonably well,[7-13] which can be advantageous in the emergency situation.[14] Reduced-lead systems will not be discussed further in this chapter.

In vectorcardiography, the sum of the heart's electrical activity in three-dimensional space throughout the cardiac cycle is traced by using only three orthogonal leads, V_x, V_y, and V_z. Vectorcardiography has been shown to have substantial potential for monitoring patients with acute myocardial infarction[15,16] and may help in identifying candidates for emergency coronary angiography.[16] It has also been shown to correlate with enzymatically estimated infarct size.[17] The use of vectorcardiography in IHD will be discussed further in subsequent parts of this chapter.

The rest of this chapter will focus on the pathophysiologic basis of ECG changes in IHD and the use of the standard 12-lead ECG for characterizing different aspects of this disease.

ECG ASPECTS OF MYOCARDIAL ISCHEMIA

■ PATHOPHYSIOLOGY OF MYOCARDIAL ISCHEMIA DUE TO DECREASED BLOOD SUPPLY

Myocardial ischemia is defined as an insufficient oxygen supply of the myocardium in relation to its oxygen demand. To put acute ischemia-related ECG changes into perspective of the serial events occurring in the myocardium in the situation of acute coronary occlusion, the following section will discuss the so-called *ischemic cascade.*[18]

Before discussing the consequences of myocardial ischemia, it is important to understand the cause of it. Blood flow to the myocardium can be partially reduced due to a coronary stenosis or completely absent due to coronary occlusion. The major pathophysiologic basis of coronary stenosis and occlusion is the formation of an atherosclerotic plaque in the coronary vessel wall. The severity of a coronary stenosis depends on the degree at which the stenosis obstructs the arterial lumen. If the atherosclerotic plaque becomes unstable and ruptures, the formation of a thrombus in situ starts, which results in occlusion of the coronary artery. Coronary occlusion can also result from embolization[19] or spasm[20,21] of the coronary artery.

■ THE ISCHEMIC CASCADE IN CORONARY OCCLUSION

A sudden coronary occlusion, in the absence of a significant coronary collateral flow, results in transmural myocardial ischemia, which is the initial step of the ischemic cascade (Fig. 7–1). The

steps of the ischemic cascade caused by sudden loss of coronary blood flow can be described as follows:

1. *Myocardial ischemia:* As the coronary artery is occluded, the perfusion to the part of the myocardium supplied by the occluded vessel is terminated, and this part of the myocardium becomes ischemic.

2. *Diastolic dysfunction:* Soon after the coronary vessel has been occluded, diastolic dysfunction can be observed in the myocardium supplied by the occluded vessel. The diastolic dysfunction is due to impaired myocardial relaxation. The relaxation is the first to be affected by the ischemia because it is the most energy-demanding process of the cardiac cycle. Normally, the myocytes relax by pumping cytosolic Ca^{2+} into the sarcoplasmatic reticulum or out of the cell. This process requires adenosine triphosphate (ATP). As the coronary artery becomes occluded, the oxygen supply to the myocardium distal to the occlusion is interrupted. The lack of oxygen results in a shift of the aerobic metabolism to anaerobic glycolysis within seconds.[22] The high-energy phosphate reserve, available predominantly as creatine phosphate, is almost completely exhausted after 30 seconds of ischemia. Thus, there is an imbalance between ATP production and consumption.[23] The latter exceeds the former, and the earliest result is dysfunctional myocyte relaxation.

3. *Systolic dysfunction:* As the ischemia persists, Ca^{2+} accumulates in the cytosol, which becomes acidotic and exhibits an increase in phosphate concentration.[24,25] This eventually causes impairment of myocyte contractility and systolic dysfunction, which is the next step in the ischemic cascade.

4. *ECG changes:* The earliest and most consistent ECG alterations due to acute transmural ischemia are increased T wave amplitude and ST-segment elevation in ECG leads above the ischemic zone. These ECG changes occur due to injury currents induced in the border zone between ischemic and nonischemic myocardium.[26-28] These ST-segment changes are discussed in detail later.

5. *Angina pectoris:* Eventually the accumulation of metabolites in the ischemic myocardium causes development of chest pain, so-called *angina pectoris.*[29] The chest pain is often experienced in conjunction with pain radiating to the arms, neck, jaw, shoulders, or back. The accumulated metabolites (including adenosine) stimulate afferent cardiac nerves that fuse with afferent nerves from the organs mentioned earlier, explaining why myocardial ischemia can be experienced as extrathoracic pain.

6. *Myocardial infarction:* If the ischemia is severe enough and persists long enough without restoration of blood flow, the ultimate fate of the myocytes supplied by the occluded vessel is irreversible injury (cell death). If ischemia persists, the myocardial infarction will evolve from the endocardial border and progress toward the epicardium in a wave-front manner.[30] If there is no restoration of blood flow, the infarction will ultimately involve the full thickness of the myocardial muscle wall, *transmural myocardial infarction.* Thus, the duration of ischemia is a major determinant of the transmural extent of infarction.[31]

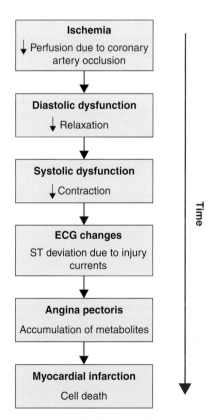

FIGURE 7–1. The ischemic cascade. The sequential events occurring after onset of myocardial ischemia are shown. ECG, electrocardiogram.

■ TRANSMURAL ISCHEMIA DUE TO CORONARY OCCLUSION: ST-SEGMENT DEVIATION

The ST-segment coincides with and is the result of the plateau phase of the ventricular transmembrane action potential. Under normal conditions, the ST segment is isoelectric because the transmembrane voltage remains at approximately the same levels in all ventricular myocytes during that time. Ischemia can reduce the resting membrane potential, shorten the duration of the action potential, and reduce the amplitude of the action potential plateau phase. These alterations of the electrical properties in ischemic myocardium result in abnormal voltage gradients between normal and ischemic myocardium. This voltage gradient induces an injury current, seen as deviation of the ST segment on the body surface ECG. As mentioned earlier, these injury currents arise in the border zones between normal and ischemic myocardium.[26-28]

There are two types of injury currents, a *diastolic injury current* and a *systolic injury current*. In the situation of transmural ischemia, the diastolic injury current causes a negative displacement (depression) of the diastolic TQ baseline due to a reduced resting membrane potential. This can partly be explained by increased extracellular K^+ in the ischemic zone.[32] As a result, a lead overlying the ischemic myocardium will detect a negative deflection during electrical diastole.

There is evidence suggesting that ST-segment elevation partly originates from a true elevation of ST segment caused by systolic injury currents. The shortening of the action potential and the decrease in its amplitude cause injury current to flow during electrical systole and cause ST-segment elevation and hyperacute tall T waves.[33] Thus, ST-segment elevation can be explained by baseline depression or true ST-segment elevation or both,[34-37] which is illustrated in Fig. 7–2. ST-segment elevation is measured at the J point, the time where the QRS complex ends and the ST segment starts.

If the ischemic injury is transmural, the overall ST vector is directed toward an overlying lead that then exhibits ST-segment elevation. Hence, transmural ischemia can be seen as ST-segment depression in leads in which the lead axis is opposite to the leads with ST-segment elevation. This can be seen, for example, when the posterolateral left ventricular (LV) wall is subject to transmural ischemic injury, when the typical change in the standard 12-lead ECG is ST-segment depression in leads V_1 and V_2.[38] This is because the ST vector is directed away from the exploring V_1 and V_2 electrodes. Thus, in this situation, ST-segment depression should be considered indicative of transmural ischemic injury.

According to current guidelines,[39] the predetermined threshold for ST-segment elevation (age, sex, and ECG lead dependent)[40-42] should be exceeded in two or more anatomically contiguous ECG leads in order to be indicative of acute transmural myocardial ischemia. The currently recommended threshold values of ST-segment changes are listed in Table 7–1.

ST-segment elevation can also occur in the absence of myocardial ischemia. In the situation of early repolarization, ST-segment elevation is characterized by J-point elevation and rapid upslope or normal ST segment, which is considered a

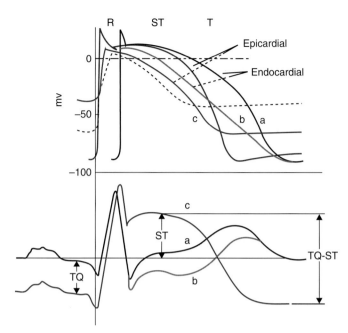

FIGURE 7–2. Typical myocardial cell action potentials (upper curves) and body surface electrocardiograms (lower curves) that represent various degrees of ischemia (b), injury (c), and cell death (necrosis). Curves labeled "a" represent the normal pattern. Reproduced with permission from Selvester et al.[46]

TABLE 7–1. Threshold Values for ST-Segment Changes

ST-Segment Elevation	ST-Segment Depression
For men 40 years of age and older, the threshold value for abnormal J-point elevation should be 0.2 mV (2 mm) in leads V_2 and V_3 and 0.1 mV (1 mm) in all other leads.	For men and women of all ages, the threshold value for abnormal J-point depression should be −0.05 mV (−0.5 mm) in leads V_2 and V_3 and −0.1 mV (−1 mm) in all other leads.
For men less than 40 years of age, the threshold values for abnormal J-point elevation in leads V_2 and V_3 should be 0.25 mV (2.5 mm).	
For women, the threshold value for abnormal J-point elevation should be 0.15 mV (1.5 mm) in leads V_2 and V_3 and greater than 0.1 mV (1 mm) in all other leads.	
For men and women, the threshold for abnormal J-point elevation in V_3R and V_4R should be 0.05 mV (0.5 mm), except for males less than 30 years of age, for whom 0.1 mV (1 mm) is more appropriate.	
For men and women, the threshold value for abnormal J-point elevation in V_7 through V_9 should be 0.05 mV (0.5 mm).	

normal variant. ST-segment elevation can also be associated with pericarditis, elevated serum potassium, acute myocarditis, Osborne waves (caused by hypothermia), and certain cardiac tumors. Thus, it can be a clinical challenge to differentiate acute transmural ischemia from other causes of ST-segment elevation. However, criteria have been suggested that can be applied to differentiate ST-segment elevation caused by acute myocardial ischemia from that resulting from other causes.[43]

CLINICAL IMPLICATIONS

The ECG is still the most important diagnostic method in the situation of suspected acute coronary occlusion. All patients who present at the emergency department with symptoms associated with myocardial ischemia should undergo an ECG examination. If ST-segment elevation above the predetermined thresholds (see Table 7–1) is seen in two or more anatomically contiguous body surface ECG leads in the situation of suspected acute coronary syndrome, the patient is likely to suffer from transmural ischemia due to a coronary occlusion and is in need of acute reperfusion therapy. Development of infarction after such an event is clinically referred to as ST-segment elevation myocardial infarction (STEMI). Patients who develop infarction with ST-segment elevation below the predetermined thresholds or without ST-segment elevation are clinically diagnosed as having non–ST-segment elevation myocardial infarction (NSTEMI).

ECG ASPECTS OF MYOCARDIAL INFARCTION

PATHOPHYSIOLOGY OF MYOCARDIAL INFARCTION

The definition of myocardial infarction is, as discussed earlier, cell death due to prolonged myocardial ischemia. Cell death can be identified pathologically by identification of specific histologic patterns such as coagulation or contraction-band necrosis. By pathology, the infarction can be localized and quantified, as well as classified, according to the timing of the infarction (acute, healing, or healed) by description of the ultrastructure of the infarction and the presence of polymorphonuclear leukocytes.

The clinical diagnosis of acute myocardial infarction is defined by a rise of cardiac biomarkers such as creatine kinase isoenzyme MB (CK-MB) and cardiac troponin T or I (cTnT or cTnI) together with evidence of myocardial ischemia with at least one of the following: (1) symptoms of ischemia; (2) ECG changes indicative of acute ischemia/infarction; (3) imaging evidence of new loss of viable myocardium or new regional wall motion abnormality.[44]

INFARCT-RELATED ECG CHANGES

The final stage of the ischemic cascade is, as previously discussed, myocardial infarction. Because the acute injury currents have subsided, the remaining ECG abnormalities are due to the resulting infarction. The infarction will affect the local activation sources of the myocardium seen as changes primarily in the QRS complex. The infarction might also cause persistent

alteration of the repolarization, resulting in remaining T wave alterations.[45] The magnitude and extent of infarct-related QRS complex changes in different leads depend on the location and extent of infarction.

The myocardial activation (depolarization) vector is the result of all parts of the myocardium that are being depolarized at a given time point. The result of the time-resolved propagation of the depolarization vector during the cardiac cycle is what causes the deflections of the QRS complex seen in different leads. The degree to which the normal depolarization vector changes after an acute myocardial infarction depends on the characteristics of the infarction such as the location, size, endocardial extent, and transmural extent.

THE PATHOLOGIC Q WAVE

If the initial depolarization forces are directed away from an exploring lead, the initial QRS deflection in that lead is negative and results in a Q wave. Presence of Q waves in leads that normally do not exhibit initial negative depolarization forces can be a sign of myocardial infarction in the underlying myocardium. Myocardial infarction can, however, result in other changes in the QRS complex depending on its location. If the infarction is isolated to the posterolateral LV wall, the alteration in the QRS complex is not the appearance of Q waves, but rather prominent R waves in leads V_1 and V_2. In fact, 10% of all infarcts are limited to the basal parts of the LV and do not produce Q waves.[46] Still, the terms Q wave myocardial infarction (QWMI) and non–Q wave myocardial infarction (non-QWMI) are well-established clinical entities, although the differences in infarct characteristics between QWMI and non-QWMI are not completely understood. Furthermore, the prognostic impact of Q wave development is still controversial.[47] Historically, the development of pathologic Q waves after acute coronary occlusion has been associated with transmural myocardial infarction. Based on animal studies, Prinzmetal et al[48] stated that transmural myocardial infarction was required for pathologic Q waves to appear. More recently, however, histopathology[49-51] studies have shown that Q waves in the ECG are not as closely related to transmural myocardial infarction as previously reported. In the past, however, it has been difficult to establish the pathologic basis for Q waves in humans due to lack of accurate in vivo methodology. Recent advances of different imaging modalities have enabled studies of the pathophysiologic basis of infarct-related ECG changes. Such studies are discussed in the last section of this chapter.

CLINICAL IMPLICATIONS

The resting standard 12-lead ECG is often used clinically to report on the presence of myocardial infarction based on infarct-related QRS and T wave changes. A newly detected pathologic Q wave is a common cause for outpatients to be referred to a cardiologist in order to rule out or confirm coronary artery disease. Thus, it is important to understand the ability and limitations of the standard 12-lead to detect and quantify myocardial infarction.

QUANTITATIVE ASSESSMENT OF MYOCARDIAL ISCHEMIA AND INFARCTION USING THE 12-LEAD ECG

■ ECG ANALYSIS OF ISCHEMIA LOCATION, SIZE, AND SEVERITY

Figure 7–3 is an illustration and mathematical characterization of solid angle theory by Holland and Arnsdorf[52] in the 1970s, produced at a time when many investigators were using epicardial and precordial ST-segment mapping to determine the *size* and *severity* of ischemia.[53,54] Holland et al[55] performed a series of experiments in pigs and showed that the amount of ST-segment elevation is affected by the size and shape of the ischemic zone in relation to the anatomic location of the ECG lead.

In the 1980s, as thrombolytic therapy moved into widespread use, investigators sought to use the 12-lead ECG to quantify the size of ischemia. In 1988, Aldrich et al[56] developed an ST-segment deviation score for use in acute anterior and inferior myocardial infarction, and later, a score was developed for posterolateral myocardial infarction.[57] The scores were developed by assessing the relationship between the predischarge ECG QRS score estimation of final infarct size and the number of leads with and the amount of ST-segment deviation on the

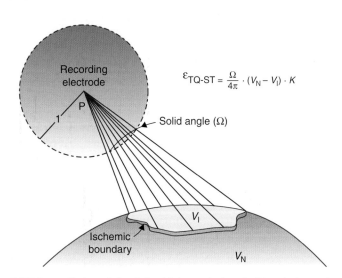

$$\varepsilon_{\text{TQ-ST}} = \frac{\Omega}{4\pi} \cdot (V_N - V_I) \cdot K$$

FIGURE 7–3. Mathematical and pictorial characterization of solid angle theory. The amount of observed ST-segment elevation is proportional to the solid angle (Ω), defined as the area of spherical surface cut off a unit sphere (inscribed about the recording electrode) by a cone formed by drawing lines from the recording electrode to every point along the ischemic boundary. The ischemic boundary is a source of electrical current flow established by differences in the transmembrane potentials of the normal (V_N) and ischemic (V_I) cells during electrical systole and diastole. Thus, the amount of observed ST-segment elevation is determined by the size and shape of the ischemic zone, along with the difference in potential between ischemic and normal cells, and a term (K) to correct for differences in conductivity between the intra- and extracellular spaces. Reprinted from Holland RP, Arnsdorf MF. Solid angle theory and the electrocardiogram: physiologic and quantitative interpretations. *Prog Cardiovasc Dis.* 1977;19:431-457, Copyright 1977, with permission from Elsevier.

presenting ECG. Because the patients did not receive reperfusion therapy, it was assumed that the entire region of ischemic myocardium at risk would infarct. The Aldrich score has been used in multiple studies to estimate myocardium at risk.[58,59] However, it did not have a strong correlation with myocardial perfusion single photon emission computed tomography (SPECT) measurements of ischemia size.[60] Simplified ECG approaches to estimate myocardium at risk are confounded by differences in distance between each LV wall and individual electrodes and by the fact that the magnitude of the ischemic vector is proportional to 1/distance[2].

In contrast to the 12-lead ECG, where the amount of ST-segment elevation in each lead is affected by the distance and location of the individual lead according to the solid angle theorem,[52] a single vector from a vectorcardiography might better correlate with the size of ischemic myocardium. Prior studies have used continuous monitoring of vectorcardiography changes to quantify myocardial ischemia and infarction.[61-65] In addition, the Frank vectorcardiography lead system[66] has been used to compare ST-vector magnitude changes to myocardial perfusion SPECT estimates of the size and severity of ischemia.[67-69] A recent study used the inverse Dower transformation to convert the 12-lead ECG to a vectorcardiogram and projected the vector to a model of the LV to localize ischemia. In addition, the ST-vector magnitude was shown to correlate with ischemia size by myocardial perfusion SPECT.[70]

The Sclarovsky-Birnbaum ischemia grading system was introduced in 1990 and is now considered to be a method for estimating the severity of ischemia.[71,72] It is based on assessment of changes in the terminal part of the QRS complex and in the ST segment. The ischemia grading system consists of three grades representing increasing severity: grade I is characterized by tall upright T waves without ST-segment elevation, grade II is characterized by ST-segment elevation in at least two adjacent leads without terminal QRS distortion, and grade III is characterized by ST-segment elevation with terminal QRS distortion in two or more adjacent leads. Observational studies have shown that patients with grade III ischemia have worse prognosis, larger myocardial infarction size, and less benefit from reperfusion therapy.[73-75]

■ ECG ACUTENESS (TIME-COURSE) OF ISCHEMIA

The Anderson-Wilkins score for estimating the acuteness of ischemia was introduced in 1995.[76,77] It describes a continuous scale from 4.0 (hyperacute) to 1.0 (subacute) based on the comparative hyperacute T waves versus abnormal Q waves in each of the leads with ST-segment elevation or tall T waves. The Anderson-Wilkins score considers each standard lead (except aVR) with at least 0.1-mV ST-segment elevation or tall T waves based on the criteria of Gambill et al.[78] Acuteness phase is designated for each of these leads based on the presence or absence of a tall T wave or an abnormal Q wave (Table 7–2), with phase 1A being the most acute (early ischemia) and phase 2B being the least acute (late ischemia/completed infarct).

TABLE 7–2. Algorithm for Designating the ECG-Time Phase

	Tall T Wave Present (A)	Tall T Wave Absent (B)
Q wave absent (1)	1A = 4 points	1B = 3 points
Q wave present (2)	2A = 2 points	2B = 1 point

ECG, electrocardiogram.

The acuteness score is calculated by the following formula:

$$\frac{4(\text{no. of leads 1A}) + 3(\text{no. of leads 1B}) + 2(\text{no. of leads 2A}) + 1(\text{no. of leads 2B})}{\text{Total no. of leads with 1A, 1B, 2A, or 2B}}$$

The Anderson-Wilkins acuteness score has demonstrated clinical prognostic value. The score was predictive of 1-year mortality after myocardial infarction ($P = .04$), whereas time from symptom onset to reperfusion was not predictive of mortality ($P = .60$).[79] In addition, ECG estimates of the relationship between ischemia size and final myocardial infarct size have suggested that the Anderson-Wilkins acuteness score predicts myocardial salvage.[79]

■ ECG CHARACTERIZATION OF INFARCTION

After the description by Pardee[80] in 1920 of the ECG changes of myocardial infarction, multiple studies looked at the ability of the ECG to detect and localize myocardial infarction with varying results.[81]

Pathology studies in the 1950s and 1960s reported a low sensitivity of conventional ECG criteria for myocardial infarction.[82-84] However, pathology studies often involved the sickest patients with multiple infarcts. In the 1970s, Savage et al[85] used detailed postmortem histologic analyses of hearts with computer digitization of infarct location in patients with single, well-circumscribed infarcts to document the relationship between ECG changes and infarct location. They showed that anteroseptal myocardial infarctions were associated with Q waves or markedly diminished R waves in V_1 to V_3; that inferior myocardial infarctions were associated with Q waves or markedly diminished R waves in II, III, and aVF; and that significant apical myocardial infarction was associated with Q waves or markedly diminished R waves in V_4 to V_6.[85] This led to the detailed testing of the so-called *Selvester QRS scoring system* to identify, localize, and quantify myocardial infarction.

Traditionally, the Minnesota coding system has been used to diagnose myocardial infarction.[86] The Minnesota coding system was developed to detect rather than quantify the amount of infarction from ECG changes. Pahlm et al[87] have shown that the Minnesota coding system correlates poorly with anatomically determined infarct size.

QRS Infarct Scoring in the Absence of ECG Confounding Factors

Based on mapping data of the electrical depolarization in isolated human hearts by Durrer et al,[88] Selvester and colleagues developed a computer simulation of the human ventricular depolarization. This computerized model was used to derive a QRS scoring system by simulating infarction in different parts of the LV.[89,90]

In the 1980s, different versions of the Selvester QRS score were evaluated.[91-96] In the 1985 version of the QRS score, it was noted that the score performed best in patients 40 to 50 years old.[95] False-positive points were most common in younger males who have increased voltages and older females who have lower voltages.[95] Later work reevaluated the specificity of the QRS score in approximately 3000 normal patients and made age and sex adjustments to the score.[97] Absolute amplitude criteria (not ratios) were normalized to age 55 by increasing them 1% per year for age 20 to 54 and decreasing them 1% per year for ages greater than 55 years. For females, duration and amplitude criteria were further decreased by 10%. In addition, some R and S amplitude criteria in the precordial leads were tightened by 0.1 to 0.2 mV.

Numerous studies have tested the potential clinical utility of QRS scoring, including the ability to predict LV ejection fraction,[98] prognosis,[99,100] and response following coronary artery bypass surgery.[101]

QRS Infarct Scoring in the Presence of Hypertrophy and Conduction Defects

Bundle branch and fascicular blocks can have multiple etiologies, including myocardial infarction, degenerative changes that occur at the base of the septum around the aortic-mitral annulus, idiopathic sclerosis of the conduction system, and increased mechanical stress and strain on the fibrous skeleton of the conduction system.[102] Fascicular blocks, bundle branch blocks, and hypertrophy have traditionally been thought to simulate or conceal the typical ECG signs of myocardial infarction.[103,104] However, computer simulations suggested that once the correct underlying activation sequence is taken into account, modified ECG criteria can be developed to detect and quantify myocardial infarction in each of these conduction/hypertrophy (ECG confounding factor) subtypes.[46,105] Until recently, the QRS scores for use in the presence of confounders had not been systematically evaluated due to the inability to collect a sufficient number of patients with infarcts and each of the conduction/hypertrophy subtypes. Using late gadolinium-enhanced (LGE) cardiovascular magnetic resonance (CMR) as a reference standard for myocardial infarction or scar, the QRS scores for use in the presence of hypertrophy and conduction defects correlated with CMR infarct/scar size ($r = 0.60$-0.80; $P < .001$).[106] Subsequent studies have shown that these QRS scores may have clinical value in predicting the risk of implantable defibrillator shocks[107] and response to cardiac resynchronization therapy.[108,109]

The following will discuss how the different conduction and hypertrophy types affect electrical activation and the ability to detect myocardial infarction or scar.

In left bundle branch block (LBBB), ventricular electrical activation begins in the endocardium of the right ventricle (RV) and proceeds through the septum to the endocardium of

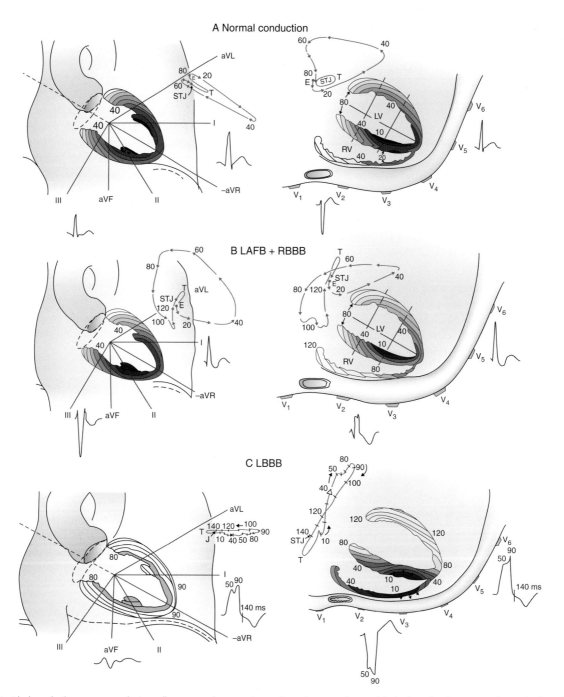

FIGURE 7–4. Ventricular activation sequences, electrocardiogram waveforms, and vector loops (vectorcardiograms) in the frontal and transverse planes. The frontal and transverse planes are shown in normal conduction (**A**), left anterior fascicular block (LAFB) + right bundle branch block (RBBB) (**B**), and left bundle branch block (LBBB) (**C**). Colored lines represent areas of myocardium activated within the same 10-ms period (isochrones). Numbers represent milliseconds since beginning of activation. Modified from Strauss DG, Selvester RH. The QRS complex–a biomarker that "images" the heart: QRS scores to quantify myocardial scar in the presence of normal and abnormal ventricular conduction. *J Electrocardiol.* 2009;42:85-96, Copyright 2009, with permission from Elsevier.

the LV (Fig. 7–4C).[46,110,111] With a septum of normal thickness, this takes approximately 40 ms, and it then takes an additional 50 ms for electrical activation to reenter the Purkinje network and propagate through the anterosuperior and inferior walls. The posterolateral wall is activated last in another 50 ms, producing a total QRS duration of at least 140 ms.[112] This is consistent with the Grant and Dodge[113] observation that the QRS duration in new-onset LBBB is consistently greater than 140

ms, and thus, patients with a QRS duration of 120 to 140 ms likely do not have LBBB, but rather a combination of LV hypertrophy (LVH) and/or left anterior fascicular block (LAFB). The criteria for LBBB QRS scoring in the limb leads (I, II, aVL, and aVF) are similar to criteria in other conduction types in that Q waves and small R waves are signs of myocardial infarction. However, the criteria are drastically different in the precordial leads, where an anteroseptal myocardial infarction causes large

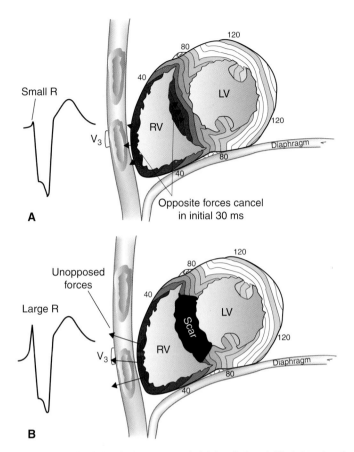

FIGURE 7–5. Electrical activation sequence in left bundle branch block (LBBB) and the effect of septal scar. **A.** LBBB conduction begins in the endocardium of the right ventricle (RV), and electrical forces from the septum and RV free wall go in opposite directions and cancel each other out, producing an isoelectric segment or small R wave in leads V_1 to V_3. However, in the presence of septal scar (**B**), the RV free wall forces are unopposed, producing large R waves in leads V_1 to V_3. LV, left ventricle. Modified from Strauss et al.[106]

the other conduction types can be applied even if LVH is present. The principal differences between the LVH and no-confounder QRS score is that QS complexes (Q waves without an R wave) in V_1 to V_3 do not always receive points, but notches in the first 40 ms of these leads do receive points.

RV hypertrophy (RVH) causes large R waves in V_1 and V_2 that can mimic posterolateral infarcts in all conduction types except LBBB, where RVH mimics anteroseptal infarcts. If large R waves are present, then the P waves should be analyzed for signs of right atrial overload (RAO), which generally accompanies RVH.[46] If the P waves suggest RAO, then large R waves in V_1 and V_2 should be assumed to be due to RVH and should not receive QRS points.

LAFB only causes 20-ms prolongation[104,117]; however, additional LVH can cause a total QRS duration of up to 140 ms or more.[46,118] Thus, patients with intermediate QRS duration between 120 and 140 ms likely have LAFB and LVH or LVH alone, and not LBBB.[113] Figure 7–4B shows combined activation of LAFB and RBBB. Left posterior fascicular block (LPFB) does not affect the scoring system because it was included in the computer simulations for inferior infarcts.[105]

MULTIMODAL IMAGING TO UNCOVER THE PATHOPHYSIOLOGIC BASIS FOR ECG CHANGES RELATED TO MYOCARDIAL ISCHEMIA AND INFARCTION

In order to understand the pathophysiologic basis for ECG changes related to myocardial ischemia and infarction, it is of great importance to have access to other diagnostic imaging modalities. The following section discusses examples of situations where multimodal imaging strategies have been applied in order to better understand the ECG mechanisms and findings in IHD.

■ MYOCARDIAL ISCHEMIA BY ECG COMPARED WITH MYOCARDIAL PERFUSION SPECT

Myocardial perfusion SPECT is considered the gold standard for quantification of myocardial perfusion defects. As mentioned earlier, the Aldrich score was shown not to have a strong correlation with myocardial perfusion SPECT.[60] Myocardial perfusion SPECT has enabled further studies of ECG measures of ischemia. Recently, Ubachs et al[119] showed that the distribution of ST-segment elevation during acute coronary occlusion can be used to locate the ischemic area depicted by myocardial perfusion SPECT (Fig. 7–6). Other approaches for localizing and quantifying the extent of myocardial ischemia during acute coronary occlusion have been proposed and compared with myocardial perfusion SPECT (Figs. 7–7 and 7–8).[120-122]

■ INFARCT CHARACTERISTICS BY ECG COMPARED WITH CMR

Currently, LGE CMR is considered the gold standard for infarct visualization in vivo. In order to determine the location of infarction based on infarct-related ECG changes, Bayes

R waves in leads V_1 and V_2, rather than Q waves as in normal conduction (Fig. 7–5).

In right bundle branch block (RBBB), ventricular activation of the LV is unaffected, but RV activation does not occur until the activation wave front proceeds through the septum. Thus, the RV free wall is activated late, producing a late positive deflection (R or R′) in leads V_1 and V_2.[46,111,114] This confounds the diagnosis of posterolateral infarcts; thus, the scoring system's R wave criteria in V_1 and V_2 are modified. In addition, there is a change in V_1 and V_2 for large anterior infarcts.

Ventricular hypertrophy and chamber enlargement frequently occur in combination with conduction defects. Although most ECG criteria for ventricular hypertrophy consider only QRS voltage changes,[115] the combined Cornell time-voltage index or QRS area measurement improves the diagnosis of LVH.[116] Consideration of the time effects of hypertrophy can be especially important when patients have combinations of hypertrophy and conduction defects.[112] The LVH QRS score should be applied to patients who have LVH (by ECG voltage criteria) without other conduction defects. The QRS score criteria for

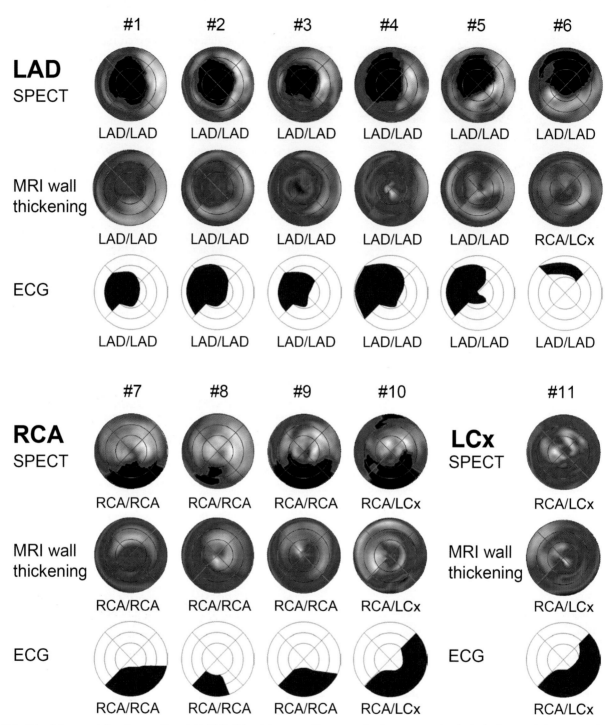

FIGURE 7–6. Polar plot representation of myocardium at risk (MaR). Polar plots generated from rest technetium 99m–tetrofosmin single photon emission computed tomography (SPECT) perfusion, cardiovascular magnetic resonance imaging (MRI) wall thickening, and electrocardiography (ECG) for all patients (patient numbers are shown) with left anterior descending artery (LAD), right coronary artery (RCA), and left circumflex artery (LCx) occlusion. Underneath each polar plot, the designated culprit arteries by the two observers are stated as observer 1/observer 2. Note the similarity in the location of MaR by the three modalities. Reproduced with permission from Ubachs et al.[119]

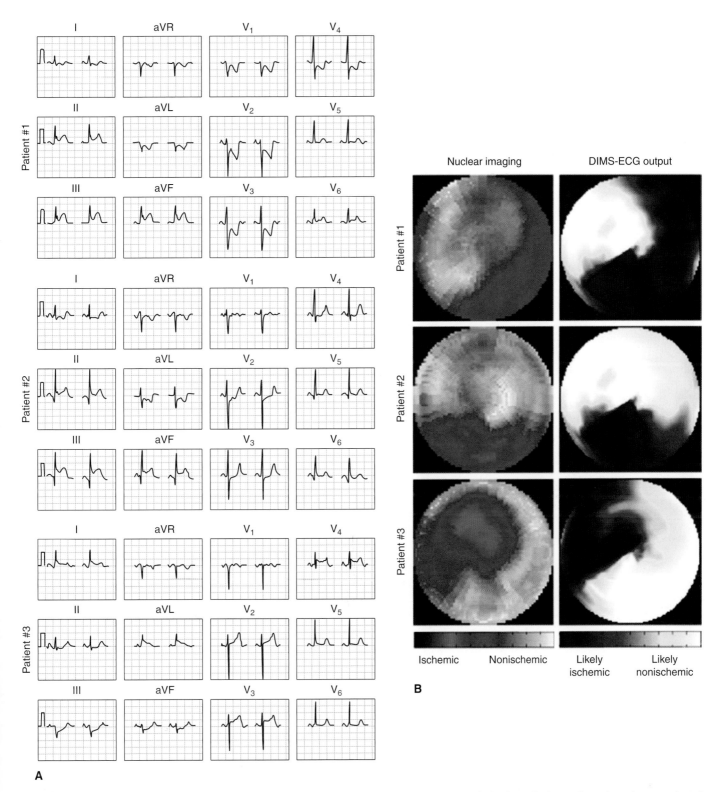

FIGURE 7–7. The display of ischemic myocardium from simulated (DIMS) electrocardiography (ECG) method. **A.** Twelve-lead ECGs for three patients who underwent prolonged coronary angioplasty. The ECGs were recorded before balloon deflation. Patient 1 had a left circumflex artery occlusion, patient 2 had a right coronary artery occlusion, and patient 3 had a left anterior descending artery occlusion. **B.** The single photon emission computed tomography (SPECT; left column) and DIMS-ECG (right column) polar plots for the same three patients. Color scales show the distribution of ischemic to nonischemic myocardium for SPECT and the predicted ischemic to nonischemic scale for DIMS-ECG. Reproduced with permission from Galeotti et al.[121]

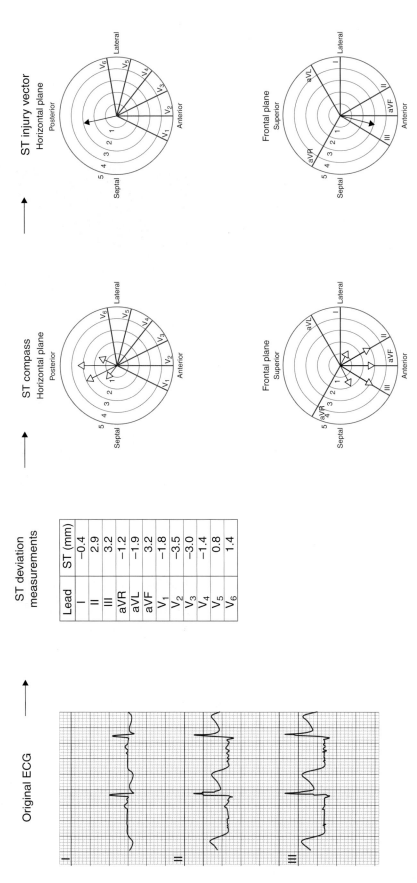

FIGURE 7-8. ST compass method. **A.** To create ST compass plots, the level of ST-segment deviation in each lead is measured automatically in the J point, and each ST measurement is plotted in the ST compass. ST-segment elevation is marked as an arrow from the center of the compass in the positive direction of the relevant lead. ST-segment depression is marked as an arrow from the center of the compass pointing in the opposite direction of the lead in question. The size of the arrow is determined by the magnitude of the ST-segment deviation. Finally, the ST injury vector that best fits all measured ST-segment deviations can be estimated.

ST deviation measurements

Lead	ST (mm)
I	−0.4
II	2.9
III	3.2
aVR	−1.2
aVL	−1.9
aVF	3.2
V1	−1.8
V2	−3.5
V3	−3.0
V4	−1.4
V5	0.8
V6	1.4

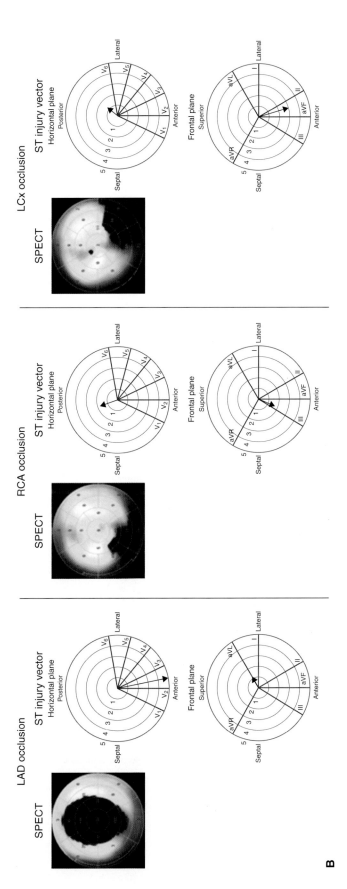

B

FIGURE 7-8. ST compass method. **B.** Examples of MPIs and ST injury vectors for three acute myocardial infarction patients with occlusion of the left anterior descending artery (LAD), right coronary artery (RCA), and left circumflex artery (LCx). There is strong agreement between the anatomic location of ischemia and the corresponding ST injury vector. The LAD patient shows apical anterior ischemia resulting in a large-magnitude anterolateral ST injury vector. The RCA patient shows inferior (slightly septal) ischemia resulting in a medium-magnitude posteroinferior (slightly septal) ST injury vector. The LCx patient has inferior (slightly lateral) ischemia, which results in a postero-inferior (slightly lateral) ST injury vector of medium magnitude. ECG, electrocardiogram; MPI, myocardial perfusion imaging; SPECT, single photon emission computed tomography. Reproduced with permission from Andersen MP, Terkelsen CJ, Sorensen JT, et al. The ST injury vector: electrocardiogram-based estimation of location and extent of myocardial ischemia. *J Electrocardiol.* 2010;43:121-131.

de Luna et al[123] suggested a novel terminology based on LGE CMR findings of infarct location in relation to the 17-segment model[124] used to standardize description of different parts of the LV (Fig. 7–9). Thus, the 17-segment model facilitates multimodal imaging approaches.

Recent imaging studies[125-128] have confirmed previous histopathology findings[49-51] that the association between pathologic Q waves and transmural myocardial infarction is weaker than previously presumed. Using CMR, it has been shown that endocardial extent of infarction seems to be more important for presence of pathologic Q waves than transmural extent of infarction (Fig. 7–10).[129] Furthermore, it was shown that the Selvester QRS scoring system can be used to estimate transmural extent of infarction in patients with early reperfused acute myocardial infarction.[127]

Recovery of infarct-related ECG changes after acute myocardial infarction has previously been described.[130-132] Until recently, however, it has been difficult to establish the anatomic correlate of these changes due to lack of an accurate in vivo method for infarct visualization. Recently, the recovery of infarct-related QRS changes in relation to infarct involution during the first year after reperfused myocardial infarction as assessed by CMR has been demonstrated.[133] This study showed that the timing and magnitude of the recovery of QRS changes was similar to that observed for infarct involution (Fig. 7–11).

Figure 7–12 shows the ECG and CMR images from a patient with LBBB and inferior and posterolateral infarcts, demonstrating how infarcts can be detected even in the presence of LBBB.

It is desirable to further develop multimodal approaches for two- and three-dimensional coregistrations of advanced ECG imaging and non-ECG imaging techniques to enable better understanding of the pathophysiologic basis of IHD and perhaps to improve management of patients suffering from IHD.

DISCLAIMER

The mention of commercial products, their sources, or their use in connection with material reported herein is not to be construed as either an actual or implied endorsement of such products by the U.S. Department of Health and Human Services.

Name	ECG pattern	Infarction area (CMR)
Septal	Q in V_1-V_2	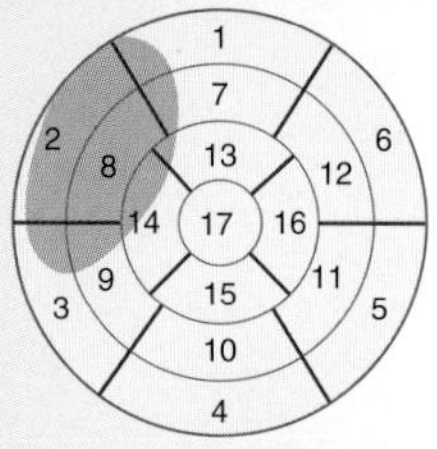
Mid-anterior	Q (qs or qr) in aVL and sometimes in I and/or V_2-V_3	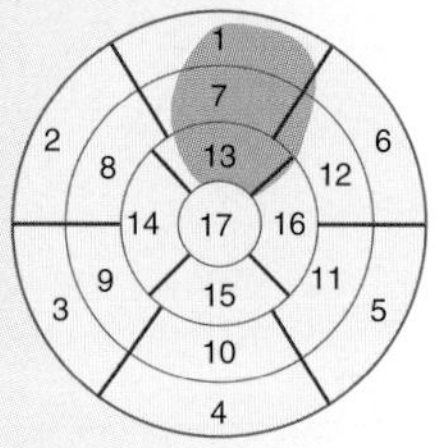
Apical-anterior	Q in V_1-V_2 to V_3-V_6	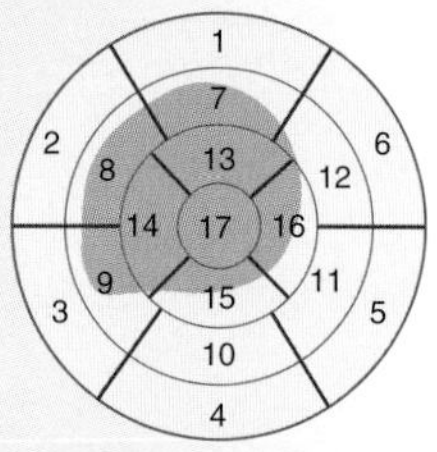
Extensive anterior	Q in V_1-V_2 to V_4-V_6, aVL, and sometimes I	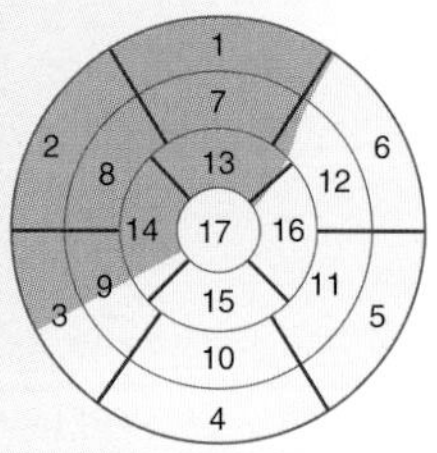
Lateral	RS in V_1-V_2 and/or Q wave in leads I, aVL, V_6, and/or diminished R wave in V_6	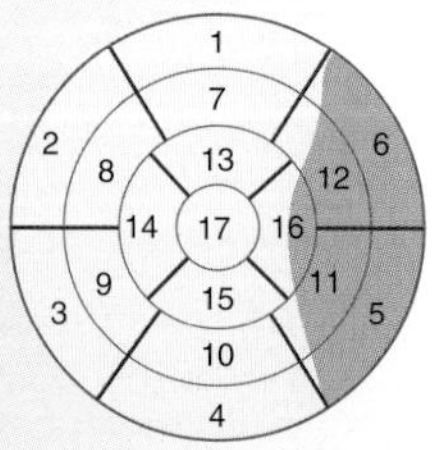
Inferior	Q in II, III, aVF	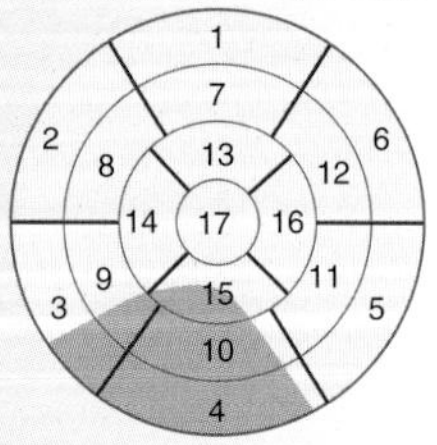

FIGURE 7–9. The electrocardiogram (ECG) patterns of Q wave myocardial infarction or Q wave equivalents with the names given to myocardial infarction and related infarction area documented by cardiovascular magnetic resonance (CMR). Purple color indicates area of infarction. Reproduced with permission from Bayes de Luna et al.[123]

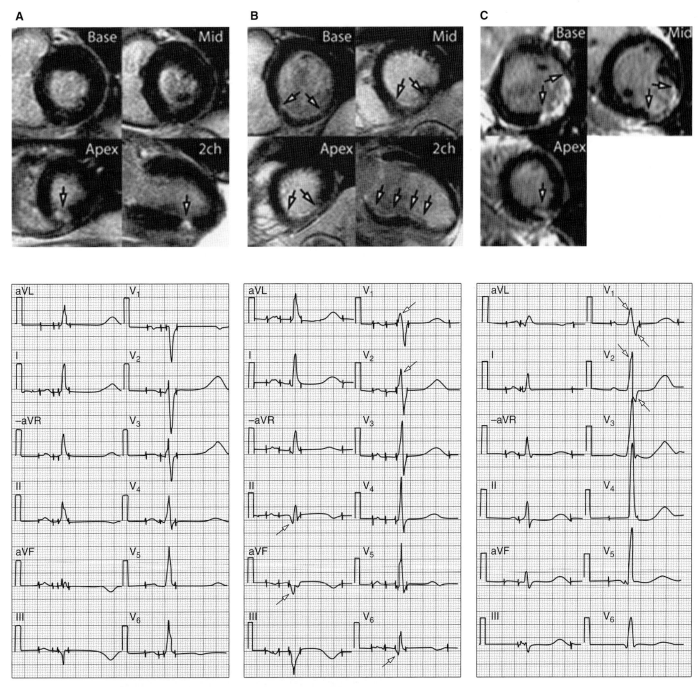

FIGURE 7-10. Three cases illustrating the importance of the endocardial extent of infarction and its location for the QRS score. **A.** A small transmural, non–Q wave myocardial infarction in the inferior left ventricular (LV) wall with a QRS score of 0 and myocardial infarction size of 2% of the LV by late gadolinium-enhanced (LGE) cardiovascular magnetic resonance (CMR). **B.** A nontransmural, Q wave myocardial infarction in the inferior LV wall with a QRS score of 8 with the following criteria met: Q duration >30 ms in lead II; Q duration >40 ms and R/Q ratio <1 in lead aVF; R duration >40 ms in lead V_1; R duration >50 ms in lead V_2; and Q duration >30 ms in lead V_6. Infarct size by LGE CMR was only 7% of the LV. The endocardial extent, however, measured 24% of the LV endocardial extent, closely resembling the QRS score of 8 (24% of the LV). **C.** A transmural, non–Q wave myocardial infarction in the posterolateral LV wall. This patient had prominent R waves and small S waves in V_1 and V_2 suggestive of posterolateral myocardial infarction. Arrows indicate either myocardial infarction by LGE CMR or QRS changes generating QRS points. 2ch, two-chamber long axis view. Reproduced with permission from Engblom et al.[127]

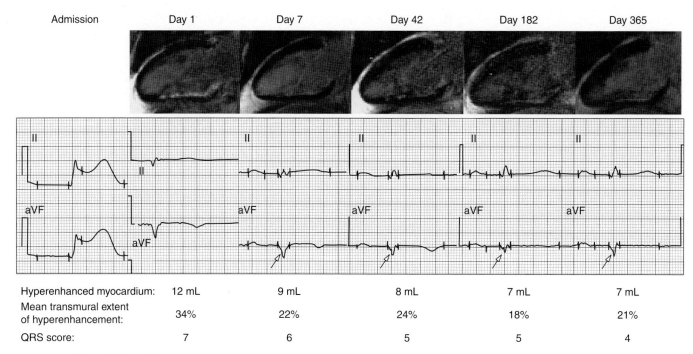

	Admission	Day 1	Day 7	Day 42	Day 182	Day 365
Hyperenhanced myocardium:		12 mL	9 mL	8 mL	7 mL	7 mL
Mean transmural extent of hyperenhancement:		34%	22%	24%	18%	21%
QRS score:		7	6	5	5	4

FIGURE 7–11. Changes in hyperenhanced myocardium in relation to changes in two representative electrocardiogram leads over time affecting the QRS score in a patient with a right coronary artery occlusion. Note the QRS notch (arrows) in the QS complex in aVF seen on days 7 to 365, indicating viable myocardium in the peri-infarction zone, which decreases the QRS score. Also note the increasing R wave amplitude and decreasing Q wave amplitude and duration over time in lead II, also affecting the QRS score. Reproduced with permission from Engblom et al.[133]

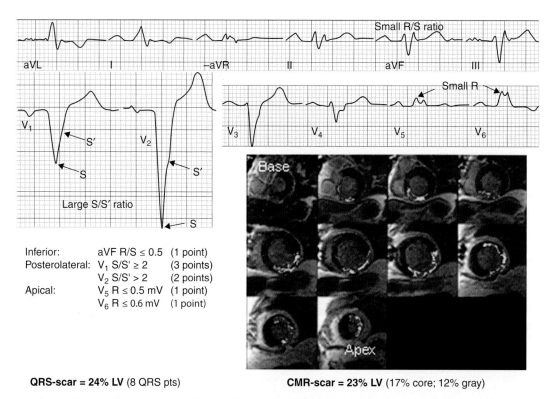

Inferior:	aVF R/S ≤ 0.5	(1 point)
Posterolateral:	V_1 S/S' ≥ 2	(3 points)
	V_2 S/S' > 2	(2 points)
Apical:	V_5 R ≤ 0.5 mV	(1 point)
	V_6 R ≤ 0.6 mV	(1 point)

QRS-scar = 24% LV (8 QRS pts)   **CMR-scar = 23% LV** (17% core; 12% gray)

FIGURE 7–12. Electrocardiogram (ECG) and short axis cardiovascular magnetic resonance (CMR) images from a patient with left bundle branch block and ischemic cardiomyopathy due to inferior and posterolateral infarcts comprising 23% of the left ventricle (LV) by CMR and that received 8 QRS points (ECG-estimated scar = 24%). Note the large S/S' ratio in V_1 and V_2, which reflects posterolateral scar. For the CMR images, the regions with solid scar ("core") are shown in red, and the regions with heterogeneous scar and live myocardium ("gray zone") are shown in yellow. For comparison with the QRS score, total CMR scar was defined as core + 1/2 gray. Reproduced with permission from Strauss et al.[106]

REFERENCES

1. Gulrajani RM, Roberge FA, Mailloux GE. The forward problem of electrocardiography. In: Macfarlane P, Lawrie T, eds. *Comprehensive Electrocardiology: Theory and Practice in Health and Disease.* Vol 1. 1st ed. New York, NY: Pergamon Press; 1989:197-236.

2. Gulrajani RM, Roberge FA, Savard P. The inverse problem of electrocardiography. In: Macfarlane P, Lawrie T, eds. *Comprehensive Electrocardiology: Theory and Practice in Health and Disease.* Vol 1. 1st ed. New York, NY: Pergamon Press; 1989:237-288.

3. Maynard SJ, Menown IB, Manoharan G, et al. Body surface mapping improves early diagnosis of acute myocardial infarction in patients with chest pain and left bundle branch block. *Heart.* 2003;89:998-1002.

4. Menown IB, Patterson RS, MacKenzie G, et al. Body-surface map models for early diagnosis of acute myocardial infarction. *J Electrocardiol.* 1998;31(Suppl):180-188.

5. Kornreich F, Rautaharju PM, Warren J, et al. Identification of best electrocardiographic leads for diagnosing myocardial infarction by statistical analysis of body surface potential maps. *Am J Cardiol.* 1985;56:852-856.

6. Menown IB, Allen J, Anderson JM, et al. Early diagnosis of right ventricular or posterior infarction associated with inferior wall left ventricular acute myocardial infarction. *Am J Cardiol.* 2000;85:934-938.

7. Drew BJ, Pelter MM, Wung SF, et al. Accuracy of the EASI 12-lead electrocardiogram compared to the standard 12-lead electrocardiogram for diagnosing multiple cardiac abnormalities. *J Electrocardiol.* 1999;32(Suppl):38-47.

8. Rautaharju PM, Zhou SH, Hancock EW, et al. Comparability of 12-lead ECGs derived from EASI leads with standard 12-lead ECGS in the classification of acute myocardial ischemia and old myocardial infarction. *J Electrocardiol.* 2002;35(Suppl):35-39.

9. Drew BJ, Adams MG, Pelter MM, et al. ST segment monitoring with a derived 12-lead electrocardiogram is superior to routine cardiac care unit monitoring. *Am J Crit Care.* 1996;5:198-206.

10. Feldman CL, MacCallum G, Hartley LH. Comparison of the standard ECG with the EASI cardiogram for ischemia detection during exercise monitoring. *Proc Comput Cardiol.* 1997;24:343-345.

11. Wehr G, Peters R, Khalife K, et al. A vector-based 5 electrode 12-lead ECG (EASI) is equivalent to the conventional 12-lead ECG for diagnosis of myocardial ischemia. *J Am Coll Cardiol.* 2002;39:122A.

12. Klein M, Key-Brothers I, Feldman C. Can the vectorcardiographically derived EASI ECG be a suitable surrogate for the standard ECG in selected circumstances? *Proc Comput Cardiol.* 1997;5:721-724.

13. Horacek BM, Warren JW, Stovicek P, et al. Diagnostic accuracy of derived versus standard 12-lead electrocardiograms. *J Electrocardiol.* 2000;33(Suppl):155-160.

14. Sejersten M, Pahlm O, Pettersson J, et al. The relative accuracies of ECG precordial lead waveforms derived from EASI leads and those acquired from paramedic applied standard leads. *J Electrocardiol.* 2003;36:179-185.

15. Dellborg M, Topol EJ, Swedberg K. Dynamic QRS complex and ST segment vectorcardiographic monitoring can identify vessel patency in patients with acute myocardial infarction treated with reperfusion therapy. *Am Heart J.* 1991;122:943-948.

16. Dellborg M, Steg P, Simoons M, et al. Vectorcardiographic monitoring to assess early vessel patency after reperfusion therapy for acute myocardial infarction. *Eur Heart J.* 1995;16:21-29.

17. Dellborg M, Herlitz J, Risenfors M, et al. Electrocardiographic assessment of infarct size: comparison between QRS scoring of 12-lead electrocardiography and dynamic vectorcardiography. *Int J Cardiol.* 1993;40:167-172.

18. Nesto RW, Kowalchuk GJ. The ischemic cascade: temporal sequence of hemodynamic, electrocardiographic and symptomatic expressions of ischemia. *Am J Cardiol.* 1987;59:23C-30C.

19. Krachmer AW. Infective endocarditis. In: Braunwald E, Zipes DP, Libby P, eds. *Heart Disease.* 6th ed. Philadelphia, PA: W.B. Saunders Company; 2001:1723-1750.

20. Gersh BJ, Bassendine MF, Forman R, et al. Coronary artery spasm and myocardial infarction in the absence of angiographically demonstrable obstructive coronary disease. *Mayo Clin Proc.* 1981;56:700-708.

21. Lip GY, Gupta J, Khan MM, et al. Recurrent myocardial infarction with angina and normal coronary arteries. *Int J Cardiol.* 1995;51:65-71.

22. Jennings RB, Murry CE, Steenbergen C Jr, et al. Development of cell injury in sustained acute ischemia. *Circulation.* 1990;82:II2-II12.

23. Jennings RB, Schaper J, Hill ML, et al. Effect of reperfusion late in the phase of reversible ischemic injury. Changes in cell volume, electrolytes, metabolites, and ultrastructure. *Circ Res.* 1985;56:262-278.

24. Camacho SA, Figueredo VM, Brandes R, et al. Ca(2+)-dependent fluorescence transients and phosphate metabolism during low-flow ischemia in rat hearts. *Am J Physiol.* 1993;265:H114-H122.

25. Meissner A, Morgan JP. Contractile dysfunction and abnormal Ca2+ modulation during postischemic reperfusion in rat heart. *Am J Physiol.* 1995;268:H100-H111.

26. Cinca J, Figueras J, Senador G, et al. Transmural DC electrograms after coronary artery occlusion and latex embolization in pigs. *Am J Physiol.* 1984;246:H475-H482.

27. Janse MJ, Cinca J, Morena H, et al. The "border zone" in myocardial ischemia. An electrophysiological, metabolic, and histochemical correlation in the pig heart. *Circ Res.* 1979;44:576-588.

28. Smith GT, Geary G, Ruf W, et al. Epicardial mapping and electrocardiographic models of myocardial ischemic injury. *Circulation.* 1979;60:930-938.

29. Sylven C. Mechanisms of pain in angina pectoris—a critical review of the adenosine hypothesis. *Cardiovasc Drugs Ther.* 1993;7:745-759.

30. Reimer KA, Jennings RB. The "wavefront phenomenon" of myocardial ischemic cell death. II. Transmural progression of necrosis within the framework of ischemic bed size (myocardium at risk) and collateral flow. *Lab Invest.* 1979;40:633-644.

31. Hedström E, Engblom H, Frogner F, et al. Infarct evolution in man studied in patients with first-time coronary occlusion in comparison to different species: implications for assessment of myocardial salvage. *J Cardiovasc Magn Reson.* 2009;11:38.

32. Kubota I, Yamaki M, Shibata T, et al. Role of ATP-sensitive K+ channel on ECG ST segment elevation during a bout of myocardial ischemia. A study on epicardial mapping in dogs. *Circulation.* 1993;88:1845-1851.

33. Goldberger AL. Hyperacute T waves revisited. *Am Heart J.* 1982;104:888-890.

34. Downar E, Janse MJ, Durrer D. The effect of acute coronary artery occlusion on subepicardial transmembrane potentials in the intact porcine heart. *Circulation.* 1977;56:217-224.

35. Kleber AG. Resting membrane potential, extracellular potassium activity, and intracellular sodium activity during acute global ischemia in isolated perfused guinea pig hearts. *Circ Res.* 1983;52:442-450.

36. Samson WE, Scher AM. Mechanism of S-T segment alteration during acute myocardial injury. *Circ Res.* 1960;8:780-787.

37. Janse MJ. ST segment mapping and infarct size. *Cardiovasc Res.* 2000;45:190-193.

38. Boden WE, Kleiger RE, Gibson RS, et al. Electrocardiographic evolution of posterior acute myocardial infarction: importance of early precordial ST-segment depression. *Am J Cardiol.* 1987;59:782-787.

39. Wagner GS, Macfarlane P, Wellens H, et al. AHA/ACCF/HRS recommendations for the standardization and interpretation of the electrocardiogram: part VI: acute ischemia/infarction: a scientific statement from the American Heart Association Electrocardiography and Arrhythmias Committee, Council on Clinical Cardiology; the American College of Cardiology Foundation; and the Heart Rhythm Society: endorsed by the International Society for Computerized Electrocardiology. *Circulation.* 2009;119:e262-e270.

40. Macfarlane PW. Age, sex, and the ST amplitude in health and disease. *J Electrocardiol.* 2001;34(Suppl):235-241.

41. Macfarlane PW, Browne D, Devine B, et al. Modification of ACC/ESC criteria for acute myocardial infarction. *J Electrocardiol.* 2004;37(Suppl):98-103.

42. Surawicz B, Parikh SR. Prevalence of male and female patterns of early ventricular repolarization in the normal ECG of males and females from childhood to old age. *J Am Coll Cardiol.* 2002;40:1870-1876.

43. Surawicz B, Knilans T. *Chou's Electrocardiography in Clinical Practice.* 5th ed. Philadelphia, PA: WB Saunders; 2001.

44. Thygesen K, Alpert JS, White HD, et al. Universal definition of myocardial infarction. *Circulation.* 2007;116(22):2634-2653.

45. Mandel WJ, Burgess MJ, Neville J Jr, et al. Analysis of T-wave abnormalities associated with myocardial infarction using a theoretic model. *Circulation.* 1968;38:178-188.

46. Selvester RH, Wagner GS, Ideker RE. Myocardial infarction. In: Macfarlane P, Lawrie T, eds. *Comprehensive Electrocardiology: Theory and Practice*

in Health and Disease. Vol. 1. 1st ed. New York, NY: Pergamon Press; 1989:566-629.

47. Phibbs B, Marcus F, Marriott HJ, et al. Q-wave versus non-Q wave myocardial infarction: a meaningless distinction. *J Am Coll Cardiol.* 1999;33:576-582.

48. Prinzmetal M, Shaw CM Jr, Maxwell MH, et al. Studies on the mechanism of ventricular activity. VI. The depolarization complex in pure subendocardial infarction: role of the subendocardial region in the normal electrocardiogram. *Am J Med.* 1954;16:469-489.

49. Phibbs B. "Transmural" versus "subendocardial" myocardial infarction: an electrocardiographic myth. *J Am Coll Cardiol.* 1983;1:561-564.

50. Pipberger HV, Lopez EA. "Silent" subendocardial infarcts: fact or fiction? *Am Heart J.* 1980;100:597-599.

51. Spodick DH. Q-wave infarction versus S-T infarction. Nonspecificity of electrocardiographic criteria for differentiating transmural and nontransmural lesions. *Am J Cardiol.* 1983;51:913-915.

52. Holland RP, Arnsdorf MF. Solid angle theory and the electrocardiogram: physiologic and quantitative interpretations. *Prog Cardiovasc Dis.* 1977;19:431-457.

53. Braunwald E, Maroko PR. The reduction of infarct size–an idea whose time (for testing) has come. *Circulation.* 1974;50:206-209.

54. Braunwald E, Maroko PR. ST-segment mapping. Realistic and unrealistic expectations. *Circulation.* 1976;54:529-532.

55. Holland RP, Brooks H, Lidl B. Spatial and nonspatial influences on the TG-ST segment deflection of ischemia. Theoretical and experimental analysis in the pig. *J Clin Invest.* 1977;60:197-214.

56. Aldrich HR, Wagner NB, Boswick J, et al. Use of initial ST-segment deviation for prediction of final electrocardiographic size of acute myocardial infarcts. *Am J Cardiol.* 1988;61:749-753.

57. Ripa RS, Holmvang L, Maynard C, et al. Consideration of the total ST-segment deviation on the initial electrocardiogram for predicting final acute posterior myocardial infarct size in patients with maximum ST-segment deviation as depression in leads V1 through V3. A FRISC II substudy. *J Electrocardiol.* 2005;38:180-186.

58. Clemmensen P, Grande P, Saunamaki K, et al. Effect of intravenous streptokinase on the relation between initial ST-predicted size and final QRS-estimated size of acute myocardial infarcts. *J Am Coll Cardiol.* 1990;16:1252-1257.

59. Clemmensen P, Ohman EM, Sevilla DC, et al. Importance of early and complete reperfusion to achieve myocardial salvage after thrombolysis in acute myocardial infarction. *Am J Cardiol.* 1992;70:1391-1396.

60. Christian TF, Gibbons RJ, Clements IP, et al. Estimates of myocardium at risk and collateral flow in acute myocardial infarction using electrocardiographic indexes with comparison to radionuclide and angiographic measures. *J Am Coll Cardiol.* 1995;26:388-393.

61. Reduction of infarct size with the early use of timolol in acute myocardial infarction. *N Engl J Med.* 1984;310:9-15.

62. Grottum P, Mohr B, Kjekshus JK. Evolution of vectorcardiographic QRS changes during myocardial infarction in dogs and their relation to infarct size. *Cardiovasc Res.* 1986;20:108-116.

63. Grottum P, Sederholm M, Kjekshus JK. Quantitative and temporal relation between the release of myoglobin and creatine kinase and the evolution of vectorcardiographic changes during acute myocardial infarction in man. *Cardiovasc Res.* 1987;21:652-659.

64. Dellborg M, Riha M, Swedberg K. Dynamic QRS and ST-segment changes in myocardial infarction monitored by continuous on-line vectorcardiography. *J Electrocardiol.* 1990;23(Suppl):11-19.

65. Dellborg M, Riha M, Swedberg K. Dynamic QRS-complex and ST-segment monitoring in acute myocardial infarction during recombinant tissue-type plasminogen activator therapy. The TEAHAT Study Group. *Am J Cardiol.* 1991;67:343-349.

66. Frank E. An accurate, clinically practical system for spatial vectorcardiography. *Circulation.* 1956;13:737-749.

67. Steg PG, Faraggi M, Himbert D, et al. Comparison using dynamic vectorcardiography and MIBI SPECT of ST-segment changes and myocardial MIBI uptake during percutaneous transluminal coronary angioplasty of the left anterior descending coronary artery. *Am J Cardiol.* 1995;75:998-1002.

68. Faraggi M, Steg PG, Francois D, et al. Residual area at risk after anterior myocardial infarction: are ST segment changes during coronary angioplasty a reliable indicator? A comparison with technetium 99m-labeled sestamibi single-photon emission computed tomography. *J Nucl Cardiol.* 1997;4:11-17.

69. Jensen SM, Karp K, Rask P, et al. Assessment of myocardium at risk with computerized vectorcardiography and technetium-99m-sestamibi-single photon emission computed tomography during coronary angioplasty. *Scand Cardiovasc J.* 2002;36:11-18.

70. Strauss DG, Olson CW, Wu KC, et al. Vectorcardiogram synthesized from the 12-lead electrocardiogram to image ischemia. *J Electrocardiol.* 2009;42:190-197.

71. Sclarovsky S, Mager A, Kusniec J, et al. Electrocardiographic classification of acute myocardial ischemia. *Isr J Med Sci.* 1990;26:525-531.

72. Billgren T, Birnbaum Y, Sgarbossa EB, et al. Refinement and interobserver agreement for the electrocardiographic Sclarovsky-Birnbaum ischemia grading system. *J Electrocardiol.* 2004;37:149-156.

73. Birnbaum Y, Kloner RA, Sclarovsky S, et al. Distortion of the terminal portion of the QRS on the admission electrocardiogram in acute myocardial infarction and correlation with infarct size and long-term prognosis (Thrombolysis in Myocardial Infarction 4 Trial). *Am J Cardiol.* 1996;78:396-403.

74. Birnbaum Y, Herz I, Sclarovsky S, et al. Prognostic significance of the admission electrocardiogram in acute myocardial infarction. *J Am Coll Cardiol.* 1996;27:1128-1132.

75. Sejersten M, Birnbaum Y, Ripa RS, et al. Influences of electrocardiographic ischaemia grades and symptom duration on outcomes in patients with acute myocardial infarction treated with thrombolysis versus primary percutaneous coronary intervention: results from the DANAMI-2 trial. *Heart.* 2006;92:1577-1582.

76. Anderson ST, Wilkins M, Weaver WD, et al. Electrocardiographic phasing of acute myocardial infarction. *J Electrocardiol.* 1992;25(Suppl):3-5.

77. Wilkins ML, Pryor AD, Maynard C, et al. An electrocardiographic acuteness score for quantifying the timing of a myocardial infarction to guide decisions regarding reperfusion therapy. *Am J Cardiol.* 1995;75:617-620.

78. Gambill CL, Wilkins ML, Haisty WK Jr, et al. T wave amplitudes in normal populations. Variation with ECG lead, sex, and age. *J Electrocardiol.* 1995;28:191-197.

79. Sejersten M, Ripa RS, Maynard C, et al. Timing of ischemic onset estimated from the electrocardiogram is better than historical timing for predicting outcome after reperfusion therapy for acute anterior myocardial infarction: a DANish trial in Acute Myocardial Infarction 2 (DANAMI-2) substudy. *Am Heart J.* 2007;154:e61-e68.

80. Pardee HEB. An electrocardiographic sign of coronary artery obstruction. *Arch Intern Med.* 1920;26:244-257.

81. Strauss DG, Selvester RH. The QRS complex—a biomarker that "images" the heart: QRS scores to quantify myocardial scar in the presence of normal and abnormal ventricular conduction. *J Electrocardiol.* 2009;42:85-96.

82. Zinn WJ, Cosby RS. Myocardial infarction; a re-evaluation of the diagnostic accuracy of the electrocardiogram. *Am J Med.* 1950;8:177-179.

83. Johnson WJ, Achor RW, Burchell HB, et al. Unrecognized myocardial infarction: a clinicopathologic study. *AMA Arch Intern Med.* 1959;103:253-261.

84. Woods JD, Laurie W, Smith WG. The reliability of the electrocardiogram in myocardial infarction. *Lancet.* 1963;2:265-269.

85. Savage RM, Wagner GS, Ideker RE, et al. Correlation of postmortem anatomic findings with electrocardiographic changes in patients with myocardial infarction: retrospective study of patients with typical anterior and posterior infarcts. *Circulation.* 1977;55:279-285.

86. Blackburn H, Keys A, Simonson E, et al. The electrocardiogram in population studies. A classification system. *Circulation.* 1960;21:1160-1175.

87. Pahlm US, Chaitman BR, Rautaharju PM, et al. Comparison of the various electrocardiographic scoring codes for estimating anatomically documented sizes of single and multiple infarcts of the left ventricle. *Am J Cardiol.* 1998;81:809-815.

88. Durrer D, van Dam RT, Freud GE, et al. Total excitation of the isolated human heart. *Circulation.* 1970;41:899-912.

89. Selvester RH, Solomon JC, Gillespie TL. Digital computer model of a total body electrocardiographic surface map. An adult male-torso simulation with lungs. *Circulation.* 1968;38:684-690.

90. Taccardi B. Distribution of heart potentials on the thoracic surface of normal human subjects. *Circ Res.* 1963;12:341-352.

91. Wagner GS, Freye CJ, Palmeri ST, et al. Evaluation of a QRS scoring system for estimating myocardial infarct size. I. Specificity and observer agreement. *Circulation.* 1982;65:342-347.

92. Ideker RE, Wagner GS, Ruth WK, et al. Evaluation of a QRS scoring system for estimating myocardial infarct size. II. Correlation with quantitative anatomic findings for anterior infarcts. *Am J Cardiol.* 1982;49:1604-1614.

93. Roark SF, Ideker RE, Wagner GS, et al. Evaluation of a QRS scoring system for estimating myocardial infarct size. III. Correlation with quantitative anatomic findings for inferior infarcts. *Am J Cardiol*. 1983;51:382-389.

94. Ward RM, White RD, Ideker RE, et al. Evaluation of a QRS scoring system for estimating myocardial infarct size. IV. Correlation with quantitative anatomic findings for posterolateral infarcts. *Am J Cardiol*. 1984;53:706-714.

95. Hindman NB, Schocken DD, Widmann M, et al. Evaluation of a QRS scoring system for estimating myocardial infarct size. V. Specificity and method of application of the complete system. *Am J Cardiol*. 1985;55:1485-1490.

96. Sevilla DC, Wagner NB, White RD, et al. Anatomic validation of electrocardiographic estimation of the size of acute or healed myocardial infarcts. *Am J Cardiol*. 1990;65:1301-1307.

97. Andresen A, Dobkin J, Maynard C, et al. Validation of advanced ECG diagnostic software for the detection of prior myocardial infarction by using nuclear cardiac imaging. *J Electrocardiol*. 2001;34:243-248.

98. Palmeri ST, Harrison DG, Cobb FR, et al. A QRS scoring system for assessing left ventricular function after myocardial infarction. *N Engl J Med*. 1982;306:4-9.

99. Bounous EP Jr, Califf RM, Harrell FE Jr, et al. Prognostic value of the simplified Selvester QRS score in patients with coronary artery disease. *J Am Coll Cardiol*. 1988;11:35-41.

100. Jones MG, Anderson KM, Wilson PW, et al. Prognostic use of a QRS scoring system after hospital discharge for initial acute myocardial infarction in the Framingham cohort. *Am J Cardiol*. 1990;66:546-550.

101. Hinohora T, Wagner NB, Cobb FR, et al. An ischemic index from the electrocardiogram to select patients with low left ventricular ejection fraction for coronary artery bypass grafting. *Am J Cardiol*. 1988;61:288-291.

102. Bharati S. Pathology of the conduction system. In: Silver MD, ed. *Cardiovascular Pathology*. Vol. 1. New York, NY: Churchill Livingstone; 2001:607-628.

103. Rosenbaum MB, Elizari MV, Lázzari LO. *The Hemiblocks*. Oldsmar, FL: Tampa Tracings; 1970.

104. Elizari MV, Acunzo RS, Ferreiro M. Hemiblocks revisited. *Circulation*. 2007;115:1154-1163.

105. Strauss DG, Selvester RH. The QRS complex: a biomarker that "images" the heart: QRS scores to quantify myocardial scar in the presence of normal and abnormal ventricular conduction. *J Electrocardiol*. 2009;42:86-97.

106. Strauss DG, Selvester RH, Lima JA, et al. ECG quantification of myocardial scar in cardiomyopathy patients with or without conduction defects: correlation with cardiac magnetic resonance and arrhythmogenesis. *Circ Arrhythm Electrophysiol*. 2008;1:327-336.

107. Strauss DG, Poole JE, Wagner GS, et al. Quantification of myocardial scar using a simple ECG tool identifies patients at risk for sudden arrhythmic death: an analysis of SCD-HeFT. *Circulation*. 2009;120:5646-5647 (abstract)

108. Sweeney MO, van Bommel RJ, Schalij MJ, et al. Analysis of ventricular activation using surface electrocardiography to predict left ventricular reverse volumetric remodeling during cardiac resynchronization therapy. *Circulation*. 2010;121:626-634.

109. Kalahasty G, Ellenbogen KA. Simpler is better: new lessons learned from the 12-lead electrocardiogram. *Circulation*. 2010;121:617-619.

110. Vassallo JA, Cassidy DM, Marchlinski FE, et al. Endocardial activation of left bundle branch block. *Circulation*. 1984;69:914-923.

111. Van Dam RT, Janse MJ. Activation of the heart. In: Macfarlane PW, Lawrie TDV, eds. *Comprehensive Electrocardiology: Theory and Practice in Health in Disease*. New York, NY: Pergamon Press; 1989:101-127.

112. Selvester RHS, Solomon JC. Computer simulation of ventricular depolarization, QRS duration and quantification of wall thickness. In: Willems JL, Van Bemmel JH, Zywitz C, eds. *Computer ECG Analysis: Toward Standardization*. Amsterdam, the Netherlands: North Holland; 1986:221-272.

113. Grant RP, Dodge HT. Mechanisms of QRS complex prolongation in man: left ventricular conduction disturbances. *Am J Med*. 1956;20:834-852.

114. Horowitz LN, Alexander JA, Edmunds LH Jr. Postoperative right bundle branch block: identification of three levels of block. *Circulation*. 1980;62:319-328.

115. Milliken JA, Macfarlane PW, Lawrie TDV. Enlargement and hypertrophy. In: Macfarlane PW, Lawrie TDV, eds. *Comprehensive Electrocardiology: Theory and Practice in Health and Disease*. New York, NY: Pergamon Press; 1989:631-670.

116. Okin PM, Roman MJ, Devereux RB, et al. Time-voltage QRS area of the 12-lead electrocardiogram: detection of left ventricular hypertrophy. *Hypertension*. 1998;31:937-942.

117. Wyndham CR, Meeran MK, Smith T, et al. Epicardial activation in human left anterior fascicular block. *Am J Cardiol*. 1979;44:638-644.

118. Selvester RH, Solomon JC. Computer simulations of ventricular depolarization, QRS duration and quantitation of wall thickness, computer ECG analysis: towards standardisations. Paper presented at the 3rd International Conference on Common Standards for Quantitative Electrocardiography, Amsterdam, the Netherlands, 1985.

119. Ubachs JF, Engblom H, Hedstrom E, et al. Location of myocardium at risk in patients with first-time ST-elevation infarction: comparison among single photon emission computed tomography, magnetic resonance imaging, and electrocardiography. *J Electrocardiol*. 2009;42:198-203.

120. Bacharova L, Mateasik A, Carnicky J, et al. The Dipolar ElectroCARdioTOpographic (DECARTO)-like method for graphic presentation of location and extent of area at risk estimated from ST-segment deviations in patients with acute myocardial infarction. *J Electrocardiol*. 2009;42:172-180.

121. Galeotti L, Strauss DG, Ubachs JF, et al. Development of an automated method for display of ischemic myocardium from simulated electrocardiograms. *J Electrocardiol*. 2009;42:204-212.

122. Andersen MP, Terkelsen CJ, Struijk JJ. The ST compass: spatial visualization of ST-segment deviations and estimation of the ST injury vector. *J Electrocardiol*. 2009;42:181-189.

123. Bayes de Luna A, Wagner G, Birnbaum Y, et al. A new terminology for left ventricular walls and location of myocardial infarcts that present Q wave based on the standard of cardiac magnetic resonance imaging: a statement for healthcare professionals from a committee appointed by the International Society for Holter and Noninvasive Electrocardiography. *Circulation*. 2006;114:1755-1760.

124. Cerqueira MD, Weissman NJ, Dilsizian V, et al. Standardized myocardial segmentation and nomenclature for tomographic imaging of the heart: a statement for healthcare professionals from the Cardiac Imaging Committee of the Council on Clinical Cardiology of the American Heart Association. *Circulation*. 2002;105:539-542.

125. Moon JC, De Arenaza DP, Elkington AG, et al. The pathologic basis of Q-wave and non-Q-wave myocardial infarction: a cardiovascular magnetic resonance study. *J Am Coll Cardiol*. 2004;44:554-560.

126. Kaandorp TA, Bax JJ, Lamb HJ, et al. Which parameters on magnetic resonance imaging determine Q waves on the electrocardiogram? *Am J Cardiol*. 2005;95:925-929.

127. Engblom H, Hedstrom E, Heiberg E, et al. Size and transmural extent of first time reperfused myocardial infarction assessed by cardiac magnetic resonance can be estimated by 12-lead electrocardiogram. *Am Heart J*. 2005;150:920.

128. Wu E, Judd RM, Vargas JD, et al. Visualisation of presence, location, and transmural extent of healed Q-wave and non-Q-wave myocardial infarction. *Lancet*. 2001;357:21-28.

129. Engblom H, Carlsson MB, Hedstrom E, et al. The endocardial extent of reperfused first-time myocardial infarction is more predictive of pathologic Q waves than is infarct transmurality: a magnetic resonance imaging study. *Clin Physiol Funct Imaging*. 2007;27:101-108.

130. Pappas MP. Disappearance of pathological Q waves after cardiac infarction. *Br Heart J*. 1958;20:123-128.

131. Albert DE, Califf RM, LeCocq DA, et al. Comparative rates of resolution of QRS changes after operative and nonoperative acute myocardial infarcts. *Am J Cardiol*. 1983;51:378-381.

132. Lyck F, Holmvang L, Grande P, et al. Effects of revascularization after first acute myocardial infarction on the evolution of QRS complex changes (the DANAMI trial). DANish Trial in Acute Myocardial Infarction. *Am J Cardiol*. 1999;83:488-492.

133. Engblom H, Hedström E, Heiberg E, et al. Rapid initial reduction of hyperenhanced myocardium after reperfused first myocardial infarction suggests recovery of the peri-infarction zone: one-year follow-up by MRI *Circ Cardiovasc Imaging*. 2009;2:47-55.

CHAPTER 8
ELECTROPHYSIOLOGIC MAPPING

Donald D. Hegland, Kevin P. Jackson, and James P. Daubert

INTRODUCTION / 146

PREPROCEDURAL EVALUATION / 146
Baseline 12-Lead ECG and Patient History / 146
Baseline 12-Lead ECG Compared With 12-Lead ECG
   in Arrhythmia / 146
Other Features to Assist With Definition of Arrhythmia
   Substrate / 147
Wide QRS Complex Tachycardia / 148
Transthoracic Echocardiography / 148
Transesophageal Echocardiography / 149
Cardiac Magnetic Resonance Imaging and Computed
   Tomography / 149
Cardiac MRI With Implanted Cardiac Devices / 151
Cardiac MRI for Left Ventricular Scar Mapping / 152
Cardiac Positron Emission Tomography / 152

**MULTIMODAL IMAGING IN THE ELECTROPHYSIOLOGY
LABORATORY / 152**
The Electrophysiology Laboratory / 153
EGM Recording / 153
The Electronic Stimulator and Fluoroscopy / 155
Analysis of Data From Electrophysiologic Mapping Catheters / 155
Tachycardia Mechanism and Location / 156
EGM Interpretation / 156
Conduction Intervals, Activation Sequence, and Refractory
   Periods / 156
Catheter Mapping of Tachycardia / 158
Characterizing Macro–Re-entrant Arrhythmias / 158
Characterizing Focal (Automatic or Triggered)
   Arrhythmias / 159
Ablation and Impedance Mapping / 160
Three-Dimensional Transesophageal Echocardiography / 161
Intracardiac Echocardiography / 161
Cardiac MRI and CT / 162
Three-Dimensional Contact Mapping / 162
Voltage Mapping (Three-Dimensional Contact Mapping
   System) / 163
Activation and Propagation Mapping (Three-Dimensional
   Contact Mapping System) / 163
Putting It All Together / 163
Limitations of Contact Mapping / 165
Three-Dimensional Electroanatomic Mapping (Three-
   Dimensional Noncontact Mapping System) / 165
Remote Catheter Navigation Systems / 166
Catheter Guidance Without Exposure to Ionizing Radiation / 167

POSTPROCEDURE EVALUATION / 167
Esophageal Evaluation / 167
Pulmonary Vein Evaluation / 167
Cardiac MRI for Assessment of Ablated Tissue / 167
Cardiac PET / 168

CONCLUSION / 168

INTRODUCTION

The purpose of cardiovascular electrophysiologic mapping is to define the anatomic sequence of myocardial activation, both at baseline and/or with arrhythmia. There have been tremendous technologic advances in this area[1] that have created fertile ground for the integration of multiple imaging modalities. High-level integration begins with preprocedural assessment of electrophysiologic properties revealed by the 12-lead surface electrocardiogram (ECG) viewed in the context of patient demographics and history.[2,3] Further information is added during invasive electrophysiologic mapping with assessment of intracardiac electrograms viewed in the context of cardiac anatomy.[4,5] The fusion of functional electrophysiologic data with anatomic data in the electrophysiology laboratory facilitates catheter navigation, data annotation, and direct visualization of target sites for therapy. Following an invasive electrophysiologic mapping procedure, there are likewise multiple imaging modalities useful for assessing response to therapy, excluding complications, and directing future diagnostic and therapeutic decisions.[6]

PREPROCEDURAL EVALUATION

■ BASELINE 12-LEAD ECG AND PATIENT HISTORY

The efficiency and effectiveness of an invasive electrophysiologic mapping procedure are dependent on the preprocedure evaluation. Patient demographics, history, and 12-lead surface ECG both at baseline and with arrhythmia help determine what diagnoses are possible and, among the possible, which are most likely. The 12-lead ECG is among the oldest and most useful imaging modalities for localizing arrhythmia origin and characterizing arrhythmia mechanism. The 12-lead ECG provides imaging by display of vectorial information contained in the body surface voltage pattern viewed from different leads, each viewing the heart from a different perspective or "angle." Tachycardia occurring in a female in her forties with a superior P wave axis, short RP interval, with a narrow QRS complex is most likely atrioventricular nodal re-entrant tachycardia.[7] A younger male with tachypalpitations originally presenting in adolescence may have an ECG that looks similar; however, based on demographics, atrioventricular re-entrant tachycardia via an accessory pathway may be more likely[8] (Fig. 8–1). A patient with a history of right atriotomy might have findings of typical right atrial flutter (ie, negative "sawtooth-shaped" flutter waves in the inferior leads and positive flutter waves in the anterior precordial leads) on the 12-lead ECG; however, the patient might also have right lateral wall atrial flutter encircling the atriotomy scar. These arrhythmias may present simultaneously or sequentially (Fig. 8–2). The probability of directing one's attention to the appropriate substrate is favored by a thoughtful preprocedure analysis.

■ BASELINE 12-LEAD ECG COMPARED WITH 12-LEAD ECG IN ARRHYTHMIA

In addition to viewing the 12-lead ECG in arrhythmia in the context of patient history, it is likewise valuable to compare the 12-lead ECG in arrhythmia with the 12-lead ECG at baseline.

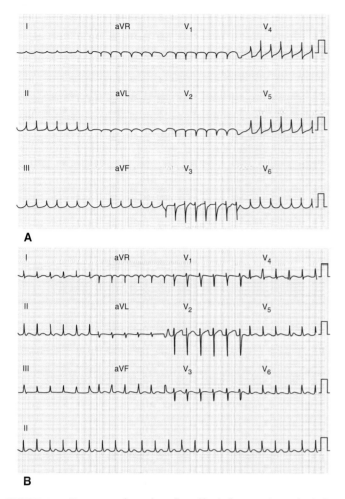

FIGURE 8–1. Narrow complex tachycardias with similar-appearing 12-lead electrocardiograms. Combining demographic information with RP interval assists with determining tachycardia mechanism. **A.** A 42-year-old woman with atrioventricular nodal reentrant tachycardia. **B.** A 22-year-old man with orthodromic atrioventricular reentrant tachycardia.

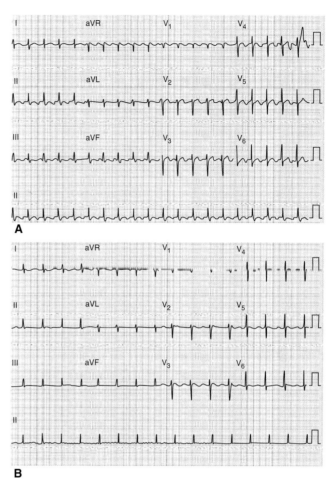

FIGURE 8–2. Substrate for more than one macro–reentrant right atrial flutter. The patient is a 53-year-old woman with previous atrial septal defect repair via a right atriotomy. **A.** Typical cavotricuspid isthmus–dependent right atrial flutter. **B.** Non–cavotricuspid isthmus–dependant flutter (encircling the right atriotomy scar) emerging during ablation across the cavotricuspid isthmus. Note the change in atrial flutter cycle length and flutter-wave morphology.

Findings present on one but not the other can be helpful in elucidating arrhythmia mechanism. The presence of ventricular pre-excitation on a baseline ECG makes a narrow complex tachycardia most likely to be secondary to atrioventricular reentrant tachycardia (orthodromic).[9] The presence of a small retrograde P wave buried in the tail of the QRS in tachycardia that is absent at baseline would be suggestive of typical atrioventricular nodal re-entrant tachycardia. The presence of a "bump" in the T wave during tachycardia that is absent at baseline or a change in the P wave morphology with tachycardia may be suggestive of atrial depolarization with a focal atrial tachycardia. The P wave axis and duration give clues to the source of the tachycardia. Narrow complex arrhythmias originating from atria that have been incised or undergone extensive linear ablation will be more likely macro–re-entrant. Atria that are not scarred (with the exception of cavotricuspid isthmus–dependent right atrial flutter) will more often be focal, usually emerging from one of many known regions of increased arrhythmogenicity (crista terminalis, superior vena cava, tricuspid valve annulus, fossa ovalis, atrial septum, coronary sinus os/body, right atrial appendage, left

atrial appendage, pulmonary veins, ligament of Marshall, mitral valve annulus, noncoronary cusp)[10] (Fig. 8–3). Knowing prior to invasive electrophysiologic mapping whether a focal tachycardia is likely to be originating from the right atrium or left atrium assists in preprocedural planning from a technical, equipment planning standpoint, as well as in assessing risks and benefits of the mapping procedure for review with the patient undergoing the procedure. Likewise, analysis of baseline P wave characteristics, including P wave duration and axis, provides information about how electrical activity is initiated and propagated through the atria, adding information about atrial structure and function that may be relevant to arrhythmia mechanism.[11]

■ OTHER FEATURES TO ASSIST WITH DEFINITION OF ARRHYTHMIA SUBSTRATE

A history of tachycardia termination with maneuvers that slow conduction through the atrioventricular node (ie, vagal maneuvers, carotid massage, adenosine, β-blockers, calcium channel blockers) suggests that the atrioventricular node may be a part

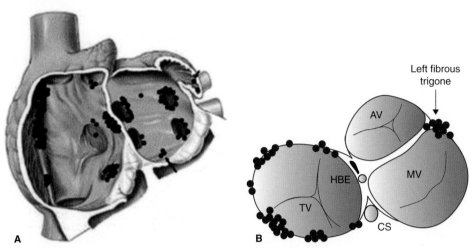

FIGURE 8–3. Anatomic distribution of focal atrial tachycardias. **A.** An oblique cut away of the atria displaying atrial tachycardia origins posterior to the atrioventricular valves. **B.** Sites of focal atrial tachycardia originating on the atrioventricular valve annuli. AV, aortic valve; CS, coronary sinus; HBE, His bundle; MV, mitral valve; TV, tricuspid valve. Reprinted from *Journal of the American College of Cardiology*, 48(5), Kistler PM, Roberts-Thomson KC, Haqqani HM, et al, P-Wave morphology in focal atrial tachycardia: development of an algorithm to predict the anatomic site of origin, Copyright 2006, with permission from Elsevier.

of the tachycardia circuit. Assessment of the PR interval and QRS duration at baseline provides a noninvasive measure of conduction through the atrioventricular node and His-Purkinje system.[12] The presence of baseline pathologic Q waves may be indicative of ischemic heart disease,[13] making a wide complex tachycardia more likely to be a "scar-related" ventricular arrhythmia. Another finding suggestive of the presence of structural heart disease (making ventricular tachycardia more likely) is the presence of low limb lead voltage with preserved (or increased) precordial voltage on the baseline ECG. This finding is frequently seen with dilated cardiomyopathy secondary to a greater proportion of the thoracic cavity being occupied by myocardium and blood pool, thus producing a smaller voltage difference in the bipolar limb leads, but maintaining the voltage measured in the unipolar precordial leads.[14,15] A prolonged QT interval (long QT syndrome), upward coved ST-segment elevation with T wave inversion in the anterior precordial leads (Brugada syndrome), epsilon waves (brief upward deflection at the J point) with T wave inversions across the anterior precordial leads (arrhythmogenic right ventricular cardiomyopathy), unexplained high voltage (hypertrophic cardiomyopathy), and frequent premature ventricular contractions with the same morphology as the clinical tachycardia (such as with an automatic or triggered ventricular tachycardia) are some of the many clues that may be seen on the baseline ECG and correlated with the ECG in tachycardia to help define the arrhythmia mechanism.

■ WIDE QRS COMPLEX TACHYCARDIA

When there is lack of clarity as to whether an arrhythmia is atrial or ventricular, evidence of ventricular pre-excitation at baseline (particularly if multiple accessory pathways are present) makes an atrioventricular reciprocating mechanism more likely. The absence of an anterograde conducting accessory pathway combined with notation of a typical bundle branch block appearance with or without presence of a "long-short"

(Ashman) phenomenon prior to the onset of a wide QRS tachycardia (right bundle branch block occurring more frequently than left bundle branch block) may indicate aberrant conduction. If the wide QRS complex is not a typical bundle branch block pattern and particularly if diagnostic features such as atrioventricular dissociation or fusion/capture beats can be identified, then attention can be focused on the ventricular chambers. The presence of a left bundle branch block pattern and inferior axis in a patient without history of structural heart disease suggests a right ventricular outflow tract origin. However, if the precordial transition occurs at V_3 or earlier, then the right coronary cusp or left ventricular outflow tract is also a possible site of origin. If a right bundle branch block morphology with inferior axis is present in the absence of structural heart disease, then the left coronary cusp, left ventricular outflow tract, aortic-mitral continuity, or superior mitral valve annulus is a likely site of origin. Left coronary cusp ventricular tachycardias often have an "M-shape" QRS complex in V_1, whereas the aortic-mitral continuity frequently demonstrates qR in V_1; are negative in V_2; and then are positive in V_3. Ventricular arrhythmias from the mitral valve annulus should have positive concordance across all precordial leads. As the site of origin moves away from the center of the heart, the QRS width should increase because it will take longer to complete ventricular depolarization moving from one side of the heart to the other rather than starting in the middle and traveling both to the left and the right simultaneously (similar to the finding of P waves in atrioventricular nodal re-entrant tachycardia being narrower than in sinus rhythm secondary to the shorter time required to activate both atria from the center of the heart).

■ TRANSTHORACIC ECHOCARDIOGRAPHY

Beyond clues provided by the history and surface ECG, transthoracic echocardiography is a useful tool to evaluate cardiac structure and function. Two-dimensional and three-dimensional echocardiography is capable of assessing chamber size, myocardial function, and valve function. Additional information relevant to electrophysiologic mapping is the ability of the transthoracic echocardiogram to exclude the presence of left ventricular thrombus as a relative contraindication to left ventricular endocardial mapping (Fig. 8–4). Transthoracic echocardiography with Doppler can also be used to estimate right ventricular systolic pressures. The presence of significant pulmonary hypertension may predict poor tolerance of sustained tachycardia and therefore may modify plans for the electrophysiologic mapping approach. Two-dimensional echocardiography findings of unexpected wall motion abnormalities

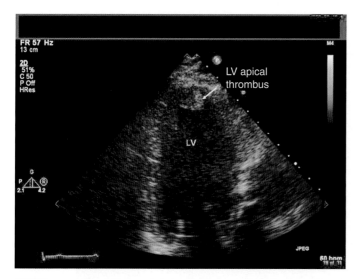

FIGURE 8–4. Left ventricular apical thrombus on two-dimensional transthoracic echocardiogram (arrow). LV, left ventricle. See Moving Image 8–4.

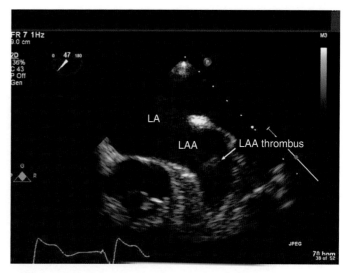

FIGURE 8–5. Transesophageal echocardiography revealing left atrial appendage thrombus despite therapeutic anticoagulation for more than 4 weeks. LA, left atrium; LAA, left atrial appendage. Image provided with permission from Patrick Hranitzky, MD, Duke University Medical Center. See Moving Image 8–5.

or worse than expected valvular heart disease may also raise points requiring further investigation prior to consideration of electrophysiologic mapping. Electrophysiologic mapping may require the use of isoproterenol and/or rapid burst pacing for arrhythmia induction. Exclusion of significant obstructive coronary artery disease may be important prior to performance of an electrophysiologic mapping procedure to avoid inducing a significant amount of ischemia with attempts at arrhythmia induction. Presence of a previously unrecognized atrial septal defect or patent foramen ovale may also be important to recognize in order to minimize risks for paradoxical embolus with right-sided procedures that would otherwise not be present with an intact atrial septum.

■ TRANSESOPHAGEAL ECHOCARDIOGRAPHY

Although transthoracic echocardiography is useful for the analysis of many cardiac structures, patients with rhythms of atrial flutter or atrial fibrillation require transesophageal echocardiography for exclusion of left atrial appendage thrombus. In the case of right atrial flutter, arrhythmia duration <48 hours or therapeutic anticoagulation (ie, warfarin with international normalized ratio ≥2.0) for ≥4 weeks is usually adequate prior to right atrial mapping and ablation. However, for patients with atrial fibrillation who require mapping catheter instrumentation of the left atrium, a more thorough investigation with transesophageal echocardiogram may be warranted to exclude the presence of left atrial appendage thrombus[16] (Fig. 8–5).

■ CARDIAC MAGNETIC RESONANCE IMAGING AND COMPUTED TOMOGRAPHY

Regarding left atrial mapping specifically, there may be much to be gained from preprocedural imaging of the left atrium and surrounding structures by either magnetic resonance imaging (MRI)[17] or computed tomography (CT).[18] Preprocedural left atrial imaging provides a road map of pulmonary vein

anatomy (normal and variant) and identifies esophageal position (Fig. 8–6). Other potential left atrial structures of interest that may be imaged with these techniques include left atrial diverticula or accessory left atrial appendices.[19] These structures have the potential to be arrhythmogenic and to be sites of increased perforation risk. MRI has the benefit of image acquisition without the use of ionizing radiation or the use of iodinated contrast. The former is of particular interest to younger patients and women. The latter is of particular interest to those with a history of iodine/contrast/shellfish allergy or renal insufficiency. In either case, both CT and MRI are able to create data sets that accurately depict left atrial anatomy in a way that can facilitate left atrial electrophysiologic mapping.

In addition to left atrial anatomy, cardiac MRI is also able to evaluate left ventricular myocardial function and obtain data regarding tissue characteristics in this region (Fig. 8–7). Although history, ECG, and echocardiogram detect the majority of patients with structural heart disease, there are patients who have myocardial abnormalities that may not be identified by techniques other than MRI,[20] particularly when the underlying disease process is in its early stages. Examples of this can be found in patients with previously unrecognized myocarditis (acute, chronic, or resolved) (Fig. 8–8), sarcoidosis,[21] hypertrophic cardiomyopathy,[22] hemochromatosis,[23] amyloidosis,[24] arrhythmogenic right ventricular cardiomyopathy,[25] or Chagas disease.[26]

In addition to anatomic and functional data, cardiac MRI is also able to obtain physiologic data including stress perfusion imaging and flow-velocity data. Both MRI and CT angiography can be useful for assessment of proximal coronary arterial anatomy, assessing systemic and pulmonary arterial and venous connections, although the ability of MRI to acquire data in a multiplanar fashion can be particularly useful in patients with complex anatomy such as patients with some forms of congenital

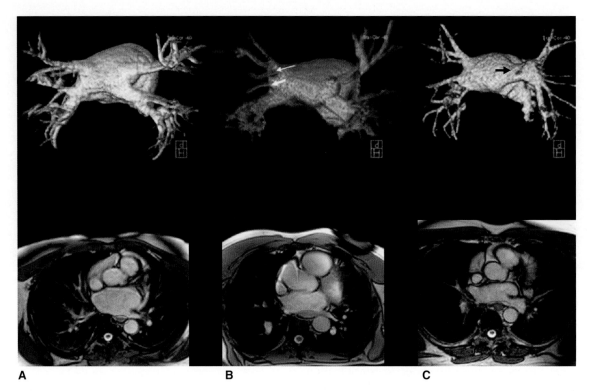

FIGURE 8–6. Cardiac magnetic resonance angiography demonstrating normal and normal variant pulmonary vein anatomy (green cube for orientation; H, head; P, posterior). **A.** All four pulmonary veins (right upper, right lower, left upper, and left lower) emerging from the left atrium in a normal fashion. **B.** Variant right pulmonary vein anatomy with a separate right middle pulmonary vein (thick white arrow) and early posterior branch off the right lower pulmonary vein (thin white arrow). **C.** Left pulmonary veins (left upper and left lower) emerging as a common trunk (black arrow). Below each left atrial image is the corresponding axial bright blood image displaying esophageal position (red ellipse around the esophagus). See Moving Images 8–6A to C.

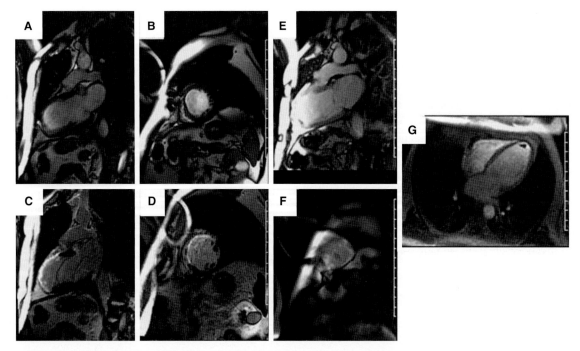

FIGURE 8–7. Cardiac magnetic resonance imaging in a patient with previous myocardial infarction and left ventricular apical thrombus. **A.** and **B.** Two-chamber and short axis cine views demonstrating focal wall thinning and hypokinesis. **C.** and **D.** Corresponding delayed-enhancement images revealing myocardial scarring/infarct. **E.** and **F.** Two-chamber and short axis, high inversion time images demonstrating thrombus in the left ventricular apex. **G.** Further confirmation of thrombus magnetic resonance angiography in a four-chamber view. See Moving Images 8–7A, B, and G.

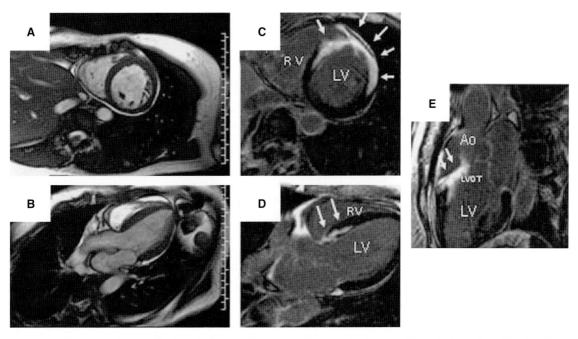

FIGURE 8–8. Cardiac magnetic resonance imaging with delayed-enhancement images revealing nonischemic myocardial scarring in a patient with outflow tract ventricular tachycardia. **A.** and **B.** Magnetic resonance cine images in short axis and three-chamber views with absence of dramatic wall motion abnormalities. **C–E.** Delayed-enhancement images revealing nonischemic extensive anterobasal myocardial scarring extending up toward the outflow tract of the left ventricle (arrows). Ao, aorta; LV, left ventricle; LVOT, left ventricular outflow tract; RV, right ventricle. See Moving Images 8–8A and B.

heart disease (Fig. 8–9). The MRI information obtained in this patient population can be useful not only for roadmapping anatomic regions of interest, but also for treatment planning (ie, exclusion of need for interventions such as baffle stenting or surgical repair that might affect the plan for electrophysiologic mapping and arrhythmia treatment).

■ CARDIAC MRI WITH IMPLANTED CARDIAC DEVICES

Cardiac MRI is useful for identifying the myocardial scar that is the substrate for ischemic ventricular tachycardia. However, most ischemic ventricular tachycardia mapping procedures are done in patients with implantable cardioverter defibrillators. The absence of a completely MRI-compatible implantable

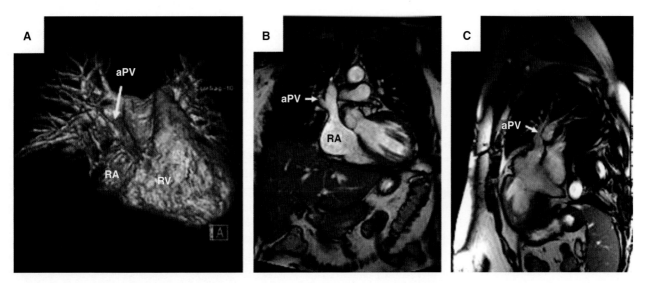

FIGURE 8–9. Magnetic resonance imaging of an anomalous pulmonary vein entering at the superior right atrium/superior vena cava. **A.** Three-dimensional magnetic resonance imaging of the heart and proximal central vasculature (green cube for orientation; A, anterior). **B.** and **C.** Bright blood magnetic resonance imaging in oblique views to visualize the region of anomalous pulmonary vein connection to the superior right atrium/superior vena cava. aPV, anomalous pulmonary vein; RA, right atrium; RV, right ventricle. See Moving Images 8–9A to C.

cardioverter defibrillator (or the presence of other contraindication to MRI) is a significant barrier to the routine use of cardiac MRI in this setting. This barrier, however, does not completely exclude the possibility of performing cardiac MRI with a defibrillator in situ. MRI protocols for some implanted cardiac devices have been published with documentation of points of concern as well as statements that MRIs can be obtained without prohibitive image compromise and without adverse effects to the patient or the device (devices implanted on or after the year 2000).[27] In the study by Nazarian and Halperin,[27] emphasis was placed on the preprocedural review of the chest x-ray to assess all used and abandoned hardware. Lead length and loops were noted to increase current and therefore create heat. A specific absorption rate (SAR) of ≤2.0 W/kg was recommended with the noted caveat that the SAR-to-heat correlation is not consistent among different MRI scanners. Recommendations were also made for the use of the largest acceptable field of view, longest repetition time, minimal flip angle, and minimal acquisition bandwidth. There was notation that magnetic fields can flip reed switches, which may affect the function of certain devices. A full device interrogation was recommended before MRI scanning (checking battery voltage, sensing, impedance, pacing threshold, and programmed parameters) and after MRI scanning to assure stability. Tachycardia detection and tachycardia therapy were programmed off prior to MRI to prevent filling tachycardia counters with noise and to prevent inappropriate tachycardia therapies for electromechanical interference associated with performance of the cardiac MRI. For pacemakers, pacing parameters were programmed to an asynchronous mode (if pacemaker dependent) or VVI/DDI (if underlying rhythm was stable) to avoid inhibition of pacing or tracking of noise, respectively (MRI scanning was not recommended for implantable cardioverter-defibrillator patients if pacemaker dependent). All magnet response features were disabled. Recommendations were made for blood pressure, ECG, oxygen saturation, and symptom monitoring with physicians and advanced cardiac life support equipment present. Imaging planes perpendicular to the device generator with shortened echo time and use of spin-echo and fast spin-echo spoiled gradient recall echo cine were used to reduce qualitative device artifacts. Implantable loop recorders are MRI safe; however, the data recorded on these devices must be downloaded prior to MRI and the memory must be cleared after MRI to avoid overwriting previous useful electrogram data with electromechanical interference and to avoid maintaining arrhythmia logs filled with electromechanical interference, respectively. Temporary pacing wires, abandoned leads, and epicardial leads are not MRI safe. MRI should not be performed within the first 6 weeks after device implant. Although the total number of patients in this study was relatively small, the combination of imaging success and absence of adverse outcomes is encouraging. Underreporting of adverse consequences, however, remains a concern; therefore, prior to attempting MRI with a pacemaker or defibrillator in situ, consideration must be given to the risk-benefit analysis of this endeavor. For further investigation of questions regarding

MRI compatibility, useful information can be obtained from the following Website: http://www.mrisafety.com/.

CARDIAC MRI FOR LEFT VENTRICULAR SCAR MAPPING

Incorporation of cardiac MRI–defined ventricular scar-specific data into a three-dimensional electroanatomic map has been described.[28] Although Desjardins et al[28] showed a good correlation between MRI scar data and information obtained electroanatomically, the transfer of scar data from the MRI to the electroanatomic map was somewhat laborious, and when imported into the electroanatomic mapping system, the ventricular scar was not able to be represented with the level of detail achievable on the original MRIs. Nevertheless, this basic concept shows great potential. Most of the technology required to bring these MRIs into the electrophysiologic mapping laboratory is available. When defibrillators become fully MRI compatible to ease the safety concerns and logistic challenges of performing cardiac MRI in patients with implantable cardioverter-defibrillators, it is likely that preprocedural scar imaging data will make a rapid leap into the electrophysiologic laboratory. Bringing these multiple imaging modalities together in a three-dimensional, merged/fused fashion will likely facilitate efficiency, safety, and efficacy in the treatment of ischemic ventricular tachycardia.

CARDIAC POSITRON EMISSION TOMOGRAPHY

In addition to cardiac MRI and CT, cardiac positron emission tomography (PET) may hold promise for the assessment of metabolic abnormalities relevant to arrhythmogenesis.[29] Evaluating abnormalities of metabolism, such as those that occur with inflammation, may provide insight into the status of myocardium not measurable by other techniques. The ability to visualize these abnormalities may be particularly useful in the investigation of cardiac sarcoidosis or myocarditis. In these disease processes, systemic markers of disease activity may be variably present and may not accurately represent disease activity in the myocardium. Identification of cardiac-specific metabolic abnormalities may be one area where cardiac PET can provide useful information (Fig. 8–10). At times of active myocardial inflammation, treatments targeting the suppression of inflammation[30] (or consequences of inflammation) may be more effective for improving long-term outcomes than using mapping and catheter-based therapies on a dynamic substrate.

MULTIMODAL IMAGING IN THE ELECTROPHYSIOLOGY LABORATORY

Electrophysiologic mapping of complex arrhythmias requires integration of multiple imaging techniques to achieve the best possible safety and efficacy profile. Multiple techniques for assessing static and real-time representations of cardiac anatomy and myocardial electrical activity are displayed simultaneously, in digital, two-dimensional, three-dimensional, and merged formats to provide well-validated information about target anatomy and target electrophysiology.

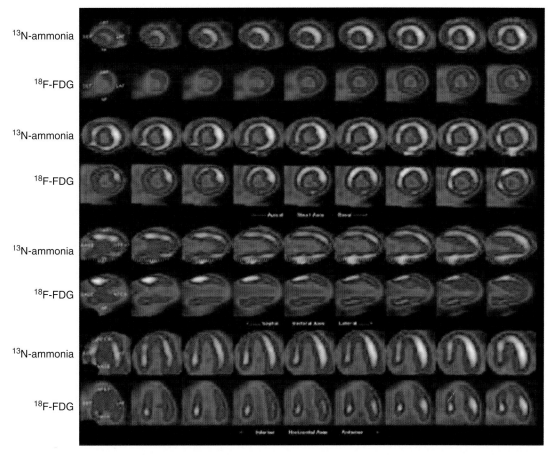

FIGURE 8–10. Cardiac positron emission tomography (cPET). A clinical picture of myocarditis accompanied by ventricular tachycardia and complete heart block was investigated by cPET following a 16-hour period of fasting. In this unusual case, a heterogeneous pattern of glucose uptake is present with increased ^{18}F-FDG uptake in the mid to basal left ventricle compared with relatively little uptake in the apical left ventricle. It is conceivable that these findings represent local metabolic abnormalities relevant to myocardial disease activity and arrhythmogenesis. ^{13}N-ammonia, nitrogen-13 ammonia.

■ THE ELECTROPHYSIOLOGY LABORATORY

A typical electrophysiologic laboratory is divided into two rooms, the control room and the patient room. The control room contains displays for real-time electrograms (EGMs), a review screen for assessment of static EGMs, fluoroscopy displays, an electronic stimulator display, three-dimensional electroanatomic mapping display, and additional monitor screens as needed for viewing real-time echocardiography, preprocedure studies, and/or a procedure room camera display. Lead glass and a doorway separate the control room from the patient room. The patient room is equipped with multiple monitor booms to display the multiple imaging modalities needed for guiding catheter manipulation during the electrophysiologic mapping procedure (Figs. 8–11 and 8–12).

■ EGM RECORDING

Within the electrophysiologic laboratory, the EGM recording system measures and displays electrical signals from both surface leads and intracardiac catheters. The timing and morphology of surface ECG leads provide the starting point for EGM interpretation and arrhythmia analysis. Three or four surface ECG leads are displayed at the top of the live EGM recording screen. The leads selected are most frequently orthogonal in the frontal plane (ie, leads I and aVF) with one or two precordial leads, usually including V_1 (V_1 is particularly useful to differentiate right bundle branch block and left bundle branch block QRS morphologies). Displayed below the surface ECG leads are the intracardiac EGMs (Fig. 8–13). Intracardiac EGMs are amplified and filtered to produce sharp deflections used to indicate timing of local electrical activity. The presentation of these EGMs on the live screen scrolls from left to right at an adjustable speed depending on operator preference (eg, 100 mm/s or 200 mm/s). There is also an audible beep that can be programmed to sound for ventricular sensed events that changes in tone for paced events in order to alert all in the electrophysiologic laboratory to the heart rate without looking at the EGM screen. Next to the live EGM screen is most frequently a review screen. When a pacing train is complete, the EGM screen shot at the end of the train is directed to the review screen for analysis. If there is a spontaneous event of interest, a single-button stroke can transmit the EGMs from the live screen to the review screen for analysis.

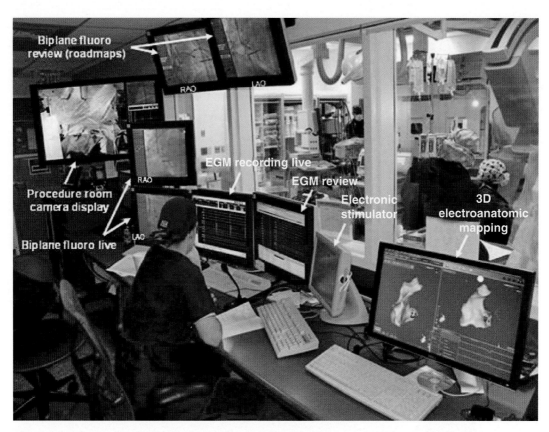

FIGURE 8–11. Electrophysiology control room. 3D, three-dimensional; EGM, electrogram; fluoro, fluoroscopy; LAO, left anterior oblique; RAO, right anterior oblique.

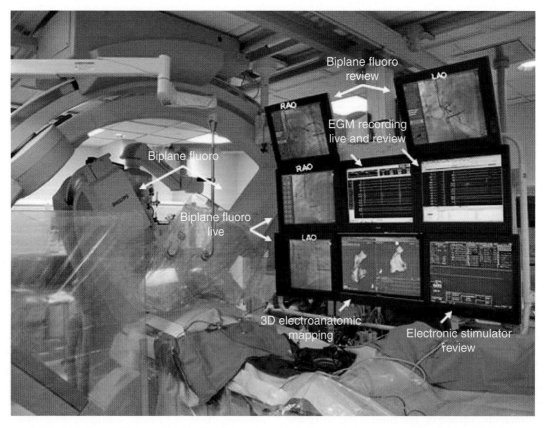

FIGURE 8–12. Electrophysiology laboratory procedure room. 3D, three-dimensional; EGM, electrogram; fluoro, fluoroscopy, LAO, left anterior oblique; RAO, right anterior oblique.

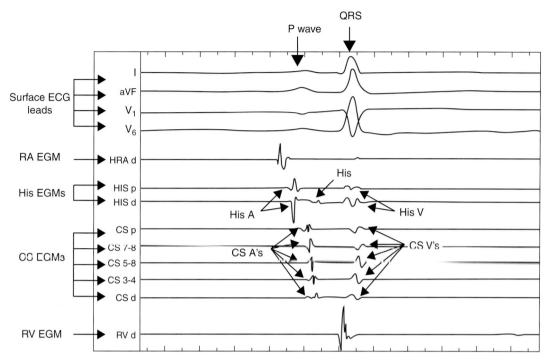

FIGURE 8–13. Electrogram recording system demonstrating surface electrocardiogram leads at the top of the screen with intracardiac electrograms (EGMs) below. Coronary sinus (CS) and His catheters have proximity to both the atrium and the ventricular and therefore detect both atrial and ventricular signals. A, atrial EGM; d, distal; HRA, high right atrium; p, proximal; RA, right atrium; RV, right ventricle; V, ventricular EGM.

The EGM recording screens (live and review) are displayed in the control room, as well as at the bedside in the patient room to allow for EGM analysis during catheter manipulation.

■ THE ELECTRONIC STIMULATOR AND FLUOROSCOPY

The EGM recording system monitors (live and review) in the control room are positioned next to the stimulator. The electronic stimulator is used to deliver pacing signals from the control room to intracardiac catheters for the purpose of electrophysiologic study and mapping. The indwelling catheters are placed in strategic positions in and around the cardiac chambers. Fluoroscopy is used to guide diagnostic catheter placement (Fig. 8–14). One limitation of fluoroscopy is its two-dimensional nature. For this reason, use of orthogonal views to represent three-dimensional anatomy is important (Fig. 8–15). In addition to the use of orthogonal views to assess location in three-dimensional space, intravascular contrast can be used to provide more detailed information about the vascular structure in question. Contrast may also be required to assist with visualizing structures such as the interatrial septum in preparation for transseptal puncture (Fig. 8–16) or epicardial tenting in preparation for epicardial access, for defining coronary anatomy that may be in close proximity to an arrhythmogenic

focus (Fig. 8–17), for identifying coronary sinus diverticula that may mark the site of an accessory pathway,[31] for opacifying structures to clarify catheter position (Fig. 8–18), or for identifying right ventricular wall motion abnormalities in patients with suspected arrhythmogenic right ventricular cardiomyopathy.

■ ANALYSIS OF DATA FROM ELECTROPHYSIOLOGIC MAPPING CATHETERS

With diagnostic catheters in place, the electrophysiologic substrate can be characterized before and after arrhythmia induction

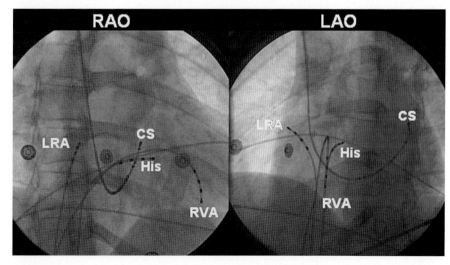

FIGURE 8–14. Four-catheter setup for evaluation of supraventricular tachycardia. CS, coronary sinus; His, His bundle; LAO, left anterior oblique; LRA, lateral right atrium; RAO, right anterior oblique; RVA, right ventricular apex.

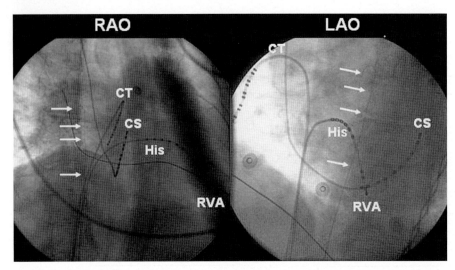

FIGURE 8–15. Use of orthogonal fluoroscopic views to identify guidewire position. Using the RAO view, the guidewire (arrows) appears to be in the inferior vena cava with J-tip in the right atrium; however, the orthogonal LAO view reveals the guidewire is too leftward to be in the inferior vena cava or right atrium. Guidewire position is behind the heart in the hemiazygos vein. CS, coronary sinus; CT, crista terminalis; His, His bundle; LAO, left anterior oblique; RAO, right anterior oblique; RVA, right ventricular apex.

to help define arrhythmia mechanism. Diagnostic and mapping catheters are positioned to obtain as much information as possible with the minimum number of catheters. A four-catheter setup such as that displayed in Figure 8–14 can be used to investigate supraventricular tachycardia. From these four catheters, information can be obtained regarding patient-specific electrophysiologic characteristics. These catheters (along with surface ECG analysis) provide information about the relative location of the tachycardia origin (ie, right or left, high or low, anterior or posterior) by EGM timing (ie, right atrial catheter is RIGHT, distal coronary sinus catheter is LEFT, the atrial EGM on the His bundle is HIGH and ANTERIOR in the middle of the heart, the proximal coronary sinus catheter is LOW and POSTERIOR in the middle of the heart). Additional multipolar catheters

and mapping systems may be applied to further assist in tachycardia localization; however, the principle of using EGM location and time-specific information to define arrhythmia mechanism is the same. The likely arrhythmia mechanism is suggested by analysis of the surface ECG and baseline conduction properties and is confirmed with mapping and pacing maneuvers in tachycardia.

■ TACHYCARDIA MECHANISM AND LOCATION

Tachycardias are generally either focal (emerging from a discrete location, spreading out in a centrifugal manner in all available directions) or macro–re-entrant (following a head-meets-tail propagation) (Fig. 8–19). The origin is either supraventricular (right atrial vs left atrial vs atrioventricular node vs coronary sinus vs noncoronary cusp) or ventricular (right ventricular vs left ventricular [endocardial vs epicardial, scar related vs non–scar related] vs pulmonary artery vs left/right coronary cusps) or dependent on an accessory pathway between the atrium and ventricles that allows for atrioventricular reciprocating tachycardia.

■ EGM INTERPRETATION

Morphologic analysis of intracardiac EGMs is useful for such things as distinguishing atrial EGMs from ventricular EGMs when obtaining electrical information near the atrioventricular groove, distinguishing far-field from near-field signals, and analysis of low-amplitude high-frequency aspects of EGM signals that may be suggestive of tissue anisotropy at an arrhythmogenic focus; otherwise, the majority of the information obtained from diagnostic catheters is from EGM timing. For this reason, EGM recording systems time-synchronize intracardiac EGMs and surface ECGs. Electronic calipers can then be used to quickly and accurately perform conduction interval measurements that are reproducible to within a few milliseconds.

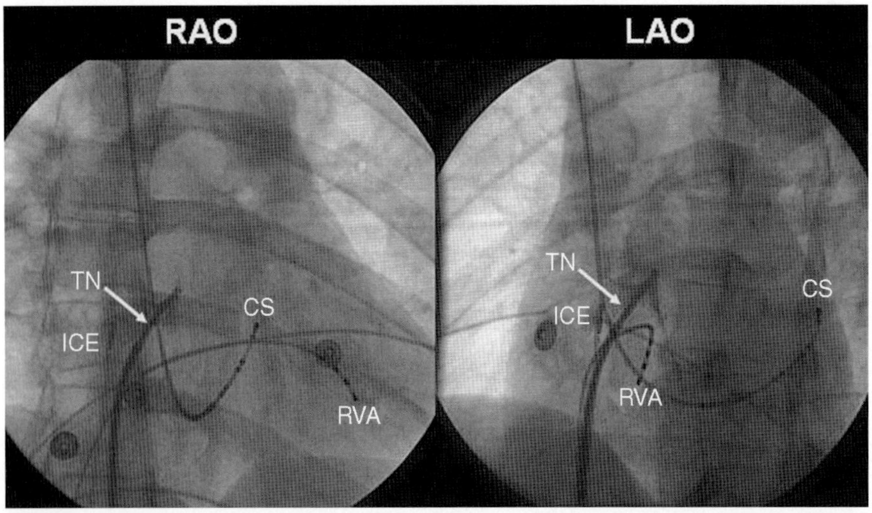

■ CONDUCTION INTERVALS, ACTIVATION SEQUENCE, AND REFRACTORY PERIODS

An electrophysiologic study begins with the measurement of baseline conduction intervals. In addition to the standard surface PR, QRS, QT, and RR intervals, intracardiac EGMs allow for the measurement of the AH (time from the local atrial EGM on the His catheter to the onset of the His EGM on

FIGURE 8–16. Use of intravenous contrast to demonstrate tenting of the interatrial septum during transseptal access. CS, coronary sinus; ICE, intracardiac echocardiography probe; LAO, left anterior oblique; RAO, right anterior oblique; RVA, right ventricular apex; TN, transseptal needle via SL1 sheath and dilator.

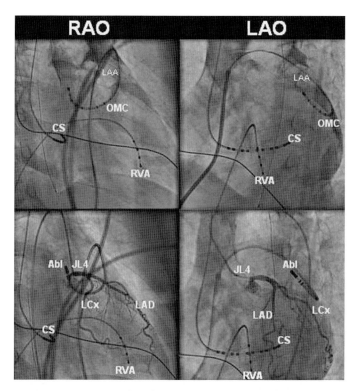

FIGURE 8–17. Coronary angiography during epicardial mapping of a focal atrial tachycardia emerging from the region of the ligament of Marshall (arrhythmia focus located between the left atrial appendage and the left pulmonary veins). Biplane fluoroscopic views demonstrate adequate distance between coronary arterial system and mapping catheter to allow safe delivery of radiofrequency energy. Abl, ablation; CS, coronary sinus; JL4, left coronary artery catheter; LAA, left atrial appendage; LAD, left anterior descending artery; LAO, left anterior oblique; LCx, left circumflex coronary artery; OMC, octapolar mapping catheter; RAO, right anterior oblique; RVA, right ventricular apex. Images provided with permission from Patrick Hranitzky, MD, Duke University Medical Center. See Moving Images 8–17A (left anterior oblique epicardial ablation catheter/ angiography), 8–17B (left anterior oblique octapolar contrast around left atrial appendage), 8–17C (right anterior oblique epicardial ablation catheter/angiography), and 8–17D (right anterior oblique octapolar contrast around left atrial appendage).

the His catheter) and HV (time from the onset of the His EGM on the His catheter to the first sign of ventricular activation, usually with the imitation of the QRS complex on the surface ECG). While measuring conduction intervals, Wenckebach cycle lengths, and refractory periods, parameters such as ventriculoatrial activation can also be assessed. Ventriculoatrial activation is determined by pacing from the ventricular catheter and observing the timing of atrial signals on diagnostic catheters in the right atrium, His bundle region, and throughout the length of the coronary sinus. Normal ventriculoatrial conduction in the absence of an accessory pathway should only occur through the atrioventricular node and therefore should be concentric (earliest at the center of the heart with earliest atrial EGMs on the His bundle catheter). Although this does not exclude a septal accessory pathway, it makes the presence of a rapidly conducting lateral (eccentric) accessory pathway less likely. If there is no ventriculoatrial conduction at baseline, then there is no retrogradely conducting accessory pathway, and the diagnosis of orthodromic reciprocating tachycardia is excluded. If there is suspicion of a septal accessory pathway, additional diagnostic maneuvers can

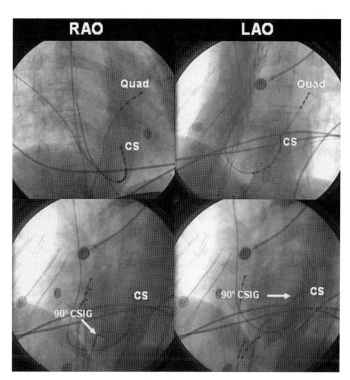

FIGURE 8–18. Use of intravenous contrast to identify catheter position. A quadripolar catheter initially intended for the right ventricle is seen crossing the spine in the LAO projection suggesting a position in the left atrium. Potential explanations include the presence of an atrial septal defect, unroofed coronary sinus, or persistent left superior vena cava. Injection of contrast reveals presence of the latter. 90° CSIG, coronary sinus inner guide; CS, coronary sinus mapping catheter; LAO, left anterior oblique; Quad, quadripolar mapping catheter; RAO, right anterior oblique. Images courtesy of Kevin Jackson, MD, Duke University Medical Center. See Moving Image 8–18.

be performed to evaluate this possibility (ie, parahisian pacing and/or comparing ventriculoatrial conduction times when pacing from the ventricular base vs the ventricular apex).

Following the assessment of ventriculoatrial conduction, assessment of atrioventricular conduction can be made. This provides information about atrioventricular node function and allows for assessment of atrioventricular conduction at rapid rates that might uncover anterograde conduction across a previously unrecognized accessory pathway as atrioventricular nodal conduction becomes decremental. If ventricular pre-excitation is suspected, additional maneuvers such as differential pacing (pacing from different locations in the atria in an attempt to identify ventricular pre-excitation by comparing QRS morphology pacing close to vs far away from the location of the suspected accessory pathway) can be used to support this hypothesis. Likewise,

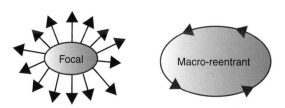

FIGURE 8–19. Focal versus macro–reentrant tachycardia mechanisms.

administration of adenosine can be used to block atrioventricular nodal conduction, noting that some accessory pathways (particularly slowly conducting accessory pathways with decremental "atrioventricular node–like" properties) may also block with adenosine. Following these pacing maneuvers, programmed electrical stimulation can then be performed in the atrium. The presence of an "AH jump" (defined as a prolongation of the AH interval >50 ms with an S_1/S_2 coupling interval decrease of only 10 ms) implies the presence of dual atrioventricular nodal physiology, with fast pathway (fast conduction velocity, but relatively long effective refractory period) and slow pathway (slow conduction velocity, but relatively short effective refractory period) inputs to the atrioventricular node creating the substrate for atrioventricular nodal re-entrant tachycardia. Additional extra stimuli may be applied (ie, atrial for supraventricular tachycardia and ventricular for ventricular tachycardia) or rapid burst pacing may be pursued with and without pharmacologic agents such as the adrenergic agonist isoproterenol (burst pacing during isoproterenol initiation, upward titration, plateau, and washout) to increase automaticity/triggered activity, increase conduction velocity, shorten refractory periods, and/or increase the dispersion of refractoriness in hopes of creating suitable substrate for tachyarrhythmia initiation and maintenance.

◼ CATHETER MAPPING OF TACHYCARDIA

In addition to the four cardiac chambers (right atrium, right ventricle, left atrium, and left ventricle), there are additional regions surrounding these chambers relevant to electrophysiologic mapping (ie, coronary sinus, coronary cusps, epicardial space). It is important to consider each of these regions as a potential site for arrhythmia origin. For example, a ventricular tachycardia may be identifiable as emerging from the right ventricular outflow tract region using only the surface ECG. This arrhythmia may be mapped in great detail positioning the mapping catheter in numerous regions throughout the right ventricular outflow tract; however, if the true origin is from the right coronary cusp, this region cannot be assessed from the right ventricle. Likewise, an atrial tachycardia may have points of earliest activation mapped from the right atrium, as well as the left atrium along the anterior interatrial septum; however, if the arrhythmia is from the noncoronary cusp, the true origin cannot be confirmed with the mapping catheter anywhere other than the proximal aorta.

If mapping of a focal tachycardia is not performed in the correct location, the origin of the arrhythmia will not be discovered, and attempts at treatment will be frustrating. The importance of mapping in the correct location is also seen with macro–re-entrant arrhythmias. Left atrial flutters that encircle the mitral annulus often use muscular bands residing in the coronary sinus. Effective linear ablation of the mitral isthmus frequently requires ablation in the coronary sinus to achieve conduction block in the tissue between the inferolateral mitral valve annulus and the inferolateral aspect of the left lower pulmonary vein.[32] Likewise, accessory atrioventricular pathways residing in the coronary sinus or middle cardiac vein will not be detected unless the mapping catheter is placed in these structures. The presence of a negative delta wave in lead II on the surface ECG suggests an

epicardial location of a posteroseptal accessory pathway.[33] When evaluating ventricular arrhythmias, consideration may also need to be given to whether the focus of the arrhythmia is epicardial or endocardial. There are some clues identifiable prior to invasive mapping that indicate that the source of a ventricular arrhythmia may be epicardial such as the underlying disease process (eg, sarcoidosis, Chagas, arrhythmogenic right ventricular cardiomyopathy), and surface ECG QRS morphology (eg, slurred upstroke to a late peaking QRS, more than one negative to positive QRS transition in the anterior precordial leads).[34] However, in many cases, requirement for epicardial access may not be apparent until subendocardial approaches have failed. With requirement for epicardial access, the need for multiple imaging modalities becomes apparent because fluoroscopy, EGMs, and three-dimensional electroanatomic maps may require additional information from intravenous contrast injection and coronary angiography to ensure that the epicardium is entered safely and to confirm that ablation energy is delivered at a safe distance from the coronary arterial tree, as illustrated in Figure 8–17.

◼ CHARACTERIZING MACRO–RE-ENTRANT ARRHYTHMIAS

If tachycardia can be initiated and maintained, additional diagnostic maneuvers can be performed to define the mechanism of the arrhythmia. The primary pacing maneuver used to define a re-entrant mechanism is entrainment. By pacing from a given sight at a paced cycle length that is slightly faster than the tachycardia cycle length (ie, entrainment pacing cycle length = tachycardia cycle length – 20 to 30 ms) and then measuring the time it takes for the local EGM in tachycardia to return to the pacing electrode after cessation of pacing, the return cycle length or postpacing interval (PPI) can be measured. Likewise, additional information can be obtained by looking for diastolic potentials, assessing EGM timing, and comparing the surface ECG morphology both while pacing and in tachycardia. Among other cardinal features, entrainment is heralded by acceleration of the tachycardia to the paced cycle length prior to cessation of pacing without termination of tachycardia. Entrainment can be attempted from any region of paceable myocardium; however, success will depend on the ability of the pacing stimulus to enter the excitable gap of the re-entrant arrhythmia (excitable gap = tachycardia cycle length – effective refractory period) without extinguishing tachycardia. If entrainment is successful, a shorter PPI will indicate that the pacing catheter is closer to the tachycardia circuit. The longer the PPI, the further away the pacing catheter is from the circuit. When the PPI equals the tachycardia cycle length (without change in EGM activation sequence or change in surface ECG morphology), the pacing catheter is in the circuit.

Additional information is obtained by incorporation of known anatomic structures serving as portals of conduction (ie, the atrioventricular node, the His-Purkinje system, accessory pathways) and areas of conduction block (ie, atrioventricular valves, the eustachian ridge, the crista terminalis) and knowledge of relatively narrow regions of conducting tissue between structures of known anatomic block (eg, the cavotricuspid isthmus lying between the eustachian ridge and the tricuspid valve annulus). Which of these structures are relevant to the tachycardia circuit needs to be determined, and these hypotheses can be tested with assessment of EGM timing, use of pharmacologic agents such as adenosine to produce atrioventricular block, and pacing maneuvers designed to test participation of a given chamber or pathway in tachycardia (ie, pacing from the ventricle during narrow complex tachycardia to produce tachycardia termination at a time of His refractoriness demonstrating participation of the ventricle in the tachycardia circuit with orthodromic reciprocating tachycardia). A single observation or response to a pacing maneuver may not be adequate to determine arrhythmia mechanism conclusively; however, reproducible observations during multiple pacing maneuvers are usually able to clarify arrhythmia mechanism.[9]

■ CHARACTERIZING FOCAL (AUTOMATIC OR TRIGGERED) ARRHYTHMIAS

For tachyarrhythmias that do not have a re-entrant mechanism (eg, focal atrial tachycardia or focal right ventricular outflow tract tachycardia secondary to increased automaticity or triggered activity), entrainment is not possible. Pacing at rates faster than the tachycardia cycle length results in overdrive suppression of these arrhythmias however, stable manifest fusion will not be achievable, and the return cycle length or PPI analysis will often yield variable results that will not provide reliable information about the proximity of the pacing catheter to the focus of the arrhythmia. One pacing tool that can be useful for defining the origin of an automatic or triggered ventricular arrhythmia is pacemapping. Pacemapping is achieved by positioning the mapping catheter in a region of suspected arrhythmia origin and pacing the local myocardium at 1.5 to 2 times the pacing threshold and then comparing the paced 12-lead surface ECG to the 12-lead surface ECG morphology of the clinical arrhythmia (Fig. 8–20). The presence of a "12-out-of-12" lead pacemap match is supportive of the catheter position being at the origin of the tachycardia. Additional information of critical importance to include with information obtained by maneuvers such as pacemapping is assessment of the local EGMs at the suspected site of arrhythmia origin. Whether the arrhythmia is atrial or ventricular, the local

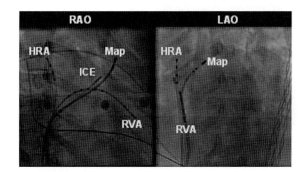
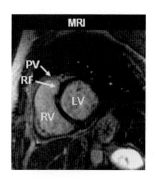
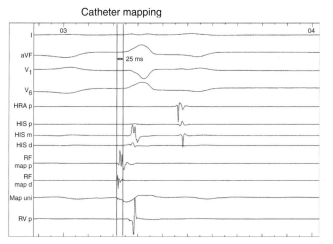
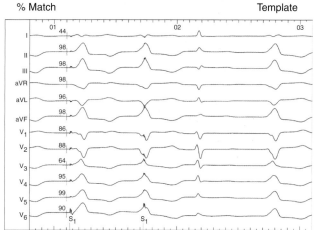

FIGURE 8–20. Catheter mapping and pacemapping of a right ventricular outflow tract tachycardia. **Top left.** Biplane fluoroscopic views of intracardiac catheters. Mapping catheter is directed at the superior-septal aspect of the right ventricular outflow tract at the site of arrhythmia origin. **Top right.** Cardiac magnetic resonance imaging (MRI) with delayed enhancement at the site of radiofrequency ablation along the septal aspect of the right ventricular outflow tract just below the pulmonary valve. **Bottom left.** Catheter electrograms at the site of arrhythmia origin demonstrating local bipolar electrograms preceding the onset of the QRS complex in the surface leads by 25 ms and a QS on unipolar electrogram. **Bottom right.** Pacing from the mapping catheter produces a QRS complex that matches the clinical QRS complex (Template) in all 12 leads. HRA, high right atrium; ICE, intracardiac echocardiography probe; LAO, left anterior oblique; LV, left ventricle; Map, mapping catheter; PV, pulmonary valve; RAO, right anterior oblique; RF, region of radiofrequency energy delivery; RV, right ventricle; RVA, right ventricular apex; Uni, unipolar.

EGM at the site of arrhythmia origin should precede the surface ECG deflection by 25 to 45 ms. If the local EGM is not sufficiently early, then additional mapping will usually be required to identify the true origin of the arrhythmia. In addition to timing of this EGM, features such as low-amplitude, highly fractionated (high-frequency) bipolar EGMs and a QS pattern (indicative of all electrical activity moving away from the catheter tip) on unipolar EGMs are usually present at the origin of a focal arrhythmia. As with integration of multiple imaging modalities to achieve an accurate depiction of cardiovascular anatomy, the accuracy of electrophysiologic mapping is improved when multiple ways of identifying arrhythmia mechanism and/or arrhythmia origin are all supportive of the same conclusion.

■ ABLATION AND IMPEDANCE MAPPING

In addition to pacing maneuvers and EGM characteristics, delivery of radiofrequency energy itself can be useful for mapping. Whether the ablation catheter is on a critical isthmus

of a re-entrant circuit or the origin of an automatic or triggered focal tachycardia, delivery of radiofrequency energy to this area that results in termination (usually preceded by prolongation of the tachycardia cycle length if the mechanism is macro-reentrant or tachycardia acceleration if mechanism is automatic or triggered) and subsequent noninducibility of that arrhythmia provides further proof of mechanism. Additional data provided by the ablation catheter include impedance information.[35] When mapping in pulmonary veins and/or other cardiac vascular structures, marked increase in impedance may indicate catheter position that lacks myocardial tissue and therefore lacks the substrate to serve as a source for arrhythmia. During pulmonary vein isolation for the treatment of atrial fibrillation, catheter position is viewed under fluoroscopy, compared with fluoroscopic road maps from pulmonary venograms, and combined with analysis of local EGMs and catheter impedance to help direct catheter position out of the pulmonary vein and to the pulmonary vein antrum (Fig. 8–21). By ablating and isolating antral tissue, procedural efficacy is improved. By preventing delivery of

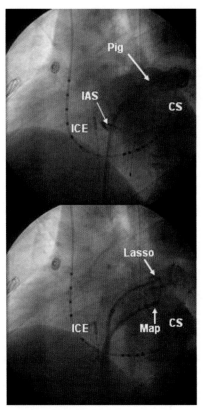
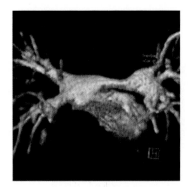
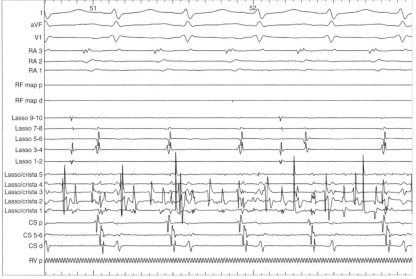

FIGURE 8–21. Pulmonary vein antral mapping in normal sinus rhythm with isolated pulmonary vein antra. **Left.** Fluoroscopic images in a left anterior oblique projection: top image with pigtail catheter in the left common pulmonary vein trunk (LCPVT); and bottom image with double transseptal with the mapping catheter and circular mapping catheter in the LCPVT. CS, coronary sinus; IAS, interatrial septum stained with contrast; ICE, intracardiac echocardiography probe; Lasso, circular mapping catheter; Map, mapping catheter; Pig, pigtail catheter for contrast injection creating venogram of the LCPVT. **Top right.** Three-dimensional magnetic resonance angiography of the left atrium. **Bottom right.** Tracing from the electrogram (EGM) recording system revealing sinus rhythm (see RA and CS EGMs) with isolated pulmonary vein potentials in the right upper pulmonary vein (RUPV) and isolated fibrillation of the left antrum. CS, coronary sinus EGMs; Lasso, RUPV EGMs (RUPV lasso not included in fluoroscopic image); Lasso/Crista, LCPVT EGMs; RA, right atrial EGMs. Images provided with permission from Patrick Hranitzky, MD, Duke University Medical Center. See Moving Image 8–21.

Patient A   Patient B

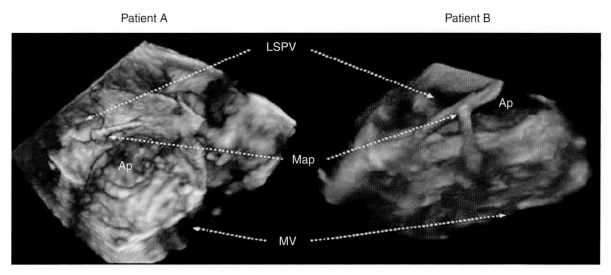

FIGURE 8–22. Three-dimensional transesophageal echocardiography–guided catheter manipulation along the ligament of Marshall (LOM). Patient A has a relatively thick LOM. Patient B has a relatively thin LOM. Ap, left atrial appendage; LSPV, left superior pulmonary vein; Map, mapping/ablation catheter; MV, mitral valve. Image provided with permission from Tristram Bahnson, MD, Duke University Medical Center. See Moving Images 8–22A to C.

radiofrequency energy outside of the pulmonary vein, complications such as pulmonary vein stenosis are reduced.

THREE-DIMENSIONAL TRANSESOPHAGEAL ECHOCARDIOGRAPHY

In addition to EGM, fluoroscopic, and impedance data, information during electrophysiologic mapping can be obtained by the use of echocardiography. Three-dimensional transesophageal echocardiography (TEE) can guide mapping and ablation in regions of the left atrium where complex left atrial topography may present challenges in achieving reliable, reproducible, and predictable catheter position.[36] Three-dimensional TEE produces heat as well as some degree of mechanical compression between the mid esophagus and posterior wall of the left atrium, and therefore, TEE is relatively contraindicated if

radiofrequency energy is being delivered to the posterior wall of the left atrium. In regions of complex anatomy, however, that are more anterior, such as the ligament of Marshall region, three-dimensional TEE provides high-resolution images of both the mapping catheter and intracardiac contours to guide catheter positioning (Fig. 8–22).

INTRACARDIAC ECHOCARDIOGRAPHY

Intracardiac echocardiography (ICE) has taken a central role in numerous aspects of electrophysiologic mapping. For procedures where transseptal access of the left atrium is required, ICE allows direct visualization of the interatrial septum, access needle, and sheath apparatus to confirm a crossover point in the region of the fossa ovalis, as well as to provide real-time visualization of the passage of this equipment into the left atrium (Fig. 8–23),

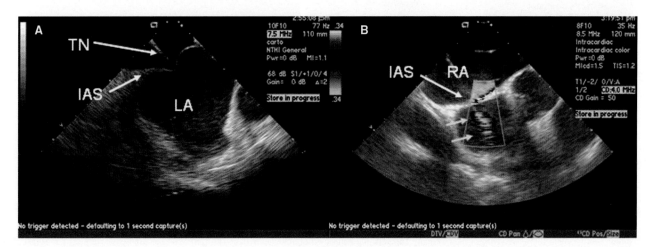

FIGURE 8–23. Intracardiac imaging of the interatrial septum. **A.** Engagement of the interatrial septum with the transseptal needle guided by an SL1 sheath and dilator. IAS, interatrial septum; LA, left atrium; TN, brock transseptal needle. **B.** Doppler analysis across the atrial septum demonstrating right to left shunting after sheath removal from the left atrium in a patient with pulmonary hypertension. RA, right atrium. Images provided with permission from Patrick Hranitzky, MD, Duke University Medical Center. See Moving Images 8–23A and B.

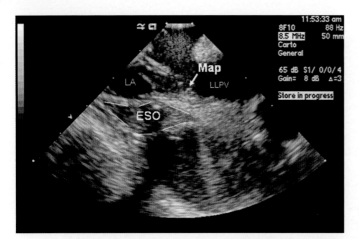

FIGURE 8–24. Intracardiac echocardiography (ICE) with ICE probe in the left atrium for visualization of mapping catheter contact with the pulmonary vein antrum and assessment of position in relation to structures of importance such as the esophagus. ESO, esophagus; LA, left atrium; LLPV, left lower pulmonary vein; Map, mapping catheter. Image provided with permission from Tristram Bahnson, MD, Duke University Medical Center. See Moving Image 8–24.

In addition to use during transseptal access, ICE can also be used to assess cardiac anatomy, confirming absence of pericardial fluid before, during, and after the procedure. The ICE catheter can also be passed directly into the left atrium for visualization of catheter position and its relation to important structures such as the pulmonary vein (to confirm good catheter-tissue contact at the pulmonary vein antrum) and esophageal tissue (Fig. 8–24). ICE can also play an important role in electrophysiologic mapping

through its use in the three-dimensional electroanatomic mapping system CARTO-sound (Biosense Webster, Diamond Bar, CA) (Fig. 8–25). One frontier in electrophysiologic mapping assisted by multiple imaging modalities is pending the development of real-time, multiplanar three-dimensional ICE. If such imaging can be achieved in a probe of acceptable size, the current requirements for mental integration of multiple sources of information (eg, biplane fluoroscopy, pulmonary venogram road maps, mapping catheter impedance data, EGMs) to reliably identify catheter position and tissue contact may be greatly simplified.

■ CARDIAC MRI AND CT

In lieu of three-dimensional real-time multiplanar ICE, the most detailed representations of intracardiac anatomy are provided by integration of images obtained by cardiac MRI or CT with imaging data obtained using a three-dimensional electroanatomic mapping system. The integration of these imaging modalities has been most useful for electrophysiologic mapping of the left atrium.

■ THREE-DIMENSIONAL CONTACT MAPPING

The application of imaging data obtained by CT or MRI is more fully appreciated in the electrophysiologic laboratory when integrated with a three-dimensional electroanatomic mapping system. The two contact mapping systems used most commonly are ESI (Endocardial Solutions Incorporated, St. Paul, MN) and CARTO (Biosense Webster). The mapping catheter (and additional diagnostic catheters) is viewed under fluoroscopy in the

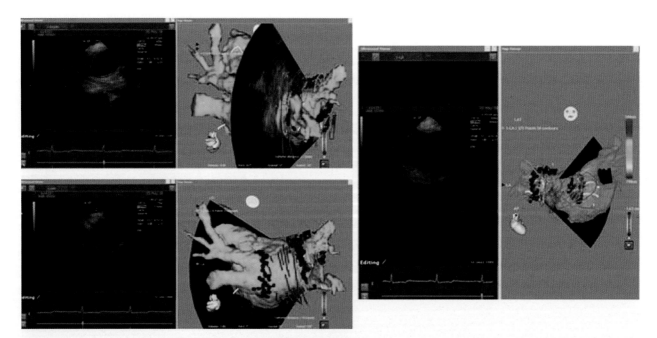

FIGURE 8–25. CARTO-sound (Biosense Webster) map building. **Top left.** Intracardiac echocardiography (ICE) fan from Soundstar (Biosense Webster) ICE catheter sweeps through the mid-left portion of the left atrium to annotate esophageal position. **Bottom left.** ICE fan sweeps through the left anterior left atrium for annotation of left atrial appendage position. **Right.** ICE fan sweeps through the left posterior left atrium for annotation of left pulmonary vein and position of the carina between the left upper and left lower pulmonary veins. See Moving Images 8–25A (CARTO-sound drawing of esophagus), 8–25B (CARTO-sound drawing of left atrial appendage), 8–25C (CARTO-sound drawing of left pulmonary veins), and 8–25D (sound map created with vessel tags).

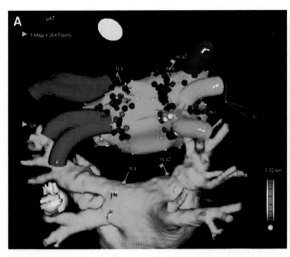
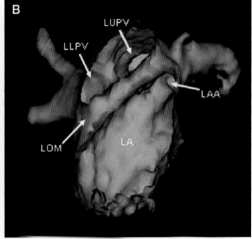

FIGURE 8–26. Bringing electroanatomic maps and magnetic resonance angiograms of the left atrium together. **A.** Landmark registration of three-dimensional CARTO (Biosense Webster) electroanatomic map and three-dimensional magnetic resonance angiogram of the left atrium brought together with CARTO-merge software. **B.** With the images merged, the electroanatomic map can fade into the background, a sagittal clipping plane can be applied, and the image can be rotated on end to create a "virtual endoscopic view" of the pulmonary vein antra. LA, left atrium; LAA, left atrial appendage; LLPV, left lower pulmonary vein; LOM, ligament of Marshall; LUPV, left upper pulmonary vein. Images provided with permission from Tristram Bahnson, MD, Duke University Medical Center. See Moving Images 8–26A and B.

most basic electrophysiologic mapping setup; however, additional information can be obtained by annotating EGM characteristics and catheter tip position in three-dimensional space by use of a three-dimensional electroanatomic mapping system. Annotation of points where catheter contacts myocardium can then be used to create an anatomic shell representing the walls of the cardiac chamber of interest. This three-dimensional electroanatomic image can then be combined with other forms of imaging, such as that obtained by CT or MRI, to improve the depiction of target the anatomy (Fig. 8–26). In addition to creation of an anatomic shell, analysis of the EGMs obtained at tissue contact points can be used to provide information about the electrophysiologic properties of the tissue at that point to create voltage maps and activation maps.

■ VOLTAGE MAPPING (THREE-DIMENSIONAL CONTACT MAPPING SYSTEM)

Local EGM amplitude (measured in millivolts in regions where myocardial contact is unimpeded by fat or other barrier to myocardial tissue contact) can be assessed to provide information about tissue viability. Voltage measurements >1.5 mV are indicative of viable myocardium. Low-voltage measurements (ie, <0.3 mV) are more indicative of myocardium with limited viability or scar tissue. Tissue with low-amplitude (or absent) EGMs that cannot be paced even with high output (ie, 10 mA) may represent dense scar or "electrically unexcitable scar." Assigning various colors to represent variations in EGM voltage allows for creation of a voltage map (Figs. 8–27 and 8–28). Macro–re-entrant scar-related ventricular arrhythmias, for example, frequently use heterogeneous regions of limited viability at the border zone of myocardial scar or regions of viable tissue between electrically unexcitable scar to create a critical isthmus of slowed conduction that allows for arrhythmia perpetuation.[37] These regions are of

particular interest because they often represent the therapeutic target for elimination of the arrhythmia circuit.[38]

■ ACTIVATION AND PROPAGATION MAPPING (THREE-DIMENSIONAL CONTACT MAPPING SYSTEM)

In addition to voltage data, additional useful information can be obtained using a three-dimensional electroanatomic mapping system by annotating local EGM timing. By comparing the timing of EGMs detected at the tip of a mapping catheter to a stable reference and representing the difference with a colorimetric scale to highlight the area of earliest activation (such as that which would be of interest with a focal tachycardia) or to identify points where early activation meets late activation (such as that which would be of interest with a macro–re-entrant circuit), the arrhythmia mechanism can be displayed anatomically. This activation data can likewise be viewed dynamically to demonstrate wave-front propagation (Fig. 8–29).

■ PUTTING IT ALL TOGETHER

Invasive electrophysiologic mapping often requires a combination of the following processes: fluoroscopy for catheter positioning to allow safe and effective catheter manipulation; EGMs for determination of electrical activity at tissue contact points (timing: early vs late diastolic potentials; morphologic: amplitude, frequency); three-dimensional electroanatomic maps to allow data annotation for creating a multipoint anatomic shell with or without merged/fused images from other modalities (CT angiography/MRI) incorporating voltage (surrogate marker for determining myocardial viability) and activation/propagation data (timing sequence); validating data with techniques such as extrainment and pacemapping; and using tools such as ICE to survey anatomy and assist with catheter navigation.

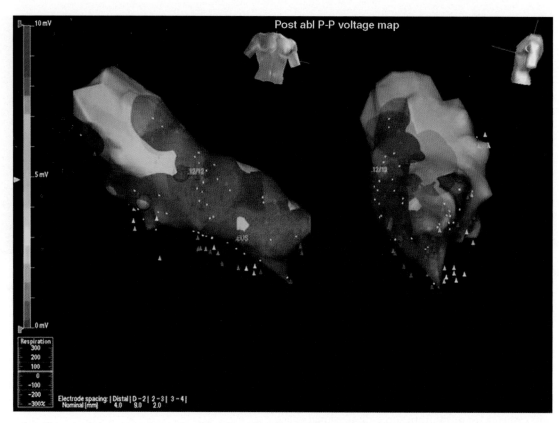

FIGURE 8–27. Contact three-dimensional electroanatomic mapping of the left ventricle with colorimetric annotation of endocardial voltage using ESI-NavX system (Endocardial Solutions Incorporated) in a patient with a large anteroseptal myocardial infarct. Note red color assigned to regions of low voltage (scar) and green, blue, and purple colors assigned to larger amplitude electrograms of viable myocardium. Thoracic models are above colorimetric maps for orientation. Image provided with permission from Patrick Hranitzky, MD, Duke University Medical Center.

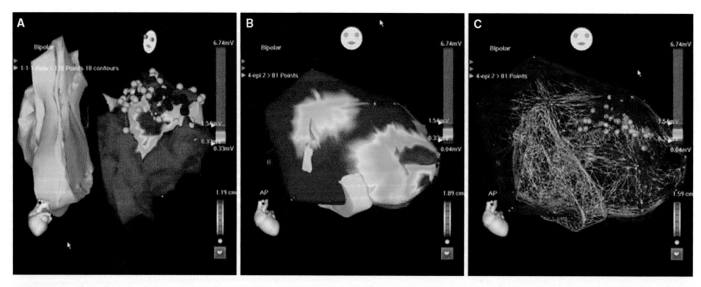

FIGURE 8–28. Three-dimensional electroanatomic mapping of both the right and left ventricles with colorimetric annotation of endocardial and epicardial voltage using CARTO and CARTO-sound systems (Biosense Webster). **A.** Three-dimensional voltage maps of the right ventricle and left ventricle endocardial surface. **B.** Three-dimensional voltage map of the epicardial surface of the ventricles. **C.** Mesh of endocardial and epicardial three-dimensional voltage maps. Gray heart model (at the bottom left of each image) and the face structure (at the top of each image) are provided for orientation. Images provided with permission from Patrick Hranitzky, MD, Duke University Medical Center. See Moving Images 8–28 A to C.

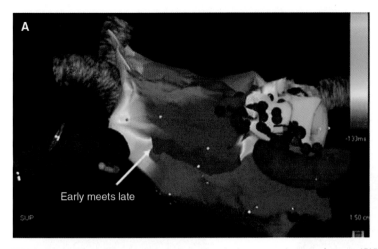
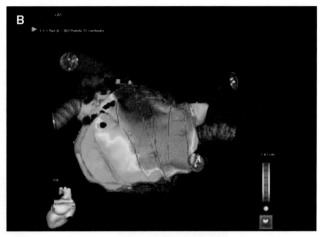

FIGURE 8–29. Three-dimensional electroanatomic activation map and propagation map (CARTO; Biosense Webster) of a left atrial macro-reentrant flutter (note the "early meets late" at the roof of the left atrium). **A.** Superior view of the left atrium. **B.** Posterior view of the left atrium. Red indicates earliest left atrial activation. Purple indicates latest left atrial activation. Tubes represent pulmonary veins (color of tubes not related to endocardial activation). See Moving Image 8–29.

■ LIMITATIONS OF CONTACT MAPPING

One limitation of activation mapping using the contact mapping method described earlier is a requirement for sustained (or at least frequently recurring) arrhythmia to provide activation data. This limitation can prevent successful characterization of nonsustained or infrequently occurring arrhythmias, such as may be the case with many automatic or triggered tachycardias, which may have a tendency to occur in bursts that are symptomatic outside the electrophysiology laboratory but occur less frequently under conditions in the electrophysiology laboratory (eg, in the presence of sedation, alteration in environmental stimuli). Despite efforts to minimize sedation and specifically to avoid sedative agents known to suppress automatic tachyarrhythmias, and even with the addition of provoking agents such as isoproterenol or atropine, a paucity of arrhythmia may be a significant limitation to the point-by-point contact mapping approach discussed earlier. An additional limitation of contact mapping may be experienced if the clinical arrhythmia has a tendency to degenerate into a disorganized rhythm, such as atrial tachycardia degenerating into atrial fibrillation or ventricular tachycardia degenerating into ventricular fibrillation. Point-by-point mapping is also limited if the clinical arrhythmia is not hemodynamically tolerated, such as with rapid ventricular tachycardia in the setting of poor left ventricular function. Unless a perfusing blood pressure can be maintained in tachycardia with the addition of vasopressors, hemodynamic support with an intraaortic balloon pump, or ventricular assist device, activation mapping using a contact mapping system in this scenario may not be possible.

■ THREE-DIMENSIONAL ELECTROANATOMIC MAPPING (THREE-DIMENSIONAL NONCONTACT MAPPING SYSTEM)

Some of the limitations of contact mapping described earlier can be overcome by use of a noncontact mapping system. The EnSite multielectrode array (MEA; Endocardial Solutions) uses a 7.5-cc balloon to expand a woven braid of 64 wires mounted on a 9-French catheter to detect far-field electrical potentials from the cardiac chamber of interest. These far-field electrical potentials are used to reconstruct "virtual" unipolar endocardial EGMs over more than 3000 points. This reconstruction is accomplished by using inverse-solution mathematics to create an instantaneous endocardial isopotential map superimposed onto a computer-simulated model of the endocardium during a single heartbeat. Electrodes are created at specified regions of disrupted insulation in the woven braid of wires. There is a ring electrode on the proximal shaft to serve as a reference. While moving the mapping catheter around the endocardial surface, the MEA detects and determines locator signal angles to create a three-dimensional computer model of the endocardium. The inverse-solution method considers how a signal detected at a remote point would have appeared at its source by noting how the potential field at any one electrode is influenced to a degree by potentials from the entire endocardium. The degree of influence is inversely proportional to the distance between the electrode and each endocardial point. Accuracy of this mapping system decreases with distance from the endocardial source and with increasing chamber complexity[39,40] (Fig. 8–30). To assure accurate mapping data, the array position must be stable and ideally within 1.5 cm of the substrate being assessed. Movement of the MEA will invalidate previously obtained data.[41] An additional limitation of this technique is the large size of the balloon, which may limit maneuverability of the balloon itself as well as the mapping catheter being used in concert with the balloon. Additionally, when mapping relatively small regions, such as the right ventricular outflow tract, the MEA may contact endocardium, producing ectopy that can be confused with the clinical arrhythmia. The balloon may be partially deflated to assist with some of these limitations. The MEA also has potential thrombogenicity that must be abrogated with concurrent use of intravenous heparin.

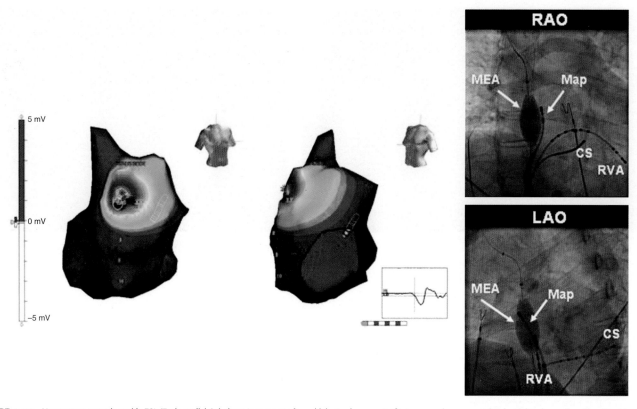

FIGURE 8–30. Noncontact mapping with ESI (Endocardial Solutions Incorporated) multielectrode array. **Left.** Images of a nonsustained atrial tachycardia with white identifying point of earliest activation surrounded by red, then yellow, then green, then blue, then purple as the focal tachycardia spreads out in a centrifugal fashion. Three-dimensional thoracic images are provided for orientation. **Right.** Corresponding fluoroscopic images showing position of array and surrounding catheters. CS, coronary sinus; Map, mapping catheter; MEA, multielectrode array; RVA, right ventricular apex. See Moving Image 8–30.

■ REMOTE CATHETER NAVIGATION SYSTEMS

In addition to mechanistic challenges of mapping complex arrhythmias, there are also logistic challenges presented by long procedure times, radiation exposure, and operator standing time while wearing lead. The toll of these undesirable aspects of electrophysiologic mapping accumulate with time and may significantly reduce the number of procedures a single operator may perform in his or her lifetime.[42] In hopes of addressing these issues as well as aiming to continue improvements in safety, effectiveness, and reproducibility of electrophysiologic mapping procedures, there has been interest in the development of automated electrophysiologic mapping techniques.

The first step in this process has been the development of remote catheter navigation systems. Remote catheter navigation systems using MRI-like large magnets to manipulate catheter position have been developed and continue to be refined (Stereotaxis, St. Louis, MO).[43] Limitations of this system have included room requirements to safely accommodate the Stereotaxis magnets (ie, large size of magnets requires large room size, large weight of magnets requires floor reinforcement, and powerful magnetic fields require magnetic shielding and nonmagnetic ancillary equipment). Additional limitations have included mapping catheter compatibility (special catheter construction required to respond to magnetic field manipulation). Specific benefits of the Stereotaxis system have included a theoretical reduction in perforation risk due to a decreased likelihood of a calculable

magnetic pull leading to perforation as opposed to mechanical push that may be less able to perceive force at the tissue contact interface. An unfortunate consequence of decreased tissue contact force occurs with attempts at arrhythmia treatment, as force of tissue contact is a key determinant of ablation lesion depth.[44] Inadequate lesion depth may prevent procedural success.

A second commercially available remote catheter navigation system has been created using a mechanical/robotic platform rather than magnetic force to manipulate catheter position (Hansen Medical, Mountain View, CA).[45] Attributes of the Hansen remote catheter navigation system include compatibility with a broad range of catheters and improved catheter-tissue contact pressure. The improved catheter-tissue contact pressure requires management to minimize risk of perforation; however, it provides significant benefits in maintaining catheter stability and increasing ablation lesion depth. To provide operator feedback to facilitate safe and effective catheter navigation, tissue contact pressure is displayed for the operator both graphically and via tactile feedback provided by the Intellisense algorithm (Sensei; Hansen Medical).[42,46] Whether the remote catheter navigation system is magnetic or mechanical, an attribute of both is the creation of a workstation environment that concentrates multiple imaging modalities in a relatively compact area (Fig. 8–31).[47] Level I multimodal imaging (MMI) is demonstrated by adding information from one two-dimensional fluoroscopic view to a second orthogonal fluoroscopic view.

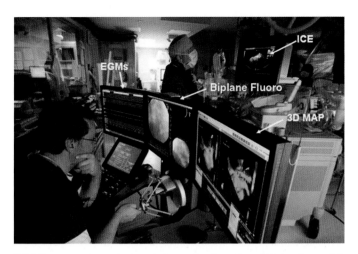

FIGURE 8–31. Hansen robotic navigation workstation with multiple imaging modalities displayed to facilitate catheter navigation. 3D MAP, three-dimensional mapping; EGM, electrogram; fluoro, fluoroscopy; ICE, intracardiac echocardiography. Image provided with permission from Tristram Bahnson, MD, Duke University Medical Center.

Level II MMI is seen when comparing the fluoroscopic view of catheter position in the pulmonary venogram to the ICE image to assure catheter position with good tissue contact at the pulmonary vein antrum. Level III MMI is represented by both the three-dimensional electroanatomic map and the three-dimensional MRI image of the left atrium and proximal pulmonary veins. Level IV MMI is achieved when the images in two dimensions are represented side by side. Level V MMI is achieved when the three-dimensional electroanatomic image is merged/fused with the three-dimensional MRI (or CT) image.

■ CATHETER GUIDANCE WITHOUT EXPOSURE TO IONIZING RADIATION

Additional opportunities for multimodal imaging in electrophysiologic mapping may be present with use of MRI, rather than fluoroscopy, to guide catheter manipulation.[48,49] Catheter guidance with MRI has several benefits over fluoroscopy. One benefit is the decreased radiation exposure for the operator and the patient. In addition, cardiac MRI has the ability to represent three-dimensional anatomy with particular imaging sequences used to depict tissue characteristics such as tissue viability; cardiac MRI also has the ability to provide detailed display of cardiac structures such as heart valves and papillary muscles that are not visible with fluoroscopy. There are several barriers to the use of MRI-guided techniques, including image acquisition speed and resolution, as well as requirement for MRI-compatible catheters effective for mapping and ablation with imaging characteristics allowing catheter visibility without marked distortion. Patient physiologic stability and tolerance of prolonged procedure times in the bore of a magnet are also important issues; however, many of these patient-related challenges may be overcome with use of anesthesia support. Development of MRI-compatible pacemakers and defibrillators will also facilitate this process by broadening the population of candidates for MRI.

Ultrasound has been shown to be a useful tool to guide catheter manipulation for the purpose of electrophysiologic

mapping.[50] Currently, ultrasound use is primarily as an adjunct to images obtained using conventional fluoroscopy. However the absence of radiation exposure with ultrasound imaging makes it an attractive candidate for reducing procedural radiation exposure. As three-dimensional ultrasound technology improves, the possibility of ultrasound-only guided catheter navigation may become a viable strategy.

POSTPROCEDURE EVALUATION

The requirement for multimodal imaging continues beyond the completion of the electrophysiologic mapping procedure. The ICE probe is useful for a survey of cardiac structures to confirm stable function and anatomy. Specifically, analysis to exclude an unexpected pericardial fluid collection prior to removal of catheters from the heart may be useful. Following departure from the electrophysiologic laboratory, telemetry analysis is used for monitoring heart rate and rhythm. Postprocedure 12-lead ECGs are useful for establishment of electrophysiologic properties after the procedure and for investigation of any concerns regarding ischemia for cases involving myocardium with ablation performed in close proximity to coronary vasculature.

■ ESOPHAGEAL EVALUATION

For patients who have undergone ablation along the posterior left atrial wall, there may be concern about thermal esophageal injury. Features concerning for risk of atrioesophageal fistula may be investigated early with esophagogastroduodenoscopy without insufflation (noting that absence of insufflation may limit endoscopic visualization within the esophagus); however, if it is more than 48 hours after the procedure, overt atrioesophageal connection is best evaluated by imaging modalities such as chest CT and, to a lesser extent, echocardiography.[51,52]

■ PULMONARY VEIN EVALUATION

Imaging modalities that have been particularly useful for evaluation after pulmonary vein procedures include both CT and cardiac MRI. Cardiac MRI in particular allows not only depiction of the pulmonary vein in three dimensions, but also en-face analysis of pulmonary vein ostia for direct measurement and flow-velocity analysis. In addition to flow-velocity information, the variation in circumference at the pulmonary vein os can also be observed throughout the cardiac cycle. A significant reduction in pulmonary vein contraction after circumferential pulmonary vein isolation may correlate with electrical isolation of the pulmonary vein (Fig. 8–32). Likewise, notation of pulmonary vein contraction that is not significantly reduced following an attempt at pulmonary vein isolation may correlate with absence of electrical isolation.

■ CARDIAC MRI FOR ASSESSMENT OF ABLATED TISSUE

Additional magnetic resonance–based techniques are being developed to assist with imaging regions of ablated tissue after percutaneous arrhythmia treatment. Ablated myocardium,

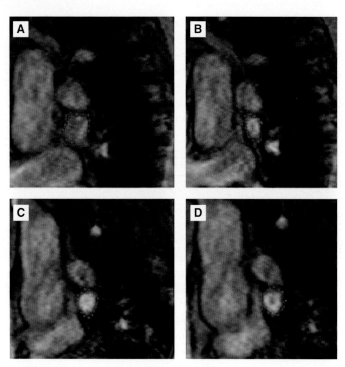

FIGURE 8–32. En-face evaluation of pulmonary vein contraction before and after pulmonary vein isolation. **A.** and **B.** Preablation outline (purple) of the right lower pulmonary vein during atrial diastole (A) and atrial systole (B). **C.** and **D.** The same right lower pulmonary vein in the same patient after undergoing pulmonary vein isolation during atrial diastole (C) and atrial systole (D). Note the absence of pulmonary vein contraction with successful electrical isolation. Images courtesy of Brett Atwater, MD, Duke University Medical Center.

including regions of delayed gadolinium enhancement, and acute changes such as "no reflow" (regions of contrast void secondary to vasculature disruption preventing tissue delivery of gadolinium contrast) can be clearly seen in cases of focal ventricular tachycardia ablation (Fig. 8–33). Barriers to imaging atrial myocardium in

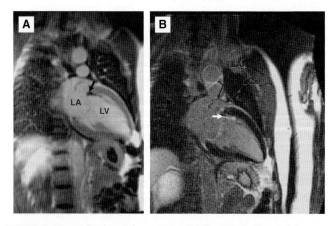

FIGURE 8–33. Cardiac magnetic resonance imaging (CMRI) after radiofrequency ablation of a focal ventricular tachycardia. CMRIs in a two-chamber view. **A.** Contrast void (black arrow) of "no reflow" after radiofrequency ablation. **B.** Conventional delayed gadolinium enhancement sequence revealing bright white region (white arrow) of ablated myocardium outside the region of no reflow. LA, left atrium; LAA, left atrial appendage; LCx, left circumflex coronary artery; LV, left ventricle. Images provided with permission from Patrick Hranitzky, MD, Duke University Medical Center.

this same manner can be attributed to the relatively thin nature of the atrial myocardium, surrounded on both sides by bright structures such as blood pool or fat. Development of dark blood delayed-enhancement images may provide promise in overcoming some of these issues. Additional means that may improve imaging in the thin-walled atria include use of techniques to track respiratory motion and adjust image analysis so that gated images can be obtained for times greater than could be achieved by breath-holding techniques alone. Successful depiction of delayed enhancement in the thin-walled atrium not only has applications for follow-up of electrophysiologic procedures, but also has the potential to be applied to other regions of the heart where identification of small regions of delayed enhancement might have substantial clinical relevance (ie, arrhythmogenic right ventricular cardiomyopathy).

■ CARDIAC PET

Additional imaging modalities under investigation in arrhythmia management include use of cardiac PET. Metabolic markers of arrhythmogenic substrate are incompletely defined; however, cardiac PET has found a useful role in individual cases. An example of cardiac PET utility after left atrial ablation was found after an initial successful treatment of atrial fibrillation with pulmonary vein isolation was followed by recurrent, incessant, drug-refractory atrial fibrillation. Antiarrhythmic medications that before the procedure had been at least partially efficacious were no longer able to maintain sinus rhythm even for a short period of time with or without electrical cardioversion. Transesophageal echocardiographic images performed for the purpose of excluding left atrial appendage thrombus were notable for marked thickening of the left atrial wall. This was evaluated in greater detail with cardiac MRI, which confirmed the presence of extensive left atrial thickening having the appearance of a rind around the left atrium. Cardiac PET imaging found this rind to be metabolically active, consistent with inflammatory tissue. The patient had no history or current evidence of malignancy. There was no lymphadenopathy or mass on chest CT. The patient was treated empirically with steroids for left atrial pericarditis reactive to the ablation process. Following steroid taper, a repeat cardiac PET scan revealed resolution of left atrial inflammation. Reinstitution of antiarrhythmic medication followed by cardioversion resulted in sustained sinus rhythm (Fig. 8–34).

CONCLUSION

For successful electrophysiologic mapping to be achieved, all available information must be integrated to explain arrhythmia mechanism. The multiple imaging modalities obtained by two-dimensional techniques such as fluoroscopy and ultrasound must be incorporated with three-dimensional representations of cardiac anatomy obtained both by preprocedure cardiac CT and cardiac MRI, as well as data obtained in the electrophysiologic laboratory with the use of three-dimensional electroanatomic mapping systems. At times, there are automated techniques to bring these imaging modalities together (eg, CARTO-merge,

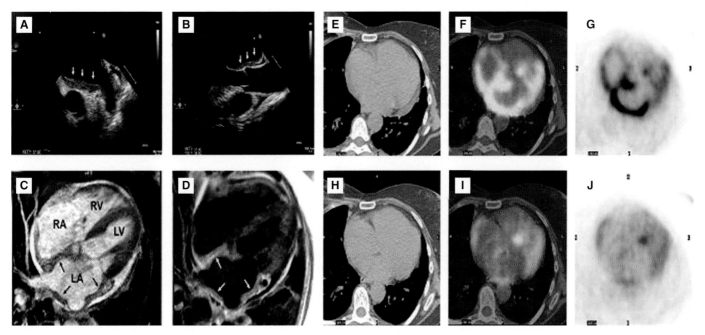

FIGURE 8–34. Left atrial inflammation following pulmonary vein isolation. **A.** and **B.** Transesophageal echocardiographic images of the left atrium showing marked left atrial thickening (arrows). **C.** and **D.** Diffuse left atrial wall thickening seen in four-chamber view magnetic resonance imaging (bright blood and dark blood imaging). Maximum left atrial wall thickness of 7 mm. T2-weighted fast spin-echo imaging (dark blood image) reveals the left atrial wall as hyperintense compared with left ventricular myocardium, consistent with higher water content such as that which would be seen with inflammation. **E–G.** Fasting cardiac fluorodeoxyglucose (FDG) positron emission tomography (PET) scan with increased metabolic activity diffusely throughout the left atrium (**E:** computed tomography [CT] image; **F:** fused PET/CT image; **G:** PET). **H–J.** Repeat cardiac FDG-PET demonstrating resolution of atrial inflammation (and resolution of pericardial effusion). LA, left atrium; LV, left ventricle; RA, right atrium; RV, right ventricle. Images provided with permission from Patrick Hranitzky, MD, Duke University Medical Center. See Moving Images 8-34A and B.

Biosense Webster; NavX Fusion, Endocardial Solutions); however, much of the coalescence of information required to achieve level V MMI integration is still done mentally by the primary operator of the electrophysiology mapping procedure. As real-time, multiplanar, three-dimensional imaging modalities that do not depend on registration for accurate depiction of anatomy are developed, the level of mental processing to provide an understanding of the relationship between cardiovascular electrophysiology, cardiac anatomy, and catheter position will be decreased and relevant procedural outcomes of safety, efficacy, and reduced procedure times will likely follow.

Moving Image Legends

All moving images are located on the complementary DVD.

REFERENCES

1. Schilling RJ, Davies DW, Peters NS. Clinical developments in cardiac activation mapping. *Eur Heart J.* 2000;21:801-807.
2. Riley MP, Marchlinski FE. ECG clues for diagnosing ventricular tachycardia mechanism. *J Cardiovasc Electrophysiol.* 2008;19:224-229.
3. Delacretaz E. Clinical practice. Supraventricular tachycardia. *N Engl J Med.* 2006;354:1039-1051.
4. Marchlinski FE, Leong-Sit P. Learning before burning: the importance of anatomy to the electrophysiologist. *Heart Rhythm.* 2009;6:1199-1201.
5. Nakagawa H, Lazzara R, Khastgir T, et al. Role of the tricuspid annulus and the eustachian valve/ridge on atrial flutter. Relevance to catheter ablation of the septal isthmus and a new technique for rapid identification of ablation success. *Circulation.* 1996;94:407-424.
6. Calkins H, Brugada J, Packer DL, et al. HRS/EHRA/ECAS expert consensus statement on catheter and surgical ablation of atrial fibrillation: recommendations for personnel, policy, procedures and follow-up. A report of the Heart Rhythm Society (HRS) Task Force on Catheter and Surgical Ablation of Atrial Fibrillation. *Heart Rhythm.* 2007;4:816-861.
7. Ganz LI, Friedman PL. Supraventricular tachycardia. *N Engl J Med.* 1995;332:162-173.
8. Tada H, Oral H, Greenstein R, et al. Analysis of age of onset of accessory pathway-mediated tachycardia in men and women. *Am J Cardiol.* 2002;89:470-471.
9. Knight BP, Ebinger M, Oral H, et al. Diagnostic value of tachycardia features and pacing maneuvers during paroxysmal supraventricular tachycardia. *J Am Coll Cardiol.* 2000;36:574-582.
10. Kistler PM, Roberts-Thomson KC, Haqqani HM, et al. P-wave morphology in focal atrial tachycardia: development of an algorithm to predict the anatomic site of origin. *J Am Coll Cardiol.* 2006;48:1010-1017.
11. Hancock EW, Deal BJ, Mirvis DM, et al. AHA/ACCF/HRS recommendations for the standardization and interpretation of the electrocardiogram: part V: electrocardiogram changes associated with cardiac chamber hypertrophy: a scientific statement from the American Heart Association Electrocardiography and Arrhythmias Committee, Council on Clinical Cardiology; the American College of Cardiology Foundation; and the Heart Rhythm Society. Endorsed by the International Society for Computerized Electrocardiology. *J Am Coll Cardiol.* 2009;53:992-1002.
12. Surawicz B, Childers R, Deal BJ, et al. AHA/ACCF/HRS recommendations for the standardization and interpretation of the electrocardiogram: part III: intraventricular conduction disturbances: a scientific statement from the American Heart Association Electrocardiography and Arrhythmias Committee, Council on Clinical Cardiology; the American College of Cardiology Foundation; and the Heart Rhythm Society. Endorsed by the International Society for Computerized Electrocardiology. *J Am Coll Cardiol.* 2009;53:976-981.
13. Wagner GS, Macfarlane P, Wellens H, et al. AHA/ACCF/HRS recommendations for the standardization and interpretation of the electrocardiogram: part

VI: acute ischemia/infarction: a scientific statement from the American Heart Association Electrocardiography and Arrhythmias Committee, Council on Clinical Cardiology; the American College of Cardiology Foundation; and the Heart Rhythm Society. Endorsed by the International Society for Computerized Electrocardiology. *J Am Coll Cardiol.* 2009;53:1003-1011.

14. Brody DA. A theoretical analysis of intracavitary blood mass influence on the heart-lead relationship. *Circ Res.* 1956;4:731-738.

15. Wellens HJ, Gorgels AP. The electrocardiogram 102 years after Einthoven. *Circulation.* 2004;109:562-564.

16. Wallace TW, Atwater BD, Daubert JP, et al. Prevalence and clinical characteristics associated with left atrial appendage thrombus in fully anticoagulated patients undergoing catheter-directed atrial fibrillation ablation. *J Cardiovasc Electrophysiol.* February 11, 2010 [Epub ahead of print].

17. Oakes RS, Badger TJ, Kholmovski EG, et al. Detection and quantification of left atrial structural remodeling with delayed-enhancement magnetic resonance imaging in patients with atrial fibrillation. *Circulation.* 2009;119:1758-1767.

18. Tops LF, van der Wall EE, Schalij MJ, Bax JJ. Multi-modality imaging to assess left atrial size, anatomy and function. *Heart.* 2007;93:1461-1470.

19. Killeen RP, O'Connor SA, Keane D, Dodd JD. Ectopic focus in an accessory left atrial appendage: radiofrequency ablation of refractory atrial fibrillation. *Circulation.* 2009;120:e60-e62.

20. Bayes de Luna A, Wagner G, Birnbaum Y, et al. A new terminology for left ventricular walls and location of myocardial infarcts that present Q wave based on the standard of cardiac magnetic resonance imaging: a statement for healthcare professionals from a committee appointed by the International Society for Holter and Noninvasive Electrocardiography. *Circulation.* 2006;114:1755-1760.

21. Patel MR, Cawley PJ, Heitner JF, et al. Detection of myocardial damage in patients with sarcoidosis. *Circulation.* 2009;120:1969-1977.

22. Choudhury L, Mahrholdt H, Wagner A, et al. Myocardial scarring in asymptomatic or mildly symptomatic patients with hypertrophic cardiomyopathy. *J Am Coll Cardiol.* 2002;40:2156-2164.

23. Wood JC, Ghugre N. Magnetic resonance imaging assessment of excess iron in thalassemia, sickle cell disease and other iron overload diseases. *Hemoglobin.* 2008;32:85-96.

24. Vogelsberg H, Mahrholdt H, Deluigi CC, et al. Cardiovascular magnetic resonance in clinically suspected cardiac amyloidosis: noninvasive imaging compared to endomyocardial biopsy. *J Am Coll Cardiol.* 2008;51:1022-1030.

25. Kayser HW, de Roos A, Schalij MJ, Bootsma M, Wellens HJ, Van der Wall EE. Usefulness of magnetic resonance imaging in diagnosis of arrhythmogenic right ventricular dysplasia and agreement with electrocardiographic criteria. *Am J Cardiol.* 2003;91:365-367.

26. Rochitte CE, Oliveira PF, Andrade JM, et al. Myocardial delayed enhancement by magnetic resonance imaging in patients with Chagas' disease: a marker of disease severity. *J Am Coll Cardiol.* 2005;46:1553-1558.

27. Nazarian S, Halperin HR. How to perform magnetic resonance imaging on patients with implantable cardiac arrhythmia devices. *Heart Rhythm.* 2009;6:138-143.

28. Desjardins B, Crawford T, Good E, et al. Infarct architecture and characteristics on delayed enhanced magnetic resonance imaging and electroanatomic mapping in patients with postinfarction ventricular arrhythmia. *Heart Rhythm.* 2009;6:644-651.

29. Bengel FM, Higuchi T, Javadi MS, Lautamaki R. Cardiac positron emission tomography. *J Am Coll Cardiol.* 2009;54:1-15.

30. Tadamura E, Yamamuro M, Kubo S, et al. Images in cardiovascular medicine. Multimodality imaging of cardiac sarcoidosis before and after steroid therapy. *Circulation.* 2006;113:e771-e773.

31. Schumacher B, Tebbenjohanns J, Pfeiffer D, Omran H, Jung W, Luderitz B. Prospective study of retrograde coronary venography in patients with posteroseptal and left-sided accessory atrioventricular pathways. *Am Heart J.* 1995;130:1031-1039.

32. Jais P, Hocini M, Hsu LF, et al. Technique and results of linear ablation at the mitral isthmus. *Circulation.* 2004;110:2996-3002.

33. Takahashi A, Shah DC, Jais P, Hocini M, Clementy J, Haissaguerre M. Specific electrocardiographic features of manifest coronary vein posteroseptal accessory pathways. *J Cardiovasc Electrophysiol.* 1998;9:1015-1025.

34. Valles E, Bazan V, Marchlinski FE. ECG criteria to identify epicardial ventricular tachycardia in non-ischemic cardiomyopathy. *Circ Arrhythm Electrophysiol.* 2010;3:63-71.

35. Zheng X, Walcott GP, Hall JA, et al. Electrode impedance: an indicator of electrode-tissue contact and lesion dimensions during linear ablation. *J Interv Cardiol Electrophysiol.* 2000;4:645-654.

36. Mackensen GB, Hegland D, Rivera D, Adams DB, Bahnson TD. Real-time 3-dimensional transesophageal echocardiography during left atrial radiofrequency catheter ablation for atrial fibrillation. *Circ Cardiovasc Imaging.* 2008;1:85-86.

37. Haqqani HM, Marchlinski FE. Electrophysiologic substrate underlying postinfarction ventricular tachycardia: characterization and role in catheter ablation. *Heart Rhythm.* 2009;6:S70-S76.

38. Aliot EM, Stevenson WG, Almendral-Garrote JM, et al. EHRA/HRS Expert Consensus on Catheter Ablation of Ventricular Arrhythmias: developed in a partnership with the European Heart Rhythm Association (EHRA), a Registered Branch of the European Society of Cardiology (ESC), and the Heart Rhythm Society (HRS); in collaboration with the American College of Cardiology (ACC) and the American Heart Association (AHA). *Heart Rhythm.* 2009;6:886-933.

39. Schilling RJ, Peters NS, Davies DW. Simultaneous endocardial mapping in the human left ventricle using a noncontact catheter: comparison of contact and reconstructed electrograms during sinus rhythm. *Circulation.* 1998;98:887-898.

40. Higa S, Tai CT, Lin YJ, et al. Focal atrial tachycardia: new insight from noncontact mapping and catheter ablation. *Circulation.* 2004;109:84-91.

41. Chinitz LA, Sethi JS. How to perform noncontact mapping. *Heart Rhythm.* 2006;3:120-123.

42. Schmidt B, Tilz RR, Neven K, Julian Chun KR, Furnkranz A, Ouyang F. Remote robotic navigation and electroanatomical mapping for ablation of atrial fibrillation: considerations for navigation and impact on procedural outcome. *Circ Arrhythm Electrophysiol.* 2009;2:120-128.

43. Katsiyiannis WT, Melby DP, Matelski JL, Ervin VL, Laverence KL, Gornick CC. Feasibility and safety of remote-controlled magnetic navigation for ablation of atrial fibrillation. *Am J Cardiol.* 2008;102:1674-1676.

44. Avitall B, Mughal K, Hare J, Helms R, Krum D. The effects of electrode-tissue contact on radiofrequency lesion generation. *Pacing Clin Electrophysiol.* 1997;20:2899-2910.

45. Wazni OM, Barrett C, Martin DO, et al. Experience with the Hansen robotic system for atrial fibrillation ablation-lessons learned and techniques modified: Hansen in the real world. *J Cardiovasc Electrophysiol.* 2009;20:1193-1196.

46. Saliba W, Cummings JE, Oh S, et al. Novel robotic catheter remote control system: feasibility and safety of transseptal puncture and endocardial catheter navigation. *J Cardiovasc Electrophysiol.* 2006;17:1102-1105.

47. Schmidt B, Chun KR, Tilz RR, Koektuerk B, Ouyang F, Kuck KH. Remote navigation systems in electrophysiology. *Europace.* 2008;10(Suppl 3):iii57-iii61.

48. Kramer CM, Narula J. Interventional CMR: great promise, but a long road ahead. *JACC Cardiovasc Imaging.* 2009;2:1337-1338.

49. Saikus CE, Lederman RJ. Interventional cardiovascular magnetic resonance imaging: a new opportunity for image-guided interventions. *JACC Cardiovasc Imaging.* 2009;2:1321-1331.

50. Singh SM, Heist EK, Donaldson DM, et al. Image integration using intracardiac ultrasound to guide catheter ablation of atrial fibrillation. *Heart Rhythm.* 2008;5:1548-1555.

51. D'Avila A, Ptaszek LM, Yu PB, et al. Images in cardiovascular medicine. Left atrial-esophageal fistula after pulmonary vein isolation: a cautionary tale. *Circulation.* 2007;115:e432-e433.

52. Cummings JE, Schweikert RA, Saliba WI, et al. Brief communication: atrial-esophageal fistulas after radiofrequency ablation. *Ann Intern Med.* 2006;144:572-574.

CHAPTER 9

NUCLEAR CARDIOLOGY APPLIED TO ELECTROPHYSIOLOGY

Philippe Chevalier, Roland Itti, and Laurence V. Bontemps

SPECIFIC TECHNICAL BACKGROUND OF NUCLEAR IMAGING IN ARRHYTHMIAS / 171

PERFUSION, VIABILITY, INNERVATION, AND MECHANICAL FUNCTION / 171

CARDIAC CYCLE SELECTION IN THE GATING PROCESS / 172

PLANAR AND THREE-DIMENSIONAL RIGHT VENTRICULAR IMAGING / 172

CONTRACTION CHRONOLOGY USING TEMPORAL FOURIER ANALYSIS / 172

PHASE HISTOGRAM DESCRIPTIVE VALUES: MEAN AND STANDARD DEVIATION / 173

INTERPRETATION OF MYOCARDIAL SYMPATHETIC INNERVATION IMAGING USING MIBG / 174

APPLICATIONS IN DISEASES WITH ISOLATED INTERVENTRICULAR DYSSYNCHRONY / 174
Wolff-Parkinson-White Syndrome / 174

APPLICATIONS IN DISEASES WITH BOTH INTER- AND INTRAVENTRICULAR DYSSYNCHRONY / 176
Arrhythmogenic Right Ventricular Dysplasia / 176
Resynchronization in Cardiac Heart Failure / 176

APPLICATION TO ASSESS MYOCARDIAL SYMPATHETIC HETEROGENEITY / 178

CONCLUSION / 178

The electrophysiologist needs precise electromechanical investigation tools to quantify the electrical propagation and its impact through the heart muscle. Analysis of the timing of the myocardial contraction based on Fourier phase histograms allows mapping of the kinetics of the different ventricular segments from functional phase pictures and, by extrapolation, mapping of the electrical activity of the heart. Nuclear cardiology combines mechanical and electrical analysis in real time. In this chapter, we report on our experience of gated blood pool scintigraphy combined with phase analysis and myocardial innervation imaging in various diseases with electrical disorders.

SPECIFIC TECHNICAL BACKGROUND OF NUCLEAR IMAGING IN ARRHYTHMIAS

Radionuclide functional imaging of the heart addresses multiple aspects of cardiac function.[1] Although most applications of nuclear cardiology are focused on coronary artery disease, in which the combination of stress/rest myocardial perfusion and/or viability imaging plays a major clinical role, many other less common cardiac diseases may benefit from this noninvasive diagnostic approach.

PERFUSION, VIABILITY, INNERVATION, AND MECHANICAL FUNCTION

Perfusion and viability imaging modalities are based on cellular uptake of a radioactive molecule such as thallium-201 (^{201}Tl), which presents an active transport comparable to that of potassium cation (K^+), or sestamibi or tetrofosmin labeled with technetium 99m (^{99m}Tc), which are larger cations whose cellular penetration is passive due to concentration gradient.

Imaging is usually performed in tomographic mode (SPECT) and is a two-step procedure that combines stress imaging (shortly after physical exercise or pharmacologic coronary vasodilation) with resting imaging after stress-injected tracer redistribution with time (thallium) or a second resting administration (technetium-labeled molecules). The first set of images describes coronary perfusion reserve at stress, whereas the second set reflects cellular viability.

In addition to single photon (gamma ray) methods, positron emission tomography (PET) may also be a choice for a comparable approach, but PET uses specific positron-emitting radiopharmaceuticals such as the generator-produced rubidium-82 for perfusion and fluorine 18–labeled fluorodeoxyglucose.

Myocardial sympathetic innervation imaging is based on the presynaptic uptake of catecholamines. The gamma-emitting tracer is meta-iodobenzyl guanidine (MIBG) labeled with iodine 123. Comparable positron-emitting tracers are used as well. Image acquisition can be planar or SPECT. Innervation defects appear as hypoactive areas, which have to be compared with perfusion defects using an adequate perfusion agent.

Imaging the mechanical contraction of the heart needs a dynamic acquisition of the periodic motion of the myocardium. Electrocardiographically (R wave) triggered acquisitions can be performed on myocardial perfusion SPECT images. Another option consists of blood pool labeling using an intravascular tracer such as albumin or red blood cells, both labeled with ^{99m}Tc. Gated blood pool pictures can be acquired in planar mode as well as in SPECT, but in any case, one single cardiac cycle is unable to provide a sufficient number of counts. Therefore, a high number of successive cardiac cycles (≥ 100) have to be superimposed for an adequate image (Fig. 9–1). Measurement of left ventricular ejection fraction is the most common variable obtained by these studies, but as will be shown later in this chapter, several other variables can be of special interest in the context of arrhythmias.

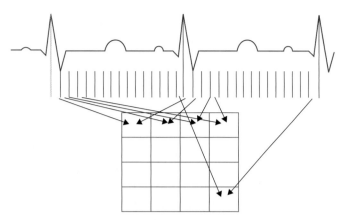

FIGURE 9–1. Principle of gating: sampling of the cardiac cycle as a sequence of successive frames during the R-R interval and superimposition in synchronism of the frames acquired from a large number of individual cycles.

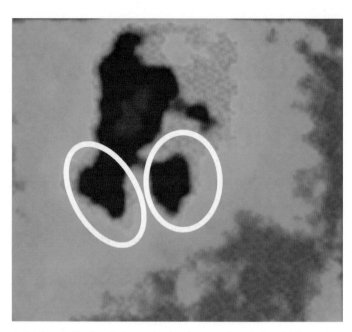

FIGURE 9–2. Blood pool pictures showing the separation of left and right ventricles in the optimal left anterior oblique view.

CARDIAC CYCLE SELECTION IN THE GATING PROCESS

The reliability of gating is the key to adequate imaging of cardiac contraction. In patients with a stable heart rate, superimposition of multiple cardiac cycles in electrocardiogram (ECG)-triggered synchronism is not a crucial problem. However, this is far from true in a patient population with cardiac rhythm abnormalities. More or less sophisticated technical approaches may be able to at least partially solve this problem. Their common principle consists in selecting the acquired cardiac cycles based on the R-R interval duration.

Cycle selection can be made a priori after acquiring for a given time a series of successive cardiac cycles and construction of the R-R histogram. By defining a temporal window on the desired part of the histogram, only the cycles matching inside the window will be accepted for final image acquisition. The R-R histogram may present a continuous variation around an average value (eg, in atrial fibrillation) or may show distinct peaks (eg, in extrasystoles where the average peak of sinusal cycles can be surrounded by a peak of shorter cycles—extrasystoles—and a second peak of longer cycles—postextrasystoles).

The option of "a posteriori" gating is more flexible because cardiac cycles are then acquired in "list mode," which means without immediate superimposition. Cycle combination is performed in a second time, when acquisition has been completed, which allows changes in R-R windowing as well as multiple window acquisitions.

PLANAR AND THREE-DIMENSIONAL RIGHT VENTRICULAR IMAGING

Diagnosis of coronary artery disease is mainly focused on the left ventricle. Perfusion tracers, as well as thallium and technetium-labeled molecules, show a very low uptake in the right ventricular wall, which is difficult to see on the images. Only in right ventricular hypertrophy can the right ventricle be clearly visualized, but it is always visualized with a lower intensity than the

left ventricle. Therefore, myocardial SPECT is a limited tool for assessment of right ventricular diseases.

Blood pool imaging does not present the same limitations, and the labeling of the circulating blood allows adequate visualization of all of the heart chambers and thoracic vessels. The drawback of this global imaging of cardiac structures is the risk of superimposition of different cavities, and technical solutions have to be found in order to minimize these overlaps.

For planar imaging, the projection must be performed in the anterior oblique view with optimization of the angle for each individual patient with regard to the orientation of the interventricular septum in order to obtain the best separation between the right and left ventricles (Fig. 9–2).

The gated blood pool SPECT approach is another option for selection of the right ventricle and evaluation of its functional variables. Measurements of ejection fractions, whether left or right, presuppose proportionality of labeled blood volumes with collected gamma counts in selected regions of interest. After adequate correction for extracardiac background activity, the end-diastolic and end-systolic counts are representative of the corresponding blood volumes.

CONTRACTION CHRONOLOGY USING TEMPORAL FOURIER ANALYSIS

The ECG gating process provides a series of images covering an average cardiac cycle over the R-R interval. The temporal course of the blood contents within the ventricles (ie, the corresponding radioactive counts) evolves from end-diastole to end-systole during the contraction phase and from end-systole again to end-diastole during the filling phase. This periodic change can be approximated by a single sinus function (Fig. 9–3); a better model of the real time/volume curve, including the faster and

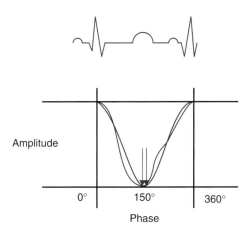

FIGURE 9–3. Sinus modeling of the left ventricular time/activity curve and definition of the phase as the time of the minimum of this curve. Phases are expressed in degrees on a scale ranging from 0° to 360° and covering the R-R interval. The blue curve is the actual time/activity curve and the red curve is its modeling by a first harmonic sinus function.

slower parts of the filling phase, may require more sinus functions (eg, three harmonics).

Temporal Fourier analysis, mostly limited to the first harmonic only, consists of mapping pixel by pixel the two variables, amplitude and phase, that characterize the sinus function, which describes the time course of the pixel activity during the R-R interval. The phases are expressed either in time units or in angular degrees. When phases are in milliseconds, they correspond to the time between the cardiac cycle origin (R wave) and the time of end-systole. The total cycle length is highly dependent on the heart rate (1000 ms for 60 beats per minute).

The use of degrees allows some independence with regard to the heart rate because a cardiac cycle is always scaled between 0° and 360° (a complete "turn") regardless of its duration. The value of the phase is somewhere in the middle of the cycle (180°), with a value usually lower because the systolic part of the cycle is shorter than the diastolic part. Nevertheless, a correction (like the Bazett correction for the QT interval) is possible to take

into account the heart rate changes. Amplitude images show the amplitude of the diastolic-systolic activity change and indicate the contraction intensity.

Phase images present for every pixel the time when the sinus function is at its minimum (nadir of the curve), which is a good approximation of the time of end-systole. A color scale gives the correspondence with the phase values and displays the time of mechanical contraction from the earliest area to the latest area. It is important to note that the phase picture is a pattern of contraction and not an activation map, even if in many cases, in absence of contraction abnormalities or delays, the contraction pattern is close to the activation map (eg, in Wolff-Parkinson-White syndrome with normal contraction and ejection fraction).

PHASE HISTOGRAM DESCRIPTIVE VALUES: MEAN AND STANDARD DEVIATION

Two characteristic values describe the phase histograms: the mean value of the phase distribution and the standard deviation of the distribution. From the phase mapping, the statistics of the phase distribution within a given ventricle (separately for left and right) can be displayed and quantified as phase histograms. The colors of the histogram bars match the colors of the phase display (green is early and red is delayed; Figs. 9–4 and 9–5).

Normal limits acquired from our personal experience with a given methodology are as follows:

Left ventricular ejection fraction (LVEF) >55%

Right ventricular ejection fraction (RVEF) >26%

Left ventricular phase standard deviation (LVSD) <28°

Right ventricular phase standard deviation (RVSD) <36°

Interventricular asynchronism (phase difference) (IVA) <14°

Values can vary substantially between scintigraphy centers due to changes in acquisition or processing modalities.

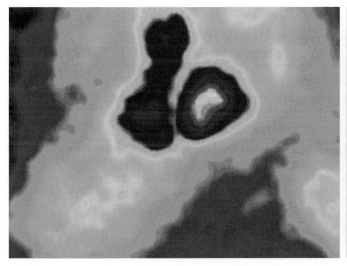
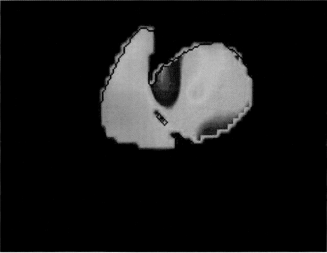

FIGURE 9–4. Left and right ventricles are shown on the left, and corresponding phase mapping is shown on the right. The earliest phases are displayed in green, and the latest phases are displayed in red; yellow and orange indicate-in between phases. This case shows a delayed left ventricular contraction due to left bundle branch block.

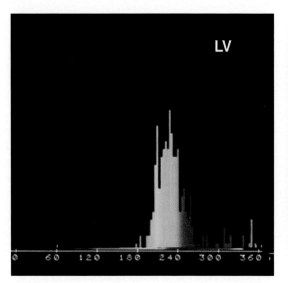
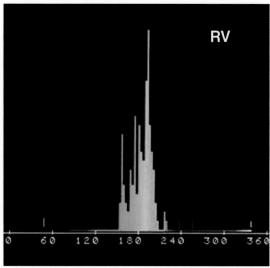

FIGURE 9–5. Phase histograms related to the case of left bundle branch block shown in Fig. 9–4 showing interventricular dyssynchrony (delayed left ventricular [LV] contraction: mean LV phase = 223° and mean right ventricular [RV] phase = 184°; interventricular dyssynchrony = 39°) and also some intraventricular dyssynchrony (enlargement of the LV histogram).

INTERPRETATION OF MYOCARDIAL SYMPATHETIC INNERVATION IMAGING USING MIBG

MIBG images can be acquired in planar mode or in SPECT mode. From planar pictures, the relative myocardial tracer uptake can be quantified as the ratio between cardiac uptake and mediastinal activity (Fig. 9–6). Normal ratios are in the range of 1.8 to 2.0. SPECT data have to be analyzed by comparing perfusion and innervation. When both studies show a concordant defect (same localization, extent, and severity), the conclusion should be the presence of a fixed myocardial lesion (probably necrosis) without any particular sign suggesting a special risk for arrhythmias. On the contrary, finding a perfusion/innervation mismatch (normal perfusion in the area of decreased MIBG uptake) indicates a significant abnormality related to risk of arrhythmias and bad prognosis (Fig. 9–7).

APPLICATIONS IN DISEASES WITH ISOLATED INTERVENTRICULAR DYSSYNCHRONY

■ WOLFF-PARKINSON-WHITE SYNDROME

For over 20 years, radionuclide ventriculography has been used to localize the atrioventricular accessory pathways associated with Wolff-Parkinson-White syndrome. So far, studies in this field have only included a limited number of patients. Moreover, the phenomenon of successful radiofrequency ablation accessory pathways is not fully understood, and the exact mechanisms leading to disappearance of pre-excitation still have not been worked out. Using scintigraphic imaging techniques, we have assessed the effects of atrioventricular accessory pathways radiofrequency ablation[2] and found that the concordance of scintigraphy and endocardial mapping for localizing accessory pathways was broadly confirmed (Fig. 9–8). In addition, the ipsilateral ventricular ejection fraction could be improved following radiofrequency ablation, particularly in patients with left-sided accessory pathways. However, the main finding was that, despite successful ablation of the accessory pathways, unexpected persistence of local ventricular pre-excitation was occasionally unveiled by scintigraphy. The persistence of a zone of premature

FIGURE 9–6. Example of planar (anterior thoracic view) meta-iodobenzyl guanidine (MIBG) scintigram. Red indicates very high activity in the liver; lungs (and thyroid) are in green whereas the cardiac uptake is mainly yellow. This study shows a heterogeneous uptake in the heart with a defect in the left ventricular apical area. Globally the cardiac MIBG uptake is decreased (heart/mediastinum ratio = 1.3) in this patient with acquired long QT syndrome. Arrow denotes the left ventricular apex.

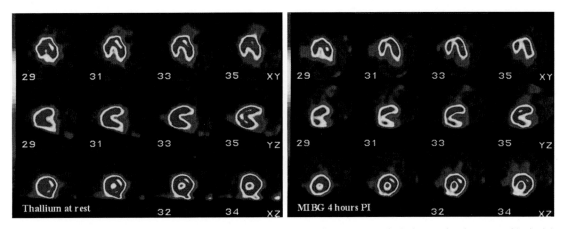

FIGURE 9–7. Case of perfusion (left) and innervation (right) mismatch. Meta-iodobenzyl guanidine (MIBG) uptake is decreased at the apex and in the inferoposterior areas, whereas the thallium-201 distribution reflecting perfusion and viability is totally normal. PI, postinjection.

ventricular contraction as shown by scintigraphy, despite the disappearance of the delta wave on the surface ECG, has never been described. Such a phenomenon may indicate a persisting aborted conduction via the accessory pathway. One must postulate that the atrial insertion of the accessory connection is, at least partly, undamaged. However, it is apparent that the site of anterograde block as a result of ablation occurred near the ventricular interface.

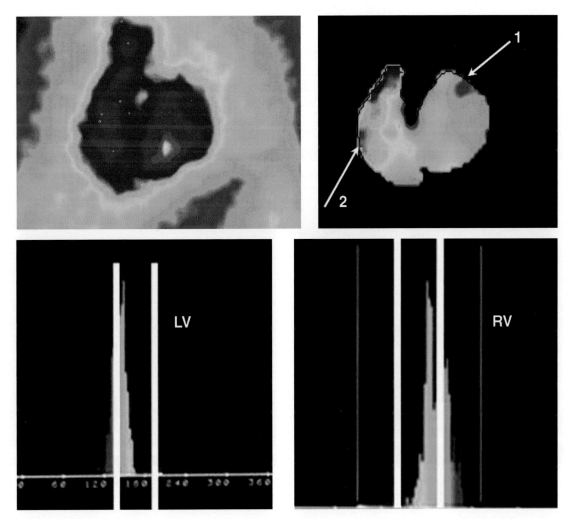

FIGURE 9–8. Typical case of Wolff-Parkinson-White syndrome. The earliest contraction takes place in the left ventricular (LV) laterobasal region (1). The contraction spreads out to the whole LV before entering the right ventricle (RV). The most delayed area is in the RV lateral wall (2). Phase histograms are both narrow with normal standard deviations. The important feature in this case is the isolated interventricular delay, which corresponds to mean values of 143° for the LV versus 163° for the RV. Pre-excitation of the LV is quantified as 20°.

APPLICATIONS IN DISEASES WITH BOTH INTER- AND INTRAVENTRICULAR DYSSYNCHRONY

■ ARRHYTHMOGENIC RIGHT VENTRICULAR DYSPLASIA

Recent clinical studies demonstrated that sudden death may be the first manifestation of arrhythmogenic right ventricular dysplasia (ARVD) and underscored the need for early diagnosis of this genetically determined heart muscle disease. The diagnosis of ARVD is based on the presence of mixed criteria established by the International Society and Federation of Cardiology (task force criteria).[3] Most of the functional parameters used to diagnose ARVD can be measured by planar radionuclide angiography.[4,5] In our hospital, we routinely use scintigraphy in patients with suspicion of ARVD (Figs. 9–9 and 9–10).

■ RESYNCHRONIZATION IN CARDIAC HEART FAILURE

The criteria for selection of heart failure patients for cardiac resynchronization therapy (CRT) (ie, ejection fraction, New York Heart Association class, and QRS width) have been

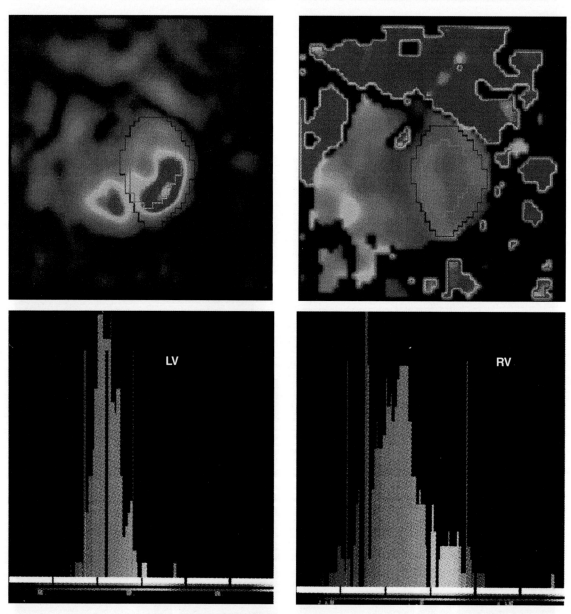

FIGURE 9–9. Example of a confirmed case of arrhythmogenic right ventricular dysplasia (ARVD). Blood pool images are on top left and phase images are on top right. Left ventricular (LV) ejection fraction measured using end-diastolic and end-systolic areas of interest (delineated on the upper row images) is normal (63%), whereas the right ventricular (RV) ejection fraction measured using one single end-diastolic region of interest (not shown in the images) is severely reduced (15%). Analysis of the phase histograms (LV is bottom left and RV is bottom right) demonstrate that there is no interventricular dyssynchrony (mean phases are 132° for LV and 137° for RV), and the phase standard deviation for the LV is within the normal limits (22°). The most characteristic result in this disease is an important and isolated RV intraventricular dyssynchrony (RV phase standard deviation = 50°) with early phases in the septal area and delayed phases in the lateral part of the RV.

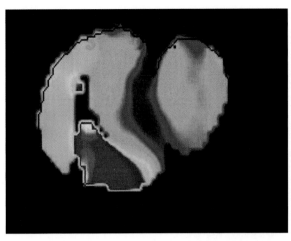
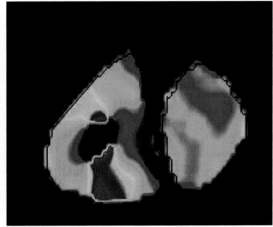

FIGURE 9–10. Two examples of severe cases of arrhythmogenic right ventricular (RV) dysplasia with pronounced intraventricular RV dyssynchrony. On the left, the standard deviation of phases is 59° for the RV versus 14° for the left ventricle (LV). On the right, the RV phase standard deviation is 84° versus 14° for the LV phase standard deviation. In both cases, there are localized areas of dyskinetic myocardium.

validated by large-scale randomized studies. However, identification of the precise determinants of the resynchronization reserve (ie, the extent and the origin of the response to biventricular pacing) is lacking. Despite thorough investigation of

electrical and mechanical dyssynchrony, identification of good candidates for biventricular therapy is still unsatisfactory. In addition, the confusion caused by the multiple Doppler measurement technique is increased by the use of different

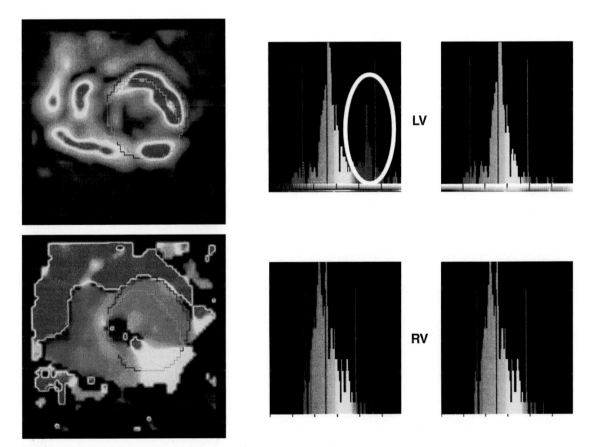

FIGURE 9–11. Patient with severe heart failure investigated prior to resynchronization therapy. Global left ventricle (LV) and right ventricle (RV) phase analysis shows a significant interventricular dyssynchrony (mean phases are 183° for LV vs 153° for RV, which corresponds to an interventricular delay of 30°). Nevertheless, the LV presents a large dyskinetic area in the apical and inferolateral region, which results in a second and delayed peak on the LV phase histogram responsible for a false increase of the mean value of the phase histogram. Excluding this aneurismal area for the phase measurement reduces the interventricular dyssynchrony considerably (LV mean phase is 160°, which compared with the 153° for RV, yields a delay of only 7°).

end points for defining response to CRT. Invasive and non-invasive electroanatomic investigations (mapping) are very informative in patients with intramyocardiac conductive disorders.[6,7] We have used planar radionuclide ventriculography with phase analysis to identify the scintigraphic markers of improved cardiac function after triple-chamber stimulation. Another goal was to improve understanding of the electromechanical mechanisms underlying the effect of biventricular pacing. We found that all of the radionuclide cardiac dyssynchronism and contraction parameters improved following implantation in responder patients. In the nonresponder group, phase standard deviation, a marker of left ventricular dyssynchronism (Fig. 9–11), did not change during follow-up despite an improvement in interventricular dyssynchrony. Interventricular dyssynchrony was identified as an independent predictive factor of good clinical response with a practical cutoff value of 25.5°, a sensitivity of 91.4%, and a specificity of 84.4%. New scintigraphic markers of cardiac dyssynchrony for tailored therapy in heart failure patients and a better comprehension of how resynchronization works may be acquired in the future using high-resolution and high-sensitivity SPECT imaging with the most recent cameras for multiple slice analysis.

APPLICATION TO ASSESS MYOCARDIAL SYMPATHETIC HETEROGENEITY

A regional disparity in myocardial sympathetic innervation has been found in patients with congenital long QT syndrome (LQTS), using iodine 123–MIBG.[8] We have also used MIBG scintigraphy in patients with acquired LQTS.[9] The heart/mediastinum activity ratio was calculated using an anterior view, 4 hours after injection of the isotope. In this way, we were able to demonstrate that patients with acquired LQTS had a reduction in sympathetic innervation (see Fig. 9–6). Indeed, much clinical and experimental evidence has proven that ventricular electrical stability may be threatened by an imbalance in the autonomic nervous system. Heterogeneous sympathetic activity could act by amplifying existing differences in transmural dispersion of repolarization in LQTS. In this way, heterogeneous sympathetic activity could be considered as having an amplifier role able to raise the propensity toward life-threatening arrhythmia and could partially explain the distinct severity of the disease within a family.

CONCLUSION

In the near future, new technical developments in nuclear imaging may help to improve the understanding of most of the heart electrical disorders. Further clinical studies are needed to evaluate the exact interest of gated blood pool SPECT global and local systolic measurements, compared with more traditional planar imaging, in the long-term follow-up of patients.

REFERENCES

1. Klocke FJ, Baird MG, Lorell BH, et al. ACC/AHA/ASNC guidelines for the clinical use of cardiac radionuclide imaging–executive summary: a report of the American College of Cardiology/American Heart Association Task Force on Practice Guidelines (ACC/AHA/ASNC Committee to Revise the 1995 Guidelines for the Clinical Use of Cardiac Radionuclide Imaging). *Circulation.* 2003;108:1404-1418.
2. Chevalier P, Bontemps L, Fatemi M, et al. Gated blood-pool SPECT evaluation of changes after radiofrequency catheter ablation of accessory pathways: evidence for persistent ventricular preexcitation despite successful therapy. *J Am Coll Cardiol.* 1999;34:1839-1846.
3. Cox MG, van der Smagt JJ, Noorman M, et al. Arrhythmogenic right ventricular dysplasia/cardiomyopathy diagnostic task force criteria: impact of new task force criteria. *Circ Arrhythm Electrophysiol.* 2010;3:126-133.
4. Le Guludec D, Slama MS, Frank R, et al. Evaluation of radionuclide angiography in diagnosis of arrhythmogenic right ventricular cardiomyopathy. *J Am Coll Cardiol.* 1995;26:1476-1483.
5. Daou D, Lebtahi R, Faraggi M, et al. Cardiac gated equilibrium radionuclide angiography and multiharmonic Fourier phase analysis: optimal acquisition parameters in arrhythmogenic right ventricular cardiomyopathy. *J Nucl Cardiol.* 1999;6:437-449.
6. Boogers MM, Van Kriekinge SD, Henneman MM, et al. Quantitative gated SPECT-derived phase analysis on gated myocardial perfusion SPECT detects left ventricular dyssynchrony and predicts response to cardiac resynchronization therapy. *J Nucl Med.* 2009;50:718-725.
7. Eder V, Fauchier L, Courtehoux M, et al. Segmental wall motion abnormality analyzed by equilibrium radionuclide angiography and improvement in ventricular function by cardiac resynchronization therapy. *PACE.* 2007;30(Suppl 1):S58-S61.
8. Momose M, Kobayashi H, Kasanuki H, et al. Evaluation of regional cardiac sympathetic innervation in congenital long QT syndrome using 123I-MIBG scintigraphy. *Nucl Med Commun.* 1998;19:943-951.
9. Chevalier P, Rodriguez C, Bontemps L, et al. Non-invasive testing of acquired long QT syndrome: evidence for multiple arrhythmogenic substrates. *Cardiovasc Res.* 2001;50:386-398.

CHAPTER 10
OPTICAL MAPPING OF ELECTRICAL ACTIVITY

Jiashin Wu, Hiroshi Morita, and Douglas P. Zipes

INTRODUCTION / 179

ELECTROPHYSIOLOGIC HETEROGENEITY ACROSS
THE VENTRICULAR WALL / 179

ARRHYTHMOGENESIS DURING ACUTE ISCHEMIA
AND REPERFUSION / 180

SPONTANEOUS ARRHYTHMIAS IN TISSUES RECOVERED
FROM ISCHEMIA / 183

ARRHYTHMOGENESIS IN TISSUE MODELS OF BRUGADA
SYNDROME / 183

ARRHYTHMOGENESIS IN A TISSUE MODEL
OF ANDERSEN-TAWIL SYNDROME / 186

AV NODAL REENTRY / 187

LIMITATIONS AND APPLICATIONS OF OPTICAL
MAPPING / 188

SUMMARY / 189

INTRODUCTION

Current diagnostic criteria of cardiac arrhythmias are based mostly on the electrocardiogram (ECG) recorded with body surface electrodes, which register local far-field potentials generated by all cardiac myocytes. The remote body surface placement and low number of electrodes limit the information content of ECG recordings and the details in the mechanisms of arrhythmias, the regions of electrophysiologic abnormalities, and the paths of reentry that can be identified.

Recently, high spatial resolution optical-mapping systems have been developed and used in research laboratories to investigate the mechanisms of cardiac arrhythmias in animal models under controlled conditions.[1] Optical mapping uses fluorescent dyes that are sensitive to transmembrane potential or to ion concentrations as probes, optics to collect the signal-carrying fluorescence, and photon-sensing devices (eg, camera or photodiode array) to convert fluorescence to electrical signals, which are then amplified, digitized, processed, and analyzed (Fig. 10–1). The advantages of camera-based optical-mapping systems are (1) recording *high spatial resolution* movies of electrophysiologic activity in cardiac muscle; (2) reporting *transmembrane* potential, which reflects cellular electrophysiology more directly than the extracellular field potential registered by electrode-based body surface and intracardiac mapping systems; and

(3) capability of recording cytosolic *ion concentrations* (eg, Ca^{2+} transient) by using ion-sensitive fluorescent dyes. The current trend in optical mapping has been moving toward dual-camera simultaneous recording of both membrane potential and Ca^{2+} transient within the same view field. High spatial resolution optical mapping provides details in electrophysiologic heterogeneity, focal activation, and abnormal conduction in the heart and has contributed significantly to the insight and mechanistic understanding of cardiac arrhythmias in recent years.

Most of the existing optical-mapping systems use a design that optically focuses the to-be-observed tissue surface onto the sensor array of a stationary camera, thus requiring direct view of the tissue surface. The mapping area can range from a single isolated cell to the entire heart, depending on the optics mounted in front of the camera. In this design, muscle contraction can change the relative position of tissue surface, introducing motion artifacts into the recorded electrophysiologic signal. The undesired motion artifacts are commonly eliminated by tissue immobilization with pharmacologic excitation-contraction uncoupling agents, such as cytochalasin D[2,3] or blebbistatin,[4] in isolated heart or tissue preparations. Alternative methods (eg, ratiometric imaging or signal processing) can also be used to extract useful data from signals containing motion artifacts obtained in beating hearts. In creating models for investigating the mechanisms of arrhythmias in diseased human hearts, hearts from large animals are preferred over those from small animals due to their similarities to human hearts in terms of ion currents, electrophysiologic heterogeneity, conduction phenomena, anatomy, and coronary perfusion, among other characteristics. All studies presented in this chapter were performed by using a 256-channel (16 × 16 array) optical-mapping system to record electric activity on the surface (mapping field: 19.5 × 19.5 mm²) of isolated and arterially perfused canine ventricular tissues that were stained with a membrane potential–sensitive dye, 4(beta-[2-(di-n-butylamino)-6-napathy]vinyl)pyridinium (di-4-ANEPPS).

Clinically, cardiac arrhythmias occur commonly in diseased hearts and are triggered by acute events. Although the basic theory and mechanisms of the initiation and maintenance of ventricular tachycardia (VT) have been investigated intensively (eg, early and delayed afterdepolarizations [EADs] and [DADs],[5] dispersion of repolarization, reentry), their manifestation, interactions, and roles in arrhythmias in diseased hearts are less clear. This chapter presents some recent developments in understanding the mechanisms of arrhythmias in tissue models of ischemia/reperfusion; Brugada, long QT, and Andersen-Tawil syndromes; and atrioventricular (AV) nodal reentry unveiled by optical mapping in our laboratory.

ELECTROPHYSIOLOGIC HETEROGENEITY ACROSS THE VENTRICULAR WALL

We used optical mapping to elucidate the functional nature of M-cell behavior in the ventricular wall. Ventricular action potentials (APs) are heterogeneous.[6] The AP duration (APD) is longest in the mid myocardium and shortest in the epicardium across the ventricular free wall. Compared with the endocardium,

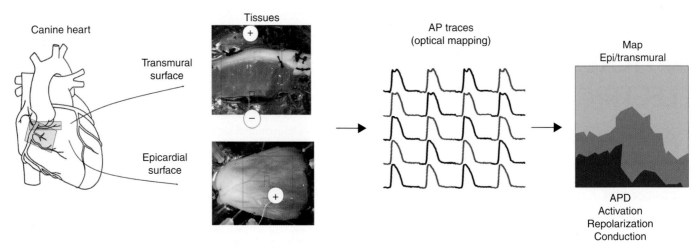

FIGURE 10–1. Optical mapping of electrical activity in cardiac muscle. Wedges of ventricular muscle are isolated and perfused via a branch of a coronary artery (left), stained with a voltage-sensitive fluorescent dye, and imaged on either a transmural or epicardial (Epi) surface with an optical-mapping system. Fluorescence movies of electrical activity are processed to obtain traces of action potentials (APs); distribution maps of activation, repolarization, and AP duration (APD); conduction sequences and velocity; and reentry pathways (right).

myocytes in the epicardium have a larger transient outward current (I_{to}); a stronger ischemia-induced K_{ATP} current; and an AP that has a larger spike and dome morphology, more pronounced rate dependency, and a higher sensitivity to ischemia. The slow delayed rectifier K$^+$ current, I_{Ks}, is lowest in the mid myocardium, whereas the density of the rapid delayed rectifier K$^+$ current, I_{Kr}, is similar across the canine left ventricle wall. The heterogeneity in ion currents causes dispersion of APs and of repolarization, which normally serves a physiologic function but can be proarrhythmic when it occurs excessively or interacts with the abnormal sequence of activation in a diseased heart.

The mid myocardium in the ventricular free wall has been shown to differ significantly from the endocardium and epicardium, with exceedingly long APDs during long cycle length (CL) activation. It was postulated that a special group of midmyocardial cells, so-called *M cells*, is responsible for the distinctive mid-myocardial electrophysiologic properties.[6-9] The M cells have been proposed to underlie the T and U waves in ECG and play major roles in the dispersion of repolarization and in the initiation of VT.[6,7] However, some studies failed to find evidence of M cells.[8,10-12] Using optical mapping, we demonstrated that instead of a separate group of cells, the M-cell behavior was functional extremes of ventricular heterogeneity that became manifest under specific conditions.[13] The mid-myocardial preferential prolongation of APDs also contributed to the formation of a transmurally asymmetric distribution of APDs in a tissue model of long QT syndrome[14] with the shortest APD in the epicardium and longest APD in the mid myocardium, upon which epicardial but not endocardial premature stimulation can easily initiate VT.[15]

We isolated and arterially perfused wedges of canine left ventricular free wall and optically mapped APDs on their cut-exposed transmural surfaces, before and after treatment with anemone toxin II (ATX-II), which delays the inactivation of membrane Na$^+$ current (I_{Na}). Before ATX-II, the row of recording sites having the longest mean APD (APD$_L$ layer) was in the (sub)endocardium. ATX-II prolonged APD heterogeneously

(mid myocardium > endocardium > epicardium) and "moved" the APD$_L$ layer progressively from the endocardium into mid myocardium (Fig. 10–2). We detected M-cell behavior (the APD$_L$ layer located at sites other than in the endocardium and epicardium with statistical significance) in 18 wedges exposed to ≥5 nmol/L of ATX-II, but not in the other 18 wedges exposed to ≤2.5 nmol/L of ATX-II. We also repeated the same experiments in wedges isolated from the canine ventricular septum. In contrast to the ventricular free wall, none of the 22 septum wedges showed M-cell behavior under the same conditions.[16,17] Therefore, M cell is a functional phenomenon in the left ventricular free wall, but not in the septum, that can become manifest under specific nonphysiologic conditions.

ARRHYTHMOGENESIS DURING ACUTE ISCHEMIA AND REPERFUSION

Acute ischemia and reperfusion are strong triggers of VT. Most ischemia-induced VTs occur during the first 10 to 15 minutes of ischemia and are due to focal activation and transmural reentry.[18-20] Both the differences in the coronary blood flow between the healthy and ischemic regions and heterogeneic tissue responses to ischemia contribute to the initiation of VT. Using optical mapping, we investigated the contributions to VT by heterogeneic tissue responses to acute global ischemia. Global ischemia eliminated the heterogeneity in coronary perfusion, thus isolating the tissue responses to ischemia.

Acute ischemia suppresses excitability faster in the epicardium than endocardium, increasing transmural dispersion of excitability in the ventricular wall.[18,21] Ischemia also slows conduction after a transient initial increase. The rapidly changing transmural dispersion of tissue excitability and velocity of conduction form a proarrhythmic substrate in which reentry can be initiated, sustained, and then abolished during acute global ischemia and reperfusion.

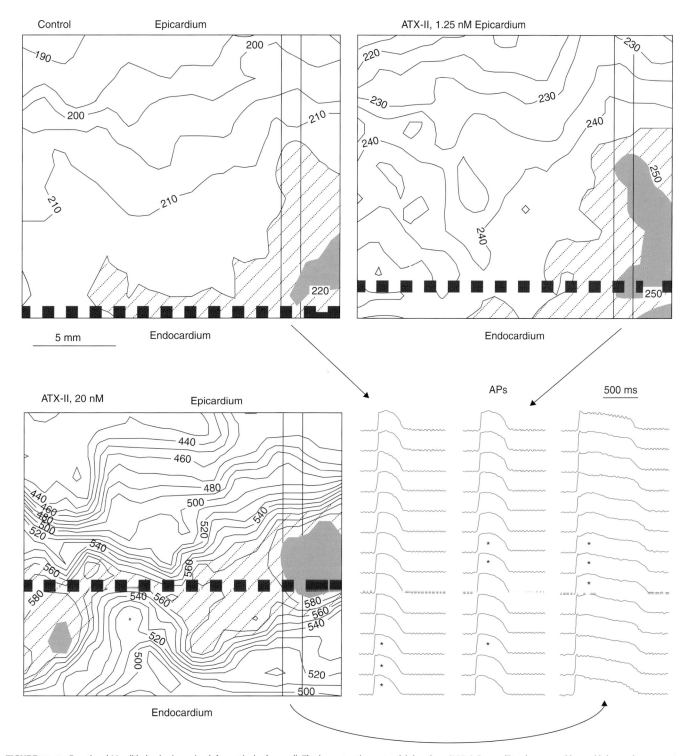

FIGURE 10–2. Functional M-cell behavior in canine left ventricular free wall. The longest action potential durations (APDs) "moved" to deeper positions with increasing concentrations of anemone toxin II (ATX-II; 0, 1.25, and 20 nmol/L). The isochronal maps show the transmural distributions of APDs (in milliseconds) with the diagonal hatched lines and solid black highlighting the regions of longer and longest APDs. The thick dashed lines indicate the APD$_L$ (longest mean APD) layer. Selected columns of APs are displayed at lower right with asterisks indicating the longest three APDs. Endocardial pacing cycle length (CL) is 1000 ms. Mapping area is 19.5 × 17.0 mm². The longest APDs are mostly in the (sub) endocardium during control and appeared as islands in the mid myocardium after 20 nmol/L of ATX-II. Reproduced with permission from Ueda N, Zipes DP, Wu J. Functional and transmural modulation of M cell behavior in canine ventricular wall. *Am J Physiol Heart Circ Physiol.* 2004;287:H2573.

We induced global ischemia and optically mapped APs on the transmural surfaces of 36 isolated wedges of canine left ventricular free wall. Before ischemia, the transmural response of the tissues was 1:1 to endocardial pacing (CL = 300 ms). Ischemia increased the transmural gradient of the refractory period, which blocked conduction unidirectionally and initiated reentry and VT after 535 ± 146 seconds (31 wedges). Multiple zones of responsiveness (1:1, 2:1, and 4:1) to endocardial pacing developed after

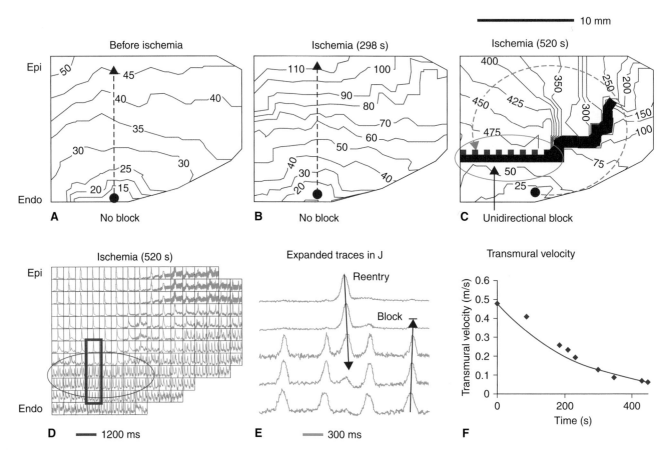

FIGURE 10–3. Unidirectional block of conduction at the transmural gradient of refractory period by endocardial stimulation during acute global ischemia. Activations were recorded on a cut-exposed transmural surface of a wedge of isolated canine left ventricular free wall that was perfused through an included diagonal branch of the left anterior descending coronary artery. Acute global ischemia was created by halting perfusion. The times of ischemia are indicated in the subtitles. The conduction sequences (**A-C**) from the endocardial sites of pacing (the black dots; cycle length [CL] = 300 ms) are shown as isochrone lines (at the times indicated by the numbers in milliseconds) moving along the directions of the thin dashed arrow-headed lines. The thick solid line and the line with one dashed side and one solid side in **C** indicate full block and unidirectional block of conduction, respectively. Grids in the action potential mosaic (**D**) separate the signals (1.2 seconds, normalized) from neighboring sensors. The framed traces in **D** are shown in **E** with an expanded time scale. The transmural velocity of conduction (**F**) is calculated from two recording sites with 11 mm of separation along a transmural line passing through the site of pacing. Epi and Endo indicate the epicardium and endocardium, respectively. Transmural conduction from the endocardial site of pacing at the CL of 300 ms was blocked in the mid myocardium in **C** and **D** by the longer refractory period. However, activation conducted along the opposite direction (toward the endocardium) penetrated the line of unidirectional block in **C** and **D**, until it collided with the refractory period of another activation initiated by the continued endocardial pacing. Reproduced with permission from Wu J, Zipes DP. Transmural reentry during global acute ischemia and reperfusion in canine ventricular muscle. *Am J Physiol Heart Circ Physiol.* 2001;280:H2719. See also Moving Image 10–3.

570 ± 165 seconds of ischemia (34 wedges). Further ischemia inactivated the epicardium and eliminated reentry and VT in 24 wedges. Therefore, heterogeneic prolongation of the refractory period and conduction slowing by early ischemia provided a proarrhythmic substrate in which reentry and VT could be induced by rapid endocardial activation (Fig. 10–3).

In contrast to endocardial pacing, epicardial pacing initiated reentry during acute ischemia by a different mechanism.[20] The transmural gradient of sensitivity to ischemia caused decremental conduction to occur first in the epicardium. At this time, epicardial stimulation failed to conduct laterally along the rim of epicardium and, instead, conducted to the more excitable endocardium, then laterally along the rim of endocardium, and finally reentered the subepicardium (in 9 of 18 wedges after 719 ± 399 seconds of ischemia). In contrast, endocardial stimulation applied right before or after the above epicardial stimulations initiated activation that conducted rapidly along

the rim of endocardium, then slowly from the endocardium toward the epicardium without initiating reentry (Fig. 10–4). In addition to these mechanisms of reentry initiation after several minutes of ischemia, we also showed that a transient prolongation of APD during the first 2 minutes of ischemia contributed to arrhythmogenesis, especially when combined with delayed I_{Na} inactivation by ATX-II.[22]

After 25 minutes of ischemia, the majority of the epicardium and mid myocardium was inexcitable, whereas the endocardium was still excitable during endocardial pacing. Reperfusion restored the perfusion flow uniformly. However, the recovery of tissue excitability was faster in the subendocardium and mid myocardium than in the deeply depressed subepicardium. During the first minute of reperfusion, the reappearance of excitability in the subepicardium was associated with APDs that were much longer than in the subendocardium. The transmural differences in reperfusion recovery produced an initial steep

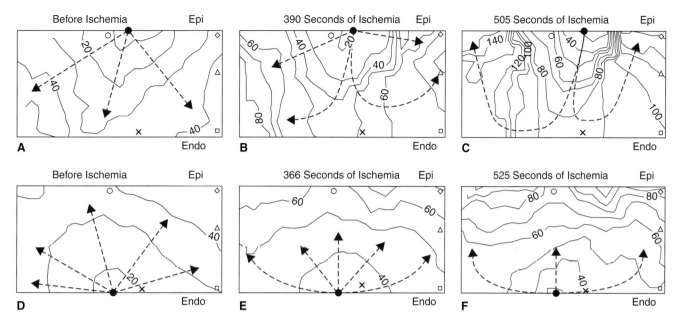

FIGURE 10-4. Unidirectional block of the epicardially initiated activation and transmural asymmetry in conduction during acute global ischemia. The isolated ventricular wedge and the recording area were similar to those in Fig. 10–3. The wedge was stimulated alternately between the epicardium (Epi) and endocardium (Endo) at the red-dotted sites. Ischemia depresses tissue excitability more rapidly in the epicardium than in endocardium. After 505 seconds of ischemia (**C**), the epicardial-initiated activation penetrated the ventricular wall transmurally while failing to conduct laterally along the epicardium, and then conducted laterally in the endocardium and mid myocardium and reentered the epicardium. Endocardial stimulation, applied 525 seconds after ischemia (**F**), initiated activation that spread quickly along the endocardium, then transmurally to the epicardium without reentry. Therefore, ischemia-induced transmural gradient of excitability provided the substrate for reentry during epicardial stimulation. The recording area is 10 (transmural) by 18 (along the epicardium) mm². Reproduced with permission from Wu J, Zipes DP. Transmural reentry triggered by epicardial stimulation during acute ischemia in canine ventricular muscle. *Am J Physiol Heart Circ Physiol*. 2002;283:H2006. See also Moving Image 10–4.

transmural gradient of APD, which was progressively reduced during further reperfusion. Unidirectional block of conduction, focal activations, and reentry occurred during the first minute of reperfusion. Sustained VT and ventricular fibrillation occurred after 93 ± 49 seconds of reperfusion (in two of the eight wedges reperfused at a quarter of the preischemia flow rate).

We concluded that transmural heterogeneity in the tissue responses to ischemia contributed to arrhythmogenesis during acute ischemia by providing steep transmural gradients of excitability and refractory period in which unidirectional block and reentry could occur easily. Transmural heterogeneity in reperfusion recovery contributed to reperfusion VT by providing a steep transmural gradient of APD and by promoting focal activation. The clinical implication is that the heterogeneic tissue responses provide a proarrhythmic substrate in which reentry appears to be a predominant mechanism of ventricular arrhythmias during and after global ischemia.

SPONTANEOUS ARRHYTHMIAS IN TISSUES RECOVERED FROM ISCHEMIA

Using optical mapping, we demonstrated a potential mechanism of arrhythmias in postischemia ventricular tissue. It is well known that myocardial ischemia can induce persistent proarrhythmic remodeling even after sufficient reperfusion. We investigated mechanisms of postischemia arrhythmogenesis in 10 isolated wedges of canine left ventricular free wall.[23] Among the 10 wedges, 8 recovered well with return of both APD and

velocity of conduction back to normal after 40 minutes of ischemia and 60 minutes of reperfusion. Subsequent perfusion with ATX-II (20 nmol/L) prolonged APDs significantly, induced EADs in all of the recovered wedges, and induced spontaneous VTs in seven of the eight recovered wedges. Focal EADs and reentry were responsible for 73% and 18% of the activations, respectively, in the VTs (Fig. 10–5). Changes in the EAD foci and conduction pathways altered the contour of the transmural ECG during VT. In comparison, a control group of eight ischemia-free wedges had less APD prolongation, less dispersion of repolarization, and no EADs or VT after the same ATX-II treatment. The exaggerated APD responses to ATX-II indicated a low repolarization reserve[24] in the postischemia wedges, which provided a proarrhythmic substrate. Therefore, a brief period of ischemia, even after sufficient reperfusion recovery of AP and conduction velocity, can persistently suppress repolarization reserve with arrhythmic consequences. Clinical implications of this study would be that patients recovered from an episode of ischemia have an increased risk of arrhythmic episodes, which can be triggered easily by an APD-prolonging event.

ARRHYTHMOGENESIS IN TISSUE MODELS OF BRUGADA SYNDROME

Brugada syndrome (BS) is characterized by ST-segment elevation and negative T waves in the right precordial ECG leads in patients.[25-28] Mutations in genes that encode the Na⁺ channel and the Ca²⁺ channel have been identified in 18% to 30%

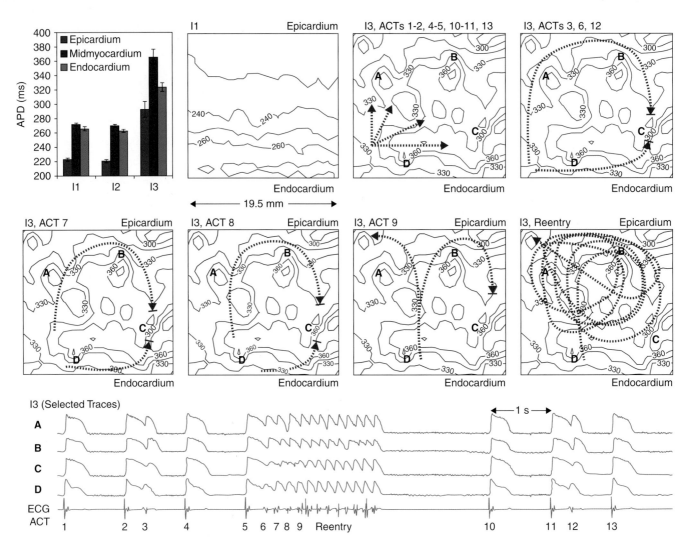

FIGURE 10–5. Prior ischemia promoted spontaneous early afterdepolarizations (EADs) and ventricular tachyarrhythmia (VT) in a canine left ventricular tissue having anemone toxin II (ATX-II)–induced long QT syndrome. The mean epicardial, mid-myocardial, and endocardial action potential durations (APDs) before ischemia (I1), after ischemia (I2), and after ATX-II (I3) are displayed at upper left. The APD contour maps (I1 and I3s) show the transmural distributions of APD (in milliseconds). Action potentials (I3, from the sites A to D) and the transmural electrocardiogram (ECG) are shown at the bottom with activations (ACTs 1-9) and reentry indicated below. The APDs in the I3 contour maps are measured from ACT 4. ACTs 3 and 12 are EADs. ACTs 6 to 9 are focal EADs that triggered VT. The first I3 map shows the paced activations (ACTs 1, 2, 4, 5, 10, 11, and 13). The other I3 maps show the conductions of focal EADs and reentry (six loops). Reproduced from Ueda N, Zipes DP, Wu J. Prior ischemia enhances arrhythmogenicity in isolated canine ventricular wedge model of long QT 3. *Cardiovasc Res.* 2004;63:69-76. See also Moving Image 10–5.

and 8% of patients with BS, respectively.[29-31] BS is temperature sensitive, and temperature elevation can lead to T wave alternans (TWAs), VT, and sudden death, especially in adult male patients. We investigated the mechanisms of VT and genotype-phenotype relationships with a series of optical-mapping studies in in vitro models of BS.[32]

In patients with BS, the right ventricular outflow tract (RVOT) is a critical area associated with prominent electrophysiologic differences and is a frequent origin of arrhythmias.[33-36] We reproduced the electrophysiologic characteristics of BS in two models, one with Na⁺ channelopathy (Na-model) and the other with Ca²⁺ channelopathy (Ca-model), using isolated canine RVOT tissues. The Na-model was induced with combinations of terfenadine, pilsicainide, and pinacidil. Pilsicainide and terfenadine reduce I_{Na}, simulating the Na⁺ channelopathy. Pinacidil deepens the phase 1 notch of the AP, which is a

major mediator of the adult male predominance of BS.[37-41] The Ca-model was induced with only verapamil, a blocker of I_{CaL}, because the involvement of other currents is still unclear in patients with the Ca²⁺ channelopathy type of BS.

We demonstrated the critical role of RVOT heterogeneity in the arrhythmogenesis in BS using the Na-model.[42] Compared with the paired right ventricular anteroinferior (RVAI) tissues, RVOT tissues have a deeper phase 1 notch of AP, especially in the epicardium, larger J wave, and higher sensitivity to the BS-inducing drugs. Induction of BS progressively deepened the phase 1 notch and delayed and enhanced the phase 2 dome initially (suprathreshold of I_{CaL} activation) and then abbreviated (due to subthreshold of I_{CaL} activation) the phase 2 dome in the RVOT epicardial AP. These changes led to the simultaneous presence of APs with and without the phase 2 dome. This created a large dispersion of repolarization in association with deep phase 1 notches in the epicardium, but not in the mid myocardium and endocardium, resulting in opposite transmural gradient of repolarization in adjacent regions (having supra- and subthreshold of I_{CaL} activation) within the RVOT. Conduction of the phase 2 dome from the epicardial region having a prominent phase 2 dome to regions without a dome led to phase 2 reentry, premature activation, and VT (Fig. 10–6). Fluctuations in the depth of the phase 1 notch around the threshold of I_{CaL} activation caused alternans in the phase 2 dome of the AP and in the T wave in the ECG, which was further promoted by bradycardia.[43]

In contrast, the same drugs had much less effect in the RVAI tissues. VTs occurred in 47% of RVOT preparations but only in 7% of the paired RVAI tissues. Blockade of I_{to} reduced the

heterogeneity of APs and prevented VT in the RVOT tissues, because I_{to} regulates the depth of phase 1 notch and the size of the phase 2 dome of AP.[44] Therefore, a high I_{to}-mediated heterogeneity in the RVOT provided a proarrhythmic substrate for the initiation of phase 2 reentry and VT in BS. Hypothermia enhanced the heterogeneity of the AP and promoted the origination of phase 2 reentry in the epicardium of the RVOT, but the prolonged APD reduced the possibility of sustained VT.[45] Hyperthermia abbreviated the AP and facilitated the maintenance of reentry and VTs, especially when combined with rapid activations.[45] Such responses occur frequently in patients with fever.[46-48] In addition, delayed epicardial activation (eg, by slowed or blocked transmural conduction in association

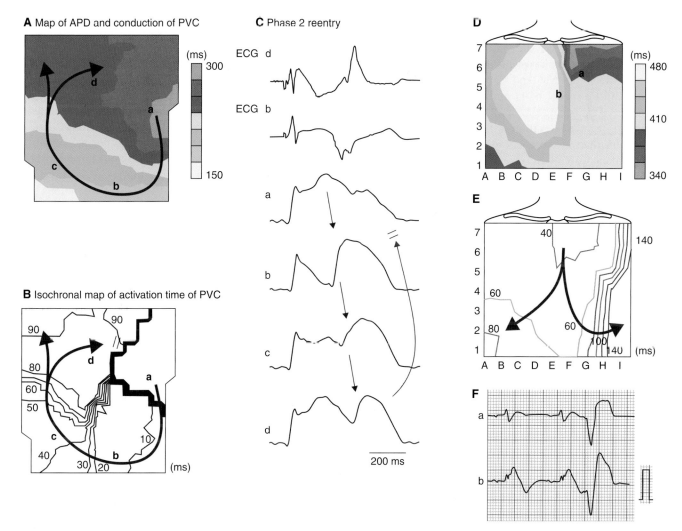

FIGURE 10–6. Ventricular arrhythmias induced by epicardial heterogeneity of action potentials (APs) in a canine right ventricular outflow tract (RVOT) model (**A-C**) and in a 48-year-old man with Brugada syndrome (BS) (**D-F**). Experiment (**A**, AP duration [APD] map; **B**, activation isochronal map; **C**, local electrocardiograms [ECGs] and APs from the sites indicated in **A** and **B**): Large phase 2 dome conducted (along the arrows) from the long APD region (site a in **A**) to the short APD region (sites b and c, light color), then reentered the long APD region (site d), and finally blocked by refractoriness (**B** and **C**). Local transmural ECGs (**C**) showed ST-segment elevation with negative T wave in the long APD region (site d) and large ST-segment elevation in the short APD region (site b). BS was induced by pinacidil (10.0 μmol/L), terfenadine (2.0 μmol/L), and pilsicainide (12.5 μmol/L). Patient (87-lead body surface map): The distribution of QT intervals in the anterior chest (**D**) shows that the upper chest (the RVOT region) had simultaneous presence of both short and long QT intervals (a and b), resembling the APD heterogeneity in the epicardium of canine RVOT model of BS (**A**). The isochronal map (**E**) shows the RVOT origin of premature ventricular contraction (PVC). J-ST elevation occurred in the local ECGs at both sites a and b (**F**). Site a had a short QT interval without negative T wave. Reproduced with permission from Morita H, Zipes DP, Ohe T, Wu J. Brugada syndrome: insights of ST elevation, arrhythmogenicity and risk stratification from experimental observations. *Heart Rhythm.* 2009;6:S40.

with a dysfunctional I_{Na}), as we simulated experimentally using separate stimulations in an additional piece of epicardial tissue staggered on the epicardium of a transmural wedge,[49] led to fragmented QRS in ECG, which is a risk marker of prognosis in BS.[50] Body surface mapping in patients with BS supported these experimental findings (see Fig. 10–6).[51] In conclusion, the AP heterogeneity within the epicardium of the RVOT contributes to the ECG characteristics, temperature sensitivity, TWA, and arrhythmias in BS.

We evaluated the efficacy of catheter ablation in eliminating VT in 17 isolated RVOT models of BS.[52] Epicardial ablation at the earliest activation site of premature ventricular complexes (PVCs) disconnected the short and long APD regions and eliminated all PVCs and VTs, although APD heterogeneity was still present in the epicardium. In contrast, endocardial ablation failed to eliminate VT. These results suggest that the most effective ablation to eliminated VT in patients with BS should be at the earliest activation sites in the epicardium of the RVOT.

We also evaluated the phenotypic differences and therapeutic effects between the Na^+ and Ca^{2+} channelopathies in BS (Na-model and Ca-model in 11 and 7 canine RVOT tissues, respectively).[53] At a pacing CL of 1000 ms, both models had coved-type ST-segment elevation in the ECG, longer APDs in the epicardium than in the endocardium, and a similar incidence of spontaneous VTs. However, the Ca-model had a higher incidence of TWA than the Na-model. At a CL of 2000 ms, the Ca-model had saddle-back–type ST-segment elevation in ECGs and shorter APDs in the epicardium than in the endocardium, whereas the Na-model had coved-type ST-segment elevation in the ECG and extensive AP heterogeneity in the epicardium. VT occurred less frequently with the Ca^{2+} than with the Na^+ channelopathy at a CL of 2000 ms. Isoproterenol normalized the ECG morphology and transmural APD gradient in both the Na^+ and Ca^{2+} channelopathy models of BS, but quinidine failed to normalize the ECG and prevent TWAs in the Ca^{2+} model, especially at the CL of 1000 ms. Both quinidine and isoproterenol eliminated epicardial AP heterogeneity and prevented VTs. We conclude that although both Na^+ and Ca^{2+} dysfunctions produced similar BS characteristic ECGs and arrhythmogenesis at 60 beats per minute (bpm), Ca^{2+} dysfunction was associated with a higher incidence of TWAs at 60 bpm, less ST-segment elevation, and fewer arrhythmias at 30 bpm compared with Na^+ dysfunction.

Our experiments suggest that patients with Ca^{2+} channelopathy–type BS are likely to have rate-dependent changes of ST-T morphology and arrhythmogenesis. The rate-dependent ECG responses and arrhythmogenicity in the Ca-model suggest that patients with Ca^{2+} channelopathy may have more arrhythmic events during the daytime, whereas cardiac events may be infrequent at night due to lower heart rates. This study demonstrated that although both quinidine and isoproterenol restored the dome in the AP and abolished arrhythmias in both Na^+ and Ca^{2+} channelopathy models, quinidine did not prevent J-ST elevation and TWA at a CL of 1000 ms in the Ca-model. Therefore, quinidine and isoproterenol can be effective in BS with either Na^+ or Ca^{2+} channelopathies, but quinidine may not fully prevent arrhythmias in patients with BS caused by Ca^{2+} channelopathy. Naturally, results from animal experiments must be applied clinically with caution.

ARRHYTHMOGENESIS IN A TISSUE MODEL OF ANDERSEN-TAWIL SYNDROME

Patients with Andersen-Tawil syndrome (ATS; also known as type 7 long QT syndrome) have mild QT prolongation, large U waves, and frequent VT.[54,55] Mutations in the gene encoding the inward rectifier K^+ channel (current: I_{K1}) have been identified in type 1 ATS (ATS1). I_{K1} plays major roles in maintaining the resting potential and in the final repolarization of the AP.[54,56,57] Patients with ATS1 were reported to have frequent bigeminal PVCs that were increased by hypokalemia[58,59] and QRS alternans in association with bidirectional VT.[60]

Using optical mapping, we investigated the mechanism of arrhythmogenesis and formation of U waves in an ATS1 model induced by I_{K1} blockade with cesium chloride (CsCl; 5-10 mmol/L) in isolated left ventricular free wall wedges.[61] To investigate the effects of sympathetic activation, we added isoproterenol (ISP; 0.05, 0.15 µmol/L) to the perfusate of 11 and 7 CsCl-treated preparations with low and normal extracellular K^+ concentration ([K^+]$_o$; 2.5 and 4.69 mmol/L), respectively. To evaluate the role of I_{CaL} in the arrhythmias in ATS1, we added verapamil (3.0 µmol/L) to the CsCl-treated preparations having VT. We mapped APs on the transmural surface of the preparations at control, after CsCl, and after adding the previously mentioned drugs.

I_{K1} blockade delayed late phase 3 repolarization and prolonged the AP, more so during low [K^+]$_o$ perfusion. The preparations were stable and free of spontaneous activity. Rapid pacing (CL = 1000 ms) induced slow phase 4 diastolic depolarization (DADs) in all low [K^+]$_o$ preparations and in 71% of normal [K^+]$_o$ preparations after CsCl treatment. Sympathetic activation (ISP: 0.05 and 0.15 µmol/L) increased the occurrence of DADs (in 86% of the normal [K^+]$_o$ preparations treated with CsCl). Prominent DADs initiated new activations. Repetitive DAD-initiated activations generated VT. VT occurrences increased with sympathetic activation (VT occurrences: 0%, 14%, and 71% at ISP concentrations of 0, 0.05, and 0.15 µmol/L, respectively). Hypokalemia promoted VT in the ATS1 preparations. DADs occurred in 0%, 25%, 100%, and 100% and VT occurred in 0%, 0%, 38%, and 100% of the low [K^+]$_o$ preparations before and after CsCl (0, 5, and 10 mmol/L) and after subsequent ISP treatment, respectively. Multiple migrating foci (with endocardial preference) caused polymorphic VT. Alternating DADs at two foci with coordinated timing resulted in bidirectional VT (Fig. 10–7), which occurred in 64% of low [K^+]$_o$ preparations having ISP, but not in the normal [K^+]$_o$ preparations. I_{CaL} blockade with verapamil shortened APD, eliminated the DADs and VT, and prevented their induction by burst pacing in all preparations. U waves appeared following the T waves in the ECG, forming a TU complex, after CsCl treatment in 75% and 29% of the low and normal [K^+]$_o$ preparations, respectively. These U

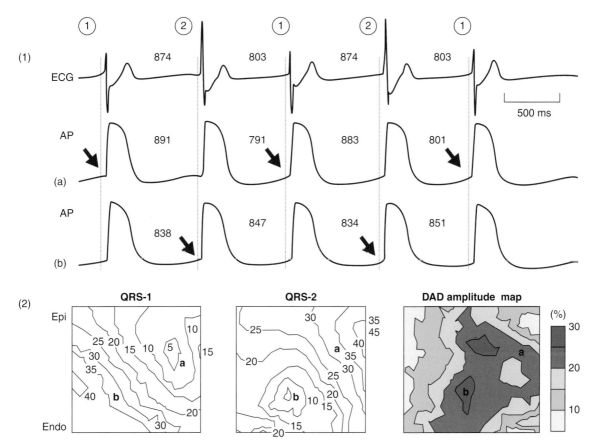

FIGURE 10–7. Bidirectional ventricular tachycardias (VTs) in an isolated wedge of canine left ventricular free wall having cesium chloride–induced (10 mmol/L) Andersen-Tawil syndrome. Traces of electrocardiogram (ECG) and action potential (AP) (at the foci) are shown in 1. The numbers in the ECG and AP traces indicate the cycle length (in milliseconds). The arrows in the AP traces indicate the earliest activations of each beat. Maps of activation isochrone (in milliseconds) and of delayed afterdepolarization (DAD) amplitude (in percentage of the phase 0 of local AP) are shown in 2. Alternating DADs from two endocardial foci (a and b) generated QRS alternans and triggered bidirectional VT. $[K^+]_o$ = 2.5 mmol/L. Endo, endocardium; Epi, epicardium. Reproduced from Morita H, Zipes DP, Morita ST, Wu J. Mechanism of U wave and polymorphic ventricular tachycardia in a canine tissue model of Andersen-Tawil syndrome. *Cardiovasc Res.* 2007;75:510-518.

waves were associated with a significant delay in the late phase 3 repolarization of the AP and with the occurrence of DADs.[5]

These results suggest the critical roles of $[K^+]_o$, heart rate, resting membrane potential, autonomic activity, and I_{CaL} in the arrhythmogenesis of ATS1. I_{K1} reduction causes instability in the resting potential and delays repolarization, which promotes I_{CaL}. ISP also increases I_{CaL}.[62] Both an unstable resting potential and an increased I_{CaL} facilitate DADs and initiation of VTs. The elimination of DADs and VT by verapamil suggested that Ca^{2+} overload was a major trigger of VT in ATS1. U waves in this ATS1 model had two origins, one from the delayed phase 3 repolarization and the other from the DADs. The dual origins provided an explanation of the polymorphism of the U wave (eg, the biphasic or enlarged U waves) observed clinically.[60] The endocardial preferences of DADs and of VT foci could be related to the longer APDs in the endocardium than epicardium. The results of this study support therapeutic strategies to manage VT in patients having ATS1 by reducing cytosolic Ca^{2+} overload, preventing and limiting excessive heart rate, controlling autonomic activity, elevating plasma K^+ concentration, and increasing the conductivity of membrane at rest.

AV NODAL REENTRY

Although dual conduction pathways have been suggested to underlie the AV nodal reentrant echo beats (EBs) and sustained AV nodal reentrant tachycardia,[63-65] newer data suggest that multiple AV nodal input pathways might exist outside the compact AV node because anterograde AV conduction remained after ablation of both the fast pathway (FP) and slow pathway (SP).[66]

Optical mapping was used to unveil the AV nodal conduction pathways and mechanisms of AV nodal reentry in arterially perfused preparations containing the AV node and surrounding atrial tissue isolated from canine hearts.[67] The isolated preparations were paced at the anterior limbus of the fossa ovalis near the FP. Electrical activity in the Koch triangle (KT) and surrounding atrial tissue was mapped optically. His bundle electrograms were also recorded.

Optical mapping identified three major *nondiscrete* AV nodal input pathways having fast (FP; 192.6 ± 17.4 cm/s), intermediate (intermediate pathway [IP]; 87.4 ± 10.2 cm/s), and slow (SP; 40.5 ± 5 cm/s) velocity of conduction in all preparations with continuous (n = 16) and discontinuous (n = 6) AV nodal function curves (AVNFCs; pacing CL = 800 ms). AV nodal EBs were induced in 12 preparations. The reentrant circuit of the slow/fast EB (n = 8) started as block in the FP, delay in the SP conduction to the compact AV node, and then exit from the AV node to the FP and rapid return to the SP through the atrial tissue at the base of KT (Fig. 10–8). The reentrant circuit of the fast/slow EB (n = 2) was in an opposite direction. In the slow/slow EB (n = 2), anterograde conduction was over the IP, and retrograde conduction was over the SP. Unidirectional conduction block occurred during short coupling intervals at the junction between the AV node and its input pathways where local transitional cells had long APDs. Conduction over the IP smoothed the transition from the FP to the SP, resulting in a continuous AVNFC. A "jump" in atrium-His bundle interval resulted from shifting of anterograde conduction from the FP to the SP (n = 4) or abrupt conduction delay within the AV node through the FP (n = 2). Transection of the SP (n = 8) eliminated all EBs. In conclusion, there were three AV nodal anterograde pathways outside the AV node without an upper common pathway; unidirectional block could occur in the transition zone between the AV node and its input pathways when the coupling interval was shorter than the local APD, and the IP could mask the FP and SP, producing continuous AVNFCs.

This study has several clinical implications. First, the involvement of the SP in all reentrant circuits provides a mechanistic explanation for the clinical success of SP ablation in terminating various types of AV nodal reentry tachycardia (AVNRT). Second, the results suggest the presence of multiple retrograde atrial exit sites in atypical AVNRT because multiple connections exist between the SP and atrial tissue near the coronary sinus ostium. Finally, the noninvolvement of FP in the reentrant circuit of slow/slow EBs explains the ineffectiveness of FP ablation in some patients with atypical AVNRT.

LIMITATIONS AND APPLICATIONS OF OPTICAL MAPPING

Although optical mapping is a powerful method to observe the spatiotemporal dynamics of electrophysiologic activity in cardiac muscle, there are several technical limitations that need to be overcome before its direct clinical applications. Most of the current optical-mapping systems use conventional lens-based optics, which require direct optical viewing of the to-be-mapped tissue surface. Miniaturization of the optics (eg, based on flexible fiber optic image conduits) and/or miniature sensor arrays need to be developed for clinical applications. Currently, most optical-mapping experiments are carried out in immobilized tissues to avoid motion artifacts. However, clinical applications require mapping in a beating heart, in which the undesired contractual distortion in the electrophysiologic signal needs to be eliminated or managed either by ratiometric imaging, which subtracts motion artifacts from the signal-carrying fluorescence, or by data processing algorithms to extract physiologic information from signals containing motion artifacts. Currently, commercially available fluorescent dyes are mostly working in the visible light spectrum, which limits the depth of tissue from where the fluorescence signal can be recorded. Long-wavelength infrared membrane potential–sensitive fluorescent dyes that enable deep tissue recording are now in active development in research laboratories. Furthermore, the safety of the dyes needs to be evaluated before clinical application. The developments in optics and in fluorescent dyes will facilitate the applications of optical mapping in clinical cardiac electrophysiology to provide real-time movies of electrical activity in heart. Optical mapping

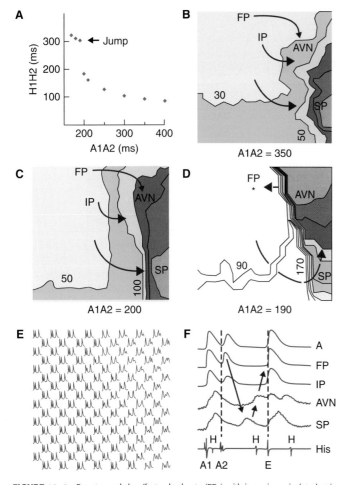

FIGURE 10–8. Reentry and slow/fast echo beats (EBs) with jump in an isolated atrioventricular (AV) nodal preparation. AV nodal function curve with jump is shown in **A.** The tissue was paced at a basic cycle length of 800 ms (A1A1). Activation maps of A2 (premature activation) at pacing coupling intervals (A1A2) of 350, 200, and 190 ms are illustrated in **B**, **C**, and **D**, respectively. **D**, **E**, and **F** were derived from the same data. Solid arrows illustrate the anterograde conduction pathways. The numbers in the maps indicate the activation times relative to the onset of A2. In **D**, the asterisk (*) and short dashed arrow represent the site of earliest retrograde atrial activation, and the longer, interrupted arrow indicates activation over the slow pathway (SP). **E.** Corresponding optical action potentials (APs) obtained during EB induced by pacing coupling interval (A1A2) of 190 ms. **F.** Selected APs from atrium (A), fast pathway (FP), intermediate pathway (IP), AV node (AVN), and SP. The time scale is indicated by A1A2 interval (190 ms) in the His bundle electrogram (His). The left and right dashed vertical lines represent the onset of A2 and earliest retrograde activation of the EB (E), respectively. The arrows indicate the SECTION sequence of A2. Reproduced with permission from Wu J, Wu J, Olgin JE, et al. Mechanisms underlying the reentrant circuit of AV nodal reentrant tachycardia in isolated canine AV nodal preparation using optical mapping. *Circ Res.* 2001;88:1189-1195.

can be very powerful when the recorded real-time movies of electrical activity are combined with anatomic and pathophysiologic imaging technologies, such as computed tomography, positron emission tomography, and magnetic resonance imaging. The complementary electrical movies and anatomic and pathophysiologic information will enable identification of the causes and their electrophysiologic consequences in a diseased heart and thus will contribute to making a more precise diagnosis and more effective treatment of cardiac arrhythmic diseases.

SUMMARY

Optical mapping has played a critical role in understanding the electrophysiologic heterogeneity in the heart and in illustrating the sites of focal activations and the mechanisms of initiation and maintenance of VT. Our optical-mapping studies demonstrated the following mechanisms. (1) Ventricular M cells are a functional expression of electrophysiologic heterogeneities under extreme conditions. (2) Transmural differences in the suppression of excitability and in the prolongation of refractoriness provide a proarrhythmic substrate in which transmural reentry can be initiated easily with either endocardial or epicardial stimulation. (3) A prior episode of ischemia can leave long-lasting suppression of repolarization reserve, providing a proarrhythmic substrate in which VT can be triggered by a repolarization delaying intervention. (4) Arrhythmogenicity in BS is caused by the following electrophysiologic sequences: a Na^+/Ca^{2+} channelopathy and an age and sex enhancement of I_{to}, a deep phase 1 notch of the AP, dispersion in the phase 2 dome and repolarization of the AP, phase 2 reentry, and VT. The presence of a large I_{to} underlies the arrhythmogenicity of the RVOT in BS. Factors that promote the increase in I_{to} and dispersion of repolarization (eg, temperature and CL) can be the triggers of arrhythmias in BS. Ablation that disconnects the long and short APD regions in the epicardium of RVOT can be effective treatment of arrhythmias in BS. (5) Arrhythmogenicity in ATS1 is an electrophysiologic consequence of I_{K1} reduction, resting membrane potential instability and repolarization delay, I_{CaL} enhancement, DADs, and VT. Both delayed repolarization and DADs cause the U wave in the ECG. Multiple DAD foci lead to polymorphism of VT and U wave in ATS1 and to bidirectional VT. (6) AV nodal reentry involves three anterograde pathways in the atrial tissue outside of the AV node.

REFERENCES

1. Efimov IR, Nikolski VP, Salama G. Optical imaging of the heart. *Circ Res.* 2004;95:21-33.
2. Wu J, Biermann M, Rubart M, Zipes DP. Cytochalasin D as excitation-contraction uncoupler for optically mapping action potentials in wedges of ventricular myocardium. *J Cardiovasc Electrophysiol.* 1998;9:1366-1374.
3. Biermann M, Rubart M, Moreno A, et al. Differential effects of cytochalasin D and 2,3 butanedione monoxime on isometric twitch force and transmembrane action potential in isolated ventricular muscle: implications for optical measurements of cardiac repolarization. *J Cardiovasc Electrophysiol.* 1998;9:1348-1357.
4. Fedorov VV, Lozinsky IT, Sosunov EA, et al. Application of blebbistatin as an excitation-contraction uncoupler for electrophysiological study of rat and rabbit hearts. *Heart Rhythm.* 2007;4:619-626.
5. Wu J, Wu J, Zipes DP. Early afterdepolarizations, U waves, and torsades de pointes. *Circulation.* 2002;105:675-676.
6. Antzelevitch C. Heterogeneity and cardiac arrhythmias: an overview. *Heart Rhythm.* 2007;4:964-972.
7. Antzelevitch C, Oliva A. Amplification of spatial dispersion of repolarization underlies sudden cardiac death associated with catecholaminergic polymorphic VT, long QT, short QT and Brugada syndromes. *J Intern Med.* 2006;259:48-58.
8. Voss F, Opthof T, Marker J, et al. There is no transmural heterogeneity in an index of action potential duration in the canine left ventricle. *Heart Rhythm.* 2009;6:1028-1034.
9. Patel C, Burke JF, Patel H, et al. Is there a significant transmural gradient in repolarization time in the intact heart? Cellular basis of the t wave: a century of controversy. *Circulation.* 2009;2:80-88.
10. Taggart P, Sutton P, Opthof T, et al. Electrotonic cancellation of transmural electrical gradients in the left ventricle in man. *Prog Biophys Mol Biol.* 2003;82:243-244.
11. Opthof T, Coronel R, Janse MJ. Is there a significant transmural gradient in repolarization time in the intact heart? Repolarization gradients in the intact heart. *Circulation.* 2009;2:89-96.
12. Coronel R, Wilms-Schopman FJG, Opthof T, et al. Dispersion of repolarization and arrhythmogenesis. *Heart Rhythm.* 2009;6:537-543.
13. Ueda N, Zipes DP, Wu J. Functional and transmural modulation of M cell behavior in canine ventricular wall. *Am J Physiol Heart Circ Physiol.* 2004;287:H2569-H2574.
14. Morita H, Wu J, Zipes DP. The QT syndromes: long and short. *Lancet.* 2008;372:750-763.
15. Ueda N, Zipes DP, Wu J. Epicardial but not endocardial premature stimulation initiates ventricular tachyarrhythmia in canine in vitro model of long QT syndrome. *Heart Rhythm.* 2004;1:684-694.
16. Morita ST, Zipes DP, Morita H, Wu J. Analysis of action potentials in the canine ventricular septum: no phenotypic expression of M cells. *Cardiovasc Res.* 2007;74:96-103.
17. Morita ST, Morita H, Zipes DP, Wu J. Acute ischemia of canine interventricular septum produces asymmetric suppression of conduction. *Heart Rhythm.* 2008;5:1057-1062.
18. Carmeliet E. Cardiac ionic currents and acute ischemia: from channels to arrhythmias. *Physiol Rev.* 1999;79:917-1017.
19. Wu J, Zipes DP. Transmural reentry during global acute ischemia and reperfusion in canine ventricular muscle. *Am J Physiol Heart Circ Physiol.* 2001;280:H2717-H2725.
20. Wu J, Zipes DP. Transmural reentry triggered by epicardial stimulation during acute ischemia in canine ventricular muscle. *Am J Physiol Heart Circ Physiol.* 2002;283:H2004-H2011.
21. Gilmour RF Jr, Zipes DP. Different electrophysiological responses of canine endocardium and epicardium to combined hyperkalemia, hypoxia, and acidosis. *Circ Res.* 1980;46:814-825.
22. Ueda N, Zipes DP, Wu J. Coronary occlusion and reperfusion promote early afterdepolarizations and ventricular tachycardia in a canine tissue model of long QT 3. *Am J Physiol Heart Circ Physiol.* 2006;290:H607-H612.
23. Ueda N, Zipes DP, Wu J. Prior ischemia enhances arrhythmogenicity in isolated canine ventricular wedge model of long QT 3. *Cardiovasc Res.* 2004;63:69-76.
24. Roden DM. Repolarization reserve: a moving target. *Circulation.* 2008;118:981-982.
25. Martini B, Nava A, Thiene G, et al. Ventricular fibrillation without apparent heart disease: description of six cases. *Am Heart J.* 1989;118:1203-1209.
26. Brugada P, Brugada J. Right bundle branch block, persistent ST segment elevation and sudden cardiac death: a distinct clinical and electrocardiographic syndrome. A multicenter report. *J Am Coll Cardiol.* 1992;20:1391-1396.
27. Morita H, Morita ST, Nagase S, et al. Ventricular arrhythmia induced by sodium channel blocker in patients with Brugada syndrome. *J Am Coll Cardiol.* 2003;42:1624-1631.
28. Antzelevitch C, Brugada P, Borggrefe M, et al. Brugada syndrome: report of the second consensus conference. *Heart Rhythm.* 2005;2:429-440.
29. Antzelevitch C, Pollevick GD, Cordeiro JM, et al. Loss-of-function mutations in the cardiac calcium channel underlie a new clinical entity characterized by ST-segment elevation, short QT intervals, and sudden cardiac death. *Circulation.* 2007;115:442-449.

30. Watanabe H, Koopmann TT, Le Scouarnec S, et al. Sodium channel beta1 subunit mutations associated with Brugada syndrome and cardiac conduction disease in humans. *J Clin Invest.* 2008;118:2260-2268.

31. Morita H, Nagase S, Miura D, et al. Differential effects of cardiac sodium channel mutations on initiation of ventricular arrhythmias in patients with Brugada syndrome. *Heart Rhythm.* 2009;6:487-492.

32. Morita H, Zipes DP, Ohe T, Wu J. Brugada syndrome: insights of ST elevation, arrhythmogenicity and risk stratification from experimental observations. *Heart Rhythm.* 2009;6:S34-S43.

33. Kurita T, Shimizu W, Inagaki M, et al. The electrophysiologic mechanism of ST-segment elevation in Brugada syndrome. *J Am Coll Cardiol.* 2002;40: 330-334.

34. Morita H, Fukushima-Kusano K, Nagase S, et al. Site-specific arrhythmogenesis in patients with Brugada syndrome. *J Cardiovasc Electrophysiol.* 2003;14:373-379.

35. Hisamatsu K, Kusano KF, Morita H, et al. Relationships between depolarization abnormality and repolarization abnormality in patients with Brugada syndrome: using body surface signal-averaged electrocardiography and body surface maps. *J Cardiovasc Electrophysiol.* 2004;15:870-876.

36. Nagase S, Kusano KF, Morita H, et al. Longer repolarization in the epicardium at the right ventricular outflow tract causes type 1 ECG in patients with Brugada syndrome. *J Am Coll Cardiol.* 2008;51:1154-1161.

37. Yan GX, Antzelevitch C. Cellular basis for the Brugada syndrome and other mechanisms of arrhythmogenesis associated with ST-segment elevation. *Circulation.* 1999;100:1660-1666.

38. Di Diego JM, Cordeiro JM, Goodrow RJ, et al. Ionic and cellular basis for the predominance of the Brugada syndrome phenotype in males. *Circulation.* 2002;106:2004-2011.

39. Aiba T, Shimizu W, Hidaka I, et al. Cellular basis for trigger and maintenance of ventricular fibrillation in the Brugada syndrome model: high-resolution optical mapping study. *J Am Coll Cardiol.* 2006;47:2074-2085.

40. Shimizu W, Matsuo K, Kokubo Y, et al. Sex hormone and gender difference—role of testosterone on male predominance in Brugada syndrome. *J Cardiovasc Electrophysiol.* 2007;18:415-421.

41. Calloe K, Cordeiro JM, Di Diego JM, et al. A transient outward potassium current activator recapitulates the electrocardiographic manifestations of Brugada syndrome. *Cardiovasc Res.* 2009;81:686-694.

42. Morita H, Zipes DP, Morita ST, Wu J. Differences in arrhythmogenicity between the canine right ventricular outflow tract and anteroinferior right ventricle in a model of Brugada syndrome. *Heart Rhythm.* 2007;4:66-74.

43. Morita H, Zipes DP, Lopshire J, Morita ST, Wu J. T wave alternans in an in vitro canine tissue model of Brugada syndrome. *Am J Physiol Heart Circ Physiol.* 2006;291:421-428.

44. Sun X, Wang HS. Role of the transient outward current (I_{to}) in shaping canine ventricular action potential—a dynamic clamp study. *J Physiol.* 2005;564:411-419.

45. Morita H, Zipes DP, Morita ST, Wu J. Temperature modulation of ventricular arrhythmogenicity in a canine tissue model of Brugada syndrome. *Heart Rhythm.* 2007;4:188-197.

46. Saura D, García-Alberola A, Carrillo P, et al. Brugada-like electrocardiographic pattern induced by fever. *Pacing Clin Electrophysiol.* 2002;25:856-859.

47. Keller DI, Rougier JS, Kucera JP, et al. Brugada syndrome and fever: genetic and molecular characterization of patients carrying SCN5A mutations. *Cardiovasc Res.* 2005;67:510-519.

48. Keller DI, Huang H, Zhao J, et al. A novel SCN5A mutation, F1344S, identified in a patient with Brugada syndrome and fever-induced ventricular fibrillation. *Cardiovasc Res.* 2006;70:521-529.

49. Morita H, Fukushima-Kusano K, Miura D, et al. Fragmented QRS as a marker of conduction abnormality and a predictor of prognosis of Brugada syndrome. *Circulation.* 2008;118:1697-1704.

50. Coronel R, Casini S, Koopmann TT, et al. Right ventricular fibrosis and conduction delay in a patient with clinical signs of Brugada syndrome: a combined electrophysiological, genetic, histopathologic, and computational study. *Circulation.* 2005;112:2769-2777.

51. Morita H, Zipes DP, Fukushima-Kusano K, et al. Repolarization heterogeneity in the right ventricular outflow tract: correlation with ventricular arrhythmias in Brugada patients and in an in vitro canine Brugada model. *Heart Rhythm.* 2008;5:725-733.

52. Morita H, Zipes DP, Morita ST, Lopshire JC, Wu J. Epicardial ablation eliminates ventricular arrhythmias in an experimental model of Brugada syndrome. *Heart Rhythm.* 2009;6:665-671.

53. Morita H, Zipes DP, Morita ST, Wu J. Genotype-phenotype correlation in tissue models of Brugada syndrome simulating patients with sodium and calcium channelopathies. *Heart Rhythm.* 2010;7:820-827.

54. Dhamoon A, Jalife J. The inward rectifier current (I_{K1}) controls cardiac excitability and is involved in arrhythmogenesis. *Heart Rhythm.* 2005;2: 316-324.

55. Tsuboi M, Antzelevitch C. Cellular basis for electrocardiographic and arrhythmic manifestations of Andersen-Tawil syndrome (LQT7). *Heart Rhythm.* 2006;3:328-335.

56. Lopatin AN, Nichols CG. Inward rectifiers in the heart: an update on IK1. *J Mol Cell Cardiol.* 2001;33:625-638.

57. Nichols CG, Makhina EN, Pearson WL, et al. Inward rectification and implications for cardiac excitability. *Circ Res.* 1996;78:1-7.

58. Tawil R, Ptacek LJ, Pavlakis SG, et al. Andersen's syndrome: potassium-sensitive periodic paralysis, ventricular ectopy, and dysmorphic features. *Ann Neurol.* 1994;35:326-330.

59. Tristani-Firouzi M, Jensen JL, Donaldson MR, et al. Functional and clinical characterization of KCNJ2 mutations associated with LQT7 (Andersen syndrome). *J Clin Invest.* 2002;110:381-388.

60. Zhang L, Benson DW, Tristani-Firouzi M, et al. Electrocardiographic features in Andersen–Tawil syndrome patients with KCNJ2 mutations: characteristic T–U-wave patterns predict the KCNJ2 genotype. *Circulation.* 2005;111:2720-2766.

61. Morita H, Zipes DP, Morita ST, Wu J. Mechanism of U wave and polymorphic ventricular tachycardia in a canine tissue model of Andersen-Tawil syndrome. *Cardiovasc Res.* 2007;75:510-518.

62. Sako H, Green SA, Kranias EG, Yatani A. Modulation of cardiac Ca^{2+} channels by isoproterenol studied in transgenic mice with altered SR Ca^{2+} content. *Am J Physiol Cell Physiol.* 1997;273:C1666-C1672.

63. Moe GK, Preston JB, Burlington H. Physiologic evidence for a dual A-V transmission system. *Circ Res.* 1956;4:357-375.

64. Denes P, Wu D, Dhingra RC, et al. Demonstration of dual A-V nodal pathways in patients with paroxysmal supraventricular tachycardia. *Circulation.* 1973;58:549-555.

65. Patterson E, Scherlag BJ. Longitudinal dissociation within the posterior AV nodal input of the rabbit, a substrate for AV nodal reentry. *Circulation.* 1999;99:143-155.

66. Hirao K, Scherlag B, Poty H, et al. Electrophysiology of atrio-AV nodal inputs and exits in the normal dog heart: radiofrequency ablation using an epicardial approach. *J Cardiovasc Electrophysiol.* 1997;8:904-915.

67. Wu J, Wu J, Olgin JE, et al. Mechanisms underlying the reentrant circuit of AV nodal reentrant tachycardia in isolated canine AV nodal preparation using optical mapping. *Circ Res.* 2001;88:1189-1195.

CHAPTER 11

DIPOLAR ELECTROCARDIO-TOPOGRAPHY IMAGING

Ljuba Bacharova and Anton Mateasik

DESCRIPTION OF THE METHOD / 191
   Vectorcardiography / 191
   Dipolar Electrocardiotopography / 191
   Normal Values for Decartograms / 192

**IMAGING CARDIAC PATHOPHYSIOLOGY
USING DECARTO / 194**
   Myocardial Infarction / 194
   Location and Extent of the Area at Risk in MI / 195
   Ventricular Hypertrophy / 195

**SIDE-BY-SIDE COMPARISON AND POSSIBLE COMBINATION
WITH OTHER IMAGING MODALITIES / 196**
   Side-by-Side Comparison of DECARTO-like Presentation
      of ST-Segment Deviations With Other ECG-Based
      Graphical Methods / 196
   Side-by-Side Comparison With Non-ECG Methods / 197
   Superimposition of the DECARTO Images Onto
      Three-Dimensional Images / 198
   Limitations of the DECARTO Method / 200

CONCLUSION / 202

DESCRIPTION OF THE METHOD

■ VECTORCARDIOGRAPHY

The vector principle is the basic principle of electrocardiography for the interpretation of the standard 12-lead electrocardiogram (ECG) as well as for teaching.[1] However, its application in the interpretation of the standard 12-lead ECG is demanding for a mental three-dimensional imagination, and the "mental image" requires linking the orientation and magnitude of the vector to the anatomy of the heart, its position in the chest, and the sequence of activation (Fig. 11–1).

Vectorcardiography partially reduces these problems. It presents the distributed electric field at every instant of time by a dipole—the equivalent dipole. This dipole is represented by a vector, defined by its magnitude and orientation, theoretically corresponding to the extent of the activation front and its location. The origin of the dipole is fixed in the center of an orthogonal coordinate system, and the trajectory of the end point of the vector during the atrial/ventricular depolarization and repolarization depicts the spatial vectorcardiographic loop. The classical graphical presentation of vectorcardiography is the planar vectorcardiogram—the planar projection of the spatial vectorcardiographic loop onto three perpendicular planes: the frontal, sagittal, and horizontal (transverse) planes.

Compared with the standard 12-lead ECG, the orthogonal ECG does not contain redundant information. The coordinate system of the orthogonal ECG/vectorcardiogram may be aligned with the geometry of the heart and to our knowledge about the sequence of atrial and ventricular activation. These characteristics make the vectorcardiogram instrumental for teaching the principles of ECG diagnosis, as well as for comparative studies with other imaging methods. However, the interpretation of vectorcardiograms is demanding for three-dimensional imagination and for good orientation in the anatomic structures and their relationships to the processes in the heart. In addition, these graphical presentations—scalar tracings of orthogonal ECG and planar vectorcardiogram—are not directly comparable with images of the heart developed from another imaging method.

In this chapter, we describe a method for graphical presentation of the orthogonal ECG/vectorcardiogram that allows the visualization of the vectors representing the cardiac electrical field comparably to other imaging methods used in cardiology. This graphical presentation of ECG is suitable for side-to-side comparisons as well as for superimposition or fusion of information from multiple imaging modalities.

■ DIPOLAR ELECTROCARDIOTOPOGRAPHY

In dipolar electrocardiotopography (DECARTO), the orthogonal ECG is transformed to areas projected on a spherical image surface. The original DECARTO model[2,3] was developed for the presentation of the QRS complex (ie, for the process of ventricular depolarization).

The mathematical model of the DECARTO transformation is based on modeling of the cardiac electrical field. A detailed description of the electric field of the excitable myocardium would require a highly complex electrodynamics model that could link the heart as electrical generator with its electrical field. In general, outputs from electrodynamics models of the heart are ill posed in relation to the structure of the cardiac generator. It means that the given distribution of the electric field around the cardiac generator can be attributed to different generators' shapes and/or spatial structure. This fact provides an opportunity to substitute a real source of the cardiac electrical field with a functionally equivalent generator with known compositions.[4]

The electrical generator of the cardiac electric field can be effectively approximated by double layers of current sources with an approximately constant density of electrical dipoles that are bounded by closed contours on the inner and outer surfaces of the ventricles. The electrostatic potential in the proximity of a double-layered object may be, in principle, calculated with any accuracy by the method of expansion in a convergent electrical multipole series describing distributions of dipoles over the double layers. The final potential is then determined by the sum of this multipole expansion.[5] The number of used multipole components in the expansion depends on the required accuracy of the potential field description. The DECARTO model is based on the double-layer representation of the field generator and uses dipole representation with minimal number of multipole components.

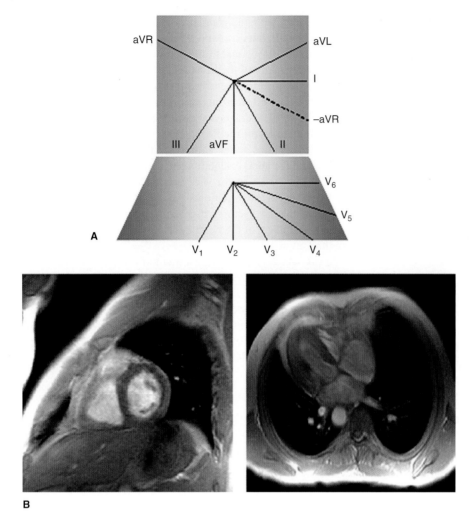

FIGURE 11–1. A. The scheme of the hexaxial coordination system of the standard 12-lead electrocardiogram (ECG). **B.** The short axis view (right) and long axis (left) view of magnetic resonance imaging (MRI). The mental three-dimensional image that would include the structural (MRI) and functional (ECG) characteristics of the heart and their temporo-spatial relations is too complicated.

where D represents the length of the instantaneous spatial VCG vector, D_{max} is the maximal spatial vector during the QRS duration, and Rs is the radius of the image sphere (Rs can be set arbitrarily; the DECARTO model uses the value of 1) (Fig. 11–2).

The activated area or activated points representing this area on the image sphere are graphically presented as maps—so-called *decartograms*. Visualization of ventricular activation can be performed by a series of decartograms calculated and displayed individually for discrete time points or by using summary maps where activations at given time points are superimposed onto one decartogram.

The image sphere is a hypothetical surface that represents the cardiac generator, and the activated areas on this image surface (decartograms) can be visualized by projecting them on a variety of shapes in two or three dimensions (Fig. 11–3). The selection of geometrical shapes aims to optimize the topographic relations of the abstract representations of the cardiac electric field to the activation process in the myocardium. Determination of the spatial localization of instantaneous vector end points enables the bridging between characteristics of myocardial activation propagation in this conceptual model and abstract representation of the cardiac electric field.

The spherical image surface can be easily transformed to any suitable analytical spatial or planar surfaces to visualize decartograms, such as polar (azimuthal) planar projection, rectangle projection, spherical projection, and parabolic projection, as well as to real heart surfaces rendered from other imaging methods.

Another simplification of the DECARTO model is the assumption that the inner and outer surfaces of the heart ventricles have a spherical form, so the double layer has a spherical shape and represents so-called *image surface*.

The basic principle of DECARTO transformation is based on the consideration that the electrical field of the generator is formed exclusively by the electrical dipoles of the double layer and delimited to its area. This activated area is projected onto the surface of a sphere called the imaged surface. The point of intersection of the vector with the image surface is considered to be the center of the activated area. Around this point, a circle with a radius proportional to the spatial magnitude of the instantaneous vector is drawn encompassing all activated elements. In particular, the radius r of the activated area is computed for a given instantaneous spatial vectorcardiogram (VCG) vector according the following formula:

$$r = Rs * \sqrt{\frac{D}{D_{max}}}$$

■ NORMAL VALUES FOR DECARTOGRAMS

The DECARTO method of graphical presentation extends the possibilities for presentation of the normal values of ECG and for its quantitative analysis. Areas of occurrence of the activated points in the normal population for decartograms were reported for the McFee-Parungao and the Frank lead systems.[6] They were constructed by indicating the areas of activation at given points of QRS duration, and the probability of being activated at the given point of time for every point of the matrix was computed. In this way, reference probability matrices of normal activation were constructed (Fig. 11–4).

Ruttkay-Nedecky[7] used these probability matrices of normal activation for application of fuzzy mathematics to quantify the normality of the QRS complex. In this method, the subset of elements in the spherical surface is regarded as a fuzzy subset with membership characteristic functions derived from objective

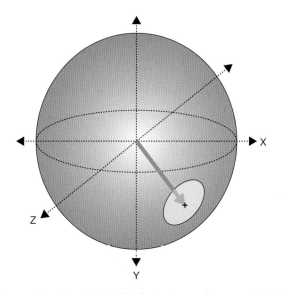

FIGURE 11–2. The basic principle of the dipolar electrocardiotopography (DECARTO) method. The ventricular surface is represented by a spherical surface, the so-called *image surface*. The origin of the QRS vector is located in the center of the image sphere, and the intersection of the spatial QRS with the image surface gives the center of the area of activated points. The radius of the area of activated points is proportional to the maximum spatial vector magnitude.

probabilities computed for the reference sample of normal subjects. In an individual case, the difference between the sum of membership function values and the mean of the reference sample at any instant of the QRS duration, or during the whole QRS, divided by the standard deviation quantifies the deviation from the reference mean value.

A similar approach was used for graphical presentation of the location and extent of the myocardium at risk in patients with acute myocardial infarction.[8] This method is based on the processing of ST-segment deviations of standard 12-lead ECG following the lines set by the DECARTO method. In this ST-DECARTO method, the center of the location of the area at risk is given by the spatial orientation of the resultant spatial ST vector, and the extent of the area at risk is derived from the Aldrich score.[10] The areas at risk are projected on a spherical image surface. On this image surface, a texture of the anatomic quadrants of the ventricular surface and the coronary artery supply are projected. The initial testing showed that the method allows a graphical presentation of estimated area at risk using clinically defined diagnostic rules. The area at risk can be displayed in images that are familiar for clinicians and can be compared with or superimposed on results of other imaging methods used in cardiology.

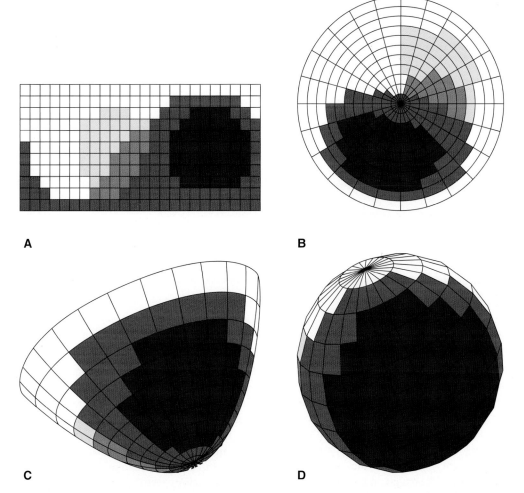

FIGURE 11–3. Examples of dipolar electrocardiotopography (DECARTO) projections onto planar and three-dimensional (3D) analytical surfaces. **A.** Planar rectangular projection; **B**, planar polar (azimuthal) projection; **C**, 3D paraboloid surface; **D**, 3D spherical surface.

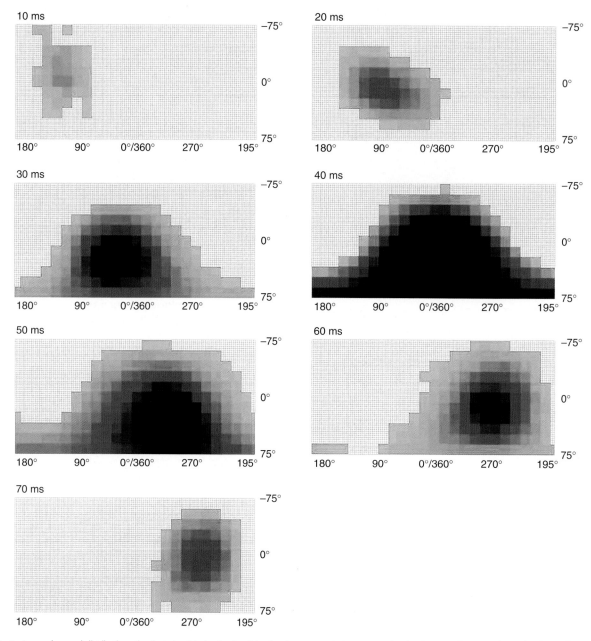

FIGURE 11–4. Areas of normal distribution of activated points for the Frank lead system, presented as rectangular decartograms for 10-ms intervals of QRS duration. The areas of activated points move during the QRS complex from the anterior middle part of the chest leftward and posteriorly. The decartograms were not corrected for the position of the heart in the chest; in this arrangement they are visually comparable with the body surface potential maps. The darker areas represent areas with higher probability of the occurrence of the activated points in the normal population.

IMAGING CARDIAC PATHOPHYSIOLOGY USING DECARTO

As mentioned earlier, the vector principle is the basic principle in the interpretation of ECGs. It follows that, in principle, the DECARTO method is applicable in any cardiac pathology. However, the most illustrative is the application in pathologies characterized by changes of the instantaneous spatial vector orientation. Here, we present examples of the application of DECARTO in visualizing the QRS changes in myocardial infarction and of the modified ST-DECARTO method for visualizing the area at risk based on ST-segment deviations.

■ MYOCARDIAL INFARCTION

Acute myocardial infarction (MI) and resulting fibrosis (scars) create regions of altered conduction. The typical signs of MI in the standard 12-lead ECG are pathologic Q waves observed in leads related to the MI location. In the VCG, the signs are manifested as changes of the instantaneous QRS vector orientation and magnitude. In decartograms, the changes in orientation and magnitude of instantaneous QRS are visible as dislocations of activated areas when compared with the normal sequence of depolarization. Figure 11–5 shows examples of instantaneous decartograms in anterior and inferior MIs and their visual comparison with the sequence of depolarization in a healthy subject.

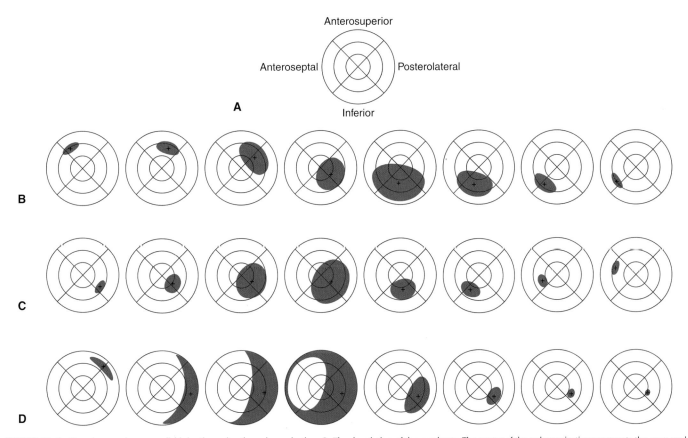

FIGURE 11–5. Decartograms in myocardial infarction using the polar projection. **A.** The description of the quadrants. The center of the polar projection represents the apex, and the outer circle represents the base of the ventricles. **B.** Series of instantaneous decartograms showing the sequence of activated areas in a normal subject in 10-ms intervals of QRS duration. **C.** Sequence of activated areas in a patient with anteroseptal myocardial infarction. The maximum differences are seen in the 10th and 20th ms of QRS duration; the activated areas are projected posteriorly. **D.** Sequence of activated areas in a patient with inferior myocardial infarction. The maximum differences are seen from the 20th and 40th ms of QRS duration; the activated areas are projected upward onto the basal segments.

The quantitative evaluation of decartograms using the fuzzy set mathematics was presented in 1994 by Ruttkay-Nedecky and Riecansky[9] in patients with coronary heart disease. They recognized the following five classes of ventricular activation taking into account the locations of the activated points with respect to the normal areas: abnormal; abnormal with normal component; normal with abnormal component; marginally normal; and normal. Thus, they demonstrated the possibility to quantify not only the abnormal decartograms, but also borderline location of the activated areas.

■ LOCATION AND EXTENT OF THE AREA AT RISK IN MI

ST-segment deviations in patients with acute MI (AMI) are associated with the location and extent of myocardium at risk, with severity of acute transmural ischemia, and with clinical outcomes.[10-14] Additionally, early resolution of ST-segment elevation correlates with myocardial salvage and better prognosis in patients with AMI treated with reperfusion therapy.[15-19]

In practical ECG diagnostics, the location of the area of myocardium at risk is estimated from the presence of ST-segment elevation and/or depression in particular leads of the 12-lead ECG.[20] For the quantification of the estimated extent of the area at risk, several formulas have been reported[10,21,22] that are,

in principle, derived from the number of leads involved and/or the ST-segment deviation amplitude. Both the location and the extent of the area at risk estimated from the ST-segment deviations are therefore easily displayable in decartograms.

However, the relationship between the areas at risk estimated from the ST-segment deviations is moderate or poor,[22-27] and the performance of the ST changes–based algorithms needs to be further validated. Because the DECARTO graphical presentation allows visualization of the location and extent of the involved area using corresponding algorithms, it enables visualization of the differences between different scores. Also, its graphical presentation is suitable for side-to-side comparison or superimposition to analyze both the agreements and disagreements with other imaging methods (Fig. 11–6).

■ VENTRICULAR HYPERTROPHY

The possibility of the DECARTO method to visualize and quantify the redistribution of activation duration over the myocardium was also demonstrated for left and right ventricular hypertrophy.[28,29] Comparing decartograms from hypertensive patients with left ventricular hypertrophy and with those from healthy subjects, differences in the redistribution of activation duration over the myocardium were seen.

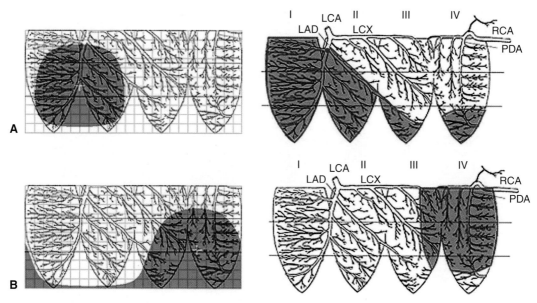

FIGURE 11–6. The side-by-side comparison of the location and extent of areas at risk estimated by two different methods based on the ST-segment deviation. Both methods—ST dipolar electrocardiotopography (DECARTO) (left) and the method developed by Ubachs et al[30] (right) used the same Mercator projection with a texture of a schematic coronary artery distribution. **A.** Patient with left anterior descending (LAD) artery occlusion. The location in both methods is similar; the area at risk is projected on the anteroseptal and anterosuperior quadrants, and using the Ubach method, it covers partly also the basal parts of the posterolateral and inferior quadrants. **B.** Patient with right coronary artery (RCA) occlusion. The area at risk estimated by both methods is projected onto the posterolateral and inferior quadrants, and the ST-DECARTO estimate is located more apically. LCA, left coronary artery; LCX, left circumflex artery; PDA, posterior descending artery.

SIDE-BY-SIDE COMPARISON AND POSSIBLE COMBINATION WITH OTHER IMAGING MODALITIES

The orthogonal coordinate system and the spherical image surface used in the DECARTO model for the QRS presentation and the DECARTO-like graphical presentation of the ST segment are convenient for further data processing and sufficiently flexible in adapting the decartograms to suitable graphical forms for combination with other imaging modalities. The possibilities for the combination are demonstrated by the example of the DECARTO-like presentation of ST-segment deviations compared with other graphical presentation of ST-segment deviations that can be used for the estimation of the area and extent of myocardium at risk in patients with AMI, and with other non-ECG imaging methods that can serve as reference or complementary methods.

■ SIDE-BY-SIDE COMPARISON OF DECARTO-LIKE PRESENTATION OF ST-SEGMENT DEVIATIONS WITH OTHER ECG-BASED GRAPHICAL METHODS

Several methods for the graphical presentation of the location and extent of the area of myocardium at risk have been recently reported.[8,30-33] The methods use different approaches for the estimation of the location and extent of the area at risk, but because these graphical methods are using basically identical or similar graphical presentation, their results can be easily visually compared side by side.

The method described by Andersen et al,[33] the ST Compass, is based on the standard 12-lead configuration of the traditional coordination system. It calculates the planar ST vectors for the frontal and horizontal planes from the ST-segment deviations of the 12-lead ECG, and the resultant planar vectors are drawn on the two perpendicular planes with hexaxial lead coordinates of the standard 12-lead ECG. These planes are displayed as circles with additional spatial and/or anatomic description. This method recommends calculating the spatial vector magnitude as a surrogate for the extent of the myocardium at risk because despite the limitation of this estimation, the ST-vector spatial magnitude corresponds better with the spatial character of the injured myocardium. Thus, this method represents a useful bridging from the evaluation of the individual ST-segment deviations of the 12-lead ECG to the vector analysis and visualization of the spatial ST-segment deviations. However, mentally visualizing the relationship of the planar vectors with the anatomic structures of the heart and the coronary artery distribution still requires a great deal of a three-dimensional mental imaging.

Strauss et al[31] developed a graphical method that synthesizes a VCG from the 12-lead ECG. The ST-segment vector direction is projected on two image surfaces of the heart—the Mercator surface with a schematic average coronary artery distribution and the polar plot. This approach provides the location of the center of the area at risk with respect to the coronary artery distribution and/or to the anatomic segments of the left ventricle. This method also gives the value of the spatial ST-vector magnitude as an estimate of the extent of the area at risk; however, similarly to the previous method, the extent is not graphically displayed.

TABLE 11–1. Comparison of Methods Developed for the Graphical Presentation of ST-Segment Deviations

	Location Estimation	Extent Estimation	Image Surface[a]
ST-DECARTO[8]	Orientation of the spatial ST vector (Frank lead, or Dower[34] transformation of 12-lead ECG)	Aldrich score (flexible to apply other methods for the extent estimation)	Basically spherical, analytically defined, transformable into any 2D or 3D surface; possible application of any texture
Strauss et al[31]	Orientation of the spatial ST vector (Dower transformation of 12-lead ECG)	A numerical value of the spatial vector magnitude, not displayed	Mercator, polar projections; texture of coronary artery distribution
Andersen et al[33]	Orientation of two planar vectors (horizontal and frontal planes) (calculated from 12-lead ECG)	A numerical value of the spatial vector magnitude, not displayed	Two perpendicular planes of 12-lead ECG (frontal, horizontal) with schematic delineation of lead axes of the standard 12-lead ECG and basic description of directions/anatomic structure; no texture
Galeotti et al[32]	Model based[35]	Model based[35]	Polar projection, with the texture of coronary artery distribution; Mercator projection with the texture of coronary artery distribution
Ubachs et al[30]	Model based[36,37]	Model based[36,37]	Polar and Mercator projections; texture of coronary artery distribution in the Mercator projection

[a]The summarized image surfaces of individual methods are in principle mutually transformable. This table summarizes the surface images that were used in the referenced publications.
2D, two dimensional; 3D, three dimensional; ECG, electrocardiogram.

The polar image surface suitable for side-by-side comparison with single photon emission computed tomography (SPECT) images was used also by Galeotti et al,[32] and the location and extent of the myocardium at risk are estimated from the similarities of the ST-segment deviation of a real patient's ECG with a database of simulated ECGs with known location and extent of ischemia.

A different approach was used by Ubachs et al.[30] They estimated the location and extent of the area at risk using the 12-segment model used previously for ECG infarct quantification (QRS score). For the final graphical presentation, both Mercator and polar presentations were used and thus are comparable with polar SPECT or adapted magnetic resonance imaging (MRI) images. Figure 11–6 shows a visual side-by-side comparison of two graphical methods for displaying the ST-segment deviation—the DECARTO-like method and a method described by Ubachs et al[30] showing the areas at risk in the two patients.

The methods of ST-segment visualization described here approach the estimation of the location and extent of the area at risk from different perspectives (Table 11–1). Knowing the principles and studying differences and agreement in the results of these ECG methods can contribute to understanding the roles of individual factors that influence the final ST-segment deviation in AMI. A challenge will be to move from descriptive visual comparison to analytical quantitative evaluation of agreements and disagreements between methods.

■ SIDE-BY-SIDE COMPARISON WITH NON-ECG METHODS

The non-ECG imaging methods used in cardiology include a variety of two- and three-dimensional images; however, the side-by-side comparison naturally requires the use of identical/comparable images. As was demonstrated earlier, the methods for graphical presentation of area at risk based on the ST-segment deviations tend to use polar or Mercator projections.

The polar projection is frequently used as one of the possibilities of displaying results for visual comparison with non-ECG imaging methods.[8,30-32] The advantage of using the polar projection is the direct visual comparability among different imaging methods and potential possibility for superimposition of the findings. Thus, the ECG-based images can be compared with, for example, SPECT images of perfusion (Fig. 11–7), wall motion, and wall thickening; MRI wall thickening; and echocardiographic images of dyskinesis. However, this projection suffers from a considerable deformation of the basal and apical regions, which must be taken into account in the interpretation of the results.

The Mercator projection with the texture of the coronary artery distribution reduces the deformation of the polar projection and illustrates well the anatomic segments of the heart and corresponding coronary artery distribution. This projection is not generally used for displaying results of the non-ECG imaging techniques, but it can be potentially used as the image surface of choice.

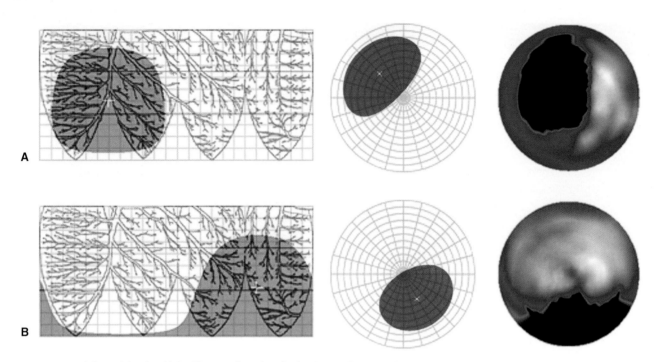

FIGURE 11-7. From left to right: The side-by-side comparison of ST dipolar electrocardiotopography (DECARTO) using Mercator and polar projections and single photon emission computed tomography (SPECT) image. **A.** A patient with the left descending artery occlusion. **B.** A patient with right coronary artery occlusion. Although the Mercator projection relates the area at risk to the coronary artery distribution, the polar projection is visually comparable with the polar SPECT image showing the perfusion defect in the corresponding area.

The common advantage of planar projections is the ability to display the whole surface, which balances the main disadvantage, which is the deformation of the shape and size of the imaged structures.

■ SUPERIMPOSITION OF THE DECARTO IMAGES ONTO THREE-DIMENSIONAL IMAGES

The planar image surfaces are not able to display accurately a three-dimensional structure or to capture the individual anatomy. DECARTO allows projection of the decartograms/activation areas onto the "realistic" individual surfaces rendered from other image methods used in cardiology. Such surfaces may be acquired from a variety of clinically available imaging techniques such as SPECT, echocardiography, and MRI. In relation to ECG, these cardiac imaging techniques are used mainly as reference methods for comparative studies. However, they bear basically different and potentially complementary information, including information on the structural characteristics of the cardiac source, which can but does not necessarily influence its function, or on the functional characteristics other than electrical properties.[38]

The transformation of ECG data into the decartograms creates a two-dimensional, image-like representation of ECG signal that is more suitable for direct comparison with imaging data. The comparison of decartograms and imaging data is done by an approximate merging of a separate coordinate system of imaging data and image sphere used in the DECARTO model, followed by the projection of decartograms onto functional and structural surfaces that were identified in imaging data.

This process is called superimposition and allows effective visualization of information about the structural and functional state of the heart and its electrical characteristics derived from the VCG signal. The identification of the surfaces in imaging data is done using standard segmentation and quantification algorithms that are based on the forming of surface according to specific iso-values in data.[39] The identified surfaces do not necessarily need to be attributed only to real structures of the heart (as in MRI or echocardiography); they can also describe a functional status of the heart muscle (eg, SPECT imaging).

The main output of data merging is a projection of the information about the spatial localization of a VCG vector end point defined by DECARTO onto the area of defined localization and size of the myocardium, and this can be used to study the relationship between electrogenesis and the myocardial structures and metabolism. However, due to several simplifications of the DECARTO model (eg, assumption about dipole content of the electrical field), the information presented by DECARTO does not need to correspond exactly to the real sequence of activation front in the myocardium. However, the visualization of ECG signal in the same context as cardiac imaging techniques offers an investigative and instructional modality for comparative studies of functional and structural changes of the heart.

The superposition of imaging data and DECARTO data provides the opportunity to study both the diagnostic and prognostic importance of agreements and disagreements of findings of both methods. In the interpretation of the superposition of DECARTO and imaging data, the same parameters embedded in the provided information inherent to both methods are considered. The first group of parameters, which influences the quality of the fusion process, has to do with the solution of merging spatial coordinates of ECG and the imaging data system. These parameters are related to the proper merging of the orthogonal ECG/VCG coordinate center with the center of the anatomic structure or the center of the geometric surface from the heart imaging data.

The second group of parameters is directly related to the diagnostic evaluation of data obtained from the fusion process. Clinically used diagnostic methods have a set of individual decision-making procedures that can differentiate between normal and pathologic findings. Fusion of two diagnostic methods thus increases the number of possible parameters suitable for diagnostic evaluation. In the case of a dynamic system such as the heart, the presence of time dimension in monitoring may lead to a dramatic increase of accessible data describing the functionality of the system. The heterogeneous parameters inherent to these diverse types of diagnostic techniques can be evaluated using multivariate statistics in order to identify new characteristics that could be useful, especially in treatment of normal and borderline pathologic findings.

The superimposition of the decartogram on the rendered three-dimensional surface positions the activated area on the anatomic structure given by the used imaging method (eg, MRI, SPECT, or coronarography). The superimposition of the QRS decartograms or ST-segment deviation decartograms can visualize, for example, the relationship between the flow in particular coronary arteries and estimated location of MI or area at risk, by superimposing the activated areas/decartograms on a three-dimensional image of the coronary artery distribution.

In the interpretation of the final superimposed images, the following key principles must be considered:

- The principles of the imaging methods (ie, what information is provided by the particular method)
- How to treat the three-dimensional images that are rendered in the case of a fuzzy border (eg, in the case of low signal as demonstrated in a case of a perfusion defect in SPECT; Fig. 11–8)
- What anatomic structure is visualized (eg, the left ventricle or the whole heart)
- How to visualize a structure located intramurally with respect to the surface (eg, a case of a scar in an MRI image that is located intramurally while the DECARTO image is projected on the surface of the heart)

The side-by-side comparison of different imaging methods and the superimposition of methods providing different primary information on the structure and function of the heart can thus complement the view of the pathologic process/disease. Imaging ECG signals will contribute to the process of moving from using the ECG as a surrogate to understand better the processes behind particular ECG changes/patterns and their clinical or prognostic relevance.

The superimposition of the decartogram on the SPECT three-dimensional image is an example of a graphical presentation of two methods that provide two complementary sets

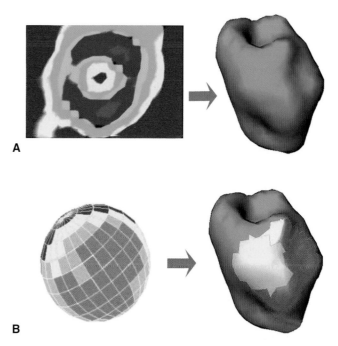

FIGURE 11–8. A. The surface representation of the heart rendered from the 2D SPECT image cross-sections. **B.** The spherical image surface with a decartogram is projected on the rendered surface. In this way, the decartogram is superimposed on the rendered myocardial surface displaying the relation between two functional characteristics of the heart—electrical (DECARTO) and perfusion (SPECT).

of information on the function of the heart. The decartogram visualizes depolarization as a sequence of activated points on the image surface, showing the dipolar content of the cardiac electric field. SPECT is a routinely used clinical imaging method that provides information on the function and structure of myocardium based on the retention of radioactive substances depending on cellular viability and integrity of cell membranes. By superimposing the decartogram onto the graphical imaging of viability, the relationships between the viability and electrical activity can be analyzed.

In the interpretation of the superimposition of DECARTO and SPECT, the following factors and limitations of both methods need to be considered:

- Proper definition and position of the coordinate system center of the orthogonal ECG that is used for construction of decartograms need to be ensured, with the center of the real heart surface constructed from SPECT. The image surface constructed from SPECT data can differ from the real surface, especially in cases with severe pathology.
- Differences exist between the anatomic axis/description of the heart and the electrical coordinate system. This requires approximating anatomic structures of the heart (eg, apex, interventricular septum) based on conventionally used views/terms (eg, anterior, posterior, lateral).
- In the clinical evaluation of both SPECT and DECARTO, it is assumed that they provide information mainly about the left ventricle, because it dominates in the image. In reality,

DECARTO contains an undefined proportion of information from the right ventricle.

- If the image surface is constructed based on perfusion SPECT data, the surface represents "healthy" myocardium in terms of perfusion. In cases of pronounced pathology (eg, in cases of considerable perfusion defects), the constructed surface can differ considerably from the real anatomic left ventricular surface. Moreover, the shape of the surface depends on the threshold that was used for rendering.

- The information presented by decartogram is based on the representation of the cardiac electrical field as a resultant single dipole and its projection on the selected image surface. This projection, however, does not necessarily correspond to the real sequence of depolarization. For example, the initial part of the depolarization can be projected onto the posterior wall, or the activation areas are projected during depolarization repetitively on the same place.

- DECARTO is constructed primarily from one heartbeat (ie, it visualizes the sequence of activated areas during one depolarization). In contrast, SPECT presents average information from several heartbeats.

These factors/limitations define a framework for the potential use of the superimposition of decartograms and SPECT images. Within this framework, the superimposition of these two methods creates a strong potential for their utilization as illustrative and innovative tools for comparative studies focused on the relationship between functional and structural/anatomic characteristics of the heart. This method of superimposition, including awareness of its limitations, is applicable to other methods as well, such as CT, MRI, and PET, that provide information on the source of the cardiac field from additional aspects.

■ LIMITATIONS OF THE DECARTO METHOD

The DECARTO method involves several simplifications related to the basic principles of the method. First, the cardiac electrical field is represented by a single dipole, and DECARTO and the decartograms are primarily defined as circles on the spherical image surface. Second, if the spatial vector is approximated from the standard 12-lead ECG, the result depends on the used formula. Third, the primary image surface is spherical; therefore, deformations due to the projection of this three-dimensional spherical surface onto two-dimensional surfaces (eg, Mercator, polar) can be considerable and will require further optimization of the method. Finally, the relations of the VCG orthogonal coordinate system, the 12-lead hexaxial coordinate system, and the anatomic axis of the heart are considered to be constant and do not consider interindividual variability of patients.

CONCLUSION

Despite the listed simplifications and limitations, the DECARTO method has its advantages. It allows the visualization of the sequence of depolarization and the areas at risk using clinically accepted concepts and defined formulas. As was demonstrated in the case of the DECARTO-like method for the estimation

of the area at risk in patients with AMI, the method is flexible, allowing the following modifications:

- Use of any defined formula for the estimation of area at risk; thus, the performance of different score formulas can be graphically compared

- The optimization/individualization of the spatial angle between the anatomic axis of the heart and the ECG coordinate system

- Use of any three-dimensional surface or three-dimensional image for the projection of the area at risk

- Superimposition of any texture on the image surface, including results of other imaging methods used in cardiology

The DECARTO method and its modification can be used to visualize the direction and size of the electric forces of the heart approximated by a single dipole. It contributes to understanding the electrical forces responsible for the changes in the shape of ECG tracings and associates them with pathophysiologic/disease processes.

ACKNOWLEDGEMENTS

Supported in part by grants VEGA: 1/0530/09, Slovak Republic, and by the Slovak Research and Development Agency under the contract APVV-20-05610. The data for the ST-DECARTO images were kindly provided by the Lund Cardiac MR Group, Lund, Sweden.

REFERENCES

1. Hurst JW. Methods used to interpret the 12-lead electrocardiogram: pattern memorization versus the use of vector concepts. *Clin Cardiol.* 2000;23:4-13.
2. Titomir LI, Ruttkay-Nedecky I. Chronotopocardiography: a new method for presentation of orthogonal electrocardiograms and vectorcardiograms. *Int J Biomed Comput.* 1987;20:275-282.
3. Titomir LI, Ruttkay-Nedecky I, Bacharova L. *Komplexnyj Analiz Elektrokardiogrammy v Ortogonalnych Otvedeniach [Complex Analysis of Orthogonal Electrocardiogram].* Moscow, Russia: Nauka Publishing House; 2001.
4. Wei D. Whole-heart modeling: progress, principles and applications. *Prog Biophys Molec Biol.* 1997;67:17-66.
5. Clayton RH, Panfilov AV. A guide to modelling cardiac electrical activity in anatomically detailed ventricles. *Prog Biophys Molec Biol.* 2008;96:19-43.
6. Bacharova L, Melotova J, Ruttkay-Nedecky I. Reference values of dipolar electrocardiotopogram of the QRS complex. *Bratisl Lek Listy.* 1991;92:402-409.
7. Ruttkay-Nedecky I. Decision making in boundary problems of computerized electrocardiology using fuzzy sets. In: *Proceedings of Computers in Cardiology.* Los Alamitos, CA: IEEE Computer Society Press; 1992:557.
8. Bacharova L, Mateasik A, Carnicky J, et al. The Dipolar ElectroCARdioTOpographic (DECARTO)-like method for graphic presentation of location and extent of area at risk estimated from ST-segment deviations in patients with acute myocardial infarction. *J Electrocardiol.* 2009;42:172-180.
9. Ruttkay-Nedecky I, Riecansky I. Dipolar electrocardiotopographic evaluation of ventricular activation in patients with various degrees of coronary artery disease. *J Electrocardiol.* 1994;27:149-155.
10. Aldrich HR, Wagner NB, Boswick J, et al. Use of initial ST-segment deviation for prediction of final electrocardiographic size of acute myocardial infarcts. *Am J Cardiol.* 1988;61:749-753.

11. Steg PG, Faraggi M, Himbert D. Comparison using dynamic vectorcardiography and MIBI SPECT of ST-segment changes and myocardial MIBI uptake during percutaneous transluminal coronary angioplasty of the left anterior descending coronary artery. *Am J Cardiol*. 1995;75:998-1002.

12. Nielsen BL. ST segment elevation in acute myocardial infarction: prognostic importance. *Circulation*. 1973;48:338-345.

13. Hlatky MA, Califf RM, Lee KL. Prognostic significance of precordial ST segment depression during inferior acute myocardial infarction. *Am J Cardiol*. 1985;55:325-329.

14. Hathaway WR, Peterson ED, Wagner GS, et al. Prognostic significance of the initial electrocardiogram in patients with acute myocardial infarction. GUSTO-I Investigators. Global Utilization of Streptokinase and t-PA for Occluded Coronary Arteries. *JAMA*. 1998;279:387-391.

15. Clemmensen P, Ohman EM, Sevilla DC, et al. Changes in standard electrocardiographic ST-segment elevation predictive of successful reperfusion in acute myocardial infarction. *Am J Cardiol*. 1990;66:1407-1411.

16. Pepine CJ. Prognostic markers in thrombolytic therapy: looking beyond mortality. *Am J Cardiol*. 1996;78:24-27.

17. De Lemos JA, Braunwald E. ST segment resolution as a tool for assessing the efficacy of reperfusion therapy. *J Am Coll Cardiol*. 2001;38:1283-1294.

18. Dong J, Ndrepepa G, Schmitt C, et al. Early resolution of ST-segment elevations correlates with myocardial salvage in patients with acute myocardial infarctions after mechanical or thrombolytic reperfusion therapy. *Circulation*. 2002;105:2946-2949.

19. Rakowski T, Dziewierz A, Siudak Z, et al. ST-segment resolution assessed immediately after primary percutaneous coronary intervention correlates with infarct size and left ventricular function in cardiac magnetic resonance at 1-year follow-up. *J Electrocardiol*. 2009;42:152-156.

20. Wagner GS. *Marriott's Practical Electrocardiography*. 10th ed. Philadelphia, PA: Lippincott Williams & Wilkins; 2001.

21. Ripa RS, Holmvang L, Maynard C, et al. Consideration of the total ST-segment deviation on the initial electrocardiogram for predicting final acute posterior myocardial infarct size in patients with maximum ST-segment deviation as depression in leads V1 through V3. A FRISC II substudy. *J Electrocardiol*. 2005;38:180-186.

22. Clemmensen P, Grande P, Aldrich HR, et al. Evaluation of formulas for estimating the final size of acute myocardial infarcts from quantitative ST-segment elevation on the initial standard 12-lead ECG. *J Electrocardiol*. 1991;24:77-83.

23. Boden WE, Gibson RS, Schechtman KB, et al. ST segment shifts are poor predictors of subsequent Q wave evolution in acute myocardial infarction. A natural history study of early non-Q wave infarction. *Circulation*. 1989;79:537-548.

24. Touchstone DA, Nygaard TW, Kaul S. Correlation between left ventricular risk area and clinical, electrocardiographic, hemodynamic, and angiographic variables during acute myocardial infarction. *J Am Soc Echocardiogr*. 1990;3:106-117.

25. Christian TF, Gibbons RJ, Clements IP, et al. Estimates of myocardium at risk and collateral flow in acute myocardial infarction using electrocardiographic indexes with comparison to radionuclide and angiographic measures. *J Am Coll Cardiol*. 1995;26:388-393.

26. Wilkins ML, Maynard C, Annex BH, et al. Admission prediction of expected final myocardial infarct size using weighted ST-segment, Q wave, and T wave measurements. *J Electrocardiol*. 1997;30:1-7.

27. Barbagelata A, Di Carli MF, Califf RM, et al. Electrocardiographic infarct size assessment after thrombolysis: insights from the Acute Myocardial Infarction STudy ADenosine (AMISTAD) trial. *Am Heart J*. 2005;150:659-665.

28. Titomir LI, Trunov VG, Aidu EA, et al. New approaches to the diagnosis of left and right ventricular hypertrophy by means of dipolar electrocardiotopography. *Anadolu Kardiyol Derg*. 2007;7(Suppl 1):29-31.

29. Titomir LI, Trunov VG, Aidu EA, et al. Electrocardiographic diagnosis of left ventricular hypertrophy on the basis of dipole electrocardiotopography method. *J Electrocardiol*. 2008;41:697.e1-e6.

30. Ubachs JF, Engblom H, Hedström E, et al. Location of myocardium at risk in patients with first-time ST-elevation infarction: comparison among single photon emission computed tomography, magnetic resonance imaging, and electrocardiography. *J Electrocardiol*. 2009;42:198-203.

31. Strauss DG, Olson CW, Wu KC, et al. Vectorcardiogram synthesized from the 12-lead electrocardiogram to image ischemia. *J Electrocardiol*. 2009;42:190-197.

32. Galeotti L, Strauss DG, Ubachs JF, et al. Development of an automated method for display of ischemic myocardium from simulated electrocardiograms. *J Electrocardiol*. 2009;42:204-212.

33. Andersen MP, Terkelsen CJ, Struijk JJ. The ST Compass: spatial visualization of ST-segment deviations and estimation of the ST injury vector. *J Electrocardiol*. 2009;42:181-189.

34. Dower GE, Machado HB, Osborne JA. On deriving the electrocardiogram from vectorcardiographic leads. *Clin Cardiol*. 1980;3:87-95.

35. van Oosterom A, Oostendorp TF. ECGSIM: an interactive tool for studying the genesis of QRST waveforms. *Heart*. 2004;90:165-168.

36. Selvester RH, Wagner GS, Ideker RE, et al. ECG myocardial infarct size: a gender-, age-, race-insensitive 12-segment multiple regression model. I: retrospective learning set of 100 pathoanatomic infarcts and 229 normal control subjects. *J Electrocardiol*. 1994;27(Suppl):31-41.

37. Selvester RH, Wagner GS, Hindman NB. The Selvester QRS scoring system for estimating myocardial infarct size. The development and application of the system. *Arch Intern Med*. 1995;145:1877-1881.

38. Carerj S, Zito C, Di Bella G, et al. Heart failure diagnosis: the role of echocardiography and magnetic resonance imaging. *Front Biosci*. 2009;14:2688-2703.

39. Bankman IN, ed. *Handbook of Medical Imaging*. San Diego, CA: Elsevier Academic Press; 2000.

SECTION II

Foundations of Future Methods for Cardiovascular Multimodal Imaging

12. Electrocardiographic Imaging of Epicardial Potentials 205

13. Electromechanical Modeling Applied to Cardiac Resynchronization Therapy 222

14. Computational Cardiac Electrophysiology: Modeling Tissue and Organ 233

15. Cardiac Simulation for Education: The Electrocardiogram According to ECGSIM 266

16. Graphical Analysis of Heart Rate Patterns to Assess Cardiac Autonomic Function 284

17. Development of the Heart, with Particular Reference to the Cardiac Conduction Tissues 299

CHAPTER 12

ELECTROCARDIOGRAPHIC IMAGING OF EPICARDIAL POTENTIALS

Fady Dawoud, John L. Sapp, John C. Clements, and B. Milan Horáček

INTRODUCTION / 205

BODY SURFACE POTENTIAL MAPPING / 205

FORWARD AND INVERSE PROBLEMS OF ECG / 207
Forward Problem in Terms of Epicardial Potentials / 207
Generation of Patient-Specific Torso Model / 207
Inverse Problem in Terms of Epicardial Potentials / 209

APPLICATION OF ECG IMAGING IN CLINICAL ELECTROPHYSIOLOGY / 209
Three-Dimensional Electroanatomic Mapping / 210
Case Study: Methods / 210
Case Study: Results / 210

DISCUSSION / 216

APPENDIX A: GENERALIZED SINGULAR VALUE DECOMPOSITION / 219

APPENDIX B: THE REGULARIZATION PARAMETER AND OPERATOR / 219

INTRODUCTION

Electrocardiograms (ECGs) recorded simultaneously at many body surface sites can be used to construct a sequence of body surface potential distributions that correspond to cardiac electrical activity; this technique is referred to as body surface potential mapping (BSPM).[1,2] The noninvasively acquired BSPM data can be used, in turn, along with a mathematical model that accounts for geometry and electrical properties of the thorax, to reconstruct electrical potentials on the epicardial surface. The problem of calculating epicardial potentials from recorded BSPM data constitutes one of the formulations of the *inverse problem of ECG*.[3,4]

The calculation of epicardial potentials from noninvasively acquired electrical and anatomic data is also referred to, quite aptly, as *electrocardiographic imaging*.[5,6] The procedure requires BSPM data, accurate representation of the patient's thoracic geometry, routines for calculating transfer coefficients relating epicardial and body surface potentials,[7] and reliable inverse-solution techniques for estimating epicardial potentials from BSPM data.[3,4] Patient-specific anatomic data can be obtained by computed tomography (CT) or magnetic resonance imaging (MRI).

ECG imaging has shown its potential in theoretical and experimental studies,[5,6] and it promises to find its way into routine clinical applications.[8,9]

The aim of this chapter is to illustrate the use of ECG imaging in clinical cardiac electrophysiology, in particular as an aid to radiofrequency catheter ablation of ventricular arrhythmias. In this chapter, we introduce our methodology of BSPM, with particular attention to applications in clinical cardiac electrophysiology; we deal with the mathematical formulation of the relationship between potentials on the epicardial surface and body surface and show how this relationship is used to solve the inverse problem of ECG in terms of epicardial potentials; we describe the application of ECG imaging during catheter-ablation procedures in the clinical cardiac electrophysiology laboratory; and we discusses results reported in this chapter in the context of current clinical practice.

BODY SURFACE POTENTIAL MAPPING

To obtain the BSPM data required for ECG imaging, 120 disposable radiolucent Ag/AgCl electrodes (Ref. 31.8778.26; Covidien, Dublin, Ireland) were placed on the patient's torso in 18 strips according to the standard Dalhousie configuration (Fig. 12–1). The electrode array was connected to the 128-channel Mark-6 acquisition system (BioSemi Inc., Amsterdam, the Netherlands), which was coupled via a fiber optics cable with a laptop computer. The ECG signals were displayed and stored with *MAPPER* software (Dalhousie University, Halifax, Nova Scotia, Canada).

The acquisition system amplified and filtered (bandpass, 0.025-300 Hz) analog ECG signals and sampled each channel at 2000 Hz with 16-bit resolution. The raw data were recorded typically for 15 seconds during sinus rhythm, pacing, or ventricular tachycardia (VT) and stored on a hard disk for subsequent analysis.

All ECG tracings were inspected to mark faulty leads, such as leads affected by poor skin-electrode contact, motion artifact, or inaccessibility of the chest area where the electrode was supposed to be placed (eg, the area occupied by external defibrillator pads). Such faulty leads were estimated using a three-dimensional Laplacian interpolation scheme.[13] Processing of the ECG data took into account ECG signals obtained during sinus rhythm, pacing, or VT.[14] In each case, a different semi-automated routine was written in MATLAB (Mathworks Inc, Natick, MA) to determine fiducial marks (ie, onsets/offsets of P wave, QRS complex, and T wave). For ECG data obtained during sinus rhythm, the baseline was determined by using the second derivative of the lead potential with respect to time, and the fiducial marks of ECG waves were determined by algorithm; these marks were subsequently revised, if necessary. For paced data, the pacing artifact was identified by thresholding the time derivative of the sum of all body surface ECGs, and then the beginning and end of each pacing cycle was determined by algorithm. For ECG data recorded during VT, the onset of each cycle was determined from the narrowest point between the upper and lower

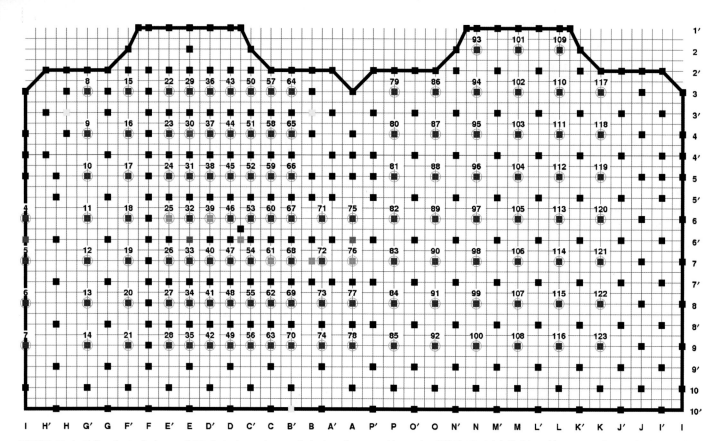

FIGURE 12–1. Dalhousie standard array of 120 electrodes on the torso for body surface potential mapping (BSPM). The left half of the grid represents the anterior chest, and the right half represents the posterior chest. Transverse levels (labeled 1′, 2,…,10′) and equiangular planes (labeled A,A′,…,P,P′) are marked after Frank,[10] with levels 1-inch apart. Potentials at 352 nodes (solid squares) are interpolated from those recorded at electrode sites (circles); green squares mark sites of precordial leads V_1 to V_6; yellow squares are sites where electrodes of Mason-Likar[11] substitution for extremity leads are placed; and red squares are sites of EASI leads.[12]

envelope of all body surface ECG tracings preceding a rapid change in their amplitudes (Fig. 12–2).

Next, each lead was averaged over a number of beats in order to improve the signal-to-noise ratio. Dynamic beat averaging was performed to include in the averaging only those beats that were similar enough to the selected template beat.

An example of four instantaneous BSPM distributions corresponding to activation/repolarization sequence initiated by epicardial pacing is shown in Fig. 12–3. Note that the color scale is adjusted to the instantaneous values of extrema; thus, spatial patterns of low-level potential distributions can be discerned as clearly as those with much higher potentials at the peak activation.

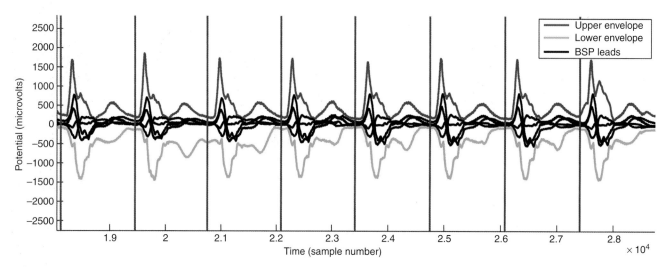

FIGURE 12–2. Detection of cycle length in body surface potential (BSP) mapping data acquired during ventricular tachycardia (VT). The upper and lower envelopes of all 120-lead electrocardiogram tracings were used to detect the onset (red line) of each VT cycle. This particular VT (marked VT A of a patient) is described in detail in the "Application of ECG Imaging in Clinical Electrophysiology" section.

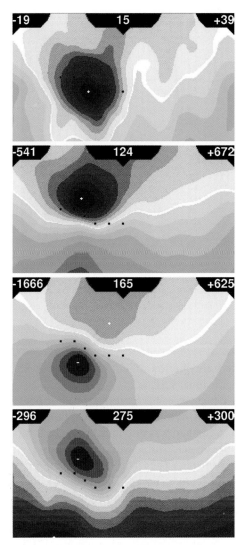

FIGURE 12–3. Body surface potential maps (BSPMs). Instantaneous BSPMs for epicardial pacing in the patient described in detail in the "Application of ECG Imaging in Clinical Electrophysiology" section are shown for the following time instants: 15 ms (early depolarization), 124 ms (advanced depolarization), 165 ms (peak depolarization), and 275 ms (early repolarization) after pacing at a basal inferior site. Each map is displayed on a cylindrical projection of the torso: the anterior chest projects on the left side of the map and posterior chest on the right side; left and right margins of each map correspond to the right mid-axillary line; top corresponds to the neck and bottom to the waist; and locations of six precordial leads of the conventional 12-lead electrocardiogram are shown as black squares. For color coding of potentials, yellow-to-red scale denotes positive potentials, and green scale denotes negative potentials. Regardless of amplitudes of extrema, there are always seven isopotential contours linearly distributed between zero and the larger of the two extrema (maximum/minimum). Amplitudes of maximum and minimum (in μV) are in the upper right and left corners, respectively, and time elapsed from the beginning of activation (in ms) is in the center of each panel.

We have shown previously[15,16] that BSPM data acquired during catheter ablation of scar-related VT can assist with the identification of VT exit sites. Patients had BSPM data recorded during episodes of VT and endocardial pacing, and the data were analyzed to assess the similarity between the BSPM sequences occurring during VT and those induced by pacing. We found that, in general, the nearer the pacing site

was to the exit site, the greater was the similarity between the VT and paced BSPM sequences. This suggested that BSPM can provide a useful adjunct to standard pace mapping. We realized, however, that additional processing—in particular, the inverse calculation of epicardial potentials/isochrones—would enhance the usefulness of the data gathered by BSPM. The rest of this chapter briefly reviews our methodology of inverse calculations and gives examples of their possible clinical use.

FORWARD AND INVERSE PROBLEMS OF ECG

The forward problem of ECG involves computation of body surface potentials from specified cardiac generators that represent the electrical activity of the heart. The problem can be formulated in different ways, depending on the assumptions regarding the equivalent sources for the cardiac electrical activity and a representation of geometric and electrical properties of the volume conductor in which these sources are embedded.[7,17,18]

Numerical methods for solving the forward problem of ECG for arbitrarily shaped domain-wise homogeneous volume conductors have been in use since the 1960s; initially, the forward solution was performed to calculate potentials on the torso surface from dipolar sources.[19-21] An alternative approach is to consider the distributed double-layer source on the epicardial surface as the equivalent generator.[22] Barr et al[7] introduced the mathematical formulation for computing linear transfer coefficients relating electric potentials on the epicardial surface and those on the body surface. This model—consisting of a homogeneous volume conductor bounded by realistically shaped surfaces of the heart and outer torso—was adopted in calculations presented in this chapter.

■ FORWARD PROBLEM IN TERMS OF EPICARDIAL POTENTIALS

Let us consider the forward problem of ECG formulated as a calculation of the electric potentials $\Phi_B = (\varphi_B^1, \ldots, \varphi_B^m)$ at m area elements (or discrete points) on the body surface, S_B, from the observed electric potentials $\Phi_H = (\varphi_H^1, \ldots, \varphi_H^n)$ at n area elements (or discrete points) on the epicardial surface, S_H. This leads to the boundary-value problem for Laplace equation in a homogeneous volume conductor that is bounded by smooth surfaces S_B and S_H.[4,7] The final result, in matrix notation, is:

$$A\Phi_H = \Phi_B, \qquad (12\text{–}1)$$

which expresses body surface potentials, Φ_B, as a linear combination of epicardial potentials, Φ_H, through the transfer matrix A. This forward relation is the basis for inverse-problem formulation in terms of epicardial potentials (see Equation 12–2).

■ GENERATION OF PATIENT-SPECIFIC TORSO MODEL

Calculation of the transfer matrix A for Equation 12–1 requires a discretized representation of surfaces S_B and S_H of the torso model; this is accomplished by defining a set of points

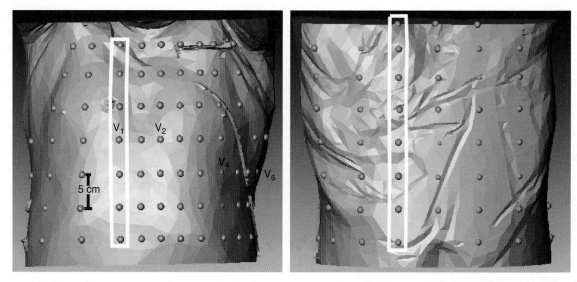

FIGURE 12–4. Dalhousie standard array of electrodes applied on the patient-specific torso surface. Anterior (left) and posterior (right) views of the torso surface with superimposed locations of 120 electrodes (yellow beads); there are 18 strips (as those in white rectangles) with four to eight electrodes in each, 12 strips on the anterior torso (extending from right to left mid-axillary line) and 6 strips on the posterior torso.

connected to form a three-dimensional mesh that represents each surface as a tessellation of planar triangles. Over the last decade, advanced imaging modalities—such as CT and MRI—have made it possible to acquire anatomic scans with high resolution, and thus, accurate patient-specific torso models can be readily generated.

We used axial CT scans (Siemens Sonata, Erlangen, Germany) acquired in supine position to generate patient-specific torso models. The location of body surface electrodes was estimated from known constraints: in-strip (5 cm) and between-strip (>2.5 cm) interelectrode distance, and correspondence with anatomic landmarks (location of precordial leads with reference to intercostal spaces). Figure 12–4 shows an example of

the estimated distribution of 120 electrodes for BSPM on the patient-specific torso surface.

The 120 patient-specific locations of electrodes were then used as vertices to create a triangulated closed surface of the outer torso. A method was developed to make this patient-specific triangulation compatible with the Dalhousie standard 352-node torso geometry. (The Dalhousie standard torso consists of 352 nodes, which are vertices of 700 triangular area elements of the body surface.) Figure 12–5 illustrates the generation of the customized 352-node torso.

Generation of the discretized epicardial surface involved two steps: segmentation and triangulation. CT images were imported into the Amira package (Mercury Computer

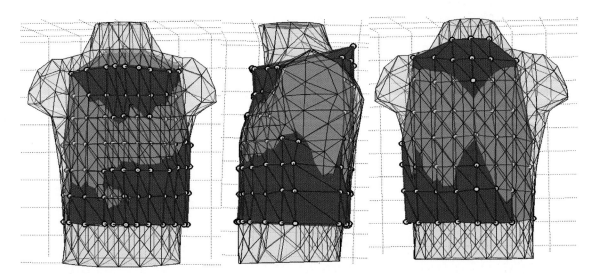

FIGURE 12–5. Patient-specific modification of the standard Dalhousie torso. From left to right are anterior, left sagittal, and posterior views of the standard Dalhousie torso before scaling (blue) aligned with the triangulated surface (red) of patient-specific locations of the 120 surface electrodes (yellow beads). After scaling, node coordinates for the 352-node patient-specific torso model were generated by means of Laplacian interpolation of the patient-specific coordinates for electrode sites.

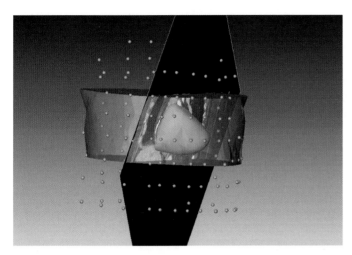

FIGURE 12–6. Segmentation and discretization of patient-specific epicardial surface. Anterior view of discretized epicardial surface (green), with selected sections of the torso (purple), oblique cut of the CT data through the coronary sinus (black), and locations of body-surface electrodes (yellow beads).

Systems, Chelmsford, MA), and an oblique slicing plane parallel to the coronary sinus was defined to facilitate segmentation of the ventricles down to the left ventricular apex. The labeled ventricles were then triangulated. Figure 12–6 shows the discretized epicardial surface, the section of the torso, and the oblique cut of the CT data through the coronary sinus to facilitate segmentation and discretization. Multiple passes of spatial filtering were applied to render a smooth surface.

■ INVERSE PROBLEM IN TERMS OF EPICARDIAL POTENTIALS

The objective of ECG imaging is to solve the inverse problem defined as the calculation of epicardial potential distributions from potential distributions acquired on the body surface (BSPM data). Whereas the mathematical solution of the forward problem of ECG is unique and depends continuously on the data (ie, the problem is "well posed"), the solution of the inverse problem may be neither unique nor depending continuously on the data (in which case, the problem is said to be "ill posed"), and small errors in the input data can generate unbound errors in the inverse solution. Thus, any attempted inverse solution usually requires that auxiliary constraints be imposed. The "ill-posedness" of the problem can be determined by examining the singular values of the transfer matrix A of Equation 12–1. Methods of mathematical regularization of ill-posed problems, most notably Tikhonov regularization,[23] provide a key to their solution. Tikhonov regularization, applied to solving the inverse problem of ECG in terms of epicardial potentials, was our method of choice.

The inverse problem is to estimate in the Equation 12–1 epicardial potentials Φ_H from the measured body-surface potentials Φ_B and the transfer matrix A. Because both Φ_B and Φ_H are functions of time (body surface ECGs and heart surface electrograms, respectively), the inverse problem has to be solved at a series of time instants. At each instant, the solution for Φ_H can be estimated by using Tikhonov regularization, which aims to solve a perturbed version of the least squares problem,

$$\min_{\Phi_H}\{||\,A\Phi_H - \Phi_B\,||^2 + \lambda^2\,||\,B\Phi_H\,||^2\,\}, \qquad (12–2)$$

where ||.|| denotes the l_2 norm, λ is the regularization parameter, and B is the regularizing operator. For a given A and appropriately selected $\lambda > 0$, a solution $\Phi_H(\lambda)$ of the perturbed minimization problem in Equation 12–2 can be obtained from the generalized form of normal equations, which is derived by means of the generalized singular value decomposition.

Given a sequence of sampled BSPM data Φ_B for a specific patient, together with the generalized singular value decomposition of the transfer matrix A and regularizing operator B for that patient (Appendix A), the solution for the epicardial potential distribution Φ_H at each time step is calculated in two steps. First the regularization parameter λ is determined by one of several possible methods (Appendix B), and then, using Equation 12–A2 in Appendix A, the corresponding epicardial potential distribution Φ_H is evaluated.

APPLICATION OF ECG IMAGING IN CLINICAL ELECTROPHYSIOLOGY

The ECG inverse solution can be applied to aid catheter ablation of scar-related VT, which is still one of the most challenging procedures in clinical electrophysiology. The majority of these tachycardias are poorly tolerated or difficult to induce, and they frequently transform to other tachycardia morphologies.[24] Successful ablation of scar-related VT requires an understanding of its mechanism and of the underlying electroanatomic substrate. Such insight can be partly achieved by percutaneous endocardial or epicardial mapping with a single catheter, which is steered to multiple sites to define the substrate for arrhythmia during sinus rhythm.[25-27] However, this alone is often not sufficient for predicting successful ablation sites; some tachycardias are "unmappable" with point-by-point mapping, and alternative methods for identifying exit sites for these tachycardias have to be sought.[28] One of the frequently used methods is pace mapping in the peri-infarct zone.[29] Our objective here was to investigate how BSPM and the ECG inverse solution, in conjunction with pace mapping, can be used to facilitate radiofrequency ablation of scar-related VT.

■ THREE-DIMENSIONAL ELECTROANATOMIC MAPPING

Catheter mapping and ablation were revolutionized by electroanatomic mapping. The CARTO electroanatomic mapping system (Biosense Webster, Inc., Diamond Bar, CA) employed in this study uses a magnetic sensor in the catheter tip to detect its location in the magnetic field created by magnets placed beneath the patient, and a triangulated ventricular surface is displayed by a system (see Fig. 12–8), allowing visualization of various electrical measurements in real time.[24,30] This system can be used to perform sinus rhythm voltage mapping, which involves sampling of the endocardial or epicardial bipolar electrograms recorded from an electrode catheter at multiple locations.[25] Low-amplitude bipolar electrograms have been shown to correspond to infarcted myocardium, with amplitudes typically less than 0.5 mV over the dense scar.[27] The CARTO system can also perform activation mapping, which annotates the anatomic construct with local activation times.[25]

The limitations of point-by-point mapping of activation sequences have led to the development of *pace mapping* methods for assessing the location of the mapping catheter relative to the reentry circuit.[31-33] The procedure involves successive stimulation at various sites and comparing the paced QRS patterns with the template pattern of the clinical VT. Distinct patterns of BSPM distributions were observed for ectopic ventricular activation sequences initiated at various endocardial pacing sites for patients with idiopathic VT,[34] as well as for patients who have had a prior myocardial infarction.[33,35]

Propagation of electrical activation in the diseased myocardium is discontinuous, and small differences in the pacing site can induce different propagation patterns and resulting QRS complexes.[31,33] Nevertheless, the pacing from a catheter located near the exit of a reentry circuit of VT usually produces a QRS morphology similar to that of VT, with a short stimulus-to-QRS delay.[36] Pacing that produces a QRS matching VT after a delay (stimulus-to-QRS interval >40 ms) has been shown to mark a site in a reentry channel within an infarct scar that is considered a good candidate for ablation.[36] Trying to approach the exit site using sequential pace mapping can be challenging and requires an intuitive interpretation of the 12-lead ECG. We hypothesized that this process could be aided by BSPM and ECG imaging.

Some intraoperative studies involving endocardial and epicardial mapping have shown that scar-related VT does not always arise in the subendocardium.[37-40] This evidence was further supported by studies using hearts explanted from patients who have had a myocardial infarction.[41] VTs in which epicardial breakthrough preceded the earliest endocardial activity were reported,[39] and some were successfully terminated by an epicardially directed procedure.[38,42,43] Sosa et al[44] described subxiphoid access to the pericardial space for mapping and ablation; this approach was used in the study reported here.

■ CASE STUDY: METHODS

The case presented here was referred for ablation of scar-related VT to the Cardiac Electrophysiology Laboratory of the Queen Elizabeth II Health Sciences Centre in Halifax. The patient (age, 64 years) had a history of severe ischemic cardiomyopathy. Previous VT storms were resistant to drug therapy and were treated with VT ablation in 2003 and 2005. Several morphologies of VT from the patient's study in 2005 suggested an epicardial origin of arrhythmia. In 2007, the patient presented with incessant slow VT (with two distinctly different morphologies, denoted VT A and VT B). A cardiac resynchronization therapy defibrillator (CONTAK RENEWAL 3 RF; Boston Scientific, Natick, MA) had been

implanted, and the patient was chronically paced. After written informed consent and detailed explanation of the procedure, the patient underwent a successful ablation of both VTs in June 2007.

The detections on the implantable cardioverter defibrillator (ICD) were deactivated prior to the ablation procedure, which was performed under general anesthesia. The groins were infiltrated with 2% lidocaine without epinephrine; 5- and 6-French sheaths were inserted percutaneously into the right femoral vein, and an 8-French sheath was inserted percutaneously into the right femoral artery. To gain access to the pericardial space, a Weiss needle was advanced below the xiphoid process to the pericardium under fluoroscopic guidance. A wire was then inserted into the pericardial space, a tract was progressively dilated with 6- and 8-French dilators, and an 8.5-French convoy sheath was advanced to the pericardial space. A 6-French hexapolar catheter was advanced to the right ventricular apex. A Navistar Thermocool F-curve catheter (Biosense Webster) was introduced into the pericardial space via the convoy sheath and used for epicardial mapping. The same catheter was later introduced into the left ventricle via the retrograde aortic approach and used for endocardial mapping and ablation.

BSPM data were collected during sinus rhythm, ICD pacing, roving catheter pacing, and VT. Multipoint catheter mapping and pacing were performed by the CARTO electroanatomic mapping system (Biosense Webster) using the Navistar Thermocool catheter. Bipolar and unipolar electrograms were recorded both by the CARTO system and by the GE Cardiolab system (GE Healthcare, Piscataway, NJ). The time delay was determined from the 12-lead ECG on the GE Cardiolab system; a stimulus-QRS interval >40 ms was referred to as *delay*.[45]

ECGs were processed as described earlier in the "Body Surface Potential Mapping" section. The patient-specific geometry of the torso and epicardial surface was extracted from the CT data, the transfer matrix, A, was calculated, and the inverse solution was obtained by means of a second-order Tikhonov regularization with the *L*-curve method used to determine the regularization parameter as described earlier in the "Forward and Inverse Problems of ECG" section and in Appendices A and B. *MAP3D* visualization software[46] was used to display potential distributions on epicardial and torso surfaces.

The gold standard for assessing the accuracy of the inverse solution was the information collected by the CARTO electroanatomic mapping system during the ablation procedure. The patient-specific CARTO geometry was registered manually and fused with the CT data, as illustrated in Fig. 12–7. The locations of the CARTO sites where pacing was delivered and the estimated locations of these sites obtained by the inverse solution were compared to determine localization accuracy. CARTO voltage mapping was performed to delineate the scar and scar margin.

■ CASE STUDY: RESULTS

Reference Maps Delineating Scar Region

Figure 12–8 shows the epicardial voltage substrate maps obtained with the CARTO system. These maps delineate electroanatomic

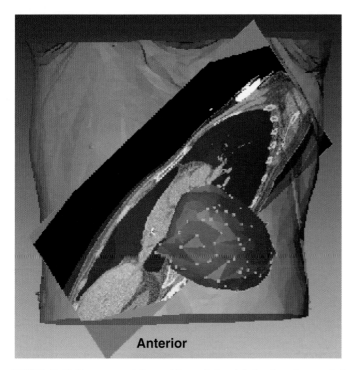

Anterior

FIGURE 12–7. Torso segmentation and image fusion. Anterior view of segmented torso shows oblique computed tomography (CT) slice cutting through the atrioventricular ring to facilitate segmentation of the ventricles; epicardial surface was identified and colored red. CARTO points (green) were incorporated into the coordinate system of the CT data, and a triangulated epicardial surface constructed from these points is shown in purple.

substrate by using color mapping to annotate bipolar signal amplitude (30-400 Hz) that distinguishes between normal myocardium, infarct scar, and border zone around scarred tissue. Regions of low-amplitude signal appear on the anterolateral left ventricle and over the lateral right ventricular wall. Moderate-size patches of confluent scar cover the midsection of the lateral left ventricle.

Localization of Epicardial Pacing Sites by Inverse Solution

Pacing on the epicardial surface initially produces epicardial potential distributions with an area of negative potentials surrounding the pacing site, along with two areas of low-level positive potentials due to conduction anisotropy at the stimulation site, as demonstrated in vivo using dense electrode arrays.[47] By using BSPM recordings obtained during epicardial pace mapping (n = 22), we tested the accuracy of the inverse solution in localizing the epicardial stimulation site by comparing the calculated location of the potential minimum with the known location of epicardial pacing determined by the CARTO system. Figure 12–9 shows, for an epicardial pacing site at the basal inferior left ventricle, computed epicardial potential maps at four instants of time, with corresponding input data (recorded body surface potential maps, also shown for both the anterior and posterior torso in Fig. 12–3). The initial minimum on the epicardial surface (of –0.96 mV, near the pacing site) with an area of negative potentials that surround it is discernible after a long delay at 124 ms after pacing stimulus. At peak depolarization, the potential minimum drifts far from the pacing site. During early repolarization, at 275 ms, a low-amplitude maximum (0.347 mV) of epicardial potentials appears again in close proximity to the pacing site. With the insight provided by epicardial maps, measured BSPM distributions (see both Fig. 12–3 and top of Fig. 12–9) seem to be compatible with epicardial-to-endocardial direction of activation initiated on the inferior wall of the left ventricle (as evidenced by the equivalent dipole pointing straight up at 124 ms).

The results for pacing site localization by means of the inverse solution for all (n = 22) epicardial pacing sites of this patient are summarized in Fig. 12–10, which shows, in four views (corresponding to electroanatomic substrate maps in Fig. 12–8), the actual pacing sites, plotted from coordinates provided by the CARTO system, and the estimates of the location of these sites obtained by the inverse solution. The electroanatomic substrate around each pacing site was characterized by the bipolar voltage detected by the CARTO system and by the delay in response to pacing.

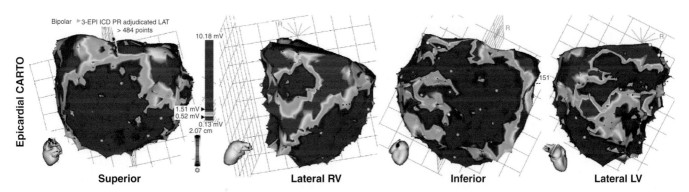

FIGURE 12–8. CARTO maps of bipolar potentials on epicardial surface delineating electroanatomic substrate in four views. The color mapping is set so that regions of bipolar amplitudes >1.5 mV, representing normal tissue, are purple; regions with amplitudes <0.5 mV are red; and regions with amplitudes between 0.5 and 1.5 mV, representing border zone between scarred and normal tissue, are yellow to blue. An image of a generic heart is shown beside each voltage map to indicate an approximate anatomic view of the heart; the color scale of bipolar potentials is the same for all four views and is indicated by a bar in the leftmost panel. LV, left ventricle; RV, right ventricle.

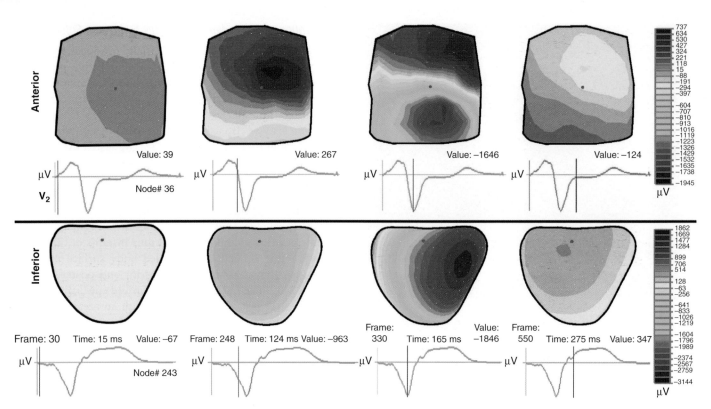

FIGURE 12–9. Calculated epicardial potential distributions with corresponding body surface potential maps (BSPMs) that were acquired during epicardial pacing. **Top row.** Anterior view of the patient-specific torso surface with recorded potential maps that were used as input data (see also Fig. 12–3, showing complete distributions for the same time instants) to calculate epicardial potentials shown in the bottom row; the electrocardiogram at the site of the precordial lead V$_2$ (pink disk) is shown in green; the bar on the right margin indicates color coding of potentials. **Bottom row.** Inferior view of the patient-specific epicardial surface with the calculated epicardial potential maps obtained by the inverse solution from BSPM data shown in the top row for time instants 15, 124, 165, and 275 ms after pacing at a basal inferior site (pink disk); the calculated electrogram at this site is shown in green. (Note that amplitude scales in top and bottom rows are different.)

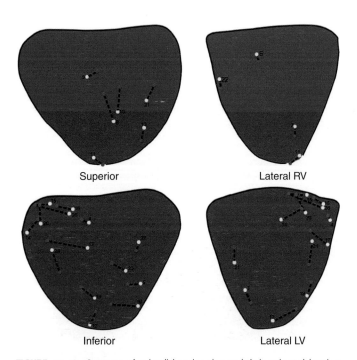

FIGURE 12–10. Summary of epicardial pacing sites and their estimated locations obtained by inverse solution. The projections of CARTO pacing sites, with the recording number, are marked by yellow disks, and the corresponding sites of early minima of epicardial potentials calculated by inverse solution are marked by blue disks; dashed lines connect corresponding yellow and blue disks. LV, left ventricle; RV, right ventricle.

We found, not surprisingly, that the electroanatomic substrate around the pacing site affected localization accuracy. For the group of pacing sites in structurally normal myocardium with no delay (n = 7), the median Euclidean distance between the actual and estimated pacing site was just 11 mm, and the potential minimum appeared after a mean interval of 29 ms following the pacing spike. For pacing in scar and scar margin—which implied involvement of the scar substrate in modifying early activation sequence—the discrepancy was larger, but it did not exceed 35 mm.

Localization of ICD Pacing Site by Inverse Solution

Localizing the paced activation initiated from the leads of the ICD device provides another approach to testing the localization accuracy of the inverse solution because the tip of the ICD lead can be accurately determined from the CT images. The BSPM recording was done during pacing from an ICD device implanted in another patient, also recruited under scar-related VT study, who had an ICD pacing electrode in the endocardial right ventricular apex.

The epicardial potential maps obtained for early activation by the inverse solution (Fig. 12–11) provided a clue for estimating the site of pacing. Because the ICD pacing site was on the right ventricular *endocardial* surface, the activation wave front propagated first across the right ventricular wall before it broke through on the epicardial surface. Thus, an area of positive potentials appeared initially near the pacing site, reflecting propagation of

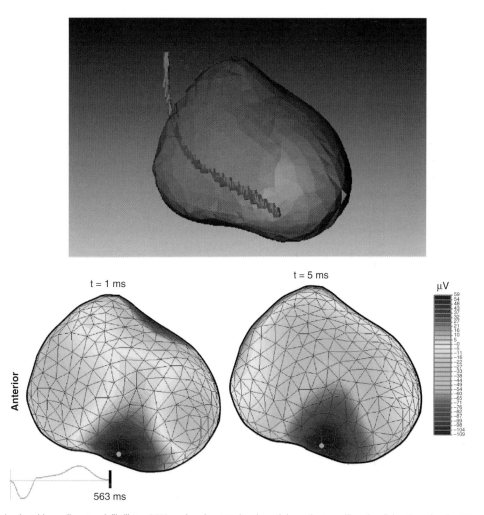

FIGURE 12–11. Localizing implantable cardioverter defibrillator (ICD) pacing site. Anterior view of the patient-specific epicardial surface showing ICD pacing lead reconstructed from computed tomography images (top) and epicardial potential maps (bottom) obtained by inverse solution at $t = 1$ ms and $t = 5$ ms, with the electrogram corresponding to the site where both the initial potential maximum and subsequent potential minimum appear (green disks). Displayed with *Map3D* visualization software.[46]

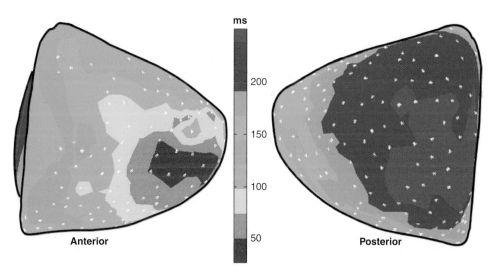

FIGURE 12–12. Isochronal maps obtained by CARTO system. Anterior and posterior views of the activation times measured by CARTO system are shown, projected, and interpolated on the patient-specific epicardial surface; white markers denote discrete sites where activation times were measured. The pacing lead was located at the endocardial right ventricular apex, just beneath the area of early activation (red) on the anterior view.

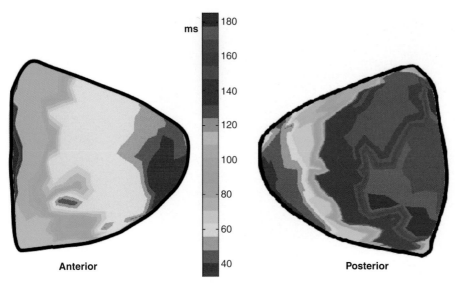

FIGURE 12–13. Isochronal maps obtained by inverse solution. Anterior and posterior views of the activation times estimated by the electrocardiographic inverse solution are shown.

the wave front toward the epicardial surface, and then, after the breakthrough, an area of negative potentials emerged and intensified throughout depolarization and was replaced by a distribution with opposite polarity during repolarization. The Euclidean distance between the actual location of an endocardial pacing electrode and the location of the early minimum on the epicardial surface was 12 mm. This small discrepancy can be attributed either to the involvement of right ventricular conduction system or to the anisotropic intramural propagation, or to both.

Activation Times Obtained by Inverse Solution

To assess the inverse solution's ability to preserve timing information, the activation time was determined by the CARTO system from bipolar electrograms at multiple points on the epicardial surface by the roving catheter, whereas the ICD device paced at the endocardial site near the right ventricular apex. The epicardial surface reconstructed from measurements made by the CARTO system was aligned with the epicardial surface reconstructed from the CT scan, and CARTO points were projected onto the nearest nodes of this patient-specific epicardial surface. Figure 12–12 shows the activation times at all nodes of this surface as estimated by three-dimensional interpolation from data provided by the CARTO system. The activation time obtained via the inverse solution was determined in each calculated epicardial electrogram by the steepest-descent criterion during depolarization; the isochronal maps obtained by this method are shown in Fig. 12–13.

The activation times yielded by the CARTO system show early depolarization of the right ventricular apex (red) and the activation wave spreading over the right ventricular anterior wall in approximately 100 ms (see Fig. 12–12, left); the latest area to activate (purple) is the basal region of the posterior left ventricle (see Fig. 12–12, right). The inverse-solution isochrones in Fig. 12–13 show a qualitatively similar spread

of activation; the early activation of the right ventricular apical region, the progression of the activation wave over the right ventricular anterior wall and then the left ventricular posterior wall, and the latest activation of the posterobasal wall are all correctly estimated by the inverse solution. However, there is some discrepancy in the time scale, which reflects inability of the steepest-descent criterion to detect the activation wave front from low-amplitude electrograms in the region with depressed conduction.

Localization of the Reentrant Circuit's Exit Site by Inverse Solution

The earliest region to depolarize during scar-related VT is the site where the reentry circuit exits the scar to reexcite normal myocardium and sustain the arrhythmia. Localizing these *exit sites* is essential during the ablation procedure to guide delivery of radiofrequency energy that interrupts the reentrant pathway. To evaluate the potential usefulness of inverse ECG in aiding radiofrequency ablation, we applied the methodology tested during paced activation to BSPM data recorded during VT.

The onset of reentrant activation can usually be determined from body surface ECGs (see Fig. 12–2), and the BSPM distribution observed during this phase can be used to estimate the locus of exit site from calculated epicardial potential distributions or activation isochrones.

Two separate morphologies of VT (denoted VT A and VT B) were recorded for this patient, and both tachycardias were successfully ablated. Figure 12–14 shows (in 20-ms increments) a sequence of body surface potential maps for VT A. Initial distributions (during the first 10 ms) have very low amplitudes; the first discernible pattern of body surface potentials with a maximum near precordial site of lead V_4 develops at 11 ms, and this distribution remains stationary until nearly 70 ms; subsequently, the maximum migrates toward the right chest. The repolarization minimum near the site of V_2 appears at approximately 250 ms and remains stationary until approximately 410 ms.

Epicardial potential distributions obtained by the inverse solution for VT A (Fig. 12–15A) show early negative potentials on the high basal inferior region (at 69 ms) near scar border zone; this area of negative potentials remains stationary during the depolarization phase (106 ms). A map of the isochrones of activation (Fig. 12–15B) shows earliest activation starting at the high inferobasal left ventricle in the region where the earliest potential minimum appeared. The isochronal map shows activation spreading in a counterclockwise direction around the area of block on the inferior epicardial surface, starting at the inferior left ventricular base and ending on the basal inferior and inferolateral right ventricle while the superior view of the isochronal map shows activation spreading globally from apex to base. The ablation site was endocardial; its projection on the epicardial

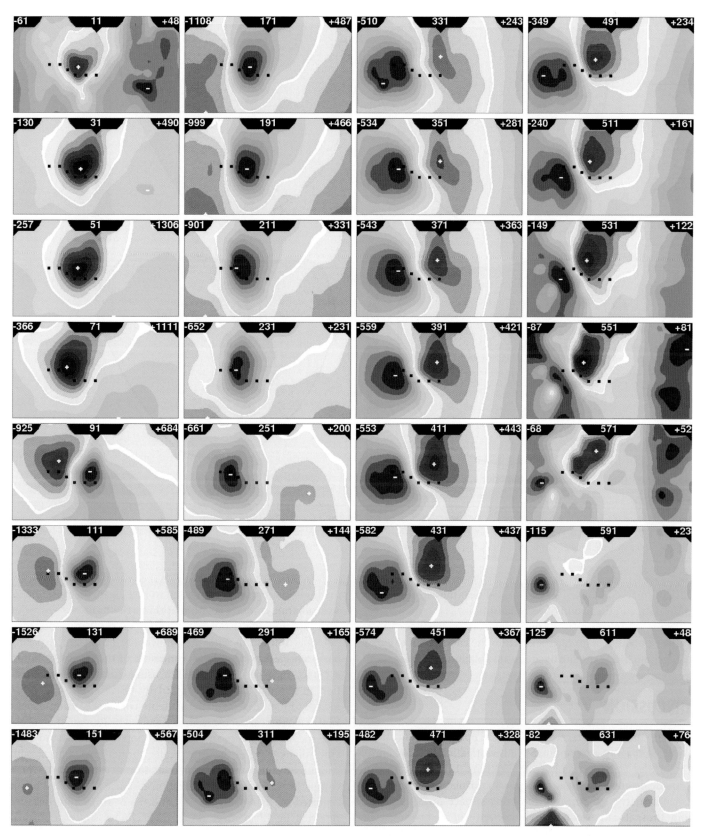

FIGURE 12–14. Body surface potential maps for ventricular tachycardia (VT A). Maps are shown in 20-ms increments of time; cycle length = 660 ms. The first 12 maps correspond to ventricular activation (with maximum peaking in 51-ms frame and minimum in 131-ms frame), followed by 16 maps corresponding to ventricular repolarization (peaking in 431-ms frame). For explanation of display of body surface potential maps, see Fig.12–3.

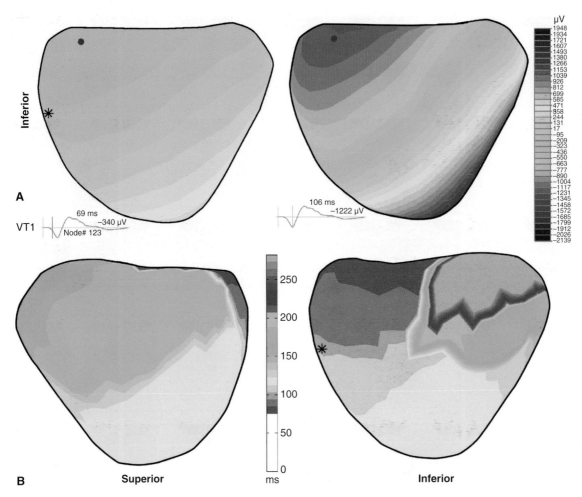

FIGURE 12–15. Inverse epicardial potential maps and isochrones of activation during ventricular tachycardia (VT A). **A.** Inferior views of the epicardial potential distribution obtained by the inverse solution at 69 and 106 ms into the VT cycle; the local electrogram is shown from a point on the basal inferior left ventricle (pink disk); the color scale of calculated potentials (μV) is on the right. **B.** Superior and inferior views of isochrones of activation (ms) obtained by inverse solution for the same VT cycle; the color scale of calculated activation times is shown in the middle. Asterisk (*) indicates the projection of endocardial ablation site that terminated VT A on epicardial surface.

surface (marked by asterisk) was located near the early potential minimum and the region of early activation.

Figure 12–16 shows (in 20-ms increments) a sequence of body surface potential maps for pacing from the endocardial site that can help to locate the site of successful ablation of VT A.

DISCUSSION

The aim of this chapter was to illustrate potential applications of ECG imaging as a noninvasive investigative tool for clinical cardiac electrophysiology applications. ECG imaging can provide detailed spatial and temporal information on the electrical activity of the heart from body surface measurements, and thus, it can become an important aid in investigating mechanisms of cardiac arrhythmias and in making their treatment more effective.

We first demonstrated the localization accuracy of ECG imaging by comparing calculated epicardial electrograms, and measures derived from them, with a gold standard provided by CARTO electroanatomic mapping. Next, we used these tested methods in recording of VT itself to investigate their usefulness in facilitating catheter ablation of this arrhythmia.

Comparing the estimated location of the early epicardial potential minimum with the known site of epicardial pacing has been used previously as a measure of the inverse-solution accuracy in experimental studies using canine heart preparation in a torso tank, as reported by Oster et al,[5] and more recently in studies involving patients with ICDs using a right ventricular apical pacing lead, as reported by Ramanathan et al.[8] The median of localization accuracy in the present study, for epicardial pacing in the structurally normal myocardium with stimulus-to-QRS delay of less than 40 ms, was 11 mm, which compares well with the localization distance of within 11 mm reported by Ramanathan et al[8] and the 6- to 29-mm distance reported by Ghanem et al[48] in their clinical study performed during open-chest surgery.

In the pace mapping recordings with stimulus-to-QRS delay of greater than 40 ms and/or those for stimuli delivered inside scar/scar margin, the effect of pacing from multiple sites around the epicardium caused clustering of early potential minima around one or two regions of the ventricular surface, in particular, in

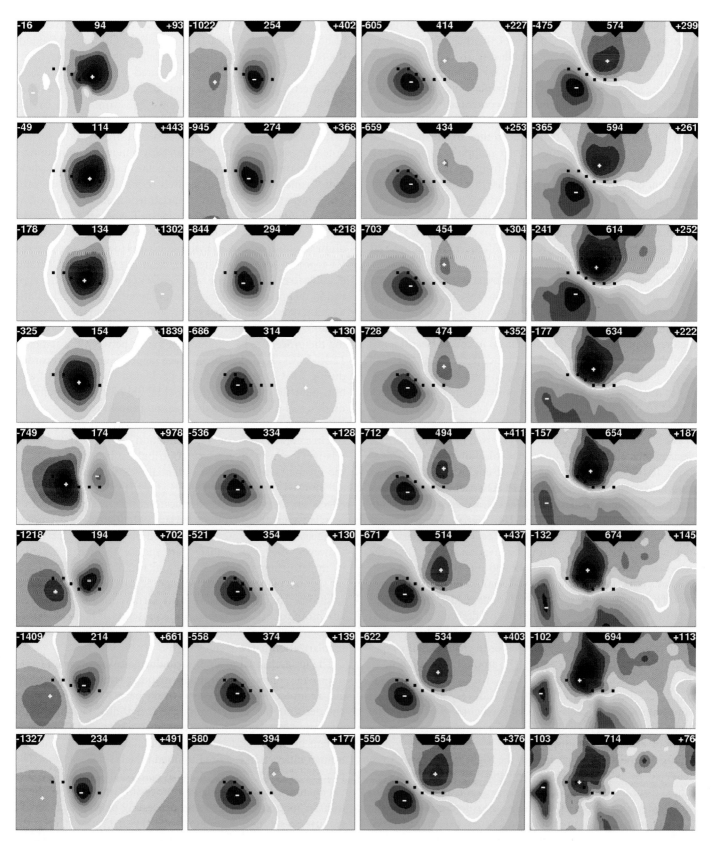

FIGURE 12–16. Body surface potential maps for pacing near endocardial exit site of ventricular tachycardia (VT A). Maps are shown in 20-ms increments of time. Compare this sequence with that of VT A itself, shown in Fig. 12–14. For explanation of conventions used in display of body surface potential maps see Fig.12–3.

the patient presented here, in the high basal inferolateral region (five sites). A possible explanation of this behavior is that in cases where pacing is delivered inside scar, the activation wave front travels with depressed velocity, taking longer to emerge out of the scar, at which point a substantial bulk of myocardial tissue activates, generating the multiple potential minima. Thus, the location of such clustering of potential minima may indicate a part of the tachycardia circuit close to the exit site that should be investigated further by the catheter mapping. In such cases, the early potential minima may be far from the pacing site. This argument is further supported by the fact that the location of the early potential minimum during recordings of VT of the same patient lies very close to the region where the early potential minima induced by pace mapping tend to cluster; these regions are also near the location where radiofrequency ablation was performed.

The display of isochrones of activation is an effective tool for visualizing propagation of the activation wave front in the ventricular myocardium. Producing the global isochronal map over the entire epicardial/endocardial surface by direct measurement requires maneuvering of the catheter tip to collect electrograms point by point and determining a time of activation for each point. This elaborate process is used in clinical electrophysiology to map sustained arrhythmias; however, the same approach cannot be used when arrhythmia is not sustained or when it is not hemodynamically tolerated. Therefore, one of our aims was to assess accuracy of activation times derived from the epicardial electrograms obtained by the inverse solution in comparison to those derived from *directly measured* epicardial electrograms collected invasively through the CARTO system. We used peak negative slope on calculated unipolar epicardial electrograms to determine the local activation time. However, in diseased hearts, there are many situations in which the peak negative derivative may not be a reliable predictor of activation time.[49] Thus, the presence of diseased tissue complicated interpretation of electrograms obtained by the inverse solution in the case presented here. The method of steepest downslope applied to electrograms obtained by the inverse solution relies on derivatives calculated from successive samples, which makes it vulnerable to measurement noise in body surface potentials or to changes in the regularization parameter that controls the amount of smoothing in the inverse calculation. In cases of electrograms with low peak amplitude, there were multiple points with very similar steepest slope values, which caused spurious assignment of activation times. This problem was partially mitigated by spatial smoothing of inverse electrograms.

During endocardial pacing at the right ventricular apex, delivered by ICD, regions of early and late activation determined from calculated epicardial electrograms agreed well with those determined from electrograms measured directly by the CARTO system. However, the isochrones determined from calculated electrograms for paced activation (see Fig. 12–13) and for VT (see Fig. 12–15) show irregularities that include compression of the total activation time range, near-instant (bulk) activation of large regions, and crowding of isochronal lines at multiple locations. These flaws are due to limitations of the inverse-solution method used here, which can only produce

unipolar electrograms that inherently contain superposition of both near- and distant-field potentials. On the other hand, the reference activation times (yielded by the CARTO system) were obtained from directly measured *bipolar* electrograms, which reflect only intrinsic near-field activity[50]; they exhibit a sharp peak when the activation wave front passes by the catheter tip.

In inverse potential maps calculated from body surface potentials recorded during VT, an early potential minimum was found on the epicardial surface near the endocardial site where radiofrequency ablation successfully terminated the arrhythmia. These observations support the argument that the early potential minimum corresponds to the location where the tachycardia reentrant pathway exits dense scar to reexcite normal myocardium to continue the arrhythmia cycle. However, because the VT reported here was not hemodynamically tolerated, it was not possible to exactly map the tachycardia's circuit using either activation mapping or prolonged entrainment mapping. Thus, the location of arrhythmia exit site was inferred from the site where radiofrequency ablation was successfully performed, aided during the procedure by goodness of match between the standard 12-lead ECG recorded during pace mapping and that recorded during VT. Comparison of Figs. 12–14 and 12–16 demonstrates how matching sequences captured by BSPM can be potentially used in real time to guide the ablation procedure.

A number of investigators have pointed out that geometric inaccuracies of the representation of the heart surface relative to the body surface contribute substantial errors in the estimates of epicardial potentials.[51-53] Recently, Cheng et al[54] showed, in an experimental study, that there are minor effects on the reconstructed epicardial potential, as measured by relative error, when body surface potentials were corrupted by measurement noise or correlated electrode displacement. However, they found that heart surface scaling, translation in three orthogonal directions, and rotation around coronal or sagittal planes resulted in significantly poorer epicardial solutions. They also noted that the *L*-curve method was generally more robust and stable in the presence of higher levels of geometric errors compared with other methods of selecting the regularization parameter.

The ultimate goal of studies conducted using inverse ECG is to provide adjunct electrical information to the electrophysiologist about local electrical events in the heart that aids diagnosis and decision making in treating the arrhythmia. Two important attributes for deployment of such an inverse ECG imaging system in the clinical setting are computational time and any human interaction required to obtain the inverse solution. The process of calculating the inverse epicardial solution involves (1) anatomic body imaging and processing of images to obtain transfer matrix; (2) BSPM and processing of recorded signals; (3) inverse-solution procedure; and (4) visualization. Currently, MRI and CT are routinely used to obtain anatomic images, and two advanced mapping systems (CARTO electroanatomic mapping and EnSite NavX mapping [Endocardial Solutions, St. Paul, MN]) allow importing of these images and segmentation of heart chamber of interest to be incorporated within the same display of data collected by these systems. The discretization of ventricular geometries and electrode locations from segmented images online is possible with current mesh generation algorithms.

Overall, it is well within the capability of current technology to perform the functions required for epicardial inverse ECG imaging during the ablation procedure. What remains to be achieved is rigorous validation of the inverse solution using physiologic data collected under clinical conditions against reference data provided by established clinical imaging tools.

APPENDIX A: GENERALIZED SINGULAR VALUE DECOMPOSITION

The generalized singular value decomposition (GSVD) of Equation 12–2 is defined as follows.[4] Let A be any $m \times n$ real matrix $(m > n)$, let B be a $p \times n (p \leq n)$ real matrix of rank $q \leq p$, and let $k+q$ be the numerical effective rank of $\binom{A}{B}$. The GSVD of A and B (representing the transfer matrix and regularization operator, respectively, in Equation 12–2) is given by

$$A = UDY^T, \quad B = VZY^T \quad (12\text{–}A1)$$

where

$$D = \begin{pmatrix} I & O \\ O & C \\ O & O \end{pmatrix}, \quad Z = \begin{pmatrix} O & S \\ O & O \end{pmatrix}.$$

Here $C = \text{diag}(\alpha_{(k+1)}, \ldots, \alpha_n)$ and $S = \text{diag}(\beta_{(k+1)}, \ldots, \beta_n)$ are diagonal matrices, O denotes the additive identity, $U_{m \times m}$ and $V_{p \times p}$ are orthogonal and $Y_{n \times n}$ is a nonsingular matrix. The generalized singular values $\mu_i = \alpha_i / \beta_i$ satisfy $0 \leq \alpha_i \leq 1$, $1 \geq \beta_i > 0$, and $\alpha_i^2 + \beta_i^2 = 1$ for $i = k+1, \ldots, n$.

The unique solution to Equation 12–2 for each $\lambda > 0$ is given by

$$\varphi_H(\lambda) = \sum_{i=1}^{k} (\boldsymbol{u}_i \cdot \boldsymbol{b}) \boldsymbol{y}_i + \sum_{i=k+1}^{n} \frac{\mu_i}{\mu_i^2 + \lambda^2} \left(\frac{1}{\beta_i} \right) (\boldsymbol{u}_i \cdot \boldsymbol{b}) \boldsymbol{y}_i \quad (12\text{–}A2)$$

where $\boldsymbol{u}_i$ are the columns of U, $\boldsymbol{y}_i$ are the columns of Y, and $\boldsymbol{b}$ stands for Φ_B.

The generalized normal equations associated with the perturbed least-square problem in Equation 12–2 can be stated as[4]

$$\Phi_H = (A^T A + \lambda B^T B)^{-1} A^T \boldsymbol{b} \quad (12\text{–}A3)$$

For each $\lambda > 0$, the residual $\| Ax(\lambda) - \boldsymbol{b} \|$ can be expressed in the form

$$\| A\Phi_H(\lambda) - \boldsymbol{b} \| = \left(\sum_{i=k+1}^{n} \left[\frac{\lambda^2}{\mu_i^2 + \lambda^2} (\boldsymbol{u}_i \cdot \boldsymbol{b}) \right]^2 + \sum_{i=n+1}^{m} (\boldsymbol{u}_i \cdot \boldsymbol{b})^2 \right)^{1/2} \quad (12\text{–}A4)$$

and for each $\lambda > 0$, the seminorm $\| B\Phi_H(\lambda) \|$ can be expressed in the form

$$\| B\Phi_H(\lambda) \| = \left(\sum_{i=k+1}^{n} \left[\frac{\mu_i}{\mu_i^2 + \lambda^2} (\boldsymbol{u}_i \cdot \boldsymbol{b}) \right]^2 \right)^{1/2}. \quad (12\text{–}A5)$$

Thus, the residual $\| A\Phi_H(\lambda) - \boldsymbol{b} \|$ and solution seminorm $\| B\Phi_H(\lambda) \|$ can be expressed simply in terms of λ, the singular values $\mu_i, i = k+1, \ldots, n$, and the scalar products $\boldsymbol{u}_i \cdot \boldsymbol{b}$, $i = k+1, \ldots, m$.

APPENDIX B: THE REGULARIZATION PARAMETER AND REGULARIZING OPERATOR

The Tikhonov regularization scheme represented by Equation 12–2 arrives at the solution by minimizing two quantities; the first is the least squares solution of Equation 12–1, and the second is a penalty function that imposes conditions on the smoothness of the solution by controlling the weighting regularization parameter λ and the regularization matrix B. Typically, the regularization matrix was chosen to be the identity matrix (I), which is called zero-order Tikhonov regularization, or a discrete approximation of the surface Laplacian matrix (L), which is referred to as second-order Tikhonov regularization. An important step in Tikhonov regularization is the choice of the regularization parameter (λ). As λ goes to zero, the solution to Equation 12–A2 tends to the least squares represented by the first term, which produces unstable epicardial potentials (underregularized solution). However, if λ is too large, the solution becomes overly smooth because the second term of Equation 12–A2 dominates the solution (overregularized solution). The optimal value of the regularization parameter provides a balance between instability and smoothness.

Several methods have been suggested in the literature for choosing the regularization parameter λ. These methods include the generalized cross-validation method,[55] the composite residual and smoothing operator (CRESO) criterion,[56] the L-curve method,[57] and the zero-crossing method.[58] We used the L-curve method of Hansen,[57] which determines the λ parameter from the plot of the seminorm of the solution $\| B\Phi_H \|$ versus the norm of the residual $\| A\Phi_H - \Phi_B \|$. Choosing the regularization parameter in the vertical segment of the L-curve puts more weight on minimizing the residual, thus underregularizing the solution and making it unstable, whereas on the horizontal part of the L-curve, more weight is put on minimizing the seminorm of the solution, thus overregularizing it and smoothing out fine details. The corner of the L-curve provides a good balance between the two quantities in Equation 12–2. The corner can be defined mathematically as the point of maximum curvature and can be computed as the maximum of the function $\kappa(\lambda)$:

$$\kappa(\lambda) = \frac{x'(\lambda) y''(\lambda) - y'(\lambda) x''(\lambda)}{[(x'(\lambda))^2 + (y'(\lambda))^2]^{3/2}} \quad (12\text{–}B1)$$

where $x(\lambda) = \| A\Phi_H(\lambda) - \Phi_B \|$, $y(\lambda) = \| B\Phi_H(\lambda) \|$, with prime and double prime denoting first and second derivatives with respect to λ, respectively. Functions $x(\lambda)$ and $y(\lambda)$ can be expressed directly in terms of the regularization parameter (λ), the singular values (μ), and vector quantities $(\boldsymbol{u}$ and $\boldsymbol{b})$ by means of Equations 12–A4 and 12–A5.

Various regularization methods have been implemented in this laboratory, making use of LAPACK and BLAS linear algebra packages.[59] In this study, we used the implementation in MATLAB, making use of the Hansen's regularization toolbox.[60]

REFERENCES

1. De Ambroggi L, Musso E, Taccardi B. Body-surface mapping. In: Macfarlane PW, Lawrie TDV, eds. *Comprehensive Electrocardiology*. New York, NY: Pergamon Press; 1989:1015.

2. Lux RL. Mapping techniques. In: Macfarlane PW, Lawrie TDV, eds. *Comprehensive Electrocardiology*. New York, NY: Pergamon Press; 1989:1001.

3. Rudy Y, Messinger-Rapport BJ. The inverse problem in electrocardiography: solutions in terms of epicardial potentials. *CRC Crit Rev Biomed Eng*. 1988;16:215-268.

4. Horáček BM, Clements JC. The inverse problem of electrocardiography: a solution in terms of single- and double-layer sources on the epicardial surface. *Math Biosci*. 1997;144:119-154.

5. Oster HS, Taccardi B, Lux RL, et al. Noninvasive electrocardiographic imaging: reconstruction of epicardial potentials, electrograms, and isochrones and localization of single and multiple electrocardiac events. *Circulation*. 1997;96:1012-1024.

6. Oster HS, Taccardi B, Lux RL, et al. Electrocardiographic imaging: noninvasive characterization of intramural myocardial activation from inverse-reconstructed epicardial potentials and electrograms. *Circulation*. 1998;97:1496-1507.

7. Barr RC, Ramsey M, Spach MS. Relating epicardial to body surface potential distributions by means of transfer coefficients based on geometry measurements. *IEEE Trans Biomed Eng*. 1977;24:1-11.

8. Ramanathan C, Ghanem RN, Jia P, et al. Noninvasive electrocardiographic imaging for cardiac electrophysiology and arrhythmia. *Nat Med*. 2004;10:422-428.

9. Wilber DJ. Electrocardiographic imaging: new tool for interventional electrophysiology, or just another pretty picture? *Heart Rhythm*. 2007;4:1085-1086.

10. Frank E. The image surface of a homogeneous torso. *Am Heart J*. 1954;4:757-768.

11. Mason RE, Likar I. A new system of multiple-lead exercise electrocardiography. *Am Heart J*. 1966;71:196-205.

12. Dower GE, Yakush A, Nazzal SB, et al. Deriving the 12-lead electrocardiogram from four (EASI) electrodes. *J Electrocardiol*. 1988;21(Suppl):S182-S187.

13. Oostendorp TF, van Oosterom A, Huiskamp G. Interpolation on a triangulated 3D surface. *J Comp Physics*. 1989;80:331.

14. Dawoud F. *Noninvasive Imaging of Epicardial Potentials for Clinical Electrophysiology* [PhD thesis]. Halifax, Nova Scotia, Canada: Dalhousie University; 2009.

15. Sapp JL, Gardner MJ, Parkash R, et al. Body-surface potential mapping to aid ablation of scar-related ventricular tachycardia. *J Electrocardiol*. 2006;39(Suppl 1):S87-S95.

16. Sapp JL, Dawoud F, Clements JC, Horáček BM. Inverse solution electrocardiographic imaging of epicardial pacing correlates with three-dimensional electroanatomic mapping. In: Murray A, Swiryn S, eds. *Computers in Cardiology*. Piscataway, NJ: IEEE Computer Society Press; 2007:769.

17. Miller WT, Geselowitz DB. Simulation studies of the electrocardiogram. I. The normal heart. *Circ Res*. 1978;43:301-315.

18. Cuppen JJM. Calculating the isochrones of ventricular depolarization. *SIAM J Sci Statist Comp*. 1984;5:105.

19. Gelernter HL, Swihart JC. A mathematical-physical model of the genesis of the electrocardiogram. *Biophys J*. 1964;4:285-301.

20. Barr RC, Pilkington TC, Boineau JP, Spach MS. Determining surface potentials from current dipoles, with application to electrocardiography. *IEEE Trans Biomed Eng*. 1966;13:88-92.

21. Barnard ACL, Duck IM, Lynn MS, Timlake WP. The application of electromagnetic theory to electrocardiology. II. Numerical solution of the integral equations. *Biophys J*. 1976;7:463-491.

22. Zablow L. An equivalent cardiac generator which preserves topography. *Biophys J*. 1966;6:535-536.

23. Tikhonov AN, Arsenin VY. *Solutions of Ill Posed Problems*. New York, NY: Wiley; 1977.

24. Soejima K, Suzuki M, Maisel WH, et al. Catheter ablation in patients with multiple and unstable ventricular tachycardias after myocardial infarction. *Circulation*. 2001;104:664-669.

25. Delacretaz E, Stevenson WG. Catheter ablation of ventricular tachycardia in patients with coronary heart disease. Part I: mapping. *Pacing Clin Electrophysiol*. 2001;24:1261-1277.

26. Hsia HH, Marchlinski FE. Characterization of the electroanatomic substrate for monomorphic ventricular tachycardia in patients with nonischemic cardiomyopathy. *Pacing Clin Electrophysiol*. 2002;25:1114-1127.

27. Marchlinski FE, Callans DJ, Gottlieb CD, Zado E. Linear ablation lesions for control of unmappable ventricular tachycardia in patients with ischemic and nonischemic cardiomyopathy. *Circulation*. 2000;101:1288-1296.

28. Brunckhorst CB, Stevenson WG, Jackman WM, et al. Ventricular mapping during atrial and ventricular pacing. Relationship of multipotential electrograms to ventricular tachycardia reentry circuits after myocardial infarction. *Eur Heart J*. 2002;23:1131-1138.

29. Wilber DJ, Kopp DE, Glascock DN, et al. Catheter ablation of the mitral isthmus for ventricular tachycardia associated with inferior infarction. *Circulation*. 1995;92:3481-3489.

30. Gepstein L, Hayam G, Ben-Haim SA. A novel method for nonfluoroscopic catheter-based electroanatomical mapping of the heart: in vitro and in vivo accuracy results. *Circulation*. 1997;95:1611-1622.

31. Josephson ME, Waxman HL, Cain ME, et al. Ventricular activation during ventricular endocardial pacing. II. Role of pace-mapping to localize origin of ventricular tachycardia. *Am J Cardiol*. 1982;50:11-22.

32. Kuchar DL, Ruskin JN, Garan H. Electrocardiographic localization of the site of origin of ventricular tachycardia in patients with prior myocardial infarction. *J Am Coll Cardiol*. 1989;13:893-903.

33. SippensGroenewegen A, Spekhorst H, van Hemel NM, et al. Localization of the site of origin of postinfarction ventricular tachycardia by endocardial pace mapping. Body surface mapping compared with the 12-lead electrocardiogram. *Circulation*. 1993;88:2290-2306.

34. SippensGroenewegen A, Spekhorst H, van Hemel NM, et al. Body surface mapping of ectopic left and right ventricular activation: QRS spectrum in patients without structural heart disease. *Circulation*. 1990;82:879-896.

35. SippensGroenewegen A, Spekhorst H, van Hemel NM, et al. Body surface mapping of ectopic left ventricular activation: QRS spectrum in patients with prior myocardial infarction. *Circ Res*. 1992;71:1361-1378.

36. Brunckhorst CB, Delacretaz E, Soejima K, et al. Identification of the ventricular tachycardia isthmus after infarction by pace mapping. *Circulation*. 2004;110:652-659.

37. Kaltenbrunner W, Cardinal R, Dubuc M, et al. Epicardial and endocardial mapping of ventricular tachycardia in patients with myocardial infarction: is the origin of the tachycardia always subendocardially localized? *Circulation*. 1991;84:1058-1071.

38. Littmann L, Svenson RH, Gallagher JJ, et al. Functional role of the epicardium in postinfarction ventricular tachycardia: observations derived from computerized epicardial activation mapping, entrainment, and epicardial laser photoablation. *Circulation*. 1991;83:1577-1591.

39. Pagé PL, Cardinal R, Shenasa M, et al. Surgical treatment of ventricular tachycardia: regional cryoablation guided by computerized epicardial and endocardial mapping. *Circulation*. 1989;80(Suppl I):I124-I134.

40. Svenson RH, Littmann L, Gallagher JJ, et al. Termination of ventricular tachycardia with epicardial laser photocoagulation: a clinical comparison with patients undergoing successful endocardial photocoagulation alone. *J Am Coll Cardiol*. 1990;15:163-170.

41. de Bakker JMT, Coronel R, Tasseron S, et al. Ventricular tachycardia in the infarcted, Langendorff-perfused human heart: role of the arrangement of surviving cardiac fibers. *J Am Coll Cardiol*. 1990;15:1594-1607.

42. Sosa E, Scanavacca M, d'Avila A. Transthoracic epicardial catheter ablation to treat recurrent ventricular tachycardia. *Curr Cardiol Rep*. 2001;3:451-458.

43. Sosa E, Scanavacca M, d'Avila A. Gaining access to the pericardial space. *Am J Cardiol*. 2002;90:203-204.

44. Sosa E, Scanavacca M, d'Avila A, et al. Nonsurgical transthoracic epicardial catheter ablation to treat recurrent ventricular tachycardia occurring late after myocardial infarction. *J Am Coll Cardiol*. 2000;35:1442-1449.

45. Aliot EM, Stevenson WG, Almendral-Garrote JM, et al. EHRA/HRS Expert Consensus on Catheter Ablation of Ventricular Arrhythmias: developed in a partnership with the European Heart Rhythm Association (EHRA), a Registered Branch of the European Society of Cardiology (ESC), and the Heart Rhythm Society (HRS); in collaboration with the American College of Cardiology (ACC) and the American Heart Association (AHA). *Heart Rhythm*. 2009;6:886-933.

46. MacLeod RS. *Map3D Manual*. Salt Lake City, UT: Cardiovascular Research and Training Institute; 2006.

47. Taccardi B, Macchi E, Lux RL, et al. Effect of myocardial fiber direction on epicardial potentials. *Circulation*. 1994;90:3076-3090.

48. Ghanem RN, Jia P, Ramanathan C, et al. Noninvasive electrocardiographic imaging (ECGI): comparison to intraoperative mapping in patients. *Heart Rhythm.* 2005;2:339-354.

49. Spach MS, Dolber PC. Relating extracellular potentials and their derivatives to anisotropic propagation at a microscopic level in human cardiac muscle. Evidence for electrical uncoupling of side-to-side fiber connections with increasing age. *Circ Res.* 1986;58:356-371.

50. Blanchard SM, Damiano RJ, Asano T, et al. The effects of distant cardiac electrical events on local activation in unipolar epicardial electrograms. *IEEE Trans Biomed Eng.* 1987;34:539-546.

51. Rudy Y, Plonsey R. The eccentric spheres model as the basis for a study of the role of geometry and inhomogeneities in electrocardiography. *IEEE Trans Biomed Eng.* 1979;26:392-399.

52. Huiskamp G, van Oosterom A. Tailored versus realistic geometry in the inverse problem of electrocardiography. *IEEE Trans Biomed Eng.* 1989;36:827-835.

53. Cheng LK, Bodley JM, Pullan AJ. Comparison of potential- and activation-based formulations for the inverse problem of electrocardiology. *IEEE Trans Biomed Eng.* 2003;50:11-22.

54. Cheng LK, Bodley JM, Pullan AJ. Effects of experimental and modeling errors on electrocardiographic inverse formulations. *IEEE Trans Biomed Eng.* 2003;50:23-32.

55. Golub GH, Heath M, Wahba G. Generalized cross-validation as a method for choosing a good ridge parameter. *Technometrics.* 1979;21:215-223.

56. Colli Franzone P, Guerri L, Taccardi B, Viganotti C. Finite element approximation of regularized solutions of the inverse potential problem of electrocardiography and applications to experimental data. *Calcolo.* 1985;22:91-186.

57. Hansen PC. Analysis of discrete ill-posed problems by means of the L-curve. *SIAM Rev.* 1992;34:561-580.

58. Johnston PR, Gulrajani RM. A new method for regularization parameter determination in the inverse problem of electrocardiography. *IEEE Trans Biomed Eng.* 1997;44:19-39.

59. Anderson E, Bai Z, Bischof C, et al. *LAPACK User's Guide.* Philadelphia, PA: Society for Industrial and Applied Mathematics; 1992.

60. Hansen PC. Regularization tools, a Matlab package for analysis and solution of discrete ill-posed problems. *Numer Algorithms.* 1994;6:1-35.

CHAPTER 13

ELECTROMECHANICAL MODELING APPLIED TO CARDIAC RESYNCHRONIZATION THERAPY

Jason Constantino, Viatcheslav Gurev, and Natalia A. Trayanova

INTRODUCTION / 222
   Overview / 222
   Dyssynchronous Heart Failure / 222
   Cardiac Resynchronization Therapy / 223
   Previous Attempts to Model Cardiac Electromechanics
      and CRT / 223

**IMAGE-BASED ELECTROMECHANICAL MODEL OF THE
HEART / 224**
   Image-Based Reconstruction of the Geometry and Structure
      of DHF Hearts / 224
   Simulating Electromechanical Activity in the Normal
      and Failing Hearts / 226

RESULTS OF SIMULATIONS / 228
   The Normal Canine Ventricles / 228
   The Failing Canine Ventricles / 229

CONCLUSION / 230

INTRODUCTION

■ OVERVIEW

Heart failure is a major cause of morbidity and mortality, contributing significantly to global health expenditure. Heart failure patients often exhibit contractile dyssynchrony, which diminishes cardiac systolic function. Cardiac resynchronization therapy (CRT), a relatively new treatment modality that employs biventricular (bi-V) pacing to recoordinate the contraction of the heart, is a valuable therapeutic option for such patients. CRT has been shown to improve heart failure symptoms and reduce hospitalization, yet approximately 30% of patients fail to respond to the therapy. In the current environment, which emphasizes reducing health care costs and optimizing therapy, robust diagnostic approaches to identify patients who would and would not benefit from CRT would have a dramatic personal, medical, and economic impact on the lives of many Americans.

The poor predictive ability of current approaches to identify potential responders to CRT reflects the incomplete understanding of the complex pathophysiologic and electromechanical factors that underlie mechanical dyssynchrony. The goal of this chapter is to present the development, from magnetic resonance imaging (MRI) and diffusion tensor (DT) MRI scans, of individualized three-dimensional (3D) image-based multiscale computational models of ventricular electromechanics that incorporate the deleterious structural, mechanical, and electrophysiologic remodeling associated with dyssynchronous heart failure (DHF), from the level of the protein to that of the intact heart. We then demonstrate how this powerful predictive modeling approach could be used to provide mechanistic insight into heart failure contractile dyssynchrony and to possibly determine the optimal CRT strategy.

The development of a predictive model of ventricular electromechanics in the setting of DHF overcomes the inability of current experimental techniques to simultaneously record the 3D electrical and mechanical activity of the heart with high spatiotemporal resolution and thus to provide an understanding of dyssynchrony and CRT effectiveness. The new basic-science insights into the electromechanical behavior that can be acquired with this modeling approach will hopefully lead to rational optimization of CRT delivery and to improvements in the selection criteria for potential CRT candidates.

■ DYSSYNCHRONOUS HEART FAILURE

Heart failure is a major cardiovascular disease affecting 5 million people in the United States alone and is associated with high morbidity and mortality rates.[1] The syndrome is characterized by impaired pump function due to the deleterious remodeling of the ventricles, from the organ down to the molecular level, which significantly alters the electrical and mechanical behavior of the heart. High-resolution MRI and DTMRI scans[2] have shown that in DHF, there is a substantial remodeling of ventricular geometry and structure. At the organ level, the ventricles become dilated, and wall thickness is reduced. At the tissue level, laminar sheet angle is altered, and the transmural gradient in fiber orientation is increased. Because chamber geometry and sheet structure are major determinants of left ventricular (LV) mechanics,[3,4] the mechanical deformation of the failing heart is markedly different. Furthermore, altered heart geometry and fiber and sheet orientations directly affect 3D electrical propagation[5] in the failing heart.

Heart failure is also characterized by remodeling of the electrophysiologic and mechanical properties at the cellular and subcellular levels. Studies[6,7] have shown that the gap junctional protein connexin 43 (Cx43) is redistributed from the intercalated disk to the lateral myocyte borders and that the amount of hypophosphorylated Cx43 is increased, leading to reduced conduction velocity in heart failure. There is a considerable downregulation of the membrane potassium channels carrying the I_{to} and I_{Kl} currents[8] and of the intracellular sarcoplasmic/endoplasmic reticulum Ca^{2+} ATPase (SERCA) pump[9] and upregulation of the Na-Ca exchanger (NCX).[9] Remodeled ionic currents and Ca^{2+} handling result in altered Ca^{2+} transients, which, in turn, impair active tension development by the myofilaments in the cell. Finally, differential expression of collagen isoforms[10] and altered ratio of titin (an intrasarcomeric protein that modulates myofilament passive tension) isoforms[11] result in increased myocardial stiffness.

Because of the combined effects of chamber, contractile, and electrophysiologic remodeling, the ability of the LV to efficiently pump blood is severely compromised in heart failure patients. Furthermore, a subset of these patients exhibits abnormal electrical conduction that delays activation of one portion of the ventricle relative to another (intraventricular conduction delay due to left bundle branch block [LBBB]). This results in contractile dyssynchrony (ie, DHF), which further diminishes cardiac systolic function and energetic efficiency.

CARDIAC RESYNCHRONIZATION THERAPY

CRT is an established therapy for DHF patients. CRT typically employs bi-V pacing, with an endocardial right ventricular (RV) pacing lead and an epicardial LV pacing lead, to recoordinate contraction.[12] CRT has been shown to acutely and chronically improve systolic function[13] of the heart and to reverse the detrimental remodeling[14] associated with heart failure. Clinical trials of CRT have consistently demonstrated improvement in heart failure symptoms, exercise tolerance, and quality of life and a reduction in recurrent hospitalizations.[15]

Although CRT reduces morbidity and mortality,[16] approximately 30% of patients fail to respond to the therapy.[17] This reflects the poor predictive capability of current approaches to identify potential responders to CRT. The QRS duration (QRS ≥150 ms), which is widely used in clinical trials as a basic component of the inclusion criteria for CRT, does not provide an indication of the degree of mechanical dyssynchrony.[18] Indeed, patients with long QRS duration may not exhibit mechanical dyssynchrony, and those with short QRS complexes may present with significant dyssynchrony in contraction.[19-21] Measurements of mechanical dyssynchrony by Doppler echocardiography[22,23] reveal only local dyssynchrony, whereas the complex deformations in DHF are global. In recent clinical trials, Doppler echocardiography demonstrated lack of repeatability and low predictive value.[24,25] The poor predictive capability of the above measures indicates an incomplete understanding of the electromechanical behavior in DHF.

The presence of myocardial infarction is an additional reason for lack of response to CRT. Placement of a pacing electrode at or near the infarct scar may result in ineffective pacing and, thus, in failure of resynchronization. Because infarction modulates electromechanical interactions, it also alters the mechanism of CRT. Bleeker et al[26] documented that patients with transmural posterolateral scar have a much lower response rate to CRT than those without scar (14% vs 81%, respectively). Increased scar volume has been found to result in unfavorable response to CRT.[27] Infarct location and scar transmurality are considered important[28,29] yet unknown factors that affect the relationship between electrical activation and contraction and contribute to diminished CRT efficacy.

Finally, the location of LV pacing has been shown to play an important role in CRT efficacy.[30-33] Currently, LV pacing lead is implanted in a tributary of the coronary sinus, as in *epicardial* bi-V pacing.[19,34] However, for a small class of patients unsuitable for transvenous bi-V, a transseptal approach has been developed that allows *endocardial* bi-V pacing.[35,36] Recent studies have brought to light the potential proarrhythmic effect of epicardial bi-V pacing,[37] resulting from the reversal of the direction of electrical propagation in the LV. Furthermore, new findings indicate that endocardial bi-V pacing might be associated with improved resynchronization in canine models[38,39] and humans.[40,41]

A comprehensive characterization of the spatiotemporal electromechanical interactions in the DHF heart is paramount to any improvement in the selection criteria for viable CRT candidates and is fundamental to the effort toward improving CRT efficacy. The development of a multiscale model of ventricular electromechanics offers a powerful methodology to unravel the mechanisms by which the deleterious structural, mechanical, and electrophysiologic remodeling in DHF, from the scale of the protein to the intact organ, causes discord between electrical activation and mechanical contraction of the heart. This unique and novel tool overcomes the limitations of previous approaches to elucidating cardiac electromechanical interactions and provides insights that cannot be obtained by experiment alone.

PREVIOUS ATTEMPTS TO MODEL CARDIAC ELECTROMECHANICS AND CRT

In the last decade, simulation research in cardiac electrophysiology has made important steps forward in linking models of myocyte action potential to geometrical models of cardiac tissue and the entire organ (see review by Trayanova and Tice[42]). Although integrative multiscale models of organ behavior that incorporate detailed biophysical models of the myocyte cellular and subcellular processes[43-45] are not yet commonplace, they have nonetheless made major contributions to obtaining insight into electrical excitation[46] and the mechanisms of arrhythmogenesis[47-49] and defibrillation[50,51] in the normal and, in some cases, the diseased heart.[52] Similarly, finite element continuum models incorporating anatomy, structure, and passive mechanics have been developed,[53,54] and recently, attempts have been made to couple them to biophysical models of cellular active tension.[55,56] The development of models of these two major physical processes in the heart has occurred largely independently. However, in the last few years, coupled models of cardiac electromechanics, in which contraction is triggered by the electrical event, have also been assembled.[55-66] All of these models incorporate major simplifications in the representations of membrane dynamics,[58,60] triggering process for contraction,[57,59,61] cellular active tension,[57,60,65] and tissue/organ geometry and structure.[55,56,59] In addition, with very few exceptions,[63,66] these models represent electromechanical activity in the normal heart. Simplifications limit the models' predictive capabilities, particularly their utility in simulating the acute effects of CRT. Indeed, models addressing CRT include those representing bi-V pacing in the normal heart without accounting for cardiac mechanics[67,68] or simulating mechanics with a simple two-element rheologic model.[61] Even the most sophisticated models of CRT[62-64] use phenomenologic representations of membrane dynamics that do not incorporate remodeling in heart failure.

The multiscale electromechanical model of DHF presented here is a major step forward in representing the detailed

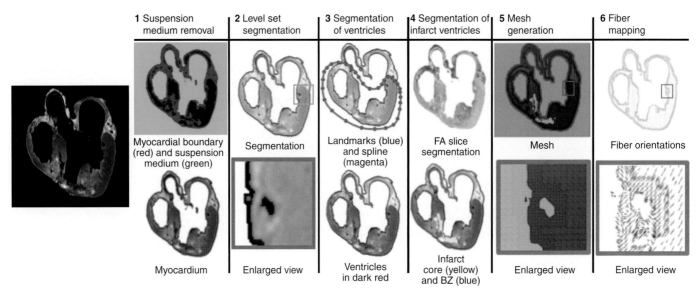

FIGURE 13–1. Pipeline for image-based heart structure and geometry reconstruction. See text for details. BZ, border zone; FA, fractional anisotropy.

electromechanical interactions in the remodeled heart, from the protein to the organ level, overcoming limitations of previous model developments. Furthermore, we incorporate, for the first time, individualized image-based organ and structure in the models, thus ensuring that the mechanistic insights that can be obtained with the model are directly applicable to the clinical setting and the clinical CRT procedure.

IMAGE-BASED ELECTROMECHANICAL MODEL OF THE HEART

■ IMAGE-BASED RECONSTRUCTION OF THE GEOMETRY AND STRUCTURE OF DHF HEARTS

Figure 13–1 illustrates the pipeline for assembling image-based models of the heart by showing the processing of an example image slice. It is important to note that the models generated in this way will retain fine structural details, such as endocardial trabeculations and papillary muscles, provided that such structural details are resolved by the ex vivo imaging method. Further details on the processing pipeline can be found in our recent publications.[69-71]

Suspension Medium Removal

The ex vivo structural MRI is processed to label and "remove" voxels corresponding to cavity content and surrounding medium. First, the image edges are detected,[72] and the myocardial boundary of the heart is extracted using a region-growing algorithm.[73] The surrounding medium is removed by assigning the background intensity to all voxels in the medium. The result is an image of the myocardium (step 1 in Fig. 13–1). In step 2, the myocardium is separated from the large coronary arteries.

Separation of Ventricles From Atria

In each slice, ventricular tissue is labeled by fitting a closed spline curve through spline points placed around the ventricles

and along the atrioventricular border. All voxels that belong to tissue inside the curve are marked as ventricular (step 3 in Fig. 13–1). Ventricles and atria are then separated.

Infarct Segmentation

Often patients with DHF also have myocardial infarction. Therefore, we included in our model reconstruction pipeline the capability to segment the zone of infarct. From the DTMRI, a 3D fractional anisotropy (FA) image is constructed.[74] FA is a measure of the directional diffusivity of water. Based on the difference in FA values,[75,76] the infarct region is separated from the normal myocardium. Next, the infarct region is subdivided into two areas, an inexcitable scar and a peri-infarct region,[75,76] which is assumed to contain excitable and contracting but pathologically remodeled tissue, by thresholding the structural MRI based on voxel intensity values[77] (step 4).

Mesh Generation

Next, a finite element tetrahedral mesh is generated from the segmented MRI for the solution of the *electrical* component of the model. The mesh requirements are based on the spatiotemporal characteristics of wave propagation in the heart; it has been shown that a spatial resolution of approximately 250 μm is appropriate for electrophysiologic finite element models of the heart.[78,79] A novel approach was recently published by our team[80] for image-based mesh generation. The electrical meshes of the heart used in the preliminary studies were generated using this methodology. Step 5 in Fig. 13–1 shows the mesh for the example slice, whereas Fig. 13–2A presents the electrical mesh of the entire canine heart. The meshing technique is automatic and produces boundary-fitted, locally refined, and smooth conformal meshes (see Fig. 13–2A, inset). The local adaptation of the resolution, as shown in Fig. 13–1 (step 5), significantly reduces the number of elements in the mesh without compromising geometric detail. Note that we typically generate electrical meshes of the heart that incorporate both ventricles and atria.

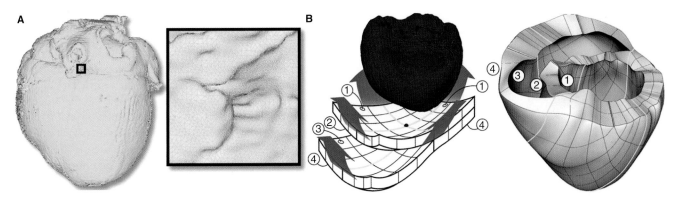

FIGURE 13–2. Computational meshes. **A.** Electrical mesh (mesh detail in inset). **B.** Mechanical mesh generation; numbers denote the various surfaces used in the mesh generation.

However, the electrical problem is effectively solved only on the ventricular portion of the mesh because atria and ventricles are electrically isolated.

The mechanical mesh consists of hexahedral elements with Hermite basis. This choice of finite elements maintains continuity of strain and is appropriate for maintaining incompressibility constraints.[81] The mechanical mesh is also generated from the segmented images and based on the electrical mesh to ensure exact match in geometries; for mechanical mesh generation, we use only the segmented ventricles. The methodology to construct image-based mechanical meshes has been recently developed by our team.[82] The mesh is constructed from a sheet with a thickness of two elements that is "wrapped around" the segmented ventricles as shown in Fig. 13–2B. Note that current mechanical meshing procedures[58,83,84] introduce an artificial hole in the LV apex; the meshing procedure described here avoids this artifact.

Fiber and Sheet Mapping

Fiber and laminar sheet organization underlie the orthotropic electrical conductivities of the tissue and the tissue mechanical properties. We recently developed a methodology to interpolate DTs from the DTMRI data onto the elements in both meshes, thus mapping the fiber and laminar sheet organization onto the meshes (ie, defining the orthotropic properties of the myocardium for the solution of the electrical and mechanical problems). To incorporate fiber and laminar sheet architecture in the model, tensors and tensor gradients were defined at each node of the finite element mesh and interpolated within the finite elements using Hermite interpolation. The eigenvectors of the tensors in the interpolated tensor field represented the fiber and laminar sheet structure in the reconstructed hearts.

Interpolation is performed in a vector space of tensors, introduced previously by Arsigny et al,[85] in the framework of which addition of two tensors, A_1 and A_2, and multiplication of a tensor A by a scalar k of the vector space were:

$$\begin{cases} A_1 \oplus A_2 = \exp(\ln(A_1) + \ln(A_2)) \\ k \otimes A = \exp(k\ln(A)) \end{cases} \qquad (13\text{--}1)$$

For positive definite symmetric matrices, these operations become:

$$\begin{cases} A_1 \oplus A_2 = A_1 A_2 \\ k \otimes A = A^k = (UDU^T)^k = UD^kU^T = U\begin{bmatrix} \lambda_1^k & 0 & 0 \\ 0 & \lambda_2^k & 0 \\ 0 & 0 & \lambda_3^k \end{bmatrix}U^T \end{cases} \qquad (13\text{--}2)$$

where U is an orthogonal matrix and D is a diagonal matrix of eigenvalues λ_1, λ_2, and λ_3. Using the operations in Equations 13-1 and 13-2, the Hermite interpolation is defined as:

$$A = \prod A_i^{\Psi_i} \qquad (13\text{--}3)$$

where Ψ_i are the Hermite basis functions described in Nielsen et al[83] and A_1 are the tensors and tensor gradients with respect to the arc lengths assigned to the nodes of each finite element.

The method for tensor fitting to the DTMRI data, which uses the least-squares method in a metric space of tensors, was similar to that of angle fitting.[83] The tensors and the tensor gradients at the nodes of the mesh were found using the least-squares method by minimizing the sum of the squared distances between the DT from the DTMRI data and the tensors from the interpolated tensor field. The log-Euclidean metric applied in the least-squares method was as follows:

$$d(A_1, A_2) = (Trace\{\ln(A_1) - \ln(A_2)\}^2)^{\frac{1}{2}} \qquad (13\text{--}4)$$

To remove artifacts that appear when voxels of MRIs represent both ventricular tissue and surrounding media at the epicardial and endocardial surfaces, the approximated tensor field was regularized. Regularization of the tensor field using the log-Euclidean metric in Equation 13–4 was performed by introducing a penalty term $Reg(s)$ to the least-squares method; the latter was derived from the norm of the tensor field gradient:

$$\begin{cases} Reg(s) = \dfrac{n_s\gamma}{V_t}\displaystyle\int s^2 dV \\ s^2 = \displaystyle\sum_j \left[Trace\left\{ \sum_i \dfrac{\partial \Psi_i}{\partial x_j}\ln(A_i) \right\}^2 \right] \end{cases}, \qquad (13\text{--}5)$$

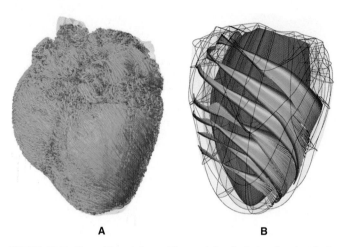

FIGURE 13–3. Fibers (**A**) and sheets (**B**) at end-diastole. Red surface in B is the endocardium. Colors in the sheets in B trace individual fibers.

where integration was performed over the volume of finite elements, n_s is the number of samples (tensors) in the DTMRI data set, V_t is the tissue volume of the ventricles, $\gamma = 1.0$ is the penalty factor, and $\frac{\partial \Psi_i}{\partial x_j}$ are the derivatives of the Hermite basis functions with respect to a fixed set of global coordinates, x_j.

Step 6 in Fig. 13–1 displays the fiber orientations for the example slice, whereas fiber and sheet organization in both meshes are shown in Fig. 13–3. It is important to note that our image-based reconstruction captures all the structural and geometrical remodeling in DHF. This approach is radically different from previous attempts at modeling heart failure,[63,64] where the ventricles were enlarged to simply approximate the increased size of the heart without representing the structural remodeling (ie, that of fibers and laminar sheets) associated with heart failure.

■ SIMULATING ELECTROMECHANICAL ACTIVITY IN THE NORMAL AND FAILING HEARTS

Structure and Modules of the Multiscale Electromechanical Model

A schematic of the model is shown in Fig. 13–4. It is composed of two coupled parts, electrical and mechanical. Physiologically, as an electrical wave propagates through the heart, the depolarization

of each myocyte initiates the release of calcium (Ca) from the intracellular Ca stores, followed by binding of Ca to troponin C and cross-bridge cycling, which forms the basis for contractile protein movement and development of active tension in the cell, ultimately resulting in contraction of the ventricles.

Accordingly, the *electrical* component of the model (see Fig. 13–4, left) simulates the propagation of a wave of transmembrane potential by solving a reaction-diffusion partial differential equation (PDE) for the transmembrane potential[79] on the electrical finite element mesh. This equation describes current flow through cardiac tissue, which has orthotropic passive electrical conductivities, the latter stemming from the cellular organization into fibers and laminar sheets. The current flow is driven by active processes of ionic exchange across myocyte membranes. These active electrical processes are represented by an *ionic model* of the myocyte membrane (see Fig. 13–4, left), where current flow through ion channels, pumps and exchangers in the myocyte membrane, and subcellular Ca cycling between cell compartments and buffers are represented by a set of ordinary differential equations (ODEs) and algebraic equations. Simultaneous solution of the PDE with the set of ionic model equations represents simulation of electrical wave propagation in the heart; a review of all the modeling details can be found in Plank et al.[79]

The intracellular Ca released during the electrical activation couples the electrical and *mechanical* components (see Fig. 13–4). It serves as an input to the cell *myofilament model* representing the generation of active tension within each myocyte, in which a set of ODEs and algebraic equations describe Ca binding to troponin C, cooperativity between regulatory proteins, and crossbridge cycling. Contraction of the ventricles arises from the active tension generated by the cardiac cells. Ventricular deformation is described by the equations of passive cardiac mechanics,[85-88] with the myocardium being an orthotropic (due to fiber and sheet organization), hyperelastic, and nearly incompressible material with passive mechanical properties defined by an exponential strain energy function. Simultaneous solution of the myofilament model equations and those representing passive cardiac mechanics on the finite element mechanical mesh constitutes simulation of cardiac contraction. During contraction, the stretch ratio (ie, the ratio of myocyte length before and after deformation) and its time derivative affect myofilament dynamics, including lengthdependent Ca sensitivity, providing a feedback loop.

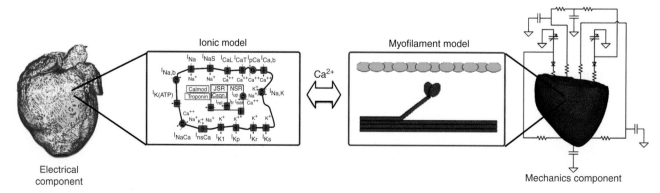

FIGURE 13–4. Schematic diagram of the electromechanical model.

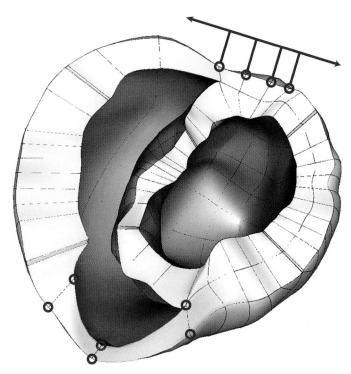

FIGURE 13–5. Boundary conditions based on cine magnetic resonance imaging. The nodes circled in blue were constrained to move only in the direction of the blue arrow, and the nodes circled in red were fixed in all directions.

To determine the appropriate boundary conditions for the mechanical component of the model, publically available animation frames of cine-MRI (INRIA, Asclepios Research Project; http://www-sop.inria.fr/asclepios/) were analyzed; they revealed that tissue near the pulmonary artery remained stationary during contraction. Additionally, tissue movement at the surface of the posterior wall was restricted to a single direction. These boundary conditions are implemented in the model by fixing the red nodes and by restricting the movement of the blue nodes to the direction indicated by the blue arrow (Fig. 13–5). In addition, the entire ventricular base movement is restricted in a fixed plane, which is perpendicular to longitudinal axis of the ventricles.

Finally, to simulate the cardiac cycle, conditions on chamber volume and pressure are imposed by a lumped-parameter model of the systemic and pulmonic circulatory systems, as shown in Fig. 13–4. The lumped-parameter model is based on the implementation by Kerckhoffs et al,[89] which we modify[82] to ensure stability of intraventricular pressure. This approach results in realistic pressure-volume loops, as shown later in Fig. 13–8C. It is important to note that unlike previous studies, the intraventricular pressures are not calculated using the penalty law, which requires the particular volume of the ventricles at each moment of cardiac cycle to be set.[58] Instead, the intraventricular pressures are set as additional unknown variables to the nonlinear system of equations of the finite element method. Such modifications simplify the algorithm of coupling the ventricular and circulatory system model and improve the stability and accuracy of the numerical calculations.

It is important to note that our electromechanical model is generic and uses any cardiac mesh (idealized-geometry or image-based); its modular structure allows for the use of ionic and myofilament models of any species. Here, we use the DHF canine heart geometry and implement ionic and myofilament models specific to the failing canine myocyte.

Choice of Species-Specific Ionic and Myofilament Models

We use the canine ionic model by Fox et al,[45] suitable for organ-level simulations,[79] which we modify to include an equation for Ca buffering by troponin C.[90] For the myofilament model, we use the Rice et al[91] comprehensive yet tractable model of cell mechanics. However, it was developed for the rabbit cell; thus, we modify it[92] to incorporate protein kinetics specific to the canine.

Modifications in the Ionic and Myofilament Models to Represent Remodeling in Heart Failure at the Cellular Level

Based on canine-specific heart failure remodeling data from the literature, we implement the following additional changes in the canine *ionic models*: K channels carrying I_{to} and I_{Kl} are downregulated by 66% and 32%, respectively[8]; SERCA pump is downregulated by 62%; and NCX is upregulated by 75%.[9] These alterations in ionic currents result in an altered shape of the canine action potential in heart failure, as shown in Fig.13–6A, as well as in a Ca transient with reduced magnitude and increased duration, as validated with experimental data.[9] Because the Ca transient serves as an input to the *myofilament model*, the profile of the active tension developed by the failing myocyte is different from that in the normal cell; it exhibits a reduced peak amplitude and a longer twitch duration (Fig. 13–6B), consistent with experimental findings.[93,94]

Electrical and Mechanical Tissue Properties in Heart Failure

Experimental data have shown lateralization and hypophosphorylation of Cx43 in heart failure.[6,7] Cx43 controls the passage of current from one cell to the next; accordingly, we decrease the values of the electrical conductivities in the tissue by 30%. To account for the heart failure changes in the tissue mechanical properties, the passive stiffness constant of the exponential strain energy function is increased by 500%, representing altered expression ratios of titin and collagen isoforms.[10,11]

Implementing Sinus Rhythm, LBBB, and bi-V Pacing

To represent activity corresponding to sinus rhythm, the model ventricles are activated at discrete locations along the endocardial

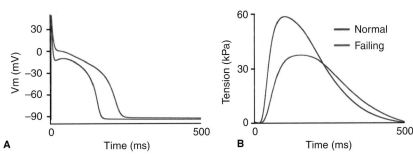

FIGURE 13–6. Epicardial canine action potentials (Vm; **A**) and single-cell twitches (**B**) for normal and failing myocytes.

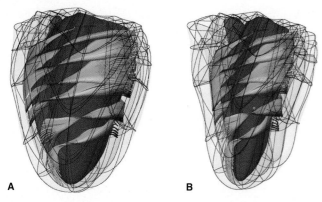

FIGURE 13–7. Fibers within laminar sheets near the endocardium of the normal canine ventricles visualized at end-diastole (**A**) and end-systole (**B**).

surface of the LV and RV free walls[95] as if activation originates from the Purkinje network. Appropriate timings and locations of the stimuli are chosen such that the resultant 3D electrical propagation matches well with experimental data.[96,97] Dyssynchronous activation in LBBB is modeled by stimulating only the RV subendocardium. Lastly, bi-V pacing during LBBB is simulated by simultaneously pacing at the RV apex endocardium and at the epicardium of the LV lateral wall near the base.

Evaluating Electromechanical Delay in the Model

To determine the 3D distribution of electromechanical delay (EMD), the local time difference between myocyte depolarization and onset of myofiber shortening is evaluated throughout the ventricles. Myocyte depolarization is defined as the instant at which the transmembrane potential exceeds 0 mV. Onset of shortening is defined as the instant when local myofiber shortening reaches 10% of its maximal value.[98]

RESULTS OF SIMULATIONS

■ THE NORMAL CANINE VENTRICLES

Using the normal canine geometry, several cardiac cycles were simulated during sinus rhythm to demonstrate the feasibility of using the model assembly pipeline to generate ventricular models of electromechanics and simulate electromechanical activity. Figure 13–7 shows the ventricles and laminar sheets near the endocardium in two stages of the cardiac cycle: end-diastole (Fig. 13–7A) and end-systole (Fig. 13–7B).

Temporal traces of transmural strain, active tension from the cardiac myofilament models, and pressure-volume relationships and torsion deformations of the ventricles during contractions are shown in Fig. 13–8. The simulated fiber strain (Fig. 13–8A),

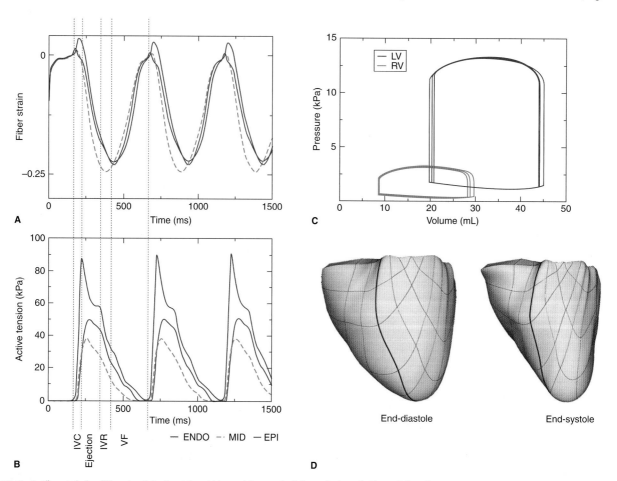

FIGURE 13–8. A. Fiber strain for different wall depths at the mid-base of the anterior left ventricular wall. The end-diastolic state of the first cycle is the reference state for the strain calculations. **B.** Active tensions at the same locations as in panel A. ENDO, endocardium; EPI, epicardium; IVC, isovolumic contraction; IVR, isovolumic relaxation; MID, midwall; VF, ventricular filling. **C.** Left ventricular (LV) and right ventricular (RV) pressure-volume loops during the cardiac cycles. **D.** End-diastolic and end-systolic states of the ventricles. Thick lines emphasize torsion deformation of the ventricles during contraction.

which was obtained from the mid-base of the ventricles at locations in the endocardium, midwall, and epicardium, demonstrated prestretching of myofibers during the isovolumic phase of contraction, which agrees with previous experimental findings.[99] The model also reproduces the experimentally observed larger amplitude of shortening at the midwall as compared with myocardial layers located closer to the wall surfaces.[99,100]

In addition to transmural strain, the model provides information about the transmural stress distribution, which is difficult to obtain experimentally. Figure 13–8B shows the active tension at the same transmural locations as in Fig. 13–8A. Maximum tension developed by myofibers at the midwall is less than that at the endocardium and epicardium due to the faster shortening during the ejection phase. The magnitude of the tension at the endocardium is the largest among the different layers due to the larger end-diastolic strain (with respect to the undeformed, stress-free reference state of the ventricles). The model also provides information about global variables of ventricular contraction such as ventricular pressure and volume. Pressure-volume loops for the LV and RV are shown in Fig. 13–8C.

The model also reproduces well-known features of the ventricular contraction such as apical twisting. Figure 13–8D shows the anterior view of ventricles during contraction and demon-

strates clearly twisting of the ventricular apex relative to the base. The angle of apical twist was roughly estimated to be 35° to 40°, which agrees with experimental data.[101]

■ THE FAILING CANINE VENTRICLES

A better understanding of the 3D spatiotemporal interactions between electrical activation and mechanical contraction in the DHF heart will ultimately lead to significant improvements in the selection criteria for CRT candidates and to rational optimization of CRT delivery. The image-based electromechanical model developed here can be used to enhance this understanding. The capabilities of the model were demonstrated in the previous section; here, we illustrate, for the first time, the application of the model to understanding the mechanism and characteristics of electromechanical function in DHF. Specifically, the electromechanical model of the DHF canine ventricles was used here to obtain insight into the electromechanical activation sequence in the DHF heart and how it is altered in bi-V pacing. To do so, we examined the distribution of EMD during LBBB and following bi-V pacing.

Figure 13–9 presents transmural maps of the electrical activation times (Fig. 13–9A) and onset of myofiber shortening times (Fig. 13–9B) during LBBB (left) and following bi-V pacing

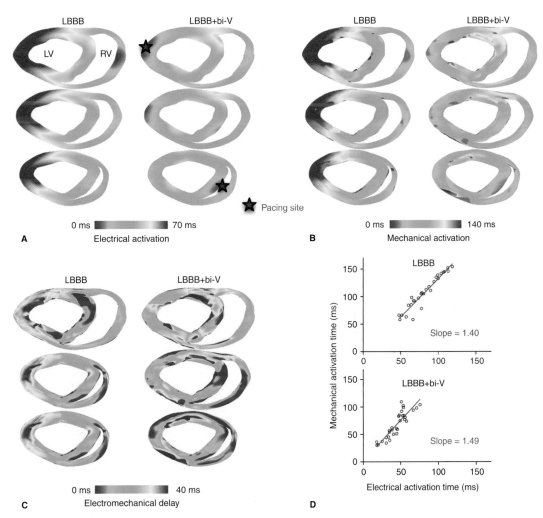

FIGURE 13–9. Transmural maps in a short axis view of electrical activation time (**A**), onset of myofiber shortening time (**B**), and electromechanical delay (**C**) during left bundle branch block (LBBB; left) and following biventricular (bi-V) pacing (right). **D.** Plots of electrical activation times versus mechanical activation times for LBBB (top) and following bi-V pacing (bottom).

(right). In LBBB, electrical and mechanical activations begin from the RV endocardium and propagate toward the LV lateral wall. Following bi-V pacing, the depolarization wave propagates from the pacing sites (the RV endocardial apex and the LV epicardial base) toward the LV anterior and posterior wall; in general, mechanical activation proceeds in the same direction.

The corresponding transmural maps of EMD are shown in Fig. 13–9C and demonstrate that the 3D distribution of EMD is heterogeneous for both LBBB and following bi-V pacing. In LBBB, EMD is longest at the late-depolarized lateral wall. Following bi-V pacing, EMD at the lateral wall was reduced and shorter than that at the anterior and posterior walls. Regression analysis of myofiber shortening onset times versus the electrical activation times is shown in Figure 13–9D. For both LBBB and bi-V, the slope of the regression lines was greater than 1, indicating that as depolarization occurred later, the onset of myofiber shortening was progressively more delayed; thus, regions that were depolarized later were characterized with a longer EMD.

Why would examining the distribution of EMD in the DHF heart be important to CRT? Previous studies have demonstrated that the LV pacing location is important for optimizing CRT response[30-33]; however, it is unclear what criteria should be used to determine the optimal pacing location. The results presented in this section suggest that minimizing the regions with extended EMD may be the approach to optimizing CRT therapy.

CONCLUSION

This chapter presents an overview of DHF, CRT, and the image-based electromechanical model developed in our lab that has demonstrated high hope for uncovering the mechanisms of electromechanical dyssynchrony, for optimization of CRT, and for possible personalized approach to the therapy. The chapter focuses, to a large extent, on the actual development of the electromechanical model and its features and, in particular, the fact that the model is developed from high-resolution MRI and DTMRI scans, allowing for an individualized approach to understanding cardiac electromechanical dysfunction. Such an image-based approach takes into account the structural remodeling of the individual failing heart and allows for seamless integration with other simulation tools such as mesh generation from segmented images and simulation of electrical and mechanical function, as presented here. The new electromechanical model presented here opens a new avenue for exploring cardiac electromechanical behavior and presents possibilities for translating the approach to patient-specific approaches to CRT optimization.

REFERENCES

1. Lloyd-Jones D, Adams R, Carnethon M, et al. Heart Disease and stroke statistics–2009 update: a report from the American Heart Association Statistics Committee and Stroke Statistics Subcommittee. *Circulation.* 2009;119:480-486.
2. Helm PA, Younes L, Beg MF, et al. Evidence of structural remodeling in the dyssynchronous failing heart. *Circ Res.* 2006;98:125-132.
3. Cheng A, Nguyen TC, Malinowski M, et al. Heterogeneity of left ventricular wall thickening mechanisms. *Circulation.* 2008;118:713-721.
4. LeGrice IJ, Takayama Y, Covell JW. Transverse shear along myocardial cleavage planes provides a mechanism for normal systolic wall thickening. *Circ Res.* 1995;77:182-193.
5. Hooks DA, Trew ML, Caldwell BJ, et al. Laminar arrangement of ventricular myocytes influences electrical behavior of the heart. *Circ Res.* 2007;101: e103-e112.
6. Akar FG, Nass RD, Hahn S, et al. Dynamic changes in conduction velocity and gap junction properties during development of pacing-induced heart failure. *Am J Physiol Heart Circ Physiol.* 2007;293:H1223-H1230.
7. Akar FG, Spragg DD, Tunin RS, et al. Mechanisms underlying conduction slowing and arrhythmogenesis in nonischemic dilated cardiomyopathy. *Circ Res.* 2004;95:717-725.
8. Kaab S, Nuss HB, Chiamvimonvat N, et al. Ionic mechanism of action potential prolongation in ventricular myocytes from dogs with pacing-induced heart failure. *Circ Res.* 1996;78:262-273.
9. O'Rourke B, Kass DA, Tomaselli GF, et al. Mechanisms of altered excitation-contraction coupling in canine tachycardia-induced heart failure. I: Experimental studies. *Circ Res.* 1999;84:562-570.
10. Marijianowski MM, Teeling P, Mann J, et al. Dilated cardiomyopathy is associated with an increase in the type I/type III collagen ratio: a quantitative assessment. *J Am Coll Cardiol.* 1995;25:1263-1272.
11. Wu Y, Bell SP, Trombitas K, et al. Changes in titin isoform expression in pacing-induced cardiac failure give rise to increased passive muscle stiffness. *Circulation.* 2002;106:1384-1389.
12. Bleeker GB, Bax JJ, Steendijk P, et al. Left ventricular dyssynchrony in patients with heart failure: pathophysiology, diagnosis and treatment. *Nat Clin Pract Cardiovasc Med.* 2006;3:213-219.
13. Nelson GS, Berger RD, Fetics BJ, et al. Left ventricular or biventricular pacing improves cardiac function at diminished energy cost in patients with dilated cardiomyopathy and left bundle-branch block. *Circulation.* 2000;102:3053-3059.
14. Sutton MG, Plappert T, Hilpisch KE, et al. Sustained reverse left ventricular structural remodeling with cardiac resynchronization at one year is a function of etiology: quantitative doppler echocardiographic evidence from the Multicenter Insync Randomized Clinical Evaluation (MIRACLE). *Circulation.* 2006;113:266-272.
15. Auricchio A, Stellbrink C, Butter C, et al. Clinical efficacy of cardiac resynchronization therapy using left ventricular pacing in heart failure patients stratified by severity of ventricular conduction delay. *J Am Coll Cardiol.* 2003;42:2109-2116.
16. Cleland JG, Daubert JC, Erdmann E, et al. The effect of cardiac resynchronization on morbidity and mortality in heart failure. *N Engl J Med.* 2005;352:1539-1549.
17. Kass DA. Cardiac resynchronization therapy. *J Cardiovasc Electrophysiol.* 2005;16(Suppl 1):S35-S41.
18. Fauchier L, Marie O, Casset-Senon D, et al. Reliability of QRS duration and morphology on surface electrocardiogram to identify ventricular dyssynchrony in patients with idiopathic dilated cardiomyopathy. *Am J Cardiol.* 2003;92:341-344.
19. Auricchio A, Stellbrink C, Block M, et al. Effect of pacing chamber and atrioventricular delay on acute systolic function of paced patients with congestive heart failure. The Pacing Therapies for Congestive Heart Failure Study Group. The Guidant Congestive Heart Failure Research Group. *Circulation.* 1999;99:2993-3001.
20. Pitzalis MV, Iacoviello M, Romito R, et al. Cardiac resynchronization therapy tailored by echocardiographic evaluation of ventricular asynchrony. *J Am Coll Cardiol.* 2002;40:1615-1622.
21. Fauchier L, Marie O, Casset-Senon D, et al. Interventricular and intraventricular dyssynchrony in idiopathic dilated cardiomyopathy: a prognostic study with Fourier phase analysis of radionuclide angioscintigraphy. *J Am Coll Cardiol.* 2002;40:2022-2030.
22. Yu CM, Chau E, Sanderson JE, et al. Tissue Doppler echocardiographic evidence of reverse remodeling and improved synchronicity by simultaneously delaying regional contraction after biventricular pacing therapy in heart failure. *Circulation.* 2002;105:438-445.
23. Bax JJ, Bleeker GB, Marwick TH, et al. Left ventricular dyssynchrony predicts response and prognosis after cardiac resynchronization therapy. *J Am Coll Cardiol.* 2004;44:1834-1840.
24. Chung ES, Leon AR, Tavazzi L, et al. Results of the Predictors of Response to CRT (PROSPECT) Trial. *Circulation.* 2008;117:2608-2616.
25. Beshai JF, Grimm RA, Nagueh SF, et al. Cardiac-resynchronization therapy in heart failure with narrow QRS complexes. *N Engl J Med.* 2007;357:2461-2471.
26. Bleeker GB, Kaandorp TA, Lamb HJ, et al. Effect of posterolateral scar tissue on clinical and echocardiographic improvement after cardiac resynchronization therapy. *Circulation.* 2006;113:969-976.

27. Adelstein EC, Saba S. Scar burden by myocardial perfusion imaging predicts echocardiographic response to cardiac resynchronization therapy in ischemic cardiomyopathy. *Am Heart J.* 2007;153:105-112.

28. White JA, Yee R, Yuan X, et al. Delayed enhancement magnetic resonance imaging predicts response to cardiac resynchronization therapy in patients with intraventricular dyssynchrony. *J Am Coll Cardiol.* 2006;48:1953-1960.

29. Choi KM, Kim RJ, Gubernikoff G, et al. Transmural extent of acute myocardial infarction predicts long-term improvement in contractile function. *Circulation.* 2001;104:1101-1107.

30. Butter C, Auricchio A, Stellbrink C, et al. Should stimulation site be tailored in the individual heart failure patient? *J Am Coll Cardiol.* 2000;86:144K-151K.

31. St John Sutton MG, Plappert T, Abraham WT, et al. Effect of cardiac resynchronization therapy on left ventricular size and function in chronic heart failure. *Circulation.* 2003;107:1985-1990.

32. Helm RH, Byrne M, Helm PA, et al. Three-dimensional mapping of optimal left ventricular pacing site for cardiac resynchronization. *Circulation.* 2007;115:953-961.

33. Ypenburg C, van Bommel RJ, Delgado V, et al. Optimal left ventricular lead position predicts reverse remodeling and survival after cardiac resynchronization therapy. *J Am Coll Cardiol.* 2008;52:1402 1409.

34. Butter C, Auricchio A, Stellbrink C, et al. Effect of resynchronization therapy stimulation site on the systolic function of heart failure patients. *Circulation.* 2001;104:3026-3029.

35. Leclercq F, Hager FX, Macia JC, et al. Left ventricular lead insertion using a modified transseptal catheterization technique: a totally endocardial approach for permanent biventricular pacing in end-stage heart failure. *Pacing Clin Electrophysiol.* 1999;22:1570-1575.

36. Ji S, Cesario DA, Swerdlow CD, et al. Left ventricular endocardial lead placement using a modified transseptal approach. *J Cardiovasc Electrophysiol.* 2004;15:234-236.

37. Fish JM, Brugada J, Antzelevitch C. Potential proarrhythmic effects of biventricular pacing. *J Am Coll Cardiol.* 2005;46:2340-2347.

38. van Deursen C, van Geldorp IE, Rademakers LM, et al. LV endocardial pacing improves resynchronization therapy in canine LBBB hearts. *Circ Arrhythm Electrophysiol.* 2009;2:580-587.

39. Rademakers LM, van Hunnik A, Lampert A, et al. Electrical and hemodynamic benefits of endocardial CRT with chronic infarction and LBBB. *Heart Rhythm.* 2009;6(Suppl 5):S237.

40. Spragg DD, Dong J, Fetics BJ, et al. Optimal LV endocardial pacing sites for CRT. *Heart Rhythm.* 2008;5(Suppl 5):S334.

41. Garrigue S, Jais P, Espil G, et al. Comparison of chronic biventricular pacing between epicardial and endocardial left ventricular stimulation using Doppler tissue imaging in patients with heart failure. *Am J Cardiol.* 2001;88:858-862.

42. Trayanova NA, Tice BM. Integrative computational models of cardiac arrhythmias: simulating the structurally realistic heart. *Drug Discov Today Dis Models.* 2009;6:85-91.

43. Luo CH, Rudy Y. A dynamic model of the cardiac ventricular action potential. II. Afterdepolarizations, triggered activity, and potentiation. *Circ Res.* 1994;74:1097-1113.

44. Mahajan A, Shiferaw Y, Sato D, et al. A rabbit ventricular action potential model replicating cardiac dynamics at rapid heart rates. *Biophys J.* 2008;94:392-410.

45. Fox JJ, McHarg JL, Gilmour RF Jr. Ionic mechanism of electrical alternans. *Am J Physiol Heart Circ Physiol.* 2002;282:H516-H530.

46. Weiss DL, Keller DU, Seemann G, et al. The influence of fibre orientation, extracted from different segments of the human left ventricle, on the activation and repolarization sequence: a simulation study. *Europace.* 2007;9(Suppl 6):vi96-vi104.

47. Arevalo H, Rodriguez B, Trayanova N. Arrhythmogenesis in the heart: multiscale modeling of the effects of defibrillation shocks and the role of electrophysiological heterogeneity. *Chaos.* 2007;17:015103.

48. Baher A, Qu Z, Hayatdavoudi A, et al. Short-term cardiac memory and mother rotor fibrillation. *Am J Physiol Heart Circ Physiol.* 2007;292:H180-H189.

49. Xie F, Qu Z, Yang J, et al. A simulation study of the effects of cardiac anatomy in ventricular fibrillation. *J Clin Invest.* 2004;113:686-693.

50. Ashihara T, Constantino J, Trayanova NA. Tunnel propagation of postshock activations as a hypothesis for fibrillation induction and isoelectric window. *Circ Res.* 2008;102:737-745.

51. Rodriguez B, Li L, Eason JC, et al. Differences between left and right ventricular chamber geometry affect cardiac vulnerability to electric shocks. *Circ Res.* 2005;97:168-175.

52. Rodriguez B, Tice BM, Eason JC, et al. Cardiac vulnerability to electric shocks during phase 1a of acute global ischemia. *Heart Rhythm.* 2004;1:695-703.

53. Legrice IJ, Hunter PJ, Smaill BH. Laminar structure of the heart: a mathematical model. *Am J Physiol Heart Circ Physiol.* 1997;272(5 Pt 2):H2466-H2476.

54. Usyk TP, Mazhari R, McCulloch AD. Effect of laminar orthotropic myofiber architecture on regional stress and strain in the canine left ventricle. *J Elasticity.* 2000;61:143-164.

55. Nickerson D, Smith N, Hunter P. New developments in a strongly coupled cardiac electromechanical model. *Europace.* 2005;7(Suppl 2):118-127.

56. Campbell SG, Howard E, Aguado-Sierra J, et al. Effect of transmurally heterogeneous myocyte excitation-contraction coupling on canine left ventricular electromechanics. *Exp Physiol.* 2009;94:541-552.

57. Usyk TP, McCulloch AD. Relationship between regional shortening and asynchronous electrical activation in a three-dimensional model of ventricular electromechanics. *J Cardiovasc Electrophysiol.* 2003;14(10 Suppl):S196-S202.

58. Usyk TP, LeGrice IJ, McCulloch AD. Computational model of three-dimensional cardiac electromechanics. *Comput Visual Sci.* 2002;4:249-247.

59. Kerckhoffs RC, Faris OP, Bovendeerd PH, et al. Timing of depolarization and contraction in the paced canine left ventricle: model and experiment. *J Cardiovasc Electrophysiol.* 2003;14(10 Suppl):S188-S195.

60. Kerckhoffs RC, Faris OP, Bovendeerd PH, et al. Electromechanics of paced left ventricle simulated by straightforward mathematical model: comparison with experiments. *Am J Physiol Heart Circ Physiol.* 2005;289:H1889-H1897.

61. Sermesant M, Delingette H, Ayache N. An electromechanical model of the heart for image analysis and simulation. *IEEE Trans Med Imaging.* 2006;25:612-625.

62. Kerckhoffs RC, Lumens J, Vernooy K, et al. Cardiac resynchronization: insight from experimental and computational models. *Prog Biophys Mol Biol.* 2008;97(2-3):543-561.

63. Usyk TP, McCulloch AD. Electromechanical model of cardiac resynchronization in the dilated failing heart with left bundle branch block. *J Electrocardiol.* 2003;36(Suppl):57-61.

64. Kerckhoffs RC, McCulloch AD, Omens JH, et al. Effects of biventricular pacing and scar size in a computational model of the failing heart with left bundle branch block. *Med Image Anal.* 2009;13:362-369.

65. Xia L, Huo M, Wei Q, et al. Analysis of cardiac ventricular wall motion based on a three-dimensional electromechanical biventricular model. *Phys Med Biol.* 2005;50:1901-1917.

66. Dou J, Xia L, Zhang Y, et al. Mechanical analysis of congestive heart failure caused by bundle branch block based on an electromechanical canine heart model. *Phys Med Biol.* 2009;54:353-371.

67. Reumann M, Osswald B, Doessel O. Noninvasive, automatic optimization strategy in cardiac resynchronization therapy. *Anadolu Kardiyol Derg.* 2007;7(Suppl 1):209-212.

68. Reumann M, Farina D, Miri R, et al. Computer model for the optimization of AV and VV delay in cardiac resynchronization therapy. *Med Biol Eng Comput.* 2007;45:845-854.

69. Vadakkumpadan F, Rantner LJ, Tice B, et al. Image-based models of cardiac structure with applications in arrhythmia and defibrillation studies. *J Electrocardiol.* 2009;42:157.e1-e10.

70. Vadakkumpadan F, Arevalo H, Prassl A, et al. Image-based models of cardiac structure in health and disease. *Wiley Interdisip Rev Syst Biol Med.* 2010;2:489-506.

71. Vigmond E, Vadakkumpadan F, Gurev V, et al. Towards predictive modelling of the electrophysiology of the heart. *Exp Physiol.* 2009;94:563-577.

72. Law MW, Chung AC. Vessel and intracranial aneurysm segmentation using multi-range filters and local variances. *Med Image Comput Comput Assist Interv.* 2007;10:866-874.

73. Adams R, Bischof L. Seeded region growing. *IEEE Trans Pattern Anal Mach Intell.* 1994;16:641-647.

74. Pierpaoli C, Basser PJ. Toward a quantitative assessment of diffusion anisotropy. *Magn Reson Med.* 1996;36:893-906.

75. Schmidt A, Azevedo CF, Cheng A, et al. Infarct tissue heterogeneity by magnetic resonance imaging identifies enhanced cardiac arrhythmia susceptibility in patients with left ventricular dysfunction. *Circulation.* 2007;115:2006-2014.

76. Wu MT, Tseng WY, Su MY, et al. Diffusion tensor magnetic resonance imaging mapping the fiber architecture remodeling in human myocardium after infarction: correlation with viability and wall motion. *Circulation.* 2006;114:1036-1045.

77. Yan AT, Shayne AJ, Brown KA, et al. Characterization of the peri-infarct zone by contrast-enhanced cardiac magnetic resonance imaging is a powerful predictor of post-myocardial infarction mortality. *Circulation.* 2006;114:32-39.

78. Pollard AE, Burgess MJ, Spitzer KW. Computer simulations of three-dimensional propagation in ventricular myocardium. Effects of intramural fiber rotation and inhomogeneous conductivity on epicardial activation. *Circ Res.* 1993;72:744-756.

79. Plank G, Zhou L, Greenstein JL, et al. From mitochondrial ion channels to arrhythmias in the heart: computational techniques to bridge the spatio-temporal scales. *Philos Transact A Math Phys Eng Sci.* 2008;366:3381-3409.

80. Prassl A, Kickinger F, Ahammer H, et al. Automatically generated, anatomically accurate meshes for cardiac electrophysiology problems. *IEEE Trans Biomed Eng.* 2009;56:1318-1330.

81. Onate E, Rojek J, Taylor RL, et al. Finite calculus formulation for incompressible solids using linear triangles and tetrahedra. *Int J Numer Meth Engng.* 2004;59:1473-1500.

82. Gurev V, Lee T, Constantino J, et al. Finite element ventricular models of cardiac mechanics based on MRI and DTMRI anatomy. *Biomech Model Mechanobiol.* June 30, 2010 [Epub ahead of print].

83. Nielsen PM, Le Grice IJ, Smaill BH, et al. Mathematical model of geometry and fibrous structure of the heart. *Am J Physiol Heart Circ Physiol.* 1991;260:H1365-H1378.

84. Bovendeerd PH, Arts T, Huyghe JM, et al. Dependence of local left ventricular wall mechanics on myocardial fiber orientation: a model study. *J Biomech.* 1992;25:1129-1140.

85. Arsigny V, Fillard P, Pennec X, et al. Log-Euclidean metrics for fast and simple calculus on diffusion tensors. *Magn Reson Med.* 2006;56:411-421.

86. Guccione JM, Costa KD, McCulloch AD. Finite element stress analysis of left ventricular mechanics in the beating dog heart. *J Biomech.* 1995; 28:1167-1177.

87. Usyk T, Legrice I, McCulloch A. Computational model of three-dimensional cardiac electromechanics. *Comput Visual Sci.* 2002;4:249-257.

88. Usyk TP, McCulloch AD. Electromechanical model of cardiac resynchronization in the dilated failing heart with left bundle branch block. *J Electrocardiol.* 2003;36(Suppl):57-61.

89. Kerckhoffs R, Neal M, Gu Q, et al. Coupling of a 3D finite element model of cardiac ventricular mechanics to lumped systems models of the systemic and pulmonic circulation. *Ann Biomed Eng.* 2007;35:1-18.

90. Solovyova O, L Katnelson, Guriev S, et al. Mechanical inhomogeneity of myocardium studied in parallel and serial cardiac muscle duplexes: experiments and models. *Chaos Solitons Fractals.* 2002;13:1685-1711.

91. Rice JJ, Wang F, Bers DM, et al. Approximate model of cooperative activation and crossbridge cycling in cardiac muscle using ordinary differential equations. *Biophys J.* 2008;95:2368-2390.

92. Campbell SG, Flaim SN, Leem CH, et al. Mechanisms of transmurally varying myocyte electromechanics in an integrated computational model. *Philos Transact A Math Phys Eng Sci.* 2008;366:3361-3368.

93. Hasenfuss G, Reinecke H, Studer R, et al. Relation between myocardial function and expression of sarcoplasmic reticulum Ca2+-ATPase in failing and nonfailing human myocardium. *Circ Res.* 1994;75:434-442.

94. del Monte F, O'Gara P, Poole-Wilson PA, et al. Cell geometry and contractile abnormalities of myocytes from failing human left ventricle. *Cardiovasc Res.* 1995;30:281-290.

95. Gurev V, Constantino J, Rice JJ, et al. Distribution of electromechanical delay in the ventricles: insights from a 3D electromechanical model of the heart. *Biophys J.* 2010;99:745-754.

96. Durrer D, van Dam RT, Freud GE, et al. Total excitation of the isolated human heart. *Circulation.* 1970;41:899-912.

97. Spach MS, Barr RC. Ventricular intramural and epicardial potential distributions during ventricular activation and repolarization in the intact dog. *Circ Res.* 1975;37:243-257.

98. Sengupta PP, Khandheria BK, Korinek J, et al. Apex-to-base dispersion in regional timing of left ventricular shortening and lengthening. *J Am Coll Cardiol.* 2006;47:163-172.

99. Ashikaga H, Coppola BA, Hopenfeld B, et al. Transmural dispersion of myofiber mechanics: implications for electrical heterogeneity in vivo. *J Am Coll Cardiol.* 2007;49:909-916.

100. Ashikaga H, Omens JH, Ingels NB JR, et al. Transmural mechanics at left ventricular epicardial pacing site. *Am J Physiol Heart Circ Physiol.* 2004;286:H2401-H2407.

101. Sengupta PP, Khandheria BK, Narula J. Twist and untwist mechanics of the left ventricle. *Heart Fail Clin.* 2008;4:315-324.

CHAPTER 14

COMPUTATIONAL CARDIAC ELECTROPHYSIOLOGY: MODELING TISSUE AND ORGAN

Martin J. Bishop, Hermenegild J. Arevalo,
Patrick M. Boyle, Natalia A. Trayanova,
Edward Vigmond, and Gernot Plank

INTRODUCTION / 233
Motivation for Using In Silico Approaches / 233
Advances in Computational Modeling
    of Cardiac Electrophysiology / 234
Future Perspectives / 235

**CONSTRUCTION OF MODELS
OF THE CARDIAC ANATOMY / 236**
Multimodal Image Acquisition / 236
Image Processing / 237
Mesh Generation / 240
Postprocessing / 240

**SIMULATING CARDIAC BIOELECTRIC ACTIVITY
AT THE TISSUE AND ORGAN LEVEL / 243**
Governing Equations / 243
Simulating the Purkinje Network / 244
Temporal Discretization / 246
Spatial Discretization / 247
Numerical Solution / 248
Performing in Silico Experiments / 249

APPLICATIONS OF THE MODELING METHODOLOGY / 253
Optimizing Defibrillation Therapy / 253
Elucidating the Role of the Purkinje Network / 257
Simulations of Postinfarction Ventricular
    Tachycardias / 260
Outlook / 261

INTRODUCTION

The heart is characterized by a complex electromechanical activity essential for the sustenance of body function. Cardiac disease is the leading cause of morbidity and mortality in the industrialized world,[1] imposing a major burden on health care systems. Current therapies rely, to a large extent, on implantable devices, administration of drugs, or the ablation of tissue. Although these therapies may improve a patient's condition significantly, they are palliative rather than curative, and undesired adverse effects of varying degrees of severity are quite common.[2-5] In the quest of devising novel, safer, and more effective therapies to reduce medical costs and treatment duration, developing a comprehensive understanding of cardiac structure and function in health and disease is the strategy most likely to succeed and, thus, is a central focus of basic and clinical heart research. Traditionally, experimental work in conjunction with clinical studies was the dominant, if not exclusive, approach for inquiries into physiological function. Today, in the postgenomic era, a wider portfolio of techniques is employed, with computational modeling being another accepted approach, either as a complement to experimental work or as a stand-alone tool for exploratory testing of hypotheses. The need for computational modeling is mainly driven by the difficulty in dealing with the vast amount of available data, obtained from various subsystems of the heart, at different hierarchical levels of organization from different species, and with the complexity involved in the dynamics of interactions between subsystems within and across levels of organization. Computational modeling plays a pivotal, if not indispensable, role in harnessing these data for further advancing our mechanistic understanding of cardiac function.

◼ MOTIVATION FOR USING IN SILICO APPROACHES

Over the past decade, impressive advances in experimental technology have generated a wealth of information across all levels of biological organization for various species, including humans, ranging from the genetic scale of the cardiac system up to the entire organ. However, attempts to translate these large quantities of experimental data into safer and more effective therapies to the benefit of patients have largely proved to be elusive. In no small part, this results from the complexity of biological systems under study. They invariably comprise multiple subsystems, interacting with each other within and across levels of organization. Although biological systems can be dissected into many subcomponents, there is now a clear recognition that the interaction within and across levels of organization may produce emergent properties that simply cannot be predicted from "reductionist" analysis. Because these emerging properties are often not intuitive and not predictable from analyzing the subsystems in isolation, detailed understanding of individual subsystems may provide little mechanistic insight into functions at the organ level.[6] Moreover, due to the highly complex nonlinear relationship between a rapidly increasing amount of disparate experimental data on an increasingly larger number of biological subsystems involved, any attempts to gain new mechanistic insights at the level of a system by deriving a qualitative understanding of all the simultaneous interactions within and between subsystems simply by reasoning are futile. Due to the complexity of the system, conclusions may even be misleading and, most likely, will not withstand thorough quantitative scrutiny. Integrative research approaches are required to address these issues, and computational modeling is a key technology to achieve such integration.

Furthermore, computer modeling can aid in overcoming the numerous limitations of current experimental techniques by complementing in vivo or in vitro experiments with matching in silico* models. The most common experimental limitations

---

*In silico refers to performed on a computer or via a computer simulation.

include the following. (1) Current experimental techniques cannot resolve, with sufficient accuracy, electrical events confined to the depth of the myocardial walls, which limits observations to the surfaces of the heart. (2) Selectively changing a single parameter in a well-controlled manner without affecting any other important parameters of cardiac function is difficult because the technology required is not available or because sufficiently selective substances have not been developed yet. (3) Certain experimental techniques require modification of the substrate or the knock-out of other physiological functions. For instance, to optically map cardiac electrical activity, first, photometric dyes are required, which modify membrane physiology and are known to be cytotoxic, and second, electromechanical uncouplers are administered to suppress mechanical contraction, further modulating physiological function. Caution is advised when interpreting such data because potentially important regulatory mechanisms are excluded.[7] (4) Experimental studies are mainly performed in animals, but species differences in the distribution and kinetics of ion channels are significant. As a result, drugs, for instance, may have significantly different effects in humans than in other species. (5) Due to the invasive nature, most advanced experimental methods are limited to animal studies and cannot be applied clinically to humans. Hence, available data from human studies are very limited, and available animal models do not adequately reflect the evolution of cardiovascular diseases in people.

■ ADVANCES IN COMPUTATIONAL MODELING OF CARDIAC ELECTROPHYSIOLOGY

Biophysically detailed cell modeling was introduced as early as 1952 in neuroscience, through the seminal modeling work of Hodgkin and Huxley on the squid giant axon.[8] Pioneered by Noble in the 1960s,[9] first models of cardiac cellular activity were proposed, but the first computer models for studying bioelectric activity at the tissue level did not emerge until the 1980s.[10] By today's standards, the level of detail in early modeling work was very limited. Computational performance was poor, efficient numerical techniques had not been fully developed, and descriptions of cellular dynamics were lacking many details. To keep simulations tractable, the cardiac geometry was approximated by geometrically very simple structures such as one-dimensional (1D) strands, two-dimensional (2D) sheets,[11,12] and three-dimensional (3D) slabs.[13] Although geometrically simple models continue to be used, due to their main advantage of simplicity, which facilitates the dissection of mechanisms, it became quickly recognized, maybe unsurprisingly, that observations made at the organ level cannot be reproduced without accounting for organ anatomy. The combined effects of structural complexity and the various functional heterogeneities in a realistic heart led to complex behavior that is hard to predict or investigate with overly simplified models. Besides computational restrictions, simple geometries were also popular because electric circuitry analogs could be used to represent the tissue as a lattice of interconnected resistors or a set of transversely interconnected core-conductor models.[11] Thus, well-established techniques for electric circuit analysis could

be applied, and simple discretization schemes based on the finite difference method became a standard due to their ease of implementation. With the advent of continuum formulations,[14] derived by homogenization of discrete tissue components,[15] and the adoption of more advanced spatial discretization techniques such as refined variants of the finite difference method,[16,17] the finite element method,[18,19] and the finite volume method,[20,21] the stage was set for anatomically realistic models of the heart. During the past few years, anatomically realistic computer simulations of electrical activity in ventricular slices,[22-24] whole ventricles,[25-28] and atria[29-31] have become accessible. Such models are considered as state-of-the-art; nonetheless, many simplifications persist:

- The geometry of the organ is represented in a stylized fashion ("one heart geometry fits all" approach)[25,26]; only parts of the heart are modeled, such as slices across the ventricles.[22]

- The computational mesh discretization is coarser than the size of the single cell (100 μm) to diminish the degrees of freedom in the model. This approach leads to (1) underrepresentation of (to the degree of fully ignoring) the finer details of the cardiac anatomy, such as endocardial trabeculations or papillary muscles and (2) the necessity to adjust, in an ad-hoc manner, the tissue conductivity tensors in order to avoid artificial scaling of the wavelength, thus compensating for the dependence of conduction velocities on grid granularity. That is, as the grid is coarsened with all other model parameters remaining unchanged, conduction velocity becomes reduced, and thus, the wavelength is diminished, with conduction block occurring above a certain spatial discretization limit.

- The myocardial mass is treated as a homogeneous continuum, without representing intramyocardial discontinuities such as vascularization, cleavage planes, or patches of fat or collagen.

- The specialized cardiac conduction system (ie, the sinoatrial node, the atrioventricular node, and the Purkinje system [PS]) is typically not represented in the whole organ simulations, although a few exceptions exist.[32-34]

- Functional gradients in the transmural[35] and apicobasal directions,[36] as well as differences between left ventricle (LV) and right ventricle (RV),[37] are often ignored.

- The conductivity tensors in the ventricles are orthotropic due to the presence of laminae.[38] Most, if not all, whole ventricular models do not account for this property. Besides, unlike the transmural rotation of fibers, the laminar arrangement cannot be described as easily by a rule because transmural variation of sheet angles appears to be spatially heterogeneous.[39]

- Myocardial membrane ion transport kinetics is modeled in a simplified fashion.[18,40] Reduced models preserve salient features such as excitability, refractoriness, and electrical restitution; these are usually represented phenomenologically at the scale of the cell (so that they can be easily manipulated).

Similar to geometrically simplified models, the fairly long list of simplifications does not restrict the utility of such models. In recent years, computational whole heart modeling has become an essential approach in the quest for integration of knowledge as evidenced by numerous contributions that led to novel insights into the electromechanical function of the heart.

FUTURE PERSPECTIVES

Despite the utility of current models, the underlying concepts and technologies are evolving at an increasingly faster pace with the aim to build the basis for comprehensive and detailed (high-dimensional) models that realistically represent as many of the known biological interactions as possible. Although this is clearly a goal worthwhile pursuing, one has to keep in mind that accounting for more and more mechanisms does not necessarily lead to deeper insights into systems behavior. Rather than accounting for all known details, modeling environments that enable researchers to flexibly choose the subsystems relevant for a particular question, as well as the level of detail for each subsystem, are sought. This flexibility helps to better balance the computational effort and to focus on specific aspects of a problem without being overwhelmed and distracted by the myriad of details. That is, some subsystems will be represented by high-dimensional models, whereas others are represented by reduced low-dimensional models, which often use nonlinear dynamics approaches to capture phenomenologically essential emergent behaviors. Although such flexibility is desirable, the involved technical challenges are formidable. Software engineering considerations begin to carry more weight to reconcile flexibility, reusability, and efficiency of increasingly more complex software stacks. The time scales and efforts involved in the development process of simulation tools as presented here are fairly substantial, at the scale of tens of man years, which complicates the implementation within an academic environment considerably and also raises sustainability issues that are not straightforward to address.

Impressive advances in imaging modalities, which provide 3D or even four-dimensional (4D) imaging data at an unprecedented resolution and quality, have led to an increased interest in using anatomically detailed, tomographically reconstructed models. Not only can anatomic parameters be quantitatively assessed with current imaging technology, but functional parameters can also be assessed. Growing access to such data sets has motivated the development of computational techniques that aim at providing a framework for the integration of data obtained from various imaging modalities into a single comprehensive computer model of an organ, which can be used for in silico experimentation. Quite often, more than one imaging modality has to be used and combined with electrocardiographic mapping techniques to complete the diagnostic picture. Although a multimodal approach complicates the model construction process, because various data sources have to be fused to precisely overlap in the same space, for the sake of biophysically accurate parametrization of in silico models, potentially relevant information is added that may improve the predictive power of the model. Further, interrelating multimodal diagnostic parameters, interpreting their relationships, and predicting the impact of procedures that modify these parameters can be challenging tasks, even for the most experienced physicians. In those cases where suitable mechanistic frameworks have been developed already to describe the relationship between diagnostic parameters and their

dependency on parameters of cardiac function, computer modeling can be used to quantitatively evaluate these relationships. There is a legitimate hope that computational modeling may contribute to better inform clinical diagnosis and guide the selection of appropriate therapies in a patient-specific manner.

Currently, the number of tomographically reconstructed anatomic models used in cardiac modeling is fairly small. This has to be attributed, to a large extent, to the technical challenges involved in image-based grid generation, which renders model generation an elaborate and time-consuming task. The small number and the lack of general availability of simulators that are sufficiently flexible, robust, and efficient to support in silico experiments using such computationally expensive models are further obstacles. However, recent technological advances have led to a simplification, facilitating model generation within a time scale approaching hours, rather than days or weeks. The speed and ease of use of image-based model generation pipelines is about to lower the barrier for using individualized models. Although heart models based on a single individual or stylized models derived from a single data set may be well suited for studying generic questions, it is important to critically question gained insights because there is clearly a danger of introducing a bias by relying on a single model that may or may not be representative for a species. Knowing that intersubject variability is quite substantial and having the ultimate aspiration of personalized medicine in mind, individualized models may prove to be of higher predictive value for specific questions because they allow representation of anatomical and functional information on a case-by-case basis in an individualized subject-specific manner.

Unlike in basic research, time constraints in a clinical context can be more restricting, and the cycle model definition, parametrization, and execution of an in silico experiment have to be seen before the background of a clinical work flow. There are obstacles to overcome that currently prevent the refinement of these cycles. First, the biophysically detailed parametrization of a subject-specific in silico heart is a nontrivial problem and will require major research efforts. Second, the computational expenses of conducting in silico experiments are substantial, which may pose a problem when fast turnaround times are key for diagnostic value. Although current simulators cannot deliver results in real time yet, dramatic improvements in numerical techniques and modeling approaches suggest that a near real-time performance with computer simulations of cardiac electromechanical activity may indeed be achievable within a time horizon of only a few years. This optimistic view is based on current developments in the high-performance computing (HPC) industry, which promise to deliver enormously increased computational power at a much higher packing density, and the capability of recent algorithmic developments that promise optimal scalability, a key feature to be able to take advantage of future HPC architectures.

The goal of this chapter is to present an overview of current state-of-the-art advances toward using anatomically detailed, tomographically reconstructed, in silico models for predictive computational modeling of the heart as developed recently by the authors of this chapter. We first outline the methodology for constructing electrophysiological models derived from imaging data sets. Further, the mathematical and numerical underpinnings required for building advanced in silico cardiac simulators are presented in detail, along with details on practical aspects of the modeling cycle in electrophysiological studies. Finally, we provide three examples that demonstrate the use of these models, focusing specifically on optimization of defibrillation therapy, the role of the specialized conduction system in the formation of arrhythmias, and finally, a very detailed model of myocardial infarction for studying arrhythmogenesis in the canine ventricles.

CONSTRUCTION OF MODELS OF THE CARDIAC ANATOMY

■ MULTIMODAL IMAGE ACQUISITION

To construct geometrically realistic models of cardiac anatomy, such information must be first obtained via various different imaging modalities and then processed and used in model construction. Depending on the specific application of the model, there is generally not a single ideal imaging modality to generate

the most complete model, and fusion of image data obtained from various different modalities is commonplace. This can involve combining structural and functional imaging data, often from modalities that probe such information at a range of different scales from the subcellular to the whole organ.

Anatomical Magnetic Resonance Imaging

In the past decade or so, efforts have been focused on developing techniques to construct 3D computational cardiac models directly from magnetic resonance (MR) data, due to the nondestructive nature of that technique.[41] However, the detail and anatomic complexity of the resulting models have been limited by the inherent resolution limits of MR data sets, often >100 μm or worse. In the last few years, the advent of stronger magnets and refined scanning protocols has significantly increased the resolution of anatomical MR scans, such that small mammalian hearts now can have MR voxel dimensions of approximately 20 to 25 μm.[42,43] An example of a high-resolution anatomic MR scan of a rabbit heart with voxel resolution of approximately 25 μm isotropic is shown in Fig. 14–1A.

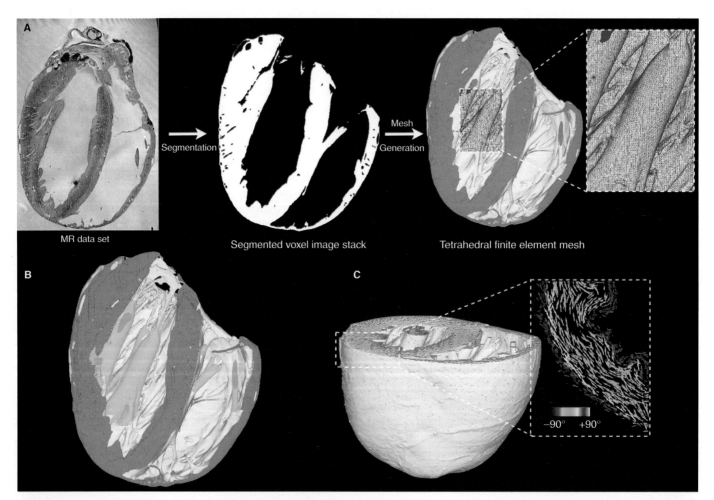

FIGURE 14–1. A. Magnetic resonance (MR)-to-model pipeline. **Left.** Longitudinal slice from a high-resolution MR image of the rabbit still heart with resolution of approximately 25 μm isotropic.[43] **Center.** Segmentation of the high-resolution MR data set to produce binary segmented voxel image stack with atria removed. **Right.** Generation of a high-resolution tetrahedral finite element mesh directly from segmented voxel stack. Highlighted region shows high quality of mesh representation of intricate endocardial surface structures. **B.** Visualization of tagged structures within the ventricular model showing papillary muscles (green) and valves (blue), generated via manually created masks prior to mesh generation. **C.** Visualization of fiber vectors incorporated into the finite element mesh using the minimum distance algorithm described in the "Assignment of Fibrous Architecture" section.

As a result of this recent increase in attainable resolution, anatomical MR imaging (MRI) is now capable of providing a wealth of information regarding fine-scaled cardiac structural complexity. Such MR data are currently allowing accurate identification of microscopic features such as the coronary vasculature, extracellular cleft spaces, and the free-running PS, as well as macroscopic structures such as trabeculations and papillary muscles. However, differentiation of different tissue types is often problematic in anatomical MR, due to the very similar signal intensities recorded from functionally different tissue regions of the preparation. Furthermore, information regarding the organization of cardiomyocytes into cardiac fibers[44] and the laminar structure of the myocardial wall[45] is unattainable with normal anatomic MRI.

Diffusion Tensor MRI

Myocardial structural information is more commonly obtained using a variation on the conventional anatomical MR protocol, called *diffusion tensor MRI* (DT-MRI). In DT-MRI, the measurement of the preferential direction of water molecule diffusion can be directly related to the underlying fiber architecture of the sample. It has been shown that the primary eigenvector from the diffusion tensor data (representing the direction of greatest water diffusion) corresponds faithfully with the cardiomyocyte direction (commonly referred to as the fiber direction), being validated with histological measurements.[46] Similar measurements also suggest that the tertiary eigenvector represents the sheet-normal direction, although this correlation is still controversially debated.[47]

Although recent advances in DT-MRI protocols have reduced voxel resolutions to approximately 100 μm isotropic for small mammalian hearts, this is still approximately an order of magnitude greater than corresponding anatomical scans,[43] which can cause problems when combining information from the two modalities. Due to this relatively low resolution, partial volume effects at tissue boundaries can also result in significant inaccuracies in predicted fiber orientation in these regions, particularly evident at epicardial/endocardial surfaces. Such effects occur when edge voxels contain a significant proportion of nontissue (where diffusion is generally isotropic) within their boundaries, meaning that the signal from these voxels does not accurately represent the underlying tissue structure in these boundary regions. This can also prove problematic close to intramural blood vessel cavities and extracellular cleft regions. Furthermore, traditional DT-MRI techniques have difficulties resolving more than one prevailing cell alignment direction in any one voxel, which can cause inaccuracies in regions such as the papillary muscle insertion site on the endocardium or where the RV and LV meet close to the septum, sites where there is known to be an abrupt change in fiber orientation. However, the development of novel DT-MRI protocols, such as Q-ball imaging,[48] have been shown in recent preliminary studies to be able to successfully locate these regions of "mixed" fiber vectors, building on the success of such techniques used previously in brain DT-MRI acquisition to delineate regions of neural fiber crossing.

■ IMAGE PROCESSING

Following the acquisition of high-resolution structural and functional imaging data sets, described earlier, such information must then be processed and transformed into a usable format to facilitate the generation of anatomically detailed computational cardiac models. One important aspect of this is that all relevant information regarding gross cardiac anatomy, histoarchitectural heterogeneity, and structural anisotropy acquired in the images must be successfully translated over to the final model, so far as resolution requirements permit. Second, the computational pipeline of technology established for the analysis and processing of the images, and the generation and parameterization of the models from the imaging data should be as automated as possible, minimizing manual interaction. The development of such an automated pipeline will facilitate its use alongside imaging atlas data sets to investigate the causal effect of intrapopulation heterogeneities on simulations of cardiac function.

Segmentation and Feature Extraction

Anatomical MR data are the most common imaging data currently being used to construct the geometric basis of computational cardiac models. The first stage of the MR-to-model pipeline is to faithfully extract all of the complex geometric information present in the MRIs, which can then be carried over and used in the computational model. This is done by the process of segmentation. Segmentation is a broad and widely used technique within medical image analysis that involves labeling voxels based on their association with different regions, objects, or boundaries within the image. In certain cases, this can be done manually, for example, a highly experienced physician may segment by hand a region of tumorous tissue within an MRI or computed tomography (CT) scan. Alternatively, computational algorithms can be developed and used, based on a priori knowledge of the image features, to automatically segment regions of interest within the image, ideally with little or no manual input. To generate a computational model from cardiac MRIs, our initial goal is simply to identify those voxels in the MR data set that belong to cardiac "tissue" and those that represent nontissue or "background." The background medium is generally identified in an MR scan as the lighter areas within the ventricular and atrial cavities, blood vessel lumens, the extracellular cleft spaces, and the medium on the exterior of the heart surrounding the preparation. Successful discrimination between background and tissue translates the gray scale MRI data set into a binary black/white (0/1) image mask.

Segmentation of the high-resolution rabbit MR data set shown in Fig. 14–1A, left[43] was conducted using a level-set segmentation approach. Level-set methods are based on a numerical regimen for tracking the evolution of contours and surfaces.[49] The contour is embedded as the zero level set of a higher dimensional function [$\Psi(\mathbf{X}, t)$], which can be evolved under the control of a differential equation. Extracting the zero level set $\Gamma(\mathbf{X}, t) = ((\mathbf{X}, t) = 0)$ allows the contour to be obtained at any time. A generic level-set equation to compute the update of the solution ψ is given by:

$$\frac{d}{dt}\Psi = -\alpha \mathbf{A}(\mathbf{x}) \cdot \nabla \Psi - \beta P(\mathbf{x})\left|\nabla \Psi\right| + \gamma Z(\mathbf{x})\kappa\left|\nabla \Psi\right| \quad (14\text{–}1)$$

where A, P, and Z are the advection, propagation, and expansion terms, respectively. The scalar constants α, β, and γ weight the relative influence of each of the terms on the movement of the surface, and thus, Equation 14–1 represents a generic structure that can be adapted to the particular characteristics of the problem. Different level-set filters use different features of an image to govern the contour propagation (eg, explicit voxel intensity or local gradient values) and can thus be combined to provide robust segmentation algorithms. Combining level-set filters in a sequential pipeline can be beneficial to provide a good initialization for filters that are prone to get trapped in local minima of the related cost function in the iterative solution to Equation 14–1. Figure 14–1A shows the final segmented voxel image stack of the rabbit MR data set following segmentation using a level-set approach.[43]

The final stage in the segmentation process involves the delineation of the ventricles from the segmented binary voxel image stack to facilitate the generation of a purely ventricular computational model. This requirement is such that the presence of an insulating layer of connective tissue that separates the ventricles from the atria (the annulus fibrosus) precludes direct electrical conduction between atrial and ventricular tissue. As a result, ventricular computational models are developed to allow the study of ventricular electrical function in isolation from the atria. Segmentation of the ventricles was performed by manual selection of 20 to 30 points in every fifth long axis slice through the MR data set along the line believed to represent the atrioventricular border. Identification of such a line was often possible because the connective tissue annulus fibrosus appeared relatively darker than the surrounding myocardium in the MR data. A smooth surface was then fitted through the landmark points to define a 2D surface, dissecting the image volume; all tissue voxels residing above the plane were subsequently removed, leaving only the ventricular tissue beneath. Figure 14–1A (center) shows the final segmented ventricular voxel image stack with atrial tissue removed.

Tissue Classification and Voxel Tagging

Following discrimination between tissue and nontissue types in the segmentation process described earlier, it is further necessary to classify tissue voxels. Classification is either based on a priori knowledge or on additional complementary image sources or features that can be used to further differentiate functional or anatomical properties, both between different tissue types and also within a particular tissue type. Identifying such differences allows variations in electrical, structural, and/or mechanical parameters to be assigned on a per-region basis to tissue throughout the model, which is vital for realistic simulations of heart function. Each voxel can have one or more classifications, and for each classification, a numerical "tag" is assigned to the voxel. Importantly, these numerical tags within the voxel image stack are retained throughout the meshing process (see later section "Mesh Generation"), becoming associated with individual finite elements that make up the computational model.

Regions may be tagged in order to assign different cellular electrical properties to different tissue types. For example, the free-running Purkinje fibers are known to have very different electrical membrane dynamics compared with normal ventricular cells, requiring the use of specialized Purkinje cell models within these structures. In addition, tags can be used to assign different structural properties to distinct regions of tissue. For example, the papillary muscles and larger trabeculae (in places where they are detached from the endocardial wall) have a very different fiber architecture than myocytes lying within the bulk of the myocardial wall, tending to align parallel to the axis of these cylindrical structures. In all of these cases, it is often not possible to discern these different regions directly from the MR data because there is usually little or no difference in voxel intensities or intensity gradients between different regions. Although it is feasible that specialized and specific shape and appearance models may be developed to segment some of these different regions (eg, the papillary muscles and free-running Purkinje fibers have very distinctive morphologies), often manually created masks are produced and convoluted with the segmented image stack to numerically tag individual regions. Such a procedure was adopted to manually delineate structures such as the papillary muscles/larger trabeculae and valves from the segmented rabbit MR data, as well as the specialized Purkinje conduction system. Figure 14–1B shows tagged regions in the finite element rabbit ventricular model of Fig. 14–A (right), delineating the papillary muscles (green) and the valves (blue). In addition, Fig. 14–2A shows the manual identification of Purkinje fibers and their respective junctions within the MRI stack. Figures 14–2B,C shows the incorporation of this information into the ventricular model, allowing the tagged Purkinje fibers to be identified with corresponding specialized electrical properties.

Furthermore, for certain applications, it may be required to delineate regions of diseased tissue, such as infarct, from the imaging data sets in order to assign the appropriate electrophysiological properties associated with such pathological conditions.[50] Infarct tissue consists of both an inexcitable scar core and a border zone, which is assumed to contain excitable but pathologically remodeled tissue. Previous experimental studies have confirmed that myocardial necrosis, the influx of inflammatory cells with a more spherical morphology, and the deposition of collagen result in less anisotropic water diffusion within the infarct region as compared with healthy myocardium.[51] Although scars cannot be discriminated from healthy myocardium in anatomical MR scans, the changes in diffusion anisotropy secondary to the structural remodeling are reflected in differences in fractional anisotropy values, which can be detected with DT-MRI scans.

The image processing procedures to generate a model of an infarcted regions are presented in Fig. 14–3 using ex-vivo MRI and DT-MRI scans of a canine heart approximately 4 weeks after infarction.[50] Using similar techniques as described earlier,[49,52] the myocardium was separated from the surrounding suspension media and segmented to obtain an accurate representation of the anatomy. Similarly, the ventricles were separated from the rest of the myocardium to account for the presence of the electrically insulating annulus fibrosus as well as to assign different electrophysiological properties (atrial vs ventricular) to the tissue on either side of this boundary. After the delineation of the ventricles, the infarct tissue is labeled. From the interpolated

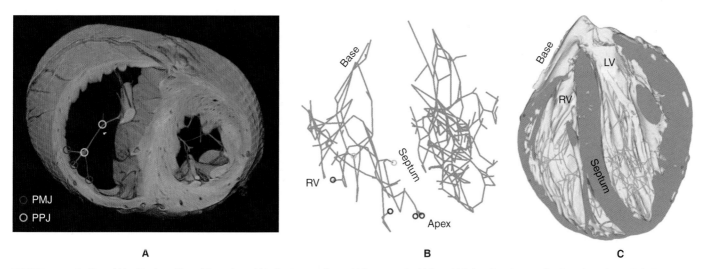

FIGURE 14–2. A. Manual identification of branching points within the free-running Purkinje system (Purkinje-Purkinje junctions [PPJ]) and points where the Purkinje fibers enter the myocardium (Purkinje-myocardial junctions [PMJ]) within the magnetic resonance image stack. **B.** and **C.** Corresponding delineation of Purkinje system within the computation ventricular model. LV, left ventricle; RV, right ventricle.

DT-MRI, the fractional anisotropy (FA) image is generated by computing the FA of the diffusion tensor at each voxel.[53] The FA of a diffusion tensor is defined as:

$$FA = \sqrt{\frac{3}{2}} \sqrt{\frac{(\lambda_1 - \lambda)^2 + (\lambda_2 - \lambda)^2 + (\lambda_3 - \lambda)^2}{\lambda_1^2 + \lambda_2^2 + \lambda_3^2}}, \quad (14\text{–}2)$$

$$\lambda = \frac{\lambda_1 + \lambda_2 + \lambda_3}{3}$$

where λ_1, λ_2, and λ_3 are the eigenvalues of the tensor. The FA is a measure of the directional diffusivity of water, and its values range from 0 to 1. A value of 0 indicates perfectly isotropic diffusion, and 1 indicates perfectly anisotropic diffusion. The infarct region is characterized by lower anisotropy, and therefore lower FA values, compared with the healthy myocardium[51] because of the myocardial disorganization in the infarct. Based on this difference in FA values, the infarct region is separated from the normal myocardium by applying a level-set segmentation to the 3D FA image. Next, the infarct region is subdivided into two areas by thresholding the structural MRI based on the intensity values. It is observed in the MRIs that the infarct region has heterogeneous image intensities. This is due to the presence of two distinct regions within the infarct: a core scar, which is assumed to contain inexcitable scar tissue, and a peri-infarct zone (PZ), which is assumed to contain excitable but pathologically remodeled tissue. The two regions are separated by thresholding the structural MRI based on the intensity values of the voxels; regions of high (>75%) and low (<25%) gray-level intensities were segmented as core scar, whereas tissue of medium intensity was segmented as PZ.[54,55] Figure 14–3 shows the final segmentation; orange identifies healthy myocardium, purple identifies the scar, and red identifies the PZ.

Alternatively, instead of a numerical tag, regions of the myocardium can be assigned quantitative information in the form of the value of a function at that particular point within the model. For example, the normalized transmural distance within the myocardial wall can be used to assign myocardial fiber orientation within the bulk of the myocardial wall (described later), as well as to modulate transmural gradients in electrophysiological cell membrane properties, with similar normalized distances

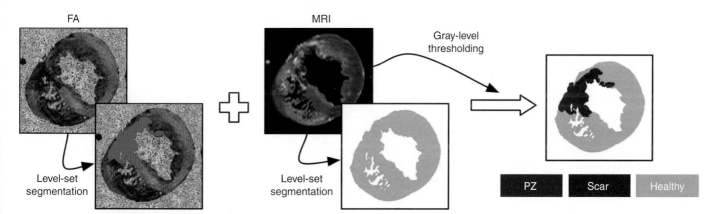

FIGURE 14–3. Construction of ventricular scar model. Left panels show results of level-set segmentation of ventricular anatomy and scar geometry. Gray-level thresholding of fractional anisotropy (FA) values was used to discriminate between scar and peri-infarct zone (PZ).

used to modulate apico-basal electrophysiological cell membrane parameter gradients. Such functional parametrizations can be assigned to the voxel image stack, but are more commonly assigned on a per-node or per-element basis within the finite element mesh as a postprocessing step following modal generation, discussed later in the "Postprocessing" section.

■ MESH GENERATION

Simulating the heart's electrical or mechanical function requires that solution be sought to the different systems of equations that are used to model these aspects of cardiac behavior. In the case of tissue or whole organ simulations, it is required that the cardiac geometry in question be discretized into a set of grid or mesh points to facilitate a numerical solution approach to these equation systems. The majority of leading cardiac electrophysiology simulators (such as the one described later under "Simulating Cardiac Bioelectric Activity at the Tissue and Organ Level") use finite element meshes as an input.[56] However, the construction of finite element meshes, representative of the particular cardiac tissue/organ preparation, is a highly nontrivial task. Previously, direct experimental measurements from ventricular preparations have provided sets of evenly spaced node points, representing the external tissue surfaces, with finite elements subsequently being assigned joining up these points. Such procedures have been used in the construction of the widely used Auckland pig[57] and canine[58] ventricular models. Recently, finite element meshes have been constructed directly from anatomic imaging modalities, such as MR. Although the exceptionally high resolution of such data sets currently being obtained can provide unprecedented insight regarding intact cardiac anatomical structure, faithfully transferring this information into a finite element mesh that is both of good quality and computationally tractable is a significant challenge.

Meshing Software

The mesh generation software of choice used by our group is Tarantula (http://www.meshing.at; CAE-Software Solutions, Eggenburg, Austria). Tarantula is an octree-based mesh generator that generates unstructured, boundary fitted, locally refined, conformal finite element meshes and has been custom designed for cardiac modeling. The underlying algorithm is similar to a recently published image-based unstructured mesh generation technique.[59] Briefly, the method uses a modified dual mesh of an octree applied directly to segmented 3D image stacks. The algorithm operates fully automatically with no requirements for interactivity and generates accurate volume-preserving representations of arbitrarily complex geometries with smooth surfaces. The smooth nature of the surfaces ensures general applicability of the meshes generated, in particular for studies involving the application of strong external stimuli, because the smooth, unstructured grids lack jagged boundaries that can introduce spurious currents due to tip effects, as is the case for structured grids. To reduce the overall computational load of the meshes, unstructured grids can be generated adaptively such that the spatial resolution varies throughout the domain. Fine

discretizations with little adaptivity can be used to model the myocardium, thus minimizing undesired effects of grid granularity on propagation velocity, while coarser elements that grow in size with distance from myocardial surfaces are generated to represent a surrounding volume conductor (eg, tissue bath or torso). Using adaptive mesh generation techniques facilitates the execution of bidomain simulations with a minimum of overhead due to the discretization of a surrounding volume conductor. Importantly with respect to model construction, Tarantula directly accepts the segmented voxel image stacks as input, which removes the need to generate tessellated representations of the cardiac surface, as required by Delaunay-based mesh generators.[60] Avoiding this additional step is a distinct advantage in the development of high-throughput cardiac model generation pipeline.[43]

Results of Mesh Generation

The final segmented and postprocessed data set was used to generate a tetrahedral finite element mesh using the meshing software Tarantula, shown in Fig. 14–1A. In addition to meshing the myocardial volume, a mesh of the volume conductor surrounding the ventricular mesh was also produced. This extracellular mesh not only consists of the space within the ventricular cavities and the vessels, but also defines an extended bath region outside of the heart, which can be used to model an in vitro situation where the heart is surrounded by a conductive bath, such as during optical mapping experiments.[61] The total mesh produced by Tarantula shown in Fig. 14–1A consisted of 6,985,108 node points, making up 41,489,283 tetrahedral elements. The intracellular mesh consisted of 4,306,770 node points making up 24,199,055 tetrahedral elements with 1,061,480 bounding triangular faces. The myocardial mesh had a mean tetrahedral edge length of 125.7 μm. The mesh took 39 minutes to generate using two Intel Xeon processors, clocked with 2.66 GHz.[43]

■ POSTPROCESSING

Whenever possible, classification and tagging operations are carried out at the preprocessing stage prior to mesh generation. In general, it is much simpler to devise algorithms that operate on perfectly regular image data sets than on fully unstructured finite element meshes. Further, due to the large and very active medical imaging community, a vast number of powerful image-processing techniques are readily available through specialized toolkits.[52] However, a subset of operations is better employed directly to the finite element mesh, because this is the computational grid that will be used for solving the biophysical problems. Although the objects, as defined by the binarized image stack on one hand and by the computational grid on the other hand, overlap fairly accurately, inevitable differences arise along the boundaries. The boundaries in the finite element mesh are smoothed representations of the object's jagged boundaries in the voxel stack. Tags assigned on a per-voxel base prior to mesh generation have to be mapped over to the finite element mesh. This processing step, referred to as voxel mapping, is nonstandard and, as such, typically not an integral part of standard mesh

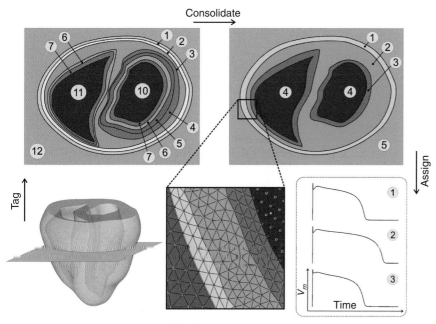

FIGURE 14–4. Tagging, consolidating, and assignment steps involved in the parametrization of biophysically detailed in silico models. Analysis of a ventricular finite element model (bottom left) provides information regarding a specialized intramural distance parameter (top left), which is then consolidated to delineate and tag within the mesh regions of the myocardial wall as subepicardial (1), mid-myocardial (2), and subendocardial (3) (top right). Such regions are then assigned different cellular ionic properties to allow experimentally observed variations in action potential dynamics to be reproduced (bottom right). This concept applies in a wider context and not only to the definition of transmural functional heterogeneity. Note that tags are assigned in a redundant manner to increase flexibility during the consolidation phase where new regions can be formed on the fly as a function of input parameters, allowing one to reuse in silico setups quickly while avoiding the time-consuming and error-prone tagging procedures. Parameters may be assigned on a per-node basis (as shown here for assigning models of cellular dynamics) or on a per-element basis (as suited for, eg, assigning tissue conductivities).

generation software. Further, by using the finite element mesh, more complex tagging strategies can be conceived based on the use of the solution of partial differential equations (PDEs). An example is given in the following section, where a Laplace problem is solved on the finite element grid. The harmonic solution to the problem, φ, is then used to provide a reference frame for assigning tags. The scalar values of φ can be used as a measure of distance, for instance, the distance to the endocardium, and $\nabla\varphi$ may provide a reference that indicates the transmural direction at every node in the grid. An example of a postprocessing tag assignment is illustrated in Fig. 14–4. Here, it is shown how different regions within a ventricular finite element model may be tagged based on their locations relative to epicardial/endocardial surfaces, allowing epicardial, endocardial, and mid-myocardial regions to be defined. Depending on the tags held by different nodes within the mesh, different cellular ionic properties may be assigned to each region replicating the experimentally observed disparity in action potential dynamics seen within subepicardial/subendocardial/mid-myocardial regions of the ventricular walls. Another important postprocessing application is the regularization of DT-MRI data along the organ surfaces. DT-MRI data are very noisy and, due to partial volume effects, tend to be inaccurate close to surfaces. Such artifacts can be corrected easily by subtracting the projection of each fiber in surface elements onto the surface normal of the element from the fiber direction

assigned to the element to ensure planarity of the fiber with the surface.

Assignment of Fibrous Architecture

The specific arrangement of cardiac myocytes within the myocardium is known to highly influence the electromechanical functioning of the heart. Specifically, the orientation of cardiac fibers is responsible for the anisotropic conduction throughout the myocardium, with electrical conduction occurring more readily along the axis of the myofiber than in the plane normal to it. Furthermore, the preferential alignment of cardiomyocytes influences the mechanical functioning of the heart, with the development of active tension that causes contraction occurring solely parallel to the fiber direction. Therefore, a realistic representation of the fibrous architecture throughout the model is paramount to faithfully simulating cardiac behavior. From histological[44] and DT-MRI[46] analysis of cardiac fiber architecture, it is known that cardiac fibers run primarily in a circumferential (or latitudinal) direction through the myocardial wall, with an additional inclination in the apico-basal (or longitudinal) direction. The inclination, or helix, angle (α) varies transmurally by approximately 120° from epi- to endocardium, being approximately zero in the mid wall.[27,44] In the following sections, we describe such experiment techniques used to measure fiber architecture within the heart, as well as mathematical rule-based methods for incorporating fiber information into cardiac models in the absence of experimentally measured data.

Experimentally Derived Fiber Architecture Information regarding cardiac fiber orientation can be obtained experimentally from either histological analysis[42,62] or DT-MRI.[46] Although the exceptional resolution of the histology data sets (up to approximately 1 μm in plane[43]) allows fiber orientation information to be readily extracted from the images through the application of simple gradient-based image analysis filters,[42] a number of problems exist. First, the physical process of cutting the sample introduces significant nonrigid deformations to the tissue. Although it is possible to use the intact geometric information obtained from a prior anatomic MR scan to register the histology slices together to recover the correct intact anatomy,[63] it is still unclear whether fully 3D information regarding cardiac fiber architecture can also be recovered from these registered data sets.

More commonly, myocardial structural information is obtained from DT-MRI recordings. Despite the potential drawbacks of DT-MRI, discussed earlier, the technique is widely used to embellish cardiac fiber orientation into computational models. There are two main ways in which DT-MRI information can be incorporated into an anatomical computational model. The first case is where the computational geometric model has been generated directly from a particular component of the DT-MRI data set; usually the intensity-based information, such as the FA or apparent diffusion coefficient values, is used. In these cases, the DT-MRI fiber vectors can be simply mapped across to the geometric finite element model using a nearest neighbor approach.[64] However, the second case involves instances in which a computational model has been generated based on a previously obtained anatomical scan from the same sample, usually following reembedding in a medium with a different contrast agent required for the anatomical scan. Alternatively, a computational model is used that has been generated from a different preparation entirely and, in some cases, from a different species. Here, the two data sets need to be geometrically registered together prior to mapping.

However, in certain instances, such DT-MRI data sets are unavailable for a particular heart preparation. In these cases, fiber architecture can be embellished into the model through the use of rule-based approaches using a priori knowledge regarding cardiac fiber structure within the heart of a particular species. The two most commonly used rule-based methods are the minimum distance algorithm and the Laplace-Dirichlet method. Both methods involve defining a smoothly varying function throughout the tissue domain and then using information regarding the variation of the function to define fiber orientation vectors. Each method is now briefly described.

Minimum Distance Algorithm The minimum distance algorithm, developed by Potse et al,[27] involves computing the minimum distance of every point within the myocardium to each of the epicardial (d_{epi}) and endocardial (d_{endo}) surfaces, respectively. This is normally performed on a node-by-node basis over a finite element mesh, describing the tissue geometry. Within the septum, in absence of an epicardial surface, d_{epi} can be taken to be the minimum distance to the endocardial surface of the RV (d_{endo}^{RV}), and d_{endo} can be taken to be the minimum distance to the endocardial surface of the LV (d_{endo}^{LV}), replicating the apparent structural continuity of the LV and septum seen in previous imaging studies.[46] With knowledge of d_{epi} and d_{endo}, a normalized thickness parameter e is computed as:

$$e = \frac{d_{endo}}{d_{endo} + d_{epi}} \tag{14–3}$$

To avoid sudden discontinuities in e at boundaries between regions, the value of e at each node is then averaged with all of its immediate neighbors (each central node of a structured mesh would have 26 neighbors). Calculation of the gradient of e within each tetrahedral element (∇e) then defines the transmural direction, u. The local circumferential direction, v, is then imposed to be perpendicular to u and the global apico-basal direction, which defines the "default" fiber vector direction with zero helix angle. To account for the widely reported transmural variation of fiber helix angle through the myocardial wall,[44] a rotation of α is then made to the fiber vector about the u-axis. The most widely used functional representations of the

variation of α through the wall are a linear or a cubic[27] variation, which is the method adopted here, giving:

$$\alpha = R(1 - 2e_{av})^3 \tag{14–4}$$

where e_{av} was taken to be the average of e of the nodal values making up the tetrahedra. Due to the reportedly less pronounced variation of fiber angles in the LV compared with the RV, R is set equal to $\pi/3$ for the LV and septum and $\pi/4$ for the RV.[27] Figure 14–1C shows the fiber vectors incorporated into the ventricular finite element model of Fig. 14–1A using the minimum distance approach.[43]

Laplace-Dirichlet Method The Laplace-Dirichlet method involves computing the solution of an electric potential φ within the tissue between two electrodes:

$$\nabla^2 \varphi = 0 \tag{14–5}$$

where isotropic conduction within the tissue is assumed. Dirichlet boundary conditions specified at the electrode positions (one ground and the other fixed voltage) produce a smoothly varying potential field between the electrodes within the tissue. The resulting potential gradient vectors can then be used to assign smoothly aligned fiber vectors that align with the underlying global and local structure of the tissue. Smoothness along the boundaries is ensured because the electric field lines only originate/terminate at electrodes due to the zero-flux boundary condition specified on all other external tissue boundaries to simulate electrical isolation; thus, the field has no component perpendicular to the tissue boundary.

However, the Laplace-Dirichlet method is highly dependent on electrode configuration with respect to the specific tissue preparation. Electrodes can be placed to produce global apico-basal (longitudinal), transmural, or circumferential (latitudinal) field directions. Computation of the gradients of such fields within each finite element of the domain gives the local orthonormal basis vectors, from which the fiber vector can be assigned in a similar manner to the minimum distance approach discussed earlier.

Histologically Derived Fiber Architecture In cases where vastly more complex geometric representations of the ventricles are constructed, simple rule-based methods cannot be used to faithfully assign fiber structure to all regions of the model. Such methods have been developed based on histological analysis of fiber vector architecture within the bulk of the ventricular free wall and therefore cannot be used to define fiber vectors in structures such as the papillary muscles or trabeculations, which are included within the next generation of cardiac models (as described earlier). Within such "tubular" endocardial structures, cardiac myocytes are known to align preferentially along the axis of the structure, because mechanically, this is the direction that facilitates the most efficient contraction. In such cases, the structure tensor method, a robust method for determining localized structure based on neighboring gradient fields, can be used to define local fiber orientation.

SIMULATING CARDIAC BIOELECTRIC ACTIVITY AT THE TISSUE AND ORGAN LEVEL

Cardiac tissue is made up of myocytes of roughly cylindrical geometry. A myocyte is approximately 100 μm long and 10 to 20 μm in diameter. The intracellular spaces of adjacent myocytes are interconnected by specialized connexins referred to as gap junctions.[65] The connexin expression over the cell is heterogeneous with a higher density of gap junctions at the intercalated discs located at the cell ends (along the long axis of the cell) and a lower density along the lateral boundaries,[66,67] and different connexins of varying conductance are expressed in different regions of the heart.[68] As a consequence of the elongated cellular geometry and the directionally varying gap junction density, current flows more readily along the longitudinal axes of the cells than transverse to it. This property is referred to as anisotropy. Cardiac tissue is composed of two spaces: an intracellular space formed by the interconnected network of myocytes, and the cleft space between myocytes referred to as interstitial space, which is made up of the extracellular matrix and the interstitial fluid. The extracellular matrix consists of networks of collagen fibers, which determine the passive mechanical properties of the myocardium. Electrically, it is assumed that the preferred directions are co-aligned between the two spaces but that the conductivity ratios between the principal axes are unequal between the two domains.[38,69-71] All parameters influencing the electrical properties of the tissue, such as density and conductance of gap junctions, cellular geometry, orientation and cell packing density, and the composition of the interstitial space, are heterogeneous and may vary at all size scales, from the cellular level up to the organ. As a consequence, direction and speed of a propagating electric wave are constantly modified by interacting with discrete spatial variations in material properties at various size scales. At a finer size scale below the space constant, λ, of the tissue (ie, <1 mm), the tissue is best characterized as a discrete network in which the electrical impulse propagates in a discontinuous manner.[72,73] At a larger more macroscopic size scale (>> λ), the tissue behaves as a continuous functional syncytium where the effects of small-scale discontinuities are assumed to play a minor role.

Theoretically, the idea of modeling an entire heart by using models of a single cell as the basic building block is conceivable. However, the associated computational costs are prohibitive with current computing hardware because a single heart consists of roughly 5 billion cells. Although a few high-resolution modeling studies have been conducted where small tissue preparations were discretized at a subcellular resolution,[38,72,74] in general, the spatial discretization steps were chosen based on the spatial extent of electrical wave fronts and not on the size scales of the tissue's microstructures. For this reason, cardiac tissue is treated as a continuum for which appropriate material parameters have to be determined that translate the discrete cellular matrix into an electrically analog macroscopic representation. In principle, this is achieved by averaging material properties over suitable length scales such that both potential and current solution match between homogenized and discrete representation.

A rigorous mathematical framework for this procedure is provided by homogenization theory, which has been applied by several authors to the bidomain problem.[15-75-77] Homogenization is a two-step process where the intracellular and interstitial domains are homogenized in a first step, and the two respective domains are spread out and overlapped to fill the entire tissue domain. This concept of interpenetrating domains states that everywhere within the entire myocardial volume intracellular space, extracellular space and the cellular membrane coexist.

■ GOVERNING EQUATIONS

Bidomain Equations

The bidomain equations[78] state that currents that enter the intracellular or extracellular spaces by crossing the cell membrane represent the sources for the intracellular, Φ_i, and extracellular potentials, Φ_e:

$$\nabla \cdot \boldsymbol{\sigma}_i \nabla \Phi_i = \beta I_m \tag{14–6}$$

$$\nabla \cdot \boldsymbol{\sigma}_e \nabla \Phi_e = -\beta I_m - I_e \tag{14–7}$$

$$I_m = C_m \frac{\partial V_m}{\partial t} + I_{\text{ion}}(V_m, \eta) - I_{\text{tr}} \tag{14–8}$$

$$\frac{\partial \eta}{\partial t} = g(V_m, \eta) \tag{14–9}$$

$$V_m = \Phi_i - \Phi_e \tag{14–10}$$

where σ_i and σ_e are the intracellular and extracellular conductivity tensors, respectively; β is the membrane surface-to-volume ratio; I_m is the transmembrane current density; I_{tr} is the current density of the transmembrane stimulus; I_e is the extracellularly applied current density; C_m is the membrane capacitance per unit area; V_m is the transmembrane voltage; and I_{ion} is the density of the total current flowing through the membrane ionic channels, pumps, and exchangers, which in turn depends on the transmembrane voltage and a set of state variables η. At the tissue boundaries, electrical isolation is assumed, which is accounted for by imposing no-flux boundary conditions on Φ_e and Φ_i.

In those cases where cardiac tissue is surrounded by a conductive medium, such as blood in the ventricular cavities or a perfusing saline solution, an additional Poisson equation has to be solved:

$$\nabla \cdot \boldsymbol{\sigma}_b \nabla \Phi_e = -I_e \tag{14–11}$$

where σ_b is the isotropic conductivity of the conductive medium and I_e is stimulation current injected into the conductive medium. In this case, no-flux boundary conditions are assumed at the boundaries of the conductive medium, whereas continuity of the normal component of the extracellular current and continuity of Φ_e are enforced at the tissue-bath interface. The no-flux boundary condition for Φ_i remains unchanged.

Equations 14–6 and 14–7 are referred to as the parabolic-parabolic form of the bidomain equations; however, the majority of solution schemes is based on the elliptic-parabolic form, which is found by adding Equations 14–6 and 14–7 and replacing Φ_i by $V_m + \Phi_e$.[79] This yields:

$$\begin{bmatrix} -\nabla \cdot (\sigma_i + \sigma_e) \nabla \Phi_e \\ -\nabla \cdot \sigma_b \nabla \Phi_e \end{bmatrix} = \begin{bmatrix} \nabla \cdot \sigma_i \nabla V_m \\ I_e \end{bmatrix} \quad (14\text{–}12)$$

$$\frac{\partial V_m}{\partial t} = \frac{1}{\beta C_m}(\nabla \cdot \sigma_i \nabla V_m + \nabla \cdot \sigma_i \nabla \Phi_e) - \frac{1}{C_m}(I_{\text{ion}}(V_m, \eta) - I_{\text{tr}}) \quad (14\text{–}13)$$

where V_m and Φ_e, the quantities of primary concern, are retained as the independent variables. Note that Equation 14–12 treats the bath as an extension of the interstitial space.

Monodomain Equations

Although the use of a bidomain formulation is preferred when effects due to extracellular stimulation,[80] defibrillation,[81,82] or bath loading[83,84] are under investigation, for studying wave propagation phenomena in cardiac tissue, the monodomain equations are by far the more popular choice due to the substantially lower computational costs. Differences between the two formulations are, relative to the inaccuracies of the overall system, fairly small.[27] Assuming that σ_i and σ_e are related by a scalar, v:

$$\sigma_e = v \sigma_i \quad (14\text{–}14)$$

the bidomain equations can be reduced to the monodomain equations:

$$C_m \frac{\partial V_m}{\partial t} + I_{\text{ion}} = \frac{v}{1+v} \nabla \cdot (\sigma_i \nabla V_m) \quad (14\text{–}15)$$

$$(1+v) \nabla \cdot (\sigma_i \nabla \Phi_e) = -\nabla \cdot (\sigma_i \nabla V_m) \quad (14\text{–}16)$$

where Equation 14–16 does not need to be solved for simulating wave propagation. However, it is widely accepted that the assumption of Equation 14–14 does not reflect biological reality. There is a large variation in reported measurements of anisotropy, ranging between 5.7 and 10.8 for $\alpha_i = \sigma_{il}/\sigma_{it}$ in the intracellular domain and between 1.5 and 2.6 $\alpha_e = \sigma_{el}/\sigma_{et}$ in the extracellular domain.[71] However, all studies unanimously agreed that the ratios between the domains, α_i/α_e, are different, ranging from 3.5 to 6.3 (ie, there is no experimental support of Equation 14–14). Furthermore, the existence of unequal anisotropy ratios is indirectly supported by the experimental observations of virtual electrodes for which the presence of unequal anisotropy ratios, according to the bidomain theory, is a necessary condition. For instance, it was theoretically postulated that the delivery of a strong unipolar point-like stimulus[85] leads to the formation of a very peculiar polarization pattern referred to as "dog bone." This prediction was experimentally confirmed by numerous labs only a few years later.

Further insights into the relationship between the two formulations are gained by considering a 1D strand. In this case, the conductivity tensors degenerate to scalar values, and bidomain and monodomain formulations are fully equivalent with

$v = \sigma_{e\zeta}/\sigma_{i\zeta}$, where ζ are the three eigendirections of the conductivity tensor.[38] This immediately reveals that V_m and Φ_e are linked by the voltage divider relationship:

$$\Phi_e = -\frac{\sigma_{i\zeta}}{\sigma_{i\zeta} + \sigma_{e\zeta}} V_m \quad (14\text{–}17)$$

Using the same choice of $v = \sigma_{e\zeta}/\sigma_{i\zeta}$ in a 3D model along the direction ζ leads to monodomain conductivities that are the harmonic mean between the two spaces along ζ. That is:

$$\sigma_{m\zeta} = \frac{\sigma_{i\zeta} \sigma_{e\zeta}}{\sigma_{i\zeta} + \sigma_{e\zeta}} \quad (14\text{–}18)$$

In this case, monodomain and bidomain formulations are equivalent in the sense that both models yield the same conduction velocities along the principal axes, which, in turn, results in very similar activation patterns. Minor deviations are expected when wave fronts are propagating in any other direction, which results in slightly different activation patterns. Differences between monodomain and bidomain simulations can be further reduced by finding an optimal v at each time step.[86]

■ SIMULATING THE PURKINJE NETWORK

The His PS is responsible for the rapid activation of the ventricles. The PS starts at the atrioventricular node as the bundle of His, extends toward the apex, and divides into the left and right Tawara branches. The branches emerge on the endocardium, continue toward the apex, and then turn and travel back toward the base (Fig. 14–5). Along the way, branches extend into the

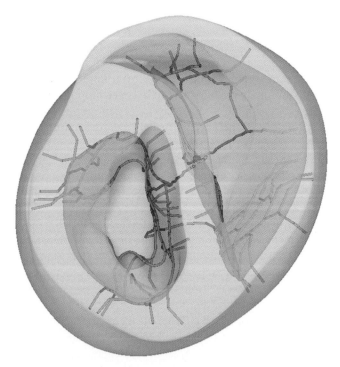

FIGURE 14–5. Superior view showing the Purkinje system on the endocardium and extending almost to the epicardium, consistent with the conduction systems of swine. The left ventricle is on the left.

myocardium and become finer, being called Purkinje fibers at that point. The Purkinje fibers travel a certain transmural distance, which is species dependent,[87] before terminating in electrical junctions with the myocardium called Purkinje-myocyte junctions (PMJs). Fibers of the PS are covered in a collagenous sheath that electrically isolates the PS from myocardium along or through which it runs.[88] Subendocardially, the PS may form a mesh-like network such that it cannot be described as an arborized structure.[88] Although the structure may appear dense, the PMJs are discrete and more sparsely distributed.[88]

Conduction within the PS is very rapid, being about four times faster than that through myocardium. Anterograde propagation of impulses from the PS to myocardium is much slower than retrograde, which has been shown to occur.

Geometrical Model

To construct the Purkinje network, a conformal approach was undertaken, meaning that the nodes representing the Purkinje network were a subset of those defining the ventricles. The ventricular endocardial surfaces were extracted, resulting in two triangularly meshed surfaces. The surfaces were flattened onto a plane using a multidimensional scaling technique,[89] which attempted to preserve geodesic distances, as computed by the classic Dijkstra algorithm.[90] A conduction system was manually laid out on each of the endocardial surfaces, based on schematics and pictures of the conduction system, text descriptions of heart anatomy, and excitation mappings of the heart,[34,91-94] taking care to preserve major features.

For each ventricle, a single cable started at the base and proceeded apically. Daughter branches were added, which ran toward the areas of early activation. The major bifurcation points were chosen to roughly correspond to published descriptions. More cables were added to provide better coverage for activation. The 2D representation of the Purkinje network was then mapped back to 3D space, the left and right Purkinje networks joined at a common point of origin, and a segment representing the bundle of His was added.

The end points of the Purkinje networks (ie, those points that make electrical contact with, and activate, the ventricular myocardium) were inserted into the ventricular wall. Each cable end was extended into the myocardium by appending elements. The new elements made an angle of approximately 45°, with the surface tangent to avoid any sharp discontinuities, and continued for several hundred micrometers into the tissue.

Mathematical Basis

Assume that the extracellular potential, Φ_e, is due to the bulk myocardium only (ie, we ignore the field produced by the PS).

The governing parabolic equation is given by:

$$\nabla \cdot \sigma_i^P \nabla \Phi_i = \beta \left(C_m \frac{\partial V_m}{\partial t} + I_{ion}\left(V_m, \eta^P\right) \right) \qquad (14\text{--}19)$$

where σ_i^P is the equivalent intracellular conductivity that homogenizes the cytoplasmic with gap junctional resistances.

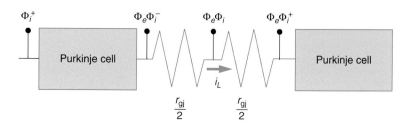

FIGURE 14-6. The intracellular potential in the gap junction is denoted by Φ_i at the midpoint, Φ_i^- on the left, and Φ_i^+ on the right. The gap junction length is so small that the extracellular potential, Φ_e, is constant across the junction. The current flowing through the junction of resistance r_{gj} is i_L.

The DiFrancesco-Noble model of the Purkinje cell[95] was used with the maximum sodium conductance increased by a factor of 3 compared with the published values. Although studies usually increase the sodium conductance by a factor of 1.5,[96,97] conductance was further augmented to increase the propagation velocity and obtain an upstroke that better agrees with experimental measurements.[98] Alternative ionic models have recently been developed.[99]

The current flowing longitudinally along each cell is given by:

$$i_L = -\pi \rho^2 \sigma_i \frac{\partial \Phi_i}{\partial x} \qquad (14\text{--}20)$$

where ρ is the radius of the Purkinje fiber, and σ_i is the intracellular conductivity. To determine V_m, we recognize that the cells are connected by gap junctions, which are represented as resistors (Fig. 14–6). Φ_i is defined as the potential midway along the gap junction, and V_m at either end of the junction can be expressed using the longitudinal current:

$$V_m^\pm = \Phi_i - \Phi_e \mp i_L \frac{r_{gj}}{2} \qquad (14\text{--}21)$$

where r_{gj} is the gap junction resistance. Thus, after determining V_m at the ends of each cell along the cable, we split the operator to isolate the ionic current term and update of V_m based on ionic current flow. Φ_i and i_L were then recomputed at each junction from:

$$\Phi_i = \frac{V_m^+ + V_m^-}{2} + \Phi_e \qquad (14\text{--}22)$$

$$i_L = \frac{V_m^+ - V_m^-}{r_{gj}} \qquad (14\text{--}23)$$

where Φ_e was computed on the myocardial grid.

To properly take into account spatial gradients, a 1D cubic Hermite formulation was used. This assumed a radially constant solution, which is justified given how small the radius is compared with the space constant. By using Equation 14–20, gradients were converted to currents. We also required the spatial and temporal derivatives of the extracellular potential (ie, $\frac{\partial \Phi_e}{\partial x}$, $\frac{\partial \Phi_e}{\partial t}$, and $\frac{\partial^2 \Phi_e}{\partial x \partial t}$). At each bifurcation, current conservation was explicitly enforced. The PS is coupled to the bulk myocardium through PMJs, which are represented as fixed resistances (R_{PMJ}). At the cable ends, current flow through the PMJ is enforced as a boundary condition. For a cable end at x_e:

$$i_L = \sum_k \frac{\Phi_i(x_e) - \Phi_i^M(x_k)}{R_{\mathrm{PMJ}}} \qquad (14\text{--}24)$$

where $\Phi_i^M(x)$ is an intracellular potential in the bulk myocardium, and k is the set of indices of the myocytes to which the Purkinje cell is connected. From the perspective of the myocardium, the current flowing through the end of the PMJ was an intracellular current injection.

TEMPORAL DISCRETIZATION

Various temporal discretization schemes have been applied to solve the cardiac bidomain equations. Initially, fully explicit schemes were popular due to their ease of implementations, but their utility was limited due to the severe restrictions imposed on the maximum possible time step, Δt, particularly when finer spatial discretizations, $h < 100 \ \mu$m, were considered. The maximum stable time step as a function of h is dictated by the Courant-Friedrich-Levy (CFL) condition. An approximation of the CFL condition can be derived by assuming equal anisotropy ratios ($\sigma_i = \nu \sigma_e$) and straight fibers:

$$\Delta t \leq \frac{\beta C_m h^2}{2(\sigma_l + \sigma_t)} \qquad (14\text{--}25)$$

where $\sigma_* = \sigma_{i*} \sigma_{e*}/(\sigma_{i*} + \sigma_{e*})$, ($* = l, t$). Despite this limitation, fully explicit schemes are still widely used, particularly with coarser meshes where accuracy constraints are the limiting factor and not so much stability. Besides, fully explicit methods are quite attractive in the context of large-scale simulations where parallel scalability plays an important role. Forward methods require only matrix-vector products, which scale very well up to high processor counts.

Fully implicit methods lift restrictions on time stepping imposed by stability constraints, allowing much larger time steps than explicit methods. With this class of methods, the choice of time step is governed by accuracy considerations. Several authors suggested fully implicit numerical schemes for solving the bidomain equations[100]; however, only simplified membrane models were used. Although it is perfectly feasible to use fully implicit time discretizations with detailed physiological cellular models, the increase in overall system size and complexity is dramatic, and the solvers required are extremely expensive due to the large nonlinear system arising at each time step. An alternative approach to circumvent this problem has been recently proposed,[101] where the ordinary differential equation (ODE) gating variables were decoupled from the PDE. The scheme was classified as fully implicit with decoupling. The underlying rationale is based on the observation that the Jacobian of a fully implicit discretization at one node of the mesh is strongly dominated by the diagonal entries, suggesting that the coupling between gating variables and potentials is weak.

Implicit-explicit (IMEX) schemes are the most widely used discretizations because they represent, from a practical point of view, a very good trade-off between stability, ease of implementation, and computational efficiency. Quite often, IMEX methods are combined with operator-splitting techniques, which is appealing from a software engineering perspective because the problem can be broken down into smaller subproblems. Moreover, on theoretical grounds, it is expected that solving two smaller problems of size N is computationally more efficient than solving a larger problem of size $2N$. In real implementations, this is not necessarily the case though.[102] The scheme preferred by our labs[103] is based on discretizing Equations 14–12 and 14–13. An operator splitting technique is applied to separate the ODE system from the PDEs (Equation 14–12 – Equation 14–13) using a θ-rule.[104-106] Depending on a choice of θ, either a first-order accurate Gudonov scheme or a second-order accurate Strang splitting scheme can be derived.[107] Solutions of the PDEs are then found by leap-frogging between the decoupled components where either V_m in Equation 14 – 12 or Φ_e in Equation 14 – 13 is considered as constant. This leads to a three-step scheme, which involves solving a parabolic PDE, an elliptic PDE, and a nonlinear system of ODEs at each time step:

$$\left[1 + \frac{1}{2}\Delta t A_i\right]V^{k*} = \left[1 - \frac{1}{2}\Delta t A_i\right]V^k - \Delta t A_i \Phi_e^k \qquad (14\text{--}26)$$

$$V^{k+1} = V^{k*} - \frac{\Delta t}{C_m}\left(I_{ion}\left(V^{k*}, \eta^k\right) - I_{\mathrm{tr}}\right) \qquad (14\text{--}27)$$

$$\eta^{k+1} = g(V_m, \eta) \qquad (14\text{--}28)$$

$$(A_i + A_e)\Phi_e^{k+1} = -A_i V^{k+1} + I_e \qquad (14\text{--}29)$$

where A_ξ is the discretized $-\nabla \cdot (\sigma_\xi \nabla)/(\beta C_m)$ operator with ξ being either i or e; Δt is the time step; and V^k, Φ_e^k, and η^k are the temporal discretizations of V_m, Φ_e, and η, respectively, at the time instant of $k\Delta t$.

Ionic Model Computation Techniques

Recent models of cellular dynamics account for increasingly more physiological detail, which increases both the overall number of state variables and the stiffness of the nonlinear system of ODEs. Evaluating the vector-valued function $g(V_m, \eta)$, where η is typically comprised of several tens of state variables, and solving the set of ODEs robustly and efficiently remain an error-prone challenges in any cardiac modeling endeavor. Equation 14–28 is written in a semidescretized form as a symbolic indication that the state vector η is being updated. A host of methods exists, and the choice of optimal method depends largely on the cellular model under consideration. Standard integration techniques include explicit (or forward) and implicit (or backward) methods. Explicit methods are popular because they are easy to implement; however, the order of this class of methods is one that often results in insufficient accuracy. Approaches to overcome this weakness include the use of several previously computed solutions (multistep methods) or additional intermediate solutions in the interval $[t; t + \Delta t]$ (Runge-Kutta methods). The more sophisticated implicit backward methods, such as backward differentiation formula (BDF) or implicit Runge-Kutta methods (eg, Rosenbrock methods[108]), have superior stability properties and allow larger time steps; however, they are computationally expensive, and in general, robust implementation of these methods is difficult. The use of BDF methods requires the solution of a linear system of equations iteratively, by either fixed-point methods or variants of the Newton-Raphson methods, which requires that Jacobian matrices are either analytically determined and repetitively evaluated or numerically approximated.[109] Many currently used integrators incorporate advanced features such as variable time stepping and error control, where a time step is chosen such that the local error per step is below a prescribed tolerance level.

Moreover, apart from the choice of integration rule, two main approaches can be distinguished: (1) standard ODE integration techniques that update the entire state vector η in one step by solving a nonlinear system; or (2) a component-wise integration approach where the vector function η is split into its components and each single state variable η_i is updated sequentially, with all other state variables η_j ($j \neq i$) held constant. Many of the ODEs comprising an ionic model, typically all gating equations in Hodgkin-Huxley–type models, but also some ODEs in Markov-state formulations, can be written in the form:

$$\frac{d\eta_i}{dt} = A_i(\overline{\eta})\eta_i + B_i(\overline{\eta}) \qquad (14\text{–}30)$$

where $\overline{\eta}$ is the subvector of state variables that are held constant when updating η_i. When using a component-wise integration approach, all variables belonging to the subvector $\overline{\eta}$ are considered constant during an integration step. Hence, the nonlinear ODE reduces to a linear ODE with constant coefficients, for which an analytic solution is given by:

$$\eta_i(t+\Delta t) = \left(\eta_i(t) + \frac{B_i}{A_i}\right)e^{A_i \Delta t} - \frac{B_i}{A_i} \qquad (14\text{–}31)$$

Numerical analysis revealed that using this analytical expression to evolve the solution to the next time step, $t+\Delta t$, offers significant stability and accuracy benefits over the forward Euler method.[110] Although many of the integration techniques summarized above have been used for solving Equation 14–28 in single cell modeling studies, in the context of tissue level simulations the technique of using the analytical solution, originally proposed by Rush and Larsen,[111] is most widely used. Those portions g_i of the vector function $g(Vm,\eta)$ that cannot be written in a linear form need to be integrated in the fully nonlinear form. In the original Rush-Larsen formulation, the forward Euler method was applied to solve the fully nonlinear form. The numerical realization of Equation 14–28 following the Rush-Larsen approach can be written as:

$$\eta_f^{k+1} = \eta_f^k e^{A_f \Delta t} + \frac{B_f}{A_f}(e^{A_f \Delta t} - 1) \qquad (14\text{–}32)$$

$$\eta_s^{k+1} = \eta_s^k + \Delta t\, \mathbf{g}(V^{k*}, \eta^k) \qquad (14\text{–}33)$$

where η_f is the linear and η_s the nonlinear portion of the state vector η. In general, the very fast acting variables that render the system stiff, such as gating variables, are in the subvector η_f, whereas slower acting variables, such as ionic fluxes, are in the subvector η_s. The Rush-Larsen scheme can be implemented to achieve high computational efficiency using various acceleration techniques. Because the physiological range of variables is well known a priori, expensive terms in the analytical solution can be conveniently precomputed and then simply looked up when required. With this scheme, one state variable can be updated with one table lookup operation, one multiplication, and one sum operation only.[112]

Several suggestions have been made to further improve the method.[110] First, for those models where fast-acting variables are in ηs, potential stability issues can be dealt with by using implicit methods.[113] Second, the integration in the component-wise form introduces an approximation error that renders the Rush-Larsen technique first-order accurate only. Recently, an important extension has been proposed that overcomes this limitation by applying a local linearization of nonlinear terms in combination with the analytical solution of the quasi-linear ODEs to obtain a second-order accurate numerical scheme.[114]

Despite the numerous benefits and the computational efficiency of accelerated Rush-Larsen techniques, for some more recent ionic models,[115] the performance may be insufficient for organ-level simulations due to the extreme stiffness of cellular subsystems such as the interactions of L-type calcium currents with ryanodine receptors. With these models, the range of time scales involved is vast, from processes occurring within a fraction of a microsecond up to processes occurring at a scale of tens of seconds. The wide range of time scales involved can be exploited in a systematic manner to devise more efficient integration schemes, where different components of the state vector are decoupled and grouped as a function of the multiple time scales involved. Each group is then integrated with the method and the time step that is appropriate for the respective time scale and stiffness of the group. Processes occurring at the tissue- and organ-level scale are unaffected by the temporal multiscale decoupling at the ODE solver stage because global quantities that link the two scales are updated synchronously at the time step chosen at the tissue level to fulfill stability and accuracy requirements.[112]

SPATIAL DISCRETIZATION

Various spatial discretization techniques have been applied to the cardiac bidomain problem, most notably the finite difference method (FDM),[27,116] the finite volume method (FVM),[20,21] and the finite element method (FEM),[18,19] although other nonstandard techniques, such as the interconnected cable model, have been used successfully as well.[11,117] In general, the FDM is easiest to implement, but the method does not accommodate complex boundaries as naturally as the FEM and the FVM do. Although suggestions were made to overcome this limitation by using the phase-field approach[16] or other generalizations,[17,118] the FDM loses its most appealing advantage, the ease of implementation. FEM and FVM are both very well suited for spatial discretizations of complex geometries with smooth representations of the boundaries, which is a key feature when polarization patterns induced via extracellularly applied currents are to be studied. Both FVM and FEM have been used to model electrical activity in anatomically realistic models of the atria[29-31,119] and the ventricles.[26-28,43] Mesh generation requirements are similar for both techniques; that is, the domain of interest has to be tessellated into a set of nonoverlapping and conformal geometric primitives. With the FVM, quadrilaterals in 2D[20] and hexahedral elements in 3D[21,29] have been preferred, whereas with the FEM, triangles and quadrilaterals were used in 2D and tetrahedral[43] or hexahedral elements were used in 3D.[31,101] Typically, monolithic meshes consisting of one element type only were used with one exception,[59] where hybrid meshes consisting of tetrahedra, hexahedra, pyramids, and prisms were used. Further, most FEM studies relied on the Galerkin FEM where linear test functions with tetrahedral elements,[19,120,121] isoparametric trilinear test functions with hexahedral elements,[101] or cubic Hermite hexahedral elements[18,122] were used.

Independently of the spatial discretization technique, the choice of space step, h, is of major importance. It has been known since very early modeling studies that the solution of the bidomain equations does depend, to a certain degree, on h, even with very fine spatial discretizations.[123] This sensitivity has to be attributed to the nonlinearity and stiffness of the reaction term, which entails an extremely fast upstroke of the cardiac action potential, lasting approximately 1 ms only. When propagating, a fast upstroke in time translates into a steep wave front in space. Depending on tissue conductivity and cellular excitability, physiological conduction velocities range between 0.2 and 0.7 m/s within the myocardium, which translates an upstroke duration of 1 ms into a wave front that extends 200 to 700 µm in space. Under physiological situations where tissue conductivity and/or excitability is reduced, conduction velocity may be substantially slower, leading to wave fronts where the spatial extent may be even below 100 µm. The spatial extent of a wave front along a direction ζ is proportional to the space constant, λ_ζ:

$$\lambda_\zeta = \sqrt{\frac{1}{\beta}\frac{\sigma_{i\zeta}\sigma_{e\zeta}}{\sigma_{i\zeta}+\sigma_{e\zeta}}} \qquad (14\text{–}34)$$

It has been shown that for sufficiently small effective discretizations, $H_\zeta = \lambda_\zeta / h_\zeta < 0.15$, solutions converge with deviations in conduction velocity <1%.[123] In practice, a trade-off has to be made between accuracy and computational tractability. A standard choice for h, or for an average discretization $\bar{h}$ when unstructured grids are considered, for modeling studies at the tissue and organ level is 250 µm, but finer[43] and coarser discretizations[26,122] have been reported as well. With very coarse discretizations, $h > 500$ µm, and physiologically realistic models of cellular dynamics, simulations deviate substantially from results obtained at finer resolutions. Conduction velocities at such coarse grids are underestimated by at least 25% or more, and even conduction block may occur as a numerical side effect due to spatial undersampling.

NUMERICAL SOLUTION

Current research in bidomain modeling aims at enabling electrophysiologists to perform in silico experiments with biophysically detailed models of the heart in the same way as in vitro experiments are performed in the wet lab. Due to the nature of the phenomenon, which requires fine spatiotemporal resolutions and long observation periods, in silico experimentation is computationally quite challenging. Typically, systems of 1 to 50 million degrees of freedom are considered, and the solution has to be evolved over several tens of thousands of time steps. Although bidomain simulations can be executed easily on current standard desktop computers, problem sizes that can be tackled have to be restricted to smaller preparations, with 10^6 degrees of freedom being roughly the upper limit beyond which simulations become quickly intractable. Larger problems, as arising when anatomically detailed models of the entire heart are discretized, lead to much larger problem sizes. The ultimate goal is to perform fine-grained exploration of parameter spaces with in silico experiments where trade-offs between anatomical and functional detail in the model on one hand and execution times on the other hand can be relaxed. Extremely efficient and complex software stacks are required that deliver the computational performance to enable this kind of research. The Cardiac Arrhythmia Research Package (CARP) simulator is considered as being one of the most efficient and versatile codes for biophysically detailed simulations of cardiac electrophysiology; nonetheless, performance lags real time by roughly a factor of 10^3 or 10^4 when running monodomain or bidomain simulations, respectively. This is clearly a limiting factor for certain applications, for instance, when simulations have to be integrated into a clinical work flow.

Performance improvements by at least one to two orders of magnitude are sought to leverage computational modeling as a complement to experimental or clinical techniques by enabling quick simulation and data analysis cycles. Two strategies are currently being investigated to provide the required performance boost. One school of thinking is to implement spatiotemporally adaptive algorithms that dramatically reduce the computational burden by reducing the overall degrees of freedom in the system and by increasing time steps in low gradient regions where tissue is quiescent or during the plateau and repolarization phase. This is achieved by dynamically refining the grid as a function of current activity, with very fine resolution along the propagating wave fronts and rather coarse resolutions elsewhere. The alternative approach is parallelization, where domain decomposition techniques are used to split the overall problem into smaller subdomains and where each subdomain is solved for in parallel. In the ideal case, computations are sped up by the number of computational cores, N_p, engaged. Unfortunately, it is not straightforward to achieve such a strong scalability (ie, a scalability where the execution times is reduced linearly with N_p).

From an algorithmic point of view, weak scalability is an important requirement to achieve good parallel performance with increasing N_p. During a weak scalability test, the problem size is increased with N_p in a way that the computational load per core remains constant. With optimal methods, weak scaling can be achieved so the execution time remains constant while increasing problem size and N_p. Multigrid and multilevel preconditioners that show weak scalability properties have been published, and the scalability has been demonstrated in implementations for problem sizes up to 135 million degrees of freedom with 2048 cores.[101] Weak scalability does not necessarily imply strong scalability because computational science aspects play an important role, which strongly depend on the specifications of a particular hardware. It can be expected that strong scalability will always break down at a sufficiently high N_p, when the ratio between computational load per core and the inevitable communication costs becomes less favorable; however, it is expected that weakly scaling implementations will scale strongly as well over a certain N_p range.

Current codes can scale up very well to a moderate number of cores in the range of 64 to 256 cores with current HPC hardware, and the available memory spaces are huge, being in the range of terabytes. The current trend in the computing industry, which moves toward many-core architectures at a fast pace, rather favors the parallelization approach, with classical sequential desktop computing, with or without spatiotemporal adaptivity, likely to lose relevance. This trend is poised to have a major impact on the design of future algorithms because parallelization and cache performance aspects are of primary concern. Future desktop computers will be very similar to HPC architectures and implementations, and algorithms that do not account for this shift in paradigm cannot deliver the high performance required for future in silico modeling studies.

The choice of methods depends largely on the problem sizes considered and the available computational resources. In general, independently of a particular algorithm or implementation, the main computational burden associated with solving the bidomain equations can be attributed to the solution of the elliptic PDE when operator splitting is applied to the diffusion part of the equation and to the set of ODEs. Typically, with simple ionic models, the elliptic problem amounts to more than 90% of the overall workload, whereas with recent ionic models involving very stiff ODEs,[115] the ODE solver time may be comparable to the elliptic solver time or even dominate computations. The ODE problem is alleviated in a parallel computing context. State variables in ionic models do not diffuse, which qualifies the ODE solve as an embarrassingly parallel problem. No communication between processors is required, and thus, the parallel scaling of the ODE portion is linear. Solving the parabolic problem is typically less of a concern. On coarser meshes, where time steps are limited by the reaction term, simple forward Euler steps can be used that do not add significantly to the overall computational expense. On finer grids, where IMEX schemes tend to perform better than explicit schemes, a linear system has to be solved. However, due to the diagonal dominance of the system, even with relatively cheap iterative solvers, the parabolic PDE is solved efficiently at a fraction of the cost of the elliptic PDE.

Solving the Linear Systems

Traditionally, with sequential computers, the linear systems of small grid problems are most efficiently solved with direct methods.[19,124] With increasing problem size, memory demands increase quickly due to fill-in arising during matrix factorization, which, in turn, significantly increases the required number of operations per solver step. For larger systems, on the order of several hundreds of thousands up to tens of millions of unknowns, direct methods are inefficient or even not feasible due to excessive memory demands, and iterative solver techniques are clearly the better choice. Furthermore, large-scale problems typically rely on parallel computing approaches to provide a sufficiently large memory space and to keep execution times reasonably short. When simulations are executed on parallel computers, iterative methods are the method of choice. Although direct methods have been implemented to perform well in parallel environments,[125,126] they are typically not competitive when using a large number of cores due to the required fine-grained parallelism that limits their parallel scalability. Among the iterative methods, Krylov subspace methods, such as the conjugate gradient (CG) method, with various preconditioners have been established as the standard technique in the field. CG scales very well in parallel, although the utility of the method depends mostly on performance and scalability of the preconditioner.

The most challenging problem is the solution of the elliptic PDE. Using an incomplete LU (ILU) or incomplete Cholesky (ICC) preconditioner for CG has been a standard choice for bidomain simulations.[19] Although the scalability of an ILU-CG iterative solver is reasonably good, at least up to a moderate number of 64 cores,[124] typically the method takes several hundreds of iterations to converge. This makes the elliptic solve substantially more expensive than the parabolic solve, which converges with the same solver configuration in less than 10 iterations. The reason for the slow converge is well studied and can be blamed on the fact that standard iterative methods are very efficient in removing the high-frequency modes from the residual, but are less efficient with the low-frequency modes. Multigrid techniques have proved to be very effective in tackling this weakness.[127] The basic idea is to project the residual onto a coarser space where the low-frequency components can be dealt with more efficiently. This has been demonstrated for the bidomain problem in several recent studies.[124,128,129] Multigrid preconditioners for CG methods significantly improve the overall performance and show reasonable parallel efficiency (better than 80%) for up to 128 processors. A generally applicable algebraic multigrid preconditioner (AMG) in conjunction with an iterative Krylov solver reduces the number of iterations per solver step by almost two orders of magnitude compared with ILU-CG. Although a single iteration with AMG is significantly more expensive than with ILU, the reduction in number of iterations clearly favors a multilevel approach. In Plank et al[124], a speedup of six-fold was reported. Using AMG-CG is, to date, the most efficient method for solving the elliptic portion of the bidomain equations.

■ PERFORMING IN SILICO EXPERIMENTS

The use of computer simulations to perform in-silico experiments has become established over the last decade, either as a complement to experimental or clinical studies[38,56,130-132] or as a standalone tool for quantitative testing of hypotheses.[26,133] Two typical scenarios are considered with in silico experiments:

1. A subset of physiological signals has been experimentally recorded at a given spatiotemporal resolution in a subdomain of interest. An in silico experiment is designed to match the in vitro setup, and model parameters are tuned to match the data. Assuming that the underlying model is mechanistically sound and that in vitro and in silico data match well, the model can be trusted with some confidence. Then the obtained results can be dissected to understand the genesis of the physiological signals recorded in vitro. The main advantages of the in silico approach are that there is almost no limitation in terms of spatiotemporal resolution and that all quantities of interest are easily accessible and can be analyzed, including those for which no suitable experimental recording technique has been devised yet. Further, it can be assumed that in silico data can be trusted in regions beyond the experimental field of view where no data could be recorded at all. For instance, optical mapping can provide high-resolution data on myocardial activation patterns, but recordings are confined to the surfaces of the heart. Such in vitro data can be complemented with in silico data on electrical activity occurring deep in the myocardial wall where experimental techniques cannot provide data at a sufficiently high spatiotemporal resolution.

2. No in vitro experimental data are available that directly match the in silico experiment. This is, by a wide margin, the more frequently encountered scenario in modeling studies. In this case, model parameters are tuned during the initial phase of a study to ensure consistency with a priori known averaged physiological observations such as conduction velocities or isochronal activation and repolarization patterns.

Although differences between experiments and simulations grow smaller, attempting to achieve a 1:1 match is a futile effort. In fact, 1:1 matches are hardly achievable between two subsequent identical in vitro experiments. Rather than striving to achieve the impossible, in silico techniques focus on reproducing the salient features of the system as a whole, rather than on creating a 1:1 digital replica of a real heart. The main reasons for discrepancies between in vitro and in silico can be attributed to the following factors:

Uncertainty in model parameters: Although very detailed measurements of many cardiac parameters are found in the literature, the variance in the reported data is quite large, which renders a very detailed model parametrization a daunting task. The reasons for the large variance are multifactorial, including both technical reasons, due to differences in measurement setups and experimental procedures, and actual biological variability, such as intersubject and interspecies variability, regional heterogeneity, sex, age, type and state of disease, and other effects secondary to cardiac memory and pacing history. The uncertainty with all relevant biological parameters is, at best, 10%, but variances of 100% or more are not uncommon. An accurate determination of all relevant model parameters for a particular in vitro experiment is virtually impossible.

Anatomical and structural differences: Recent progress in imaging and modeling techniques allows the generation of microanatomically realistic models of the heart at a paracellular resolution.[43] Such models are geometrically very detailed, accounting for fine endocardial structures and interstitial cleft spaces due to embedded connective tissue secondary to fibrosis or deposition of fat. Despite the geometric detail, information provided through current nondestructive 3D imaging techniques on fiber and laminar arrangement cannot be obtained at a sufficiently high resolution, and alternative techniques such as serial histology are destructive and too time consuming for many applications. Moreover, imaging techniques provide data only on the eigendirections of the tissue, but not on the electrical conductivities along them.

Unaccounted mechanisms: Despite the high level of structural and functional detail in current high-end modeling studies, many mechanisms remain unaccounted for because they are either unknown or poorly understood or available data are insufficient to support the formulation of a sound model. That is, with in vitro models, all mechanisms are included, whether known or not, but quite often, some of these mechanisms have to be knocked out first to facilitate experimental observation (eg, in optical mapping studies, electromechanical coupling has to suppressed to avoid movement artifacts).

Numerical inaccuracies: Stiffness and nonlinearity of the bidomain equations renders their numerical solution a computationally expensive task. Trade-offs have to be made between spatiotemporal resolution, functional and anatomical detail included, and computing time. This is particularly true with whole heart simulations where the computational burden for high-resolution models may become prohibitive. Currently, depending on the species, approximately 100 to 200 μm is the highest resolution that can be used in silico in the context of whole heart simulations. In the case of a human heart, a discretization at 200 μm results in approximately 25 million degrees of freedom, which is currently the upper limit that can be handled efficiently with turnaround cycles that are sufficiently fast to support parameter studies. However, within this range of resolutions, the solution of the bidomain equations is not only a function of the model parameters; there is also, to some extent, a dependency on the spatiotemporal discretization.[123] With discretization schemes that rely on spatially fixed grids, h and dt are chosen to keep the numerical uncertainty below a certain percentage of 5% or less. Relative to the uncertainty of model parameters, numerical uncertainty does not constitute a problem per se. Numerical uncertainties are more problematic for comparisons between modeling studies, than for comparing in silico and in vitro results. Further, for simple pacing simulations where the same sequence is repeated, numerical deviations are negligible due to the synchronizing effect of the stimulus. However, deviations are to be expected when reentrant activation patterns are simulated over prolonged periods of time at the order of seconds or longer.

The multitude of factors and their complex interplay render the performance of in silico experiments a challenging task that requires a great deal of electrophysiological and theoretical expertise to determine an appropriate set of parameters that is suitable for a particular study. In current models, there are tens to hundreds of parameters involved, where each parameter is uncertain within a fairly large range. The sensitivity of simulation outcomes to these parameters is not well known, and due to the nonlinearity of the system, it is not easily predictable either. Strategies to determine this optimal parameter set vary from lab to lab; no commonly accepted standard has been established yet for this challenging and important problem. Thus far, in the majority of modeling studies, this problem has not been addressed at all. Instead, vanilla parameters are taken directly from published reports to parametrize a model.

Despite the lack of an established protocol, parametrization procedures can be broadly subdivided into two stages—first, a cellular stage where membrane kinetics are adjusted, and second, the adjustment of tissue level parameters to match conduction velocities and activation and repolarization patterns. The two stages are performed independently and sequentially, although it is known that there is a nonnegligible bidirectional interplay between the single cell and the tissue level. That is, cellular parameters, such as upstroke velocity or shape and duration of the action potential, may change substantially when coupled in a tissue as a function of cellular location relative to stimulus site and tissue boundaries,[134] as well as due to electrotonic loading in presence of cellular heterogeneity.[135]

During the first stage, cellular parameters are modified to fit a particular scenario under a given pacing protocol. In more complex studies where cellular heterogeneities are accounted for, the procedure has to be applied to several cells to obtain a representative cell for each heterogeneous region that is included in the tissue/organ model. In a subsequent step, adjustments of tissue-level bidomain parameters are made to arrive at a good match between in silico results and experimentally observed activation and repolarization patterns. This tuning is a more evolved procedure. A minimum prerequisite to allow any comparisons between model and experiment is to match the wavelength, L, defined as the product between action potential duration (APD) and conduction velocity, ϑ:

$$L = APD \times \vartheta \qquad (14\text{-}35)$$

Since L is the decisive factor that determines the presence and distribution of excitable gap and refractory tissue, wavelength matching is of key importance when comparing theoretical and experimental observations. This is particularly important for whole heart studies, where conduction velocities cannot be estimated as easily as in geometrically simplified models. Using cellular kinetics as set up at the first stage and neglecting the dependency of cellular APD on tissue parameters, conduction velocity has to be adjusted first. Due to the orthotropic tissue properties and the complex fiber and laminae arrangements in organ-level models, auxiliary simulations are performed in thin strand models to determine conductivities that yield the desired conduction velocities, ϑ_l, ϑ_t, and ϑ_n, along the main axes of the tissue (ie, along the fibers, el, transverse to the fibers within a sheet, et, and along the sheet orthogonal direction, en).

Conduction velocity ϑ_ζ depends on tissue conductivities and surface-to-volume ratio:

$$\vartheta_\zeta \propto \sqrt{\frac{1}{\beta}\frac{\sigma_{i\zeta}\sigma_{e\zeta}}{\sigma_{i\zeta} + \sigma_{e\zeta}}}, \quad \sigma_{b\zeta} = \frac{\sigma_{i\zeta}\sigma_{e\zeta}}{\sigma_{i\zeta} + \sigma_{e\zeta}} \qquad (14\text{-}36)$$

where $\sigma_{b\zeta}$, the harmonic mean between intracellular and extracellular conductivity along ζ, are the conductivities of the tissue bulk. For tuning ϑ_ζ, the bulk conductivities $\sigma_{b\zeta}$ have to be modified because β is a global scaling factor that influences ϑ in a direction-independent way. Auxiliary simulations are run in a sufficiently long strand of length $>10\cdot\lambda_\zeta$, where one end of the strand is stimulated to initiate propagation and ϑ_ζ is measured at the center of the strand. To minimize differences due to discretization errors in ϑ between auxiliary simulations and organ model, it is advisable to use the same average spatial discretization h in both the strand and the organ model. The ratio between desired ϑ_ζ and measured conduction velocity, $\tilde{\vartheta}_\zeta$, is then used to adjust $\sigma_{b\zeta}$:

$$\sigma_{b\zeta} = \left(\frac{\vartheta_\zeta}{\tilde{\vartheta}_\zeta}\right)^2 \sigma_{b\zeta}^0 \qquad (14\text{-}37)$$

where $\sigma_{b\zeta}$ is the adjusted conductivity parameter that will be plugged into the organ model and $\sigma_{b\zeta}^0$ is a default initial value taken from the literature. For setting up monodomain studies, the choice of $\sigma_{b\zeta}^0$ does not matter. Any of the reported values can be used because the final $\sigma_{b\zeta}$ as determined via this procedure is independent of $\sigma_{b\zeta}^0$.

All reports on measured bidomain conductivities seem to be fairly consistent in terms of bulk conductivities, with σ_{bl} ranging between 0.09 and 0.13 s/m and σ_{bt} between 0.017 and 0.034 s/m.[69,70,136] The larger discrepancy reported with σ_{bt} may be partially attributed to the fact, that, unlike in recent studies,[38] transverse conductivities were estimated without knowledge of the laminar structure of the heart. Using the extremal values of bulk conductivities in a computer simulation would lead to differences in conduction velocity of 23% and 76% in the longitudinal and transverse directions, respectively.

For bidomain studies, the situation is substantially more complex. Not only do the bulk conductivities matter in this case, but also the individual bidomain conductivities $\sigma_{i\zeta}$ and $\sigma_{e\zeta}$ and, in particular, the anisotropies α_i and α_e, as well as the anisotropy ratios between the two spaces, α. However, unlike with bulk conductivities, the variability in terms of individual bidomain conductivities between the experiments is quite large. For instance, individual conductivities such as the interstitial longitudinal conductivity σ_{el} differ by a factor 5.2 between Clerc[69] and Roberts and Scher,[70] and the ratio between the longitudinal conductivities σ_{il}/σ_{el} between the lowest and highest values differs by a factor of 10.[71] Reports on anisotropies α_i range from 5.7 to 10.8 in the intracellular space and on α_e between 1.5 and 2.6 in the interstitial space. In terms of anisotropy ratios α between the domains, these values translate into a range between 3.5 and

6.3. The anisotropy ratio α is a key factor in all bidomain modeling studies, and it is desirable to change α without changing the bulk conductivities. A systematic approach to adjust the bidomain conductivities for a desired α has been described by Roth[71] for transversely isotropic tissue. A more general recipe that also covers the more general case of orthotropic conductivities has not been reported yet.

An accurate parametrization of an organ model with bidomain conductivities remains an unresolved problem. Most likely, conductivities are not constant throughout the heart. Conductivities as used in the bidomain equations are the result of a homogenization procedure where the discrete intracellular and interstitial conductivities are averaged to obtain syncytial conductivities that can be used in a continuum representation. The homogenization results depend on type and density of gap junction expression, cellular geometry, cell arrangement, packing density, and tissue composition, such as deposition of collagen or fat, within the volume over which one is averaging. Because all of these factors vary throughout the heart, not only the eigendirections of the tensor, but also the bidomain conductivities, are a function of space.

Accurate measurements of tissue conductivities are often difficult to perform, even for small tissue samples, let alone measurements of their spatial variation. As a result, faithful identification of conductivities cannot be determined by experimental means. However, to circumvent this, at the tissue level, activation and repolarization isochrones can be matched between simulations with experiments. The parameter of utmost importance is conduction velocity because most phenomena depend on the ratio between wavelength and size of a heart.[137] There are no systematic matching procedures reported yet. Currently, research relies on ad-hoc adjustments of bulk conductivities. A more systematic strategy would require the solution of an inverse problem where experimental data serve as a constraint. Such an approach has been suggested to estimate space constants for simplified eikonal diffusion models[130]; however, for biophysically detailed bidomain models, no attempt has been reported yet.

Model Setup

Preparation of an in silico experiment normally proceeds via the following steps, described here and summarized in Fig. 14–7.

Definition of model anatomy: The geometric model over which the simulations are to be performed must first be defined. This involves the extraction of anatomical information of the preparation from an imaging modality (usually MR) via the process of segmentation, as described in the "Image Processing" section. The mesh generation stage then tessellates the geometry defined in the binarized segmented image stack to produce an unstructured finite element grid, as described in the "Mesh Generation" section, where jagged boundaries of the structured stack are replaced by smooth representations of the cardiac surfaces. Structurally or functionally different anatomical features that are either manually or automatically identified and "tagged" in the segmentation stage are also mapped across to the finite element mesh.

Inclusion of fine-scale anatomical detail: Cardiac fiber directions throughout the model are assigned to each finite element within the mesh, either directly from DT-MRI measurements or from a set of rules. In the case of DT-MRI, a voxel mapping method is used to map across voxel-based DT-MRI eigenvectors onto the centroids of the finite elements. For rule-based methods, prior computation of a smoothly varying field within the mesh is used to define fiber vectors based on a priori knowledge, as described in the "Assignment of Fibrous Architecture" section. Orthotropy within the model can be accounted for by including a laminar direction to simulate the effects of cardiac sheets.

Inclusion of electrophysiological detail: The relevant ionic model of cellular membrane dynamics, matching the species of the anatomical model if possible, must be defined within the model, usually on a per-node basis. Gradients in cellular model parameters may be included based on experimentally recorded transmural or apico-basal modulations. In addition, different cell models may be assigned to different tagged regions of the mesh to represent their differing electrophysiological behavior (eg, ventricles, atria, Purkinje fibers).

Initialization of tissue conductivities: Electrical conductivity values, associated with cardiac fiber and/or sheet/sheet-normal directions, are usually assigned experimentally measured values obtained from the literature. However, only a small number of robust measurements exists for a limited number of species, and large variations between these literature values are often seen.[71] Further, simulated activation patterns also depend, to some extent, on a chosen spatial discretization. To compensate for these numerical inaccuracies, additional simulations on auxiliary grids are conducted to tune the default conductivities until simulations reproduce experimentally observed conduction velocities.

Definition of experimental protocol: Similar to an in vitro experimental setup, electrode geometry and location have to be defined. Electrodes usually include a pacing electrode (eg, located at the apex), in addition to external plate electrodes (eg, at the exterior boundaries of a surrounding conductive bath) through which stronger shocks may be delivered. Stimulation protocols are assigned to each electrode to closely replicate experimental procedures.

Definition of the initial state: During in vitro experiments, preparations are paced for several minutes to arrive at a steady-state before the actual experiment commences. In an in silico study, this protocol can be duplicated, but the computational cost of pacing a tissue preparation over several minutes may be prohibitive. In this case, one can resort to applying the desired protocol to a single cell to subsequently populate the tissue model with the final state of the single-cell experiment. Steady-state at the tissue level will be different, but the overall system is close to steady-state, which reduces computer time vastly because only a few further beats need to be simulated to arrive at the organ level steady-state.

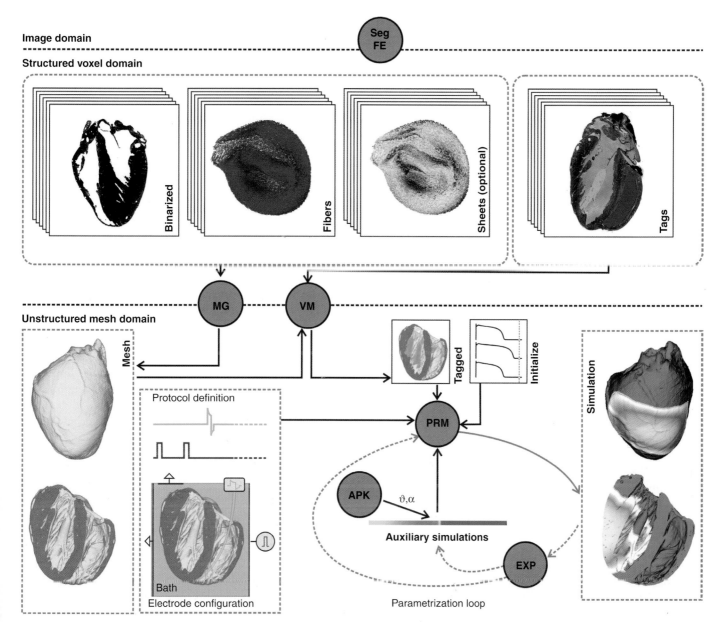

FIGURE 14–7. Basic concept of a model generation and parametrization pipeline. The image processing stage provides structured voxel stacks where each voxel has been binarized by a segmentation procedure (Seg), classified by a feature extraction procedure (FE), and a fiber direction has been assigned, either from diffusion tensor magnetic resonance imaging or on a per-rule base. Optionally, a laminar direction can be assigned as well. During the mesh generation (MG) stage, the binarized structured voxel stack is converted to an unstructured finite element mesh, and all voxel classifications are mapped over to the mesh by the voxel mapper (VM). Electrode configuration and stimulation protocols are added to define the basic setup of an in silico experiment. An initial parametrization (PRM) is found by (1) using a given set of tissue conductivities $\sigma_{\xi i}$ and $\sigma_{\zeta e}$ and (2) using a set of states for the respective tagged regions to properly initialize models of cellular dynamics, where appropriate initial states are found in a preprocessing step by pacing single cells at a given basic cycle length. A priori knowledge (APK) on experimentally observed conduction velocities and anisotropy ratios α serve as input for auxiliary simulations, using simple strand geometries that match the average discretization of the organ model, which are used to tune default conductivities in an automatic iterative procedure until the correct conduction velocities are observed in the auxiliary model. Simulations are performed then with the organ model, and the resulting activation patterns are compared against experimental observations (EXP). Subsequently, in the case of major deviations, parameters may be iteratively adjusted and simulations repeated until the required match is found.

Performing of simulations and comparison with experimental data: If available, comparisons with activation patterns from experiments (usually optical mapping) should be performed in an iterative manner, whereby conductivity parameters undergo repetitive refinements to bring a closer match with experimental observations. Sometimes, comparison may involve inclusion of the potential distortion effects of the experimental measurement technique in question.[131]

APPLICATIONS OF THE MODELING METHODOLOGY

■ OPTIMIZING DEFIBRILLATION THERAPY

Background

Several multicenter clinical trials have provided consistent evidence that implantable defibrillation therapy prolongs patient life. This convincing demonstration of efficacy has led to a nearly exponential growth, over the last decade, in the number of patients receiving implantable devices. Currently, approximately 0.2 million implantable cardioverter-defibrillators (ICDs) are implanted every year throughout the world. Although ICD therapy has proven to be efficient and reliable in preventing sudden cardiac death,[138] with success rates clearly superior to other therapeutic options such as pharmacological antiarrhythmia therapy,[139] it is far from ideal. There are several known adverse effects secondary to the administration of electrical shocks; the most prominent are linked to electroporation[140] (ie, the formation of pores in the cellular membrane that allow the free and indiscriminate redistribution of ions, enzymes, and large molecules between intracellular and interstitial space) and its aftereffects, which are indirectly caused by the high field strengths required to terminate arrhythmias such as ventricular fibrillation (VF) with sufficiently high probability. More importantly, psychological effects on patients play a nonnegligible role. Conscious patients may perceive shock delivery as extremely painful, which leads to traumatization and reduction in quality of life. Although pain may be tolerable in those cases where shock delivery terminates an otherwise lethal arrhythmia, this is less likely in those cases where inadequate shocks were delivered due to high-voltage component malfunctions of the device. A recent meta-analysis of industrial reports[3] concluded that such malfunctions are much more frequent than expected, with thousands of patients being affected. Further, clinical data from ICD trials suggested that six of seven shocks delivered can be classified as inadequate, indicating that the amount of overtreatment in the ICD population is significant.[139]

A substantial reduction in shock energy can only be achieved by full appreciation of the mechanisms by which a shock interacts with the heart and by devising novel therapeutic approaches on their basis. However, despite major advances in both experimental technology and computational modeling, our understanding of the biophysical basis of defibrillation remains incomplete. Further progress has been hampered by the inability of current experimental techniques to resolve electrical events in 3D during and after shock delivery with sufficiently high spatiotemporal resolution. Current mapping techniques are limited to record electrical activity from cardiac surfaces only and thus are incapable of detecting electrical events in the depth of the myocardium, which may exist there without any signature at the surfaces.[26] Computer models were introduced as a means to overcome experimental limitations, allowing the observation of electrical events within the depth of the myocardium. Initially, monodomain models were used, but theory and simulations predicted shock-induced changes in transmembrane voltage, ΔV_m, only along tissue boundaries and conductive discontinuities in the heart. These predictions contradicted experimental studies that had established that a critical mass of the tissue of approximately 95%[141,142] has to be affected by a sufficiently strong gradient of >5 V/cm[143,144] to be effective. Later, the "missing link"[145] that could explain shock-induced polarizations in the far field was discovered with the advent of the bidomain model, which predicted the existence of "virtual electrodes" (ie, polarizations that occur far from any physical electrode).[85]

Conceptually, defibrillation can be considered to be a two-step process. First, the applied shock drives currents that traverse the myocardium and cause complex polarization changes in transmembrane potential distribution.[81] Second, postshock active membrane reactions are invoked that eventually result either in termination of fibrillation in the case of shock success or in reinitiation of fibrillatory activity in the case of shock failure. Using computer models to analyze the etiology of "virtual electrode polarization" (VEP) patterns during the shock application phase revealed that shape, location, polarity, and intensity of shock-induced VEP are determined by both the cardiac tissue structure and the configuration of the applied field.[81,146,147] Based on theoretical considerations, VEPs can be classified either as "surface VEP," which penetrates the ventricular wall over a few cell layers, or as "bulk VEP," where polarizations arise throughout the ventricular wall.[148,149] Analysis of the bidomain equations revealed that a necessary condition for the existence of the bulk VEP is the presence of unequal anisotropies in the myocardium. Sufficient conditions include either spatial nonuniformity in applied electric field or nonuniformity in tissue architecture, such as fiber curvature, fiber rotation, fiber branching and anastomosis, and local changes in tissue conductivity due to resistive heterogeneities. A mathematical rationale supporting these notions is given in the "Theoretical Considerations for Low-Voltage Defibrillation" section.

The cellular response depends on VEP magnitude and polarity as well as on preshock state of the tissue. APD can be either extended (by positive VEP) or shortened (by negative VEP) to a degree that depends on VEP magnitude and shock timing, with strong negative VEP completely abolishing (de-exciting) the action potential, thus creating postshock excitable gaps. As demonstrated in bidomain modeling studies,[26,150] the postshock VEP pattern is also the major determinant of the origin of postshock activations. In those regions where shock-induced virtual anodes and virtual cathodes are in close proximity, a "break" excitation at shock-end (ie, the "break" of the shock) can be elicited. The virtual cathode serves as an electrical stimulus eliciting a regenerative depolarization and a propagating wave in the newly created excitable area. Whether or not break excitations arise depends on whether the transmembrane potential gradient across the border spans the threshold for regenerative depolarization.[151] The finding of break excitations, combined with the fact that positive VEP can result in "make" excitations (where "make" refers to the onset of a shock) in regions where tissue is at or near diastole, resulted in a novel understanding of how a strong stimulus can trigger the development of new activations.

According to VEP theory, mechanisms for shock success or failure are multifactorial depending mainly on postshock distribution of V_m as well as timing and speed of propagation of shock-induced wave fronts. Whether the depolarization of the postshock excitable gap is achieved in time critically depends on number and conduction velocity of postshock activations, as well as the available time window that is bounded by the instant at which refractory boundaries enclosing the excitable regions recover excitability. All factors ultimately depend on shock strength. Increasing shock strength results in higher voltage gradients across borders between regions of opposite polarity, leading to more break excitations,[151] which then start to traverse the postshock excitable gap earlier[116] and at a faster velocity,[151] as well as extending refractoriness to a larger degree.[152]

Optimization Strategies for Lowering Defibrillation Threshold

Although ICD therapy has improved over the years, no major breakthrough was achieved that would allow the lowering of defibrillation threshold (DFT) substantially. Incremental technical refinements were implemented that led to smaller, longer lasting devices and less invasive implantation procedures. Many parameters such as size, geometry, and location of coils and can relative to the heart, as well as the waveform of the delivered pulse and the timing of the shock, play an important role in determining DFT. The large number of parameters and their nontrivial relationship renders optimizing an ICD configuration a challenging task. A large body of research exists that deals with optimization of shock waveforms. It has been demonstrated that biphasic[153-155] or multiphasic[156-158] waveforms defibrillate at a lower threshold than monophasic waveforms and that truncated exponential pulses further increase the efficiency.[159] In addition to shock waveforms, optimization of lead placement has also seen increases in defibrillation efficacy. However, despite the many optimizations, shock energies delivered by current ICDs remain more than one order of magnitude too high to render defibrillation painless.

Although VEP theory provides a sound framework to describe mechanisms underlying success and failure of defibrillation shock in a high-voltage regimen, the theory does not lend itself easily to derive strategies that would facilitate defibrillation in a low-voltage regimen. Approaches to lower DFT by using more creative protocols are under examination; however, so far, only antitachycardia pacing (ATP) has gained clinical relevance. ATP is clinically applied with high success rates of 78% to 91% with VTs in the range of 188 to 200 beats/min and with similar success rates with faster VTs (200-250 beats/min).[2] Although the underlying mechanisms are not fully understood, the therapy aims at eliciting new wave fronts by pacing the excitable gap instead of trying to reset the tissue via a strong shock. For ATP to work, it is assumed that the organizing center of a reentry is accessible from a chosen pacing site. With reentries characterized by a fairly stable cycle length, a proper timing for a pacing pulse can be chosen by delivering a series of pulses at a pacing frequency that is higher than the intrinsic frequency of the circuit such that each pacing pulse is delivered progressively closer to the wave back of the reentry. Once a stimulus falls sufficiently close to the wave back, a unidirectional block occurs, and extinction of the arrhythmia is accomplished by collision with the approaching wave front. Empirically, it has been shown that success rates are highest at approximately 88% of the cycle length with ventricular rates <250 beats/min.[2] For faster activation rates or for more complex arrhythmias, ATP is more likely to fail, and a high-energy defibrillation shock has to be delivered, even if the arrhythmia has not degenerated into VF.

An alternative approach to avoid high-energy shocks has been suggested by Ripplinger et al,[160] which targets arrhythmias driven by reentrant cores attached to anatomic obstacles. The proposed therapy is based on destabilizing such a reentry by unpinning the reentrant core from the anatomic obstacle. The unpinned reentry either self-terminates when encountering a tissue boundary or repins and anchors to another heterogeneity. The unpinning mechanism relies on the formation of VEPs of opposite polarity in the far field in response to an applied electric field. As predicted by VEP theory, areas of depolarization and hyperpolarization form around tissue heterogeneities including those that anchor the core of a reentry. Depending on the timing of the pulse, the reentrant core either shifts its phase or detaches from the obstacle. Because unpinning relies on the VEP mechanism of excitation, simultaneous excitation of all reentrant cores can be achieved, independently of a chosen electrode location. In vitro studies in rabbits demonstrated that unpinning could be achieved with shock strengths ≤2.4 V/cm.[160] Success rates in terminating reentry depend critically on the timing of the unpinning pulse relative to the phase of the reentry. When unpinning shocks were applied uniformly throughout all phases of reentry, the success rate was only 13.1%. Hence, choosing the optimal phase for shock delivery is important. However, the phase of reentry is difficult to establish in vivo, and in the presence of multiple reentries, the timing of the unpinning pulse cannot be optimal for all reentrant circuits. Besides, in a whole heart model where heterogeneity is omnipresent, immediate repinning after detachment is not unlikely, which requires the repeated application of the therapy.

An alternative approach to terminate arrhythmias sustained by reentrant mechanism is to use a feedback-driven pacing protocol to control and eliminate reentry cores, by moving them until they hit inexcitable obstacles or each other, and annihilate. The mechanism used for influencing the direction of drift of the reentrant core relies on a phenomenon of resonant drift[161,162] (ie, the drift of reentrant waves when periodic, low-energy shocks are applied in resonance with the period of the reentry). A feedback algorithm[163] is required to maintain the resonance, which is implemented as a sensing electrode that serves to derive trigger signals for the pacing electrodes. A recent theoretical study that used a realistic anisotropic bidomain model of cardiac tissue with microscopic heterogeneities and realistic cellular kinetics confirmed earlier experimental and theoretical reports that were based on overly simplified models of cardiac tissue (such as the Belousov-Zhabotinsky reaction or monodomain models using a FitzHugh-Nagumo kinetics) that resonance drift pacing can be indeed used to move organizing centers of arrhythmias.[133] Simulations showed that termination can be achieved with high probability and within a sufficiently short time frame at a fraction of the conventional single-shock defibrillation strength. The direction of drift can be controlled by choosing a delay between detection of the trigger signal at the sensing electrode and delivery of a pacing pulse. For arrhythmias where the organizing center is anatomically anchored, unpinning is required first to induce drift via resonance drift pacing.

Neither ATP nor unpinning or resonance drift is likely to be efficient with more complex activation patterns (ie, in the presence of multiple anatomical or functional reentrant circuits or during fibrillatory activity). Recently, Fenton et al[132] proposed a strategy for such a scenario. A train of low-voltage field stimuli is applied at a fast rate to cause changes in polarizations, ΔV_m, in the far field along conductive discontinuities of the myocardium. Discontinuities within excitable regions at which ΔV_m is sufficiently large to be suprathreshold act as virtual electrodes, which become sites of wave-front emission. With sufficiently high field strengths, many virtual electrodes are formed, which progressively entrain the tissue until synchrony is achieved everywhere. The efficiency of the method has been demonstrated experimentally in vitro for thin-walled atrial preparations at very low field strengths of ≤1.6 V/cm. Whether the method can be applied with similarly low field strengths to ventricular arrhythmias where reentrant activity may occur within the thick ventricular walls has not yet been established.

Theoretical Considerations for Low-Voltage Defibrillation

At the very core of any attempt to understand the mechanisms underlying defibrillation shock and failure is the mechanistic link by which externally applied electric fields, $E = -\nabla\Phi_e$, transduce into changes in membrane polarization. Surface VEPs arise due to current redistribution near boundaries separating myocardium from blood in cavities or vessels or from a surrounding bath. Due to the arrangements of myocytes that tend to be aligned parallel to the organ surfaces, the attenuation of surface VEPs with distance to a boundary is governed by the transverse space constants λ_t and λ_n. That is, within a few space constants, typically <1 mm, surface VEP drops off to zero, leaving tissue unaffected by the shock, despite the presence of an extracellular potential gradient $\nabla\Phi_e$. Hence, surface VEPs alone are insufficient to affect a critical mass of the tissue, and defibrillation success depends critically on the formation of bulk VEPs. According to bidomain theory, bulk VEPs exist only in the presence of unequal anisotropy ratios. Sufficient conditions for the existence of bulk VEPs are most easily understood by rewriting Equation 14–6:

$$\beta C_m \frac{\partial V_m}{\partial t} = \underbrace{\nabla \cdot (\sigma_i \nabla \Phi_e)}_{S} + \nabla \cdot (\sigma_i \nabla V_m) - \beta I_{\text{ion}} \quad (14\text{–}38)$$

which reveals that the term S, referred to as activating function,[81,164] acts to induce changes in V_m. As shown by Sobie et al,[81] S can be decomposed into:

$$S = \underbrace{(\nabla \cdot \sigma_i) \cdot \nabla \Phi_e}_{S_1} + \underbrace{\sigma_i : \nabla(\nabla \Phi_e)}_{S_2} \quad (14\text{–}39)$$

That is, field-induced changes in V_m are driven either by the component S_1, the spatial variation in the intracellular conductivities ($\nabla \cdot \sigma_i$) weighted by the applied electric field $\nabla\Phi_e$, or by the component S_2, the spatial variation in the applied electric field $\nabla(\nabla\Phi_e)$ weighted by the intracellular conductivity tensor σi. By inspecting Equations 14–15 and 14–16, it becomes immediately evident that unequal anisotropy ratios are a necessary condition for bulk VEP because S disappears from the parabolic part of the bidomain equations.

Relevance to Low-Voltage Defibrillation Recently proposed low-voltage defibrillation strategies such as unpinning[160] or antifibrillatory pacing[132] rely on the presence of minimum field strengths

either to unpin an anatomically anchored core or to elicit a sufficiently large number of activations via VEP mechanisms that act to entrain and synchronize the tissue. With traditional single-shock defibrillation strategies, it is assumed that a minimum gradient of 5 V/cm is required to facilitate successful defibrillation.[165] With low-voltage strategies, the required minimum gradient seems to be lower, in the range between 1.6 and 2.4 V/cm. Designing an electrode configuration that ensures the required minimum gradients in an in vitro setup is easily achieved with large plate electrodes, where the field strength is constant throughout the tissue. This is clearly not the case when ICD configurations for in vivo use are under consideration. For technical reasons, size, shape, and location of the electrodes are subjected to limitations. Standard ICD configurations use fairly small coils, which lead to highly heterogeneous fields in their immediate vicinity. Further, due to the small size, field strength drops off rapidly with distance, leading to very high gradients in the near field, but the bulk of the tissue experiences much weaker field strengths below 10 V/cm,[166,167] which is also below the electroporation threshold.[168]

Quantitative investigation of shock-tissue interaction within the heart and how this depends on specific electrode configurations could lead to important advances in ICD technologies and protocols with direct clinical relevance.[169] However, predicting the exact electrical potential gradient distribution or activating function for determining changes in polarization in the presence of applied extracellular fields in vitro or in vivo in 3D at a sufficiently high spatiotemporal resolution is currently beyond the capabilities of any available clinical or experimental modality. In this scenario, computer modeling is the only choice for acquiring such information.

Indeed, the importance of predicting such factors has been recognized in earlier combined experimental and theoretical studies.[146] However, the applied experimental technique provided only a fairly small epicardial field of view, and consistent with this experimental setup, the computational model represented the cardiac structure as a 2D patch that matched the experimental field of view. More recent computational studies to quantify DFT within 3D models have been highly simplified,[169] fully relying on the critical mass hypothesis and ignoring the current view based on VEP theory. Further, these models are monodomain and disregard most structural and functional details that are known to be key determinants of shock outcome. Nonetheless, such models have been applied in a clinical study to provide metrics for relative comparison of electrode performance.[169]

Recent developments in computational cardiac modeling, as described earlier in this chapter, have significantly advanced our ability to simulate the electrical behavior of myocardial tissue within anatomically detailed whole ventricular models. Not only do such models provide us with knowledge of the response of both the extracellular and transmembrane potentials to an electrical stimulus throughout the fully 3D volume of the ventricles, but, due to the inherent detail and complexity of the models, they also allow us to assess the mechanisms by which fine-scale anatomical structures within the heart interact with

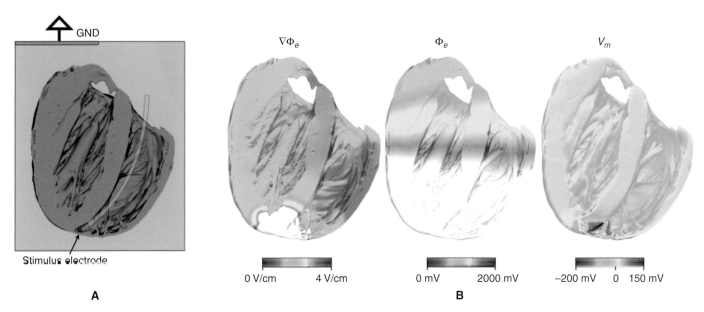

FIGURE 14–8. A. Shown is the electrode configuration corresponding to an implantable cardioverter-defibrillator (ICD) set up, with a grounding (GND) electrode at the base of the left ventricle and a catheter inserted into the right ventricular (RV) cavity, applying a stimulus directly to endocardial surface at the apex of the RV. **B.** Shown is the effect of applying a current injection stimulus of 50×10^8 A/μm^3 via the electrode configuration shown in A, with the left image showing the gradient of the extracellular potential ($\nabla\Phi_e$) within the ventricular cavities, where the color scale has been chosen to saturate at 4 V/cm; the center image showing the extracellular potential (Φ_e); and the right image showing the transmembrane potential (V_m).

strong electrical fields. Such micro-anatomically realistic models are currently being used by our groups to quantitatively predict DFT and tissue damage for clinically relevant electrode configurations and shock waveforms to rationalize placement and geometry of ICD cans and coils. Preliminary results from these investigations are presented in the following section.

Results

The anatomically highly detailed MR-based computational model of the rabbit ventricles, described previously in the "Construction of Models of the Cardiac Anatomy" section, was used to simulate a typical ICD setup, as shown in Fig. 14–8A. The stimulus catheter is inserted into the RV, applying a stimulus to the endocardial surface of the RV close to the apex. A grounding electrode is placed close to the base of the LV, in line with typical clinical configurations. A strong electrical stimulus of variable strength, in the form of a current injection, is applied to the tissue via the catheter.

Figure 14–8B shows the resulting distribution of extracellular potential gradient $\nabla\Phi_e$ (left), extracellular potential Φ_e (center), and transmembrane potential V_m (right) throughout the volume of the ventricular model following the application of a 50×10^8 A/μm^3 stimulus.

As can be seen from Fig. 14–8B, detailed information can be obtained regarding the prediction of voltage gradients for suprathreshold activations. These preliminary simulation results demonstrate, perhaps unsurprisingly, that the critical field strength isosurface (shown as 4 V/cm in Fig. 14–8B, left) is very close to the site of shock delivery, even though gradients in the immediate vicinity of the electrode are fairly high. The V_m panel also demonstrates how the model can be used to predict anatomical locations at which VEP-triggered activations arise.

Although preliminary, these initial simulations demonstrate the utility of such a modeling approach to provide a detailed analysis of electric potential distributions within the ventricular tissue during ICD protocols and to assess their dependency on specific lead placements. The flexibility of the model used here will also facilitate future investigations of novel ICD configurations to be tested in silico, providing the potential to optimize ICD configurations and protocols to improve success while reducing shock energy and tissue damage. Our initial results suggest how alterations in electrode placement may result in significant changes in distribution and heterogeneity of electric fields and activating function within the myocardial mass, which can thus be a major determinant of the DFT as well as spatial distribution and severity of tissue damage secondary to adverse shock effects. The bidomain nature of our model also allows for the computation of vulnerability grids for arrhythmia induction following shock application in order to accurately determine DFT, as well as allowing computation of the activating function to quantify shock-tissue interaction as a function of electrode configuration. Finally, the high level of anatomical detail contained within the model will provide knowledge of how anatomical heterogeneity within the ventricles influences the shock response, which is of great importance in the development of patient-specific therapies.

■ ELUCIDATING THE ROLE OF THE PURKINJE NETWORK

Background

Electrophysiological properties of PS cells are distinct from those of ventricular myocytes, with prominent variations in numerous ionic currents.[170-172] PS fibers respond to electrical fields differently from the endocardium upon which they run because of cellular differences[173] and because they are oriented in different directions than the myocardial fibers. Because the PS is a network of 1D cables, they should also be more prone to field excitation than 3D tissue.[32] Moreover, the myocardial response resulting from a particular shock depends on the orientation of the stimulating field; thus, different shocks may elicit distinct contributions from the PS, which could have implications for clinical techniques, where field direction is constrained by physical limitations.

Despite ever-accumulating evidence that the PS promotes and sustains arrhythmias[174] and is the source of postshock activations that may contribute to the failure of defibrillation,[175] no studies have directly observed the PS response to normal-strength stimuli at the organ level and the associated impact on shock outcome. Studies of field effects on papillary-Purkinje preparations[173] have used strong shocks to study electroporation but have disregarded the effects of weaker shocks on the PS-ventricular system as a whole, which are certainly clinically relevant. Measurements of PS electrical activity are difficult to obtain experimentally because fibers are fine and penetrate into the myocardium where the PMJs are situated. Optical mapping is problematic because the PS signal is overwhelmed by the myocardial signal at the organ scale. Computer modeling offers a noninvasive alternative to experimentation for ascertaining contributions of the PS to the whole heart response to defibrillation-strength shocks.

In this section, we demonstrate how the computer model developed as described in the preceding sections can be used to assess the role of the PS during defibrillation. Using our model, we will investigate the various issues raised. By applying large electric fields to the ventricles and observing behavior of the system with and without the PS, we will clearly identify its role.

We hypothesize that the PS is easily activated by electrical fields, which leads to far-field myocardial depolarizations emanating from PMJs during defibrillation. This is a distinct phenomenon from VEP effects but would produce complementary results. The strength and orientation of the applied field are expected to determine the postshock excitable gap and affect transmission characteristics; thus, shock features will mediate PS contributions. A computer model of 3D rabbit ventricles was used to study the response of quiescent tissue to various defibrillation shocks, with and without a detailed representation of the PS.

Results

Purkinje Network Activation The angle of incidence of an electric field on a fiber determines the strength of the interaction, so it was presumed that the His/Purkinje network, with its variously oriented branches, would respond differently to various fields. The ventricles with PS were subjected to 1-ms constant electric fields of 5 V/cm in the three principal directions. As expected, the excitation patterns for each of the fields were quite distinct (Fig. 14–9). The myocardium was excited in a small number of regions. For transverse shocks, the cathodal epicardial wall, the

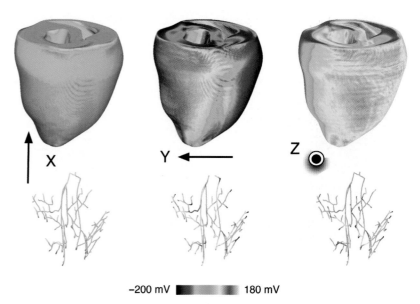

FIGURE 14–9. Electric field stimulation of the ventricles with Purkinje system. Constant electric fields were applied in the x-, y-, and z-directions. Induced transmembrane voltages are shown 1.25 ms after application of the field for the myocardium (above) and the Purkinje system (below).

septal wall nearest the cathode, and the endocardial wall nearest the anode were depolarized. For shocks along the major axis, the basal epicardium and apical endocardium were excited. Looking at the PS, many small regions were affected strongly. These regions corresponded to either endings or sharp curves, whereas straight regions were relatively unaffected, demonstrating once again that saw-tooth effects are not strong under constant electric fields. Excitation occurred downfield where there were abrupt changes in conductivities. Such changes encompassed bends in the branches and endings. Conversely, de-excitation occurred upfield, again at abrupt changes in geometry. Thus, looking at a field in the x-direction (see Fig. 14–9, left), the bottom ends of the network are hyperpolarized, whereas the tops are depolarized. For the other directions, similar patterns hold in the appropriate directions. A field along the x-direction appeared to activate more of the network than fields oriented along the other directions. There were more excitation regions in the PS than in the myocardium.

The time for the entire network to activate is given in Fig. 14–10. This time varied with the direction of the field and decreased

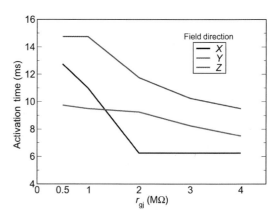

FIGURE 14–10. Time for the Purkinje tree to completely depolarize as a function of field direction and Purkinje system gap junction resistance.

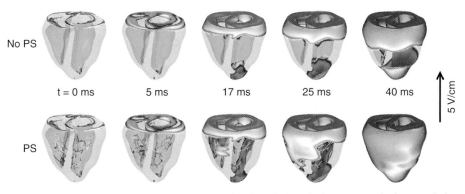

FIGURE 14–11. The Purkinje system (PS) alters shock-induced ventricular activation. A 5-V/cm shock was applied to quiescent ventricles without (top) and with (bottom) PS. With a PS, far-field excitations on the endocardial surface due to activations from the PS abbreviated total activation time by 30% compared with no PS.

with increasing gap junction resistance. Decreasing r_{gj} below 0.5 M Ω had essentially no effect. The total activation time was determined by the lengths of the branches, which were unaffected by the stimuli. The vast majority of the network was excited within 6 ms, with a particular branch being responsible for the remaining time. Such branches relied on activity to propagate into them and took considerably longer to activate than branches that were field stimulated at both ends. The activation time was reduced drastically for small increases in coupling resistance if that change in resistance resulted in field activation of a new branch; otherwise, the decrease in activation time was small with an increase in r_{gj}. Fields along the y-direction took the longest time to activate the network, whereas fields in the x-direction excited the entire network faster. For the most part, increasing the gap junction resistance had a gradual effect, reducing the activation time by slightly increasing the regions depolarized by the field. The saw-tooth potential was enough to bring a near-threshold excitation portion of the membrane above threshold. With an x-directed field, there was a drastic decrease in excitation time as the resistance was increased from 1 to 2 MΩ. This corresponded to a case where the saw-tooth effect became large enough to trigger a branch that was raised to near threshold by the field. If the field failed to trigger the branch, the branch would be activated by activity propagating through the Purkinje network.

Ventricular Activation Figure 14–11 compares the effect of shocks oriented along the long axis with and without a PS. Without a PS, initial depolarization of tissue at the ventricular base was a result of proximity to the anodal plane, which raised V_m above threshold by decreasing local Φ_e. The second source of activation was due to a VEP on the endocardial surface of the left ventricular apex, a consequence of hyperpolarization on the apical endocardium induced by the cathodal plane. Following the end of the shock, the pair of resultant wave fronts propagated gradually across the ventricles, completing activation in 59.5 ms.

Although ventricular activation immediately following the shock (0 ms) was independent of the PS, strong gradients were induced within segments of the PS. Ensuing activations emanating from these excited segments markedly affected the shock response. Initial effects of the PS on myocardial activation sequence were visible shortly after the end of the shock (5 ms); numerous ventricular locations were indirectly activated by the far field as a result of propagation from excited PMJs in PS sections excited by the shock. The resultant wave fronts propagated through the myocardial wall, giving rise to epicardial breakthroughs (right ventricular free wall, 17 ms) that did not occur in the absence of a PS, because the only sources of depolarization were wave fronts propagating from the apex and base. Later still (25 ms), several regions that remained inactive in the no PS case were completely activated in the presence of a PS. Complete activation of the ventricles with PS occurred in 39.0 ms, whereas a thick band of unexcited tissue between wave fronts remained when no PS was present (40 ms).

Full details of this study are provided in the article by Boyle et al.[176]

Contribution to Shock Induced Reentry Initiation We examined how the PS contributed to postshock arrhythmogenesis. A transmembrane pacing pulse was applied to the apex of the ventricles. At varying coupling intervals, cross-shocks were applied in the Y direction to induce reentry. When a PS was present compared with no PS, the window of vulnerability was narrower (10 vs 15 ms) because the ventricles depolarized and, hence, repolarized more quickly. The minimum shock strength to induce reentry was lower with a PS (3.3 V/cm vs 4 V/cm).

The PS was active throughout reentry and exhibited both anterograde and retrograde conduction at PMJs. PS activity contributed to reentry dynamics in three ways (Fig. 14–12). First, PS end points conducted intramural activity retrogradely, exciting distant endocardium ahead of the wave front and

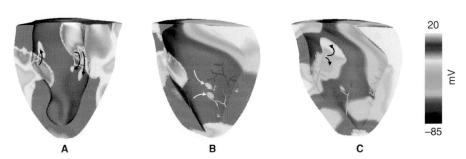

FIGURE 14–12. Purkinje system (PS) contributions during reentry. **A.** Wave fronts can be accelerated as activity is rapidly shunted ahead because of retrograde propagation through the PS, which causes breakthroughs (black arrow tips) that eventually merge with the primary front. **B.** Activity from wave fronts about to be extinguished due to refractoriness (white arrows) can "escape" annihilation by entering the PS retrogradely. **C.** Large areas of refractoriness surrounding PS end points create functional obstacles, which can cause wave fronts to fractionate (black arrows) and provide anchoring points for reentry.

effectively accelerating propagation when the original wave front merged with the new wave front. Second, retrograde activity provided an escape route for wave fronts terminating due to refractory tissue, thereby prolonging activity. Third, refractory regions surrounding PS entry points caused fractionation in wave fronts. Because PS cells have a longer intrinsic APD, this sort of wave front splitting occurred frequently.

To assess how the PS contributed to the maintenance and stabilization of reentry as time progressed, the PS was disconnected at various postshock instants. Isolating the PS immediately after the shock extinguished activity. PS disconnection at 200 ms led to reentry termination at 555 ms. In contrast, PS disconnection at later stages (≥1000 ms) did not terminate reentry. Thus, once meandering wave fronts on the epicardium and the endocardium converged into stable rotors, the PS did not appear to play a direct role.

Full details of this study are provided in the article by Deo et al.[177]

Discussion

These simulations demonstrate that the PS is a very important component in determining the response of the ventricles to defibrillation shocks and in the propagation of electrical activity in the ventricles. Thus, it is vital that the PS is included in organ-level models if fibrillation and defibrillation are to be studied.

First, the PS runs in all directions, so it will be activated in several places by electric fields regardless of the orientation of the field. The PS can be considered 1D, so it is easier to directly excite than the myocardium. Activity in the PS is widespread following shocks and spreads quickly into the myocardium to accelerate the activation of the ventricles. Compared with the myocardium, more regions were excited in the PS. In many regions where the PS was depolarized, the ventricles were not affected. The gap junction resistance played a role in determining how long it took for the entire PS to activate. Higher gap junction resistances in the PS lead to a small saw-tooth effect, which effectively increases the spatial extent of cathode make excitation.

The PS contributed to the establishment of postshock reentry. We identified several mechanisms by which this occurred. PMJs conduct both anterogradely and retrogradely, offering entry and exit points for propagating wave fronts. They effectively increase the dimensionality of the organ, leading to longer reentry times. Activity arriving through the PS was manifest on the surface as breakthroughs, which often reestablished activity after it had died out in a region. Conversely, wave fronts that appeared to be heading toward collision with refractory tissue survived by retrograde propagation. A more subtle effect led to wave-front speed up as PS wave fronts raced ahead of a myocardial wave front and emerged slightly ahead of the myocardial wave front. The longer action potential of the PS led to increased refractoriness at the PMJs, which could cause wave-front fractionation as wide wave fronts split when passing through a PMJ.

Propagation through the ventricles is complicated by the presence of the PS. Furthermore, the effects of the PS may not always be obvious or directly observable. Modeling provides a way to gauge the importance of the PS in light of experimental difficulties in measuring both global ventricular and PS behavior.

■ SIMULATIONS OF POSTINFARCTION VENTRICULAR TACHYCARDIAS

Background

Complex myocardial remodeling that occurs in postinfarcted hearts has been shown to give rise to substrates that could initiate/anchor ventricular tachycardia (VT) reentrant activity. The degree of myocardial injury in the infarcted region is dependent on tissue proximity from the site of occlusion. Tissue that experiences zero perfusion undergoes cellular necrosis and formation of scar tissue. Infarct shape analysis has demonstrated that strands of viable tissue within electrically passive scar tissue could provide alternate pathways for propagation. In addition, partial perfusion in the adjacent PZ tissue results in ion channel and gap junction remodeling that has been shown to result in slowed conduction and altered action potential morphology. The complexity of tissue remodeling within the infarct has made it difficult to elucidate the specific mechanisms that give rise to postinfarction VT and its morphology. This section will outline the application in simulation studies of an image-based 3D model of an infarcted canine heart that incorporates accurate infarct geometry and composition.

Results

The ionic kinetics in the normal and PZ myocardium were represented by the Luo-Rudy dynamic model.[178] Membrane kinetics in the PZ were modified based on data from literature. Previous studies of PZ in infarcted canine hearts have reported a reduction in peak sodium current to 38% of the normal value[179]; a reduction in peak L-type calcium current to 31% of normal[180]; and a reduction in peak potassium currents I_{Kr} and I_{Ks} to 30% and 20% of the maximum,[181] respectively. These modifications result in longer APD and decreased excitability compared with the normal myocardium. Mathematical description of current flow in cardiac tissue was based on the monodomain representation. To examine the arrhythmogenic propensity of the infarct substrate, an aggressive pacing protocol was delivered from the apex, similar to protocols used for clinical evaluation of patients with myocardial infarction. Pacing commenced at a basic cycle length of 250 ms for five beats (S1); 450 ms after the last S1, six stimuli were delivered at progressively shorter coupling intervals, starting at 190 ms and decreasing in steps of 10 ms. The induced activity was monitored for an additional 2.5 seconds.

Figure 14–13 illustrates the events that lead to VT induction. It depicts isochrones of activation times for time periods during the fourth stimulus of the aggressive pacing protocol and during the resulting VT. Images on the right present the intramural activation pattern on a slice through the heart, the location of which is indicated by the dashed white line on the epicardium. When the propagating wave front from the pacing site reaches the PZ, conduction significantly slows compared with the surrounding normal tissue. Faster wave fronts from the normal myocardium converge into the PZ laterally (white arrows)

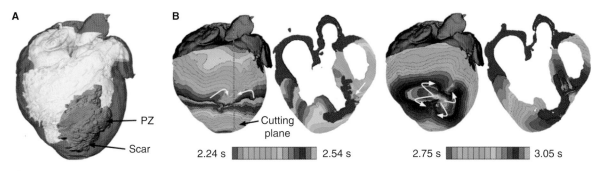

FIGURE 14–13. A. Canine ventricular model of infarction containing scar (purple) and peri-infarct zone (PZ; red) regions. **B.** Isochrones of activation times during the fourth pacing stimulus between 2.24 and 2.54 seconds (left) and 2.75 and 3.05 seconds (right) shown on the epicardial surface and within an intramural slice.

activating the entire PZ. The transmural view shows late activation of the PZ due to the wave front propagating from the normal myocardium. Because the PZ has a longer APD, it remains refractory, whereas the surrounding myocardium is fully recovered. As the pacing rate is increased, the wave front encounters refractory tissue, resulting in conduction block. This region of block later becomes the conduit for wave front propagation from the intramural PZ toward the surface. When pacing is completed, the activation from within the PZ tissue develops into an epicardial quatrefoil reentry. The reentry core remains within the PZ and is sustained throughout the simulation with a rotation frequency of 5 Hz.

Previous experimental studies of infarcted canine hearts have reported the induction of VT with epicardial reentry morphology.[182,183] The simulations revealed that decreased excitability, longer APD, and reduced conduction velocity throughout the PZ promoted conduction block and wave break that develops into epicardial reentry. Furthermore, the simulation showed that wave break and reentry formation occurred in both the epicardial and intramural portions of the PZ. Thus, this study showcased the utility of image-based computational modeling in predicting sites of reentry formation and maintenance.

■ OUTLOOK

The use of modeling techniques to complement experimental work has proved to be fruitful and has become an almost indispensable tool in many studies. Despite the many limitations, which enforce trade-offs to keep simulation studies tractable, it has become widely accepted that cardiac modeling is a viable approach to gain mechanistic insights into the electrophysiological function of the heart in health and disease. Recent advancements in various disciplines that are key to further develop modeling technology will allow for the lifting of many of these restrictions. New image acquisition techniques, such as high-field MRI and DT-MRI, provide very detailed geometrical and structural descriptions of the heart at a paracellular resolution. Image processing techniques and fully automatic mesh generation techniques are available that are capable of generating micro-anatomically accurate models of the heart directly from image stacks. The introduction of optimal multigrid and multilevel preconditioning techniques improves the performance and

parallel scalability of cardiac simulators, rendering large-scale parameter studies with anatomically realistic and biophysically detailed models feasible. Many of these very advanced solver techniques have been integrated in stable, mature, and easy to use toolkits.[184] Current developments in HPC hardware, which aim at overcoming limitations of the current CPU-centric paradigm by using accelerator technologies such as general purpose graphics processing units, promise a tremendous boost in performance at a substantially lower price. Combining all these key technologies in a robust framework that supports researchers in performing in silico experiments with ease will require major research efforts, but the basic building blocks for such simulation tools are already available today. Although current whole heart simulators lag real time by a factor of 10^3 to 10^4, next-generation HPC hardware in conjunction with novel simulation technologies will enable research to perform in silico experiments with near real-time performance, lagging real time only by a factor of 10^1 to 10^2. Such high-performance simulation tools open new and exciting applications, such as the integration of in silico techniques into a clinical work flow to support clinicians in making better informed decisions that are not feasible today.

ACKNOWLEDGMENTS

M. J. Bishop was supported by a Sir Henry Wellcome Postdoctoral Fellowship. E. Vigmond was supported by a grant from the Mathematics of Information Technology and Complex Systems. G. Plank was supported by grant no. F-3210-N18 of the Austrian Science Fund FWF.

REFERENCES

1. Rodgers A, Vaughan P. The world health report: reducing risks, promoting healthy lives. Technical Report. Geneva, Switzerland: The World Health Organization; 2002.
2. Wathen MS, DeGroot PJ, Sweeney MO, et al. Prospective randomized multicenter trial of empirical antitachycardia pacing versus shocks for spontaneous rapid ventricular tachycardia in patients with implantable cardioverter-defibrillators: Pacing Fast Ventricular Tachycardia Reduces Shock Therapies (PainFREE Rx II) trial results. *Circulation.* 2004;110:2591-2596.
3. Maisel W. Pacemaker and ICD generator reliability: meta-analysis of device registries. *JAMA.* 2006;295:1929-1934.

4. Waldo AL, Camm AJ, deRuyter H, et al. Effect of d-sotalol on mortality in patients with left ventricular dysfunction after recent and remote myocardial infarction. The SWORD Investigators. Survival With Oral d-Sotalol. *Lancet*. 1996;348:7-12.

5. Epstein AE, Hallstrom AP, Rogers WJ, et al. Mortality following ventricular arrhythmia suppression by encainide, flecainide, and moricizine after myocardial infarction. The original design concept of the Cardiac Arrhythmia Suppression Trial (CAST). *JAMA*. 1993;270:2451-2455.

6. Rudy Y, Ackerman MJ, Bers DM, et al. Systems approach to understanding electromechanical activity in the human heart: a National Heart, Lung, and Blood Institute workshop summary. *Circulation*. 2008;118:1202-1211.

7. Kohl P, Ravens U. Cardiac mechano-electric feedback: past, present, and prospect. *Prog Biophys Mol Biol*. 2003;82:3-9.

8. Hodgkin AL, Huxley AF. A quantitative description of membrane current and its application to conduction and excitation in nerve. *J Physiol*. 1952;117:500-544.

9. Noble D. Cardiac action and pacemaker potentials based on the Hodgkin-Huxley equations. *Nature*. 1960;188:495-497.

10. Spach MS, Kootsey JM. Relating the sodium current and conductance to the shape of transmembrane and extracellular potentials by simulation: effects of propagation boundaries. *IEEE Trans Biomed Eng*. 1985;32:743-755.

11. Leon LJ, Roberge FA. Directional characteristics of action potential propagation in cardiac muscle. A model study. *Circ Res*. 1991;69:378-395.

12. Beaumont J, Davidenko N, Davidenko JM, Jalife J. Spiral waves in two-dimensional models of ventricular muscle: formation of a stationary core. *Biophys J*. 1998;75:1-14.

13. Vigmond E, Leon L. Computationally efficient model for simulating electrical activity in cardiac tissue with fiber rotation. *Ann Biomed Eng*. 1999;27:160-170.

14. Hunter P, Smaill B. The analysis of cardiac function: a continuum approach. *Prog Biophys Mol Biol*. 1988;52:101-164.

15. Henriquez CS. Simulating the electrical behavior of cardiac tissue using the bidomain equations. *Crit Rev Biomed Eng*. 1993;1:1-77.

16. Fenton FH, Cherry EM, Karma A, Rappel WJ. Modeling wave propagation in realistic heart geometries using the phase-field method. *Chaos*. 2005;15:13502.

17. Buist M, Sands G, Hunter P, Pullan A. A deformable finite element derived finite difference method for cardiac activation problems. *Ann Biomed Eng*. 2003;31:577-588.

18. Rogers JM, McCulloch AD. A collocation–Galerkin finite element model of cardiac action potential propagation. *IEEE Trans Biomed Eng*. 1994;41:743-757.

19. Vigmond EJ, Aguel F, Trayanova NA. Computational techniques for solving the bidomain equations in three dimensions. *IEEE Trans Biomed Eng*. 2002;49:1260-1269.

20. Harrild DM, Henriquez CS. A finite volume model of cardiac propagation. *Ann Biomed Eng*. 1997;25:315-334.

21. Trew M, Le Grice I, Smaill B, Pullan A. A finite volume method for modeling discontinuous electrical activation in cardiac tissue. *Ann Biomed Eng*. 2005;33:590-602.

22. Hillebrenner MG, Eason JC, Trayanova NA. Mechanistic inquiry into decrease in probability of defibrillation success with increase in complexity of preshock reentrant activity. *Am J Physiol Heart Circ Physiol*. 2004;286:H909-H917.

23. Meunier J, Eason J, Trayanova N. Termination of reentry by a long-lasting AC shock in a slice of the canine heart: a computational study. *J Cardiovasc Electrophysiol*. 2002;13:1253-1262.

24. Trayanova N, Eason J. Shock-induced arrhythmogenesis in the myocardium. *Chaos*. 2002;12:962-972.

25. Xie F, Qu Z, Yang J, Baher A, Weiss JN, Garfinkel A. A simulation study of the effects of cardiac anatomy in ventricular fibrillation. *J Clin Invest*. 2004;113:686-693.

26. Ashihara T, Constantino J, Trayanova NA. Tunnel propagation of postshock activations as a hypothesis for fibrillation induction and isoelectric window. *Circ Res*. 2008;102:737-745.

27. Potse M, Dube B, Richer J, Vinet A, Gulrajani R. A comparison of monodomain and bidomain reaction-diffusion models for action potential propagation in the human heart. *IEEE Trans Biomed Eng*. 2006;53:2425-2435.

28. Ten Tusscher KH, Hren R, Panfilov AV. Organization of ventricular fibrillation in the human heart. *Circ Res*. 2007;100:e87-e101.

29. Harrild D, Henriquez C. A computer model of normal conduction in the human atria. *Circ Res*. 2000;87:E25-E36.

30. Vigmond EJ, Tsoi V, Kuo S, et al. The effect of vagally induced dispersion of action potential duration on atrial arrhythmogenesis. *Heart Rhythm*. 2004;1:334-344.

31. Seemann G, Hoper C, Sachse FB, Dossel O, Holden AV, Zhang H. Heterogeneous three-dimensional anatomical and electrophysiological model of human atria. *Philos Transact A Math Phys Eng Sci*. 2006;364:1465-1481.

32. Vigmond EJ, Clements C. Construction of a computer model to investigate sawtooth effects in the Purkinje system. *IEEE Trans Biomed Eng*. 2007;54:389-399.

33. Tusscher KH, Panfilov AV. Modelling of the ventricular conduction system. *Prog Biophys Mol Biol*. 2008;96:152-170.

34. Berenfeld O, Jalife J. Purkinje-muscle reentry as a mechanism of polymorphic ventricular arrhythmias in a 3-dimensional model of the ventricles. *Circ Res*. 1998;82:1063-1077.

35. Yan GX, Shimizu W, Antzelevitch C. Characteristics and distribution of M cells in arterially perfused canine left ventricular wedge preparations. *Circulation*. 1998;98:1921-1927.

36. Szentadrassy N, Banyasz T, Biro T, et al. Apico-basal inhomogeneity in distribution of ion channels in canine and human ventricular myocardium. *Cardiovasc Res*. 2005;65:851-860.

37. Di Diego JM, Sun ZQ, Antzelevitch C. I(to) and action potential notch are smaller in left vs. right canine ventricular epicardium. *Am J Physiol*. 1996;271:H548-H561.

38. Hooks DA, Trew ML, Caldwell BJ, et al. Laminar arrangement of ventricular myocytes influences electrical behavior of the heart. *Circ Res*. 2007;101:e103-e112.

39. Rohmer D, Sitek A, Gullberg GT. Reconstruction and visualization of fiber and laminar structure in the normal human heart from ex vivo diffusion tensor magnetic resonance imaging (DTMRI) data. *Invest Radiol*. 2007;42:777-789.

40. ten Tusscher KHWJ, Panfilov AV. Alternans and spiral breakup in a human ventricular tissue model. *Am J Physiol Heart Circ Physiol*. 2006;291:H1088-H1100.

41. Hren R, Nenonen J, Horacek BM. Simulated epicardial potential maps during paced activation reflect myocardial brous structure. *Ann Biomed Eng*. 1998;26:1022-1035.

42. Burton R, Plank G, Schneider J, et al. 3D models of individual cardiac histo-anatomy: tools and challenges. *Ann NY Acad Sci*. 2006;1380:301-319.

43. Plank G, Burton R, Hales P, et al. Generation of histo-anatomically representative models of the individual heart: tools and application. *Philos Transact A Math Phys Eng Sci*. 2009;367:2257-2292.

44. Streeter D, Spontnitz H, Patel D, Ross J, Sonnenblick E. Fiber orientation in the canine left ventricle during diastole and systole *Circ Res*. 1969;24:339-347.

45. LeGrice I, Smaill B, Chai L, Edgar S, Gavin J, Hunter P. Laminar structure of the heart: ventricular myocyte arrangement and connective tissue architecture in the dog. *Am J Physiol*. 1995;269:H571-H582.

46. Scollan D, Holmes A, Zhang J, Winslow R. Reconstruction of cardiac ventricular geometry and fiber orientation using magnetic resonance imaging. *Ann Biomed Eng*. 2000;28:934-944.

47. Helm P, Beg M, Miller M, Winslow R. Measuring and mapping cardiac fiber and laminar architecture using diffusion tensor MR imaging. *Ann NY Acad Sci*. 2005;1047:296-307.

48. Dierckx H, Benson AP, Gilbert SH, et al. Intravoxel fibre structure of the left ventricular free wall and posterior left-right ventricular insertion site in canine myocardium using q-ball imaging. In: *FIMH 2009: Proceedings of the 5th International Conference on Functional Imaging and Modeling of the Heart*. Berlin, Germany: Springer-Verlag; 2009:495-504.

49. Sethian J. *Level-Set Fash Marching Methods*. Cambridge, United Kingdom: Cambridge University Press; 2002.

50. Vadakkumpadan F, Rantner LJ, Tice B, et al. Image-based models of cardiac structure with applications in arrhythmia and defibrillation studies. *J Electrocardiol*. 2009;42:157.e1-e10.

51. Chen J, Song SK, Liu W, et al. Remodeling of cardiac fiber structure after infarction in rats quantified with diffusion tensor MRI. *Am J Physiol Heart Circ Physiol*. 2003;285:H946-H954.

52. Ibanez L, Schroeder W, Ng L, Cates J. *The Insight Segmentation and Registration Toolkit (version 1.4)*. New York, NY: Kitware Inc.; 2003.

53. Basser PJ, Pierpaoli C. Microstructural and physiological features of tissues elucidated by quantitative-diffusion-tensor MRI. *J Magn Reson B*. 1996;111:209-219.

54. Schmidt A, Azevedo CF, Cheng A, et al. Infarct tissue heterogeneity by magnetic resonance imaging identifies enhanced cardiac arrhythmia susceptibility in patients with left ventricular dysfunction. *Circulation.* 2007;115:2006-2014.

55. Wu MT, Tseng WY, Su MY, et al. Diffusion tensor magnetic resonance imaging mapping the fiber architecture remodeling in human myocardium after infarction: correlation with viability and wall motion. *Circulation.* 2006;114:1036-1045.

56. Hunter P, Pullan A, Smaill B. Modelling total heart function. *Rev Biomed Eng.* 2003;5:147.

57. Stevens C, Remme E, LeGrice I, Hunter P. Ventricular mechanics in diastole: material parameter sensitivity. *J Biomech.* 2003;36:737-748.

58. Nielsen P, Le Grice I, Smaill B, Hunter P. Mathematical model of geometry and brous structure of the heart. *Am J Physiol.* 1991;260:1365-1378.

59. Prassl AJ, Kickinger F, Ahammer H, et al. Automatically generated, anatomically accurate meshes for cardiac electrophysiology problems. *IEEE Trans Biomed Eng.* 2009;56:1318-1330.

60. Plotkowiak M, Rodriguez B, Plank G, et al. High performance computer simulations of cardiac electrical function based on high resolution MRI datasets. Paper presented at Computational Science - ICCS 2008, 8th International Conference, Kraków, Poland, June 23-25, 2008, Proceedings, Part I.

61. Efimov I, Nikolski V, Salama G. Optical imaging of the heart (review). *Circ Res.* 2004;94:21-33.

62. Vetter FJ, McCulloch A. Three-dimensional analysis of regional cardiac function: a model of rabbit ventricular anatomy. *Prog Biophys Molec Biol.* 1998;69:157-183.

63. Mansoori T, Plank G, Burton R, et al. Building detailed cardiac models by combination of histoanatomical and high-resolution MRI images. Presented at the IEEE International Symposium on Biomedical Imaging (ISBI). 2007:572-575.

64. Bishop MJ, Hales P, Plank G, Gavaghan DJ, Scheider D, Grau V. Comparison of rule-based and DTMRI-derived fibre architecture in a whole rat ventricular computational model. In: *FIMH 2009: Proceedings of the 5th International Conference on Functional Imaging and Modeling of the Heart.* Berlin, Germany: Springer-Verlag; 2009:87-96.

65. Desplantez T, Dupont E, Severs NJ, Weingart R. Gap junction channels and cardiac impulse propagation. *J Membr Biol.* 2007;218:13-28.

66. Gourdie RG, Green CR, Severs NJ. Gap junction distribution in adult mammalian myocardium revealed by an anti-peptide antibody and laser scanning confocal microscopy. *J Cell Sci.* 1991;99:41-55.

67. Hoyt RH, Cohen ML, Saffitz JE. Distribution and three-dimensional structure of intercellular junctions in canine myocardium. *Circ Res.* 1989;64:563-574.

68. Severs NJ, Bruce AJ, Dupont E, Rothery S. Remodelling of gap junctions and connexin expression in diseased myocardium. *Cardiovasc Res.* 2008;80:9-19.

69. Clerc L. Directional differences of impulse spread in trabecular muscle from mammalian heart. *J Physiol.* 1976;255:335-346.

70. Roberts DE, Scher AM. Effect of tissue anisotropy on extracellular potential fields in canine myocardium in situ. *Circ Res.* 1982;50:342-351.

71. Roth BJ. Electrical conductivity values used with the bidomain model of cardiac tissue. *IEEE Trans Biomed Eng.* 1997;44:326-328.

72. Spach MS, Heidlage JF. The stochastic nature of cardiac propagation at a microscopic level. Electrical description of myocardial architecture and its application to conduction. *Circ Res.* 1995;76:366-380.

73. Kleber AG, Rudy Y. Basic mechanisms of cardiac impulse propagation and associated arrhythmias. *Physiol Rev.* 2004;84:431-488.

74. Roberts SF, Stinstra JG, Henriquez CS. Effect of nonuniform interstitial space properties on impulse propagation: a discrete multidomain model. *Biophys J.* 2008;95:3724-3737.

75. Neu J, Krassowska W. Homogenization of syncytial tissue. *Crit Reb Biomed Eng.* 1993;21:137-199.

76. Pennacchio M, Savare G, Colli Franyone P. Multiscale modeling for the bioelectric activity of the heart. *SIAM J Math Anal.* 2006;37:1333-1370.

77. Hand PE, Griffith BE, Peskin CS. Deriving macroscopic myocardial conductivities by homogenization of microscopic models. *Bull Math Biol.* 2009;71:1707-1726.

78. Tung L. *A Bi-Domain Model for Describing Ischemic Myocardial D-C Potentials* [doctoral dissertation]. Cambridge, MA: MIT; 1978.

79. Pollard AE, Hooke N, Henriquez CS. Cardiac propagation simulation. *Crit Rev Biomed Eng.* 1992;20:171-210.

80. Roth BJ, Wikswo JP. Electrical stimulation of cardiac tissue: a bidomain model with active membrane properties. *IEEE Trans Biomed Eng.* 1994;41:232-240.

81. Sobie EA, Susil RC, Tung L. A generalized activating function for predicting virtual electrodes in cardiac tissue. *Biophys J.* 1997;73:1410-1423.

82. Trayanova N, Skouibine K, Moore P. Virtual electrode effects in defibrillation. *Prog Biophys Mol Biol.* 1998;69:387-403.

83. Henriquez C, Muzikant A, Smoak C. Anisotropy, fiber curvature, and bath loading effects on activation in thin and thick cardiac tissue preparations: simulations in a three dimensional bidomain model. *J Cardiovasc Electrophysiol.* 1996;7:424-444.

84. Trayanova NA. Effects of the tissue-bath interface on the induced transmembrane potential: a modeling study in cardiac stimulation. *Ann Biomed Eng.* 1997;25:783-792.

85. Sepulveda NG, Roth BJ, Wikswo JP Jr. Current injection into a two-dimensional anisotropic bidomain. *Biophys J.* 1989;55:987-999.

86. Nielsen B, Ruud T, Lines G, Tveito A. Optimal monodomain approximations of the bidomain equations. *Appl Math Comput.* 2007;184:276-290.

87. Coghlan H, Coghlan A, Buckberg G, Cox J. "The electrical spiral of the heart": its role in the helical continuum. The hypothesis of the anisotropic conducting matrix. *Eur J Cardiothorac Surg.* 2006;29(Suppl 1):S178-S187.

88. Oosthoek PW, Virgh S, Mayen AE, van Kempen MJ, Lamers WH, Moorman AF. Immunohistochemical delineation of the conduction system. I: the sinoatrial node. *Circ Res.* 1993;73:473-481.

89. Zigelman G, Kimmel R, Kiryati N. Texture mapping using surface flattening via multidimensional scaling. *IEEE Trans Vis Comput Graph.* 2002;8:1-10.

90. Gould R. *Graph Theory.* Reading, MA: Benjamin Cummings; 1988.

91. Durrer D, van Dam RT, Freud GE, Janse MJ, Meijler FL, Arzbaecher RC. Total excitation of the isolated human heart. *Circulation.* 1970;41:899-912.

92. Netter FH. *Atlas of Human Anatomy.* 2nd Ed. New York, NY: Saunders; 1997.

93. Pollard AE, Barr RC. The construction of an anatomically based model of the human ventricular conduction system. *IEEE Trans Biomed Eng.* 1990;37:1173-1185.

94. Simelius K, Nenonen J, Horacek M. Modeling cardiac ventricular activation. *Int J Bioelectromag.* 2001;3:51-58.

95. DiFrancesco D, Noble D. A model of cardiac electrical activity incorporating ionic pumps and concentration changes. *Philos Trans R Soc Lond B Biol Sci.* 1985;307:353-398.

96. Huelsing D, Spitzer K, Cordeiro J, Pollard A. Conduction between isolated rabbit Purkinje and ventricular myocytes coupled by a variable resistance. *Am J Physiol.* 1998;274:H1163-H1173.

97. Monserrat M, Saiz J, Ferrero J Jr, Ferrero J, Thakor N. Ectopic activity in ventricular cells induced by early afterdepolarizations developed in Purkinje cells. *Ann Biomed Eng.* 2000;28:1343-1351.

98. Lu HR, Marin R, Saels A, Clerck FD. Species plays an important role in drug-induced prolongation of action potential duration and early afterdepolarizations in isolated Purkinje fibers. *J Cardiovasc Electrophysiol.* 2001;12:93-102.

99. Aslanidi OV, Stewart P, Boyett MR, Zhang H. Optimal velocity and safety of discontinuous conduction through the heterogeneous Purkinje-ventricular junction. *Biophys J.* 2009;97:20-39.

100. Murillo M, Cai X. A fully implicit parallel algorithm for simulating the non-linear electrical activity of the heart. *Numer Linear Algebra Appl.* 2004;11:261-277.

101. Munteanu M, Pavarino L, Scacchi S. A scalable Newton-Krylov-Schwarz method for the bidomain reaction-diffusion system. *SIAM J Sci Comput.* 2009;31:3861-3883.

102. Southern JA, Plank G, Vigmond EJ, Whiteley SP. Solving the coupled system improves computational efficiency of the bidomain equations. *IEEE Trans Biomed Eng.* 2009;56:2404-2412.

103. Vigmond EJ, Hughes M, Plank G, Leon LJ. Computational tools for modeling electrical activity in cardiac tissue. *J Electrocardiol.* 2003;36(Suppl):69-74.

104. Keener J, Bogar K. A numerical method for the solution of the bidomain equations in cardiac tissue. *Chaos.* 1998;8:234-241.

105. Qu Z, Garfinkel A. An advanced algorithm for solving partial differential equation in cardiac conduction. *IEEE Trans Biomed Eng.* 1999;46:1166-1168.

106. Sundnes J, Lines GT, Tveito A. An operator splitting method for solving the bidomain equations coupled to a volume conductor model for the torso. *Math Biosci.* 2005;194:233-248.

107. Strang G. On the construction and comparision of difference scheme. *SIAM J Numerical Analysis.* 1968;5:506-517.

108. Rosenbrock HH. Some general implicit processes for the numerical solution of differential equations. *Computer J.* 1963:329-331.

109. Hairer E, Wanner G. *Solving Ordinary Differential Equations II: Stiff and Differential Algebraic Problems.* 2nd ed. Ser. Springer Series in Computational Mathematics. New York, NY: Springer; 2004.

110. Maclachlan MC, Sundnes J, Spiteri RJ. A comparison of non-standard solvers for ODEs describing cellular reactions in the heart. *Comput Methods Biomech Biomed Engin.* 2007;10:317-326.

111. Rush S, Larsen H. A practical algorithm for solving dynamic membrane equations. *IEEE Trans Biomed Eng.* 1978;25:389-392.

112. Plank G, Zhou L, Greenstein JL, et al. From mitochondrial ion channels to arrhythmias in the heart: computational techniques to bridge the spatio-temporal scales. *Philos Transact A Math Phys Eng Sci.* 2008;366:3381-3409.

113. Whiteley JP. An efficient numerical technique for the solution of the monodomain and bidomain equations. *IEEE Trans Biomed Eng.* 2006;53:2139-2147.

114. Sundnes J, Artebrant R, Skavhaug O, Tveito A. A second-order algorithm for solving dynamic cell membrane equations. *IEEE Trans Biomed Eng.* 2009;56:2546-2548.

115. Cortassa S, Aon MA, O'Rourke B, et al. A computational model integrating electrophysiology, contraction, and mitochondrial bioenergetics in the ventricular myocyte. *Biophys J.* 2006;91:1564-1589.

116. Skouibine K, Trayanova N, Moore P. Success and failure of the defibrillation shock: insights from a simulation study. *J Cardiovasc Electrophysiol.* 2000;11:785-796.

117. Wang S, Leon LJ, Roberge FA. Interactions between adjacent fibers in a cardiac muscle bundle. *Ann Biomed Eng.* 1996;24:662-674.

118. Trew ML, Smaill BH, Bullivant DP, Hunter PJ, Pullan AJ. A generalized finite difference method for modeling cardiac electrical activation on arbitrary, irregular computational meshes. *Math Biosci.* 2005;198:169-189.

119. Virag N, Jacquemet V, Henriquez CS, et al. Study of atrial arrhythmias in a computer model based on magnetic resonance images of human atria. *Chaos.* 2002;12:754-763.

120. Franzone PC, Deuflhard P, Erdmann B, Lang J, Pavarino LF. Adaptivity in space and time for reaction-diffusion systems in electrocardiology. *SIAM J Sci Comput.* 2006;28:942-962.

121. Sundnes J, Nielsen BF, Mardal KA, Cai X, Lines GT, Tveito A. On the computational complexity of the bidomain and monodomain models of electrophysiology. *Ann Biomed Eng.* 2006;34:1088-1097.

122. Saucerman JJ, Healy SN, Belik ME, Puglisi JL, McCulloch AD. Proarrhythmic consequences of a KCNQ1 AKAP-binding domain mutation: computational models of whole cells and heterogeneous tissue. *Circ Res.* 2004;95:1216-1224.

123. Pollard AE, Burgess MJ, Spitzer KW. Computer simulations of three-dimensional propagation in ventricular myocardium. Effects of intramural fiber rotation and inhomogeneous conductivity on epicardial activation. *Circ Res.* 1993;72:744-756.

124. Plank G, Liebmann M, Weber dos Santos R, Vigmond EJ, Haase G. Algebraic multigrid preconditioner for the cardiac bidomain model. *IEEE Trans Biomed Eng.* 2007;54:585-596.

125. Li X, Demmel J. SuperLU DIST: a scalable distributed-memory sparse direct solver for unsymmetric linear systems. *ACM Transact Ions Mathematical Software (TOMS).* 2003;29:110-140.

126. Amestoy P, Duff IS, L'Excellent JY, Koster J. Mumps: a general purpose distributed memory sparse solver. In: *Para 2000: Proceedings of the 5th International Workshop on Applied Parallel Computing, New Paradigms for HPC in Industry and Academia.* London, United Kingdom: Springer-Verlag; 2001:121-130.

127. Briggs WL, Henson VE, McCormick SF. *A Multigrid Tutorial.* Philadelphia, PA: SIAM Publications; 2000.

128. Weber dos Santos R, Plank G, Bauer S, Vigmond EJ. Parallel multigrid preconditioner for the cardiac bidomain model. *IEEE Trans Biomed Eng.* 2004;51:1960-1968.

129. Austin TM, Trew ML, Pullan AJ. Solving the cardiac bidomain equations for discontinuous conductivities. *IEEE Trans Biomed Eng.* 2006;53:1265-1272.

130. Sermesant M, Peyrat JM, Chinchapatnam P, et al. Toward patient-specific myocardial models of the heart. *Heart Fail Clin.* 2008;4:289-301.

131. Bishop M, Rodriguez B, Qu F, Efimov I, Gavaghan D, Trayanova N. The role of photon scattering in optical signal distortion during arrhythmia and defibrillation. *Biophys J.* 2007;93:3714-3726.

132. Fenton FH, Luther S, Cherry EM, et al. Termination of atrial fibrillation using pulsed low-energy far-field stimulation. *Circulation.* 2009;120:467-476.

133. Morgan SW, Plank G, Biktasheva IV, Biktashev VN. Low energy defibrillation in human cardiac tissue: a simulation study. *Biophys J.* 2009;96:1364-1373.

134. Sampson KJ, Henriquez CS. Electrotonic influences on action potential duration dispersion in small hearts: a simulation study. *Am J Physiol Heart Circ Physiol.* 2005;289:H350-H360.

135. Sampson KJ, Henriquez CS. Interplay of ionic and structural heterogeneity on functional action potential duration gradients: implications for arrhythmogenesis. *Chaos.* 2002;12:819-828.

136. Roberts DE, Hersh LT, Scher AM. Influence of cardiac fiber orientation on wavefront voltage, conduction velocity, and tissue resistivity in the dog. *Circ Res.* 1979;44:701-712.

137. Panfilov AV. Is heart size a factor in ventricular fibrillation? Or how close are rabbit and human hearts? *Heart Rhythm.* 2006;3:862-864.

138. Bardy GH, Hofer B, Johnson G, et al. Implantable transvenous cardioverter-defibrillators. *Circulation.* 1993;87:1152-1168.

139. A comparison of antiarrhythmic-drug therapy with implantable defibrillators in patients resuscitated from near-fatal ventricular arrhythmias. The Antiarrhythmics versus Implantable Defibrillators (AVID) Investigators. *N Engl J Med.* 1997;337:1576-1583.

140. De Bruin K, Krassowska W. Electroporation and shock-induced transmembrane potential in a cardiac fiber during defibrillation strength shocks. *Ann Biomed Eng.* 1998;26:584-596.

141. Ideker RE, Wolf PD, Alferness C, Krassowska W, Smith WM. Current concepts for selecting the location, size and shape of defibrillation electrodes. *Pacing Clin Electrophysiol.* 1991;14:227-240.

142. Adgey AAJ, Spence MS, Walsh SJ. Theory and practice of defibrillation: (2) defibrillation for ventricular fibrillation. *Heart.* 2005;91:118-125.

143. Frazier DW, Wolf PD, Wharton JM, Tang AS, Smith WM, Ideker RE. Stimulus-induced critical point. Mechanism for electrical initiation of reentry in normal canine myocardium. *J Clin Invest.* 1989;83:1039-1052.

144. Zhou X, Daubert JP, Wolf PD, Smith WM, Ideker RE. Epicardial mapping of ventricular defibrillation with monophasic and biphasic shocks in dogs. *Circ Res.* 1993;72:145-160.

145. Roth BJ, Krassowska W. The induction of reentry in cardiac tissue. The missing link: how electric fields alter transmembrane potential. *Chaos.* 1998;8:204-220.

146. Knisley SB, Trayanova N, Aguel F. Roles of electric field and fiber structure in cardiac electric stimulation. *Biophys J.* 1999;77:1404-1417.

147. Rodriguez B, Li L, Eason JC, Efimov IR, Trayanova NA. Differences between left and right ventricular chamber geometry affect cardiac vulnerability to electric shocks. *Circ Res.* 2005;97:168-175.

148. Trayanova N, Skouibine K, Aguel F. The role of cardiac tissue structure in defibrillation. *Chaos.* 1998;8:221-233.

149. Entcheva E, Trayanova NA, Claydon FJ. Patterns of and mechanisms for shock induced polarization in the heart: a bidomain analysis. *IEEE Trans Biomed Eng.* 1999;46:260-270.

150. Roth BJ. A mathematical model of make and break electrical stimulation of cardiac tissue by a unipolar anode or cathode. *IEEE Trans Biomed Eng.* 1995;42:1174-1184.

151. Cheng Y, Mowrey K, Van Wagoner D, Tchou P, Efimov I. Virtual electrode-induced reexcitation: a mechanism of defibrillation. *Circ Res.* 1999;85:1056-1066.

152. Knisley S, Smith W, Ideker R. Prolongation and shortening of action potentials by electrical shocks in frog ventricular muscle. *Am J Physiol.* 1994;266:H2348-H2358.

153. Neuzner J, Pitschner H, Huth C, Schlepper M. Effect of biphasic waveform pulse on endocardial defibrillation efficacy in humans. *Pacing Clin Electrophysiol.* 1994;17:207-212.

154. Walcott GP, Walker RG, Cates AW, Krassowska W, Smith WM, Ideker RE. Choosing the optimal monophasic and biphasic waveforms for ventricular defibrillation. *J Cardiovasc Electrophysiol.* 1995;6:737-750.

155. Matula M, Brooks M, Pan Q, Pless B, Province R, Echt D. Biphasic waveforms for ventricular defibrillation: optimization of total pulse and second phase durations. *Pacing Clin Electrophysiol.* 1997;20:2154-2162.

156. Zhang Y, Ramabadran R, Boddicker K, et al. Triphasic waveforms are superior to biphasic waveforms for 80 transthoracic defibrillation: experimental studies. *J Am Coll Cardiol.* 2003;42:568-575.

157. Dosdall D, Rothe D, Brandon T, Sweeney J. Effect of rapid biphasic shock subpulse switching on ventricular defibrillation thresholds. *J Cardiovasc Electrophysiol.* 2004;15:802-808.

158. Zhang Y, Rhee B, Davies L, et al. Quadriphasic waveforms are superior to triphasic waveforms for transthoracic defibrillation in a cardiac arrest swine model with high impedance. *Resuscitation.* 2006;68:251-258.

159. Schuder JC, Stoeckle H, West JA, Keskar PY. Transthoracic ventricular defibrillation in the dog with truncated and untruncated exponential stimuli. *IEEE Trans Biomed Eng.* 1971;18:410-415.

160. Ripplinger CM, Krinsky VI, Nikolski VP, Efimov IR. Mechanisms of unpinning and termination of ventricular tachycardia. *Am J Physiol Heart Circ Physiol.* 2006;291:H184-H192.

161. Davydov VA, Zykov VS, Mikhailov AS, Brazhnik PK. Drift and resonance of spiral waves in active media. *Radiozika.* 1988;31:574-582.

162. Agladze KI, Davydov VA, Mikhailov AS. An observation of resonance of spiral waves in distributed excitable medium. *JETP Lett.* 1987;45:767-770.

163. Biktashev VN, Holden AV. Design principles of a low voltage cardiac debrillator based on the effect of feedback resonant drift. *J Theor Biol.* 1994;169:101-112.

164. Rattay F. Analysis of models for external stimulation of axons. *IEEE Trans Biomed Eng.* 1986;33:974-977.

165. Ideker RE, Zhou X, Knisley SB. Correlation among fibrillation, defibrillation, and cardiac pacing. *Pacing Clin Electrophysiol.* 1995;18:512-525.

166. Fotuhi PC, Epstein AE, Ideker RE. Energy levels for defibrillation: what is of real clinical importance? *Am J Cardiol.* 1999;83:24D-33D.

167. Kinst TF, Sweeney MO, Lehr JL, Eisenberg SR. Simulated internal defibrillation in humans using an anatomically realistic three-dimensional finite element model of the thorax. *J Cardiovasc Electrophysiol.* 1997;8:537-547.

168. Fedorov VV, Nikolski VP, Efimov IR. Effect of electroporation on cardiac electrophysiology. *Methods Mol Biol.* 2008;423:433-448.

169. Jolley M, Stinstra J, Pieper S, et al. A computer modeling tool for comparing novel ICD electrode orientations in children and adults. *Heart Rhythm.* 2008;5:565-572.

170. Han W, Wang Z, Nattel S. A comparison of transient outward currents in canine cardiac Purkinje cells and ventricular myocytes. *Am J Physiol Heart Circ Physiol.* 2000;279:H466-H474.

171. Han W, Bao W, Wang Z, Nattel S. Comparison of ion-channel subunit expression in canine cardiac Purkinje fibers and ventricular muscle. *Circ Res.* 2002;91:790-797.

172. Han W, Zhang L, Schram G, Nattel S. Properties of potassium currents in Purkinje cells of failing human hearts. *Am J Physiol Heart Circ Physiol.* 2002;283:H2495-H2503.

173. Li HG, Jones DL, Yee R, Klein GJ. Defibrillation shocks produce different effects on Purkinje fibers and ventricular muscle: implications for successful defibrillation, refibrillation and postshock arrhythmia. *J Am Coll Cardiol.* 1993;22:607-614.

174. Dosdall DJ, Tabereaux PB, Kim JJ, et al. Chemical ablation of the Purkinje system causes early termination and activation rate slowing of long-duration ventricular 82 fibrillation in dogs. *Am J Physiol Heart Circ Physiol.* 2008;295:H883-H889.

175. Dosdall DJ, Cheng KA, Huang J, et al. Transmural and endocardial Purkinje activation in pigs before local myocardial activation after defibrillation shocks. *Heart Rhythm.* 2007;4:758-765.

176. Boyle PM, Deo M, Plank G, Vigmond EJ. Purkinje-mediated effects in the response of quiescent ventricles to defibrillation shocks. *Ann Biomed Eng.* 2010;38:456-468.

177. Deo M, Boyle P, Plank G, Vigmond E. Arrhythmogenic mechanisms of the Purkinje system during electric shocks: a modeling study. *Heart Rhythm.* 2009;6:1782-1789.

178. Luo CH, Rudy Y. A dynamic model of the cardiac ventricular action potential. I. Simulations of ionic currents and concentration changes. *Circ Res.* 1994;74:1071-1096.

179. Pu J, Boyden PA. Alterations of Na+ currents in myocytes from epicardial border zone of the infarcted heart. A possible ionic mechanism for reduced excitability and postrepolarization refractoriness. *Circ Res.* 1997;81:110-119.

180. Dun W, Baba S, Yagi T, Boyden PA. Dynamic remodeling of K+ and Ca2+ currents in cells that survived in the epicardial border zone of canine healed infarcted heart. *Am J Physiol Heart Circ Physiol.* 2004;287:H1046-H1054.

181. Jiang M, Cabo C, Yao J, Boyden PA, Tseng G. Delayed rectifier K currents have reduced amplitudes and altered kinetics in myocytes from infarcted canine ventricle. *Cardiovasc Res.* 2000;48:34-43.

182. Ashikaga H, Sasano T, Dong J, et al. Magnetic resonance-based anatomical analysis of scar-related ventricular tachycardia: implications for catheter ablation. *Circ Res.* 2007;101:939-947.

183. Ciaccio EJ, Ashikaga H, Kaba RA, et al. Model of reentrant ventricular tachycardia based on infarct border zone geometry predicts reentrant circuit features as determined by activation mapping. *Heart Rhythm.* 2007;4:1034-1045.

184. Balay S, Buschelman K, Gropp W, et al. PETSc Homepage. Accessed August 11, 2010; Available at: http://www.mcs.anl.gov/petsc.

CHAPTER 15

CARDIAC SIMULATION FOR EDUCATION: THE ELECTROCARDIOGRAM ACCORDING TO ECGSIM

Adriaan van Oosterom and Thom F. Oostendorp

INTRODUCTION / 266

THE SOURCE MODEL / 266
  The Equivalent Double Layer / 266
  Generalization of the EDL / 267
  Potentials Generated by the EDL / 268
  Dipolar Approximations of the EDL / 269

THE THORAX MODEL / 269

MATRIX FORMULATION OF THE FORWARD PROBLEM / 269

ABOUT ECGSIM / 270

THE ECG ACCORDING TO ECGSIM / 271
  The Normal ECG / 271
  Potential Field at S_h; Electrograms / 273
  Basic Statistics of the Timing Parameters / 273
  The T Wave / 275
  Changing the TMP Parameters Locally / 278
  Direct Current Recordings; ST-T Changes / 281

CONCLUSION / 283

INTRODUCTION

Most diagnostic methods used in clinical electrocardiography (ECG) are statistically based forms of pattern recognition. Over the years, the selection of the signal features used in these methods, such as timing, amplitude, and duration of wavelets, has been guided by knowledge gathered through linking clinical observations with ECG waveforms, along with insight gained from invasive electrophysiology. These methods have reached a diagnostic accuracy of up to 90% in some categories of cardiac disease. However, in other categories, the performance is much lower. Moreover, the manifestation in the ECG of some types of abnormality remains poorly understood. Examples of these problematic domains are the diagnosis of left ventricular hypertrophy, the interpretation of ST changes during acute ischemia, the electric manifestation of the Brugada syndrome, and the long QT syndrome. What these examples have in common is that the major features that play a role in the related ECG analysis are their waveforms, which are the result of the electric depolarization and repolarization processes of the membranes of cardiac myocytes, rather than rhythm abnormalities.

Since Einthoven's day (late nineteenth century/early twentieth century),[1,2] the development of diagnostic ECG criteria has been accompanied by the development of biophysical models aimed at linking the electrophysiology of cardiac function with the waveforms of the ECG signals observed on the body surface. In such an approach, two aspects of the bioelectric generator need to be specified—a *source model* of the cardiac electric activity, and a *volume conductor model*, which is a model for describing the passive effects on the observed data of the body tissues that surround the active electric sources.

This chapter focuses on these model-based explanations of ECG morphology, in particular on the ECG components that reflect the electric activity of the ventricles. It does not include an analysis of cardiac rhythm. The emphasis of the approach lies on the ventricular activity. However, it applies in a similar manner to the electric activity of the atria.

The topic is illustrated by simulations from a computer program ECGSIM,[3] which allows the user to interactively change the major source parameters: the timing of depolarization and repolarization on the ventricular surface and the local source strength. The program is available, free of charge, from the Web site http://www.ecgsim.org. The program was designed specifically to serve both as a tool in teaching the basic link between electrophysiology and ECG morphology and as an instrument in research applications.

In ECGSIM, the expression of the cardiac sources in terms of electric potential fields and signals (the handling of the so-called *forward problem*) is worked out in a realistic volume conductor model that accounts for the spreading out of the electric currents in a three-dimensional (3D) representation of the tissues surrounding the heart. Images are presented of the distribution of these parameter values over the ventricular surface as well as those of the accompanying potentials on the ventricular surface and on the body surface.

The theory behind the forward computation is outlined only briefly, focusing on the most essential part of it—a description of the nature of the source and of the source parameters that can be changed interactively. The remaining part of the chapter discusses a selection of the applications of this tool, summarized as "the ECG according to ECGSIM."

THE SOURCE MODEL

■ THE EQUIVALENT DOUBLE LAYER

The cardiac electric source in ECGSIM is the equivalent double layers (EDL) model. It expresses the entire electrical activity *within* the ventricular walls by means of a double layer source situated on the *closed* surface S_h bounding the mass of all ventricular myocytes: endocardium, epicardium, and their connection at the base. Referring to the surface as *closed* expresses the fact that any ant moving about inside such a surface would be able to reach all interior points but not be able to make its way out.

The EDL can be viewed as a generalization of the classic uniform double layer (UDL) source model, the model based on the analysis of Wilson et al[4] in 1933. This source model has been shown to be very effective in describing the sources at the

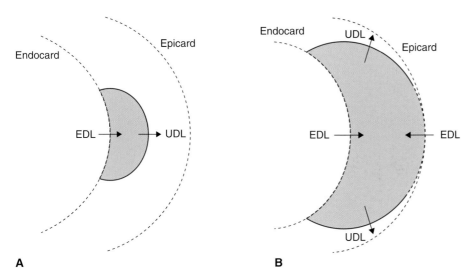

FIGURE 15–1. Schematic representation of a cross-section of the ventricular wall. The heavy solid lines mark the wave fronts–the boundaries between activated tissue (in purple) and regions that are still at rest. The wave front propagates in the direction of the local surface normals, marked by uniform double layer (UDL). **A.** Early stage, single wave front. **B.** Later stage, breakthrough has occurred at the epicardium; the wave front (in this cross-section) has split up into two parts. The intersections of the wave fronts with the tissue boundaries, marked by heavy dashed line segments, constitute the locations of active parts of the equivalent double layer (EDL) on endocardium and epicardium.

depolarization wave fronts.[5] The link between the UDL and the EDL models, explained in detail in van Oosterom,[6] is summarized here to facilitate the introduction of the EDL concept.

To this end, in Fig. 15–1, a schematic diagram is presented of the activation of the ventricular wall initiated at a single site on the endocardium, shown in a transmural cross-section. The heavy solid lines mark the wave fronts (ie, the boundaries between activated tissue [in grey] and the regions that are still at rest). The wave front propagates along the local normals, marked by UDL. The gradients of the intracellular potential of the myocytes across the wave fronts (≈100 mV/mm) act as the dominant electric forces for the potential field generated in the medium outside the myocardium. In the UDL source model, the sources are taken to be an electric double layer of uniform strength. The double layer can be viewed as an infinite number of current dipoles of uniform (infinitesimally small) strength that are evenly distributed over the activation boundary, each oriented normal to its local surface and pointing toward the tissue still at rest, the direction of the arrows marked UDL in Fig. 15–1. In an infinite medium, the potential at any point that is exterior to the myocardium generated by the UDL source is proportional to the solid angle subtended by the wave front at the observation point. The sign of the potential, with reference to the potential at infinity defined as zero, is positive if the observation point faces the approaching side of the wave front; elsewhere, it is negative.[4,7-9]

In Fig. 15–1A, the intersection between the wave front and the ventricular wall is marked by a heavy dashed line segment. This borders the depolarized zone of the (closed) ventricular surface. At an exterior observation point, the solid angle subtended by this zone is identical to the one subtended by the wave front, because their rim is identical.[10] As a consequence, instead of the source distribution at the wave front, the potential field in the

exterior medium may be described by a *virtual* double layer, acting as an equivalence surface source distribution all over S_h. In order to apply this to the situation shown in panel A, the strength of the EDL over the depolarized part of S_h is taken to be nonzero, equal to the UDL strength at the wave front. Over the remaining part of S_h, the strength is zero. Note that for an exterior observation point close to the depolarized zone, the sign of the potential is negative, in agreement with measured electrophysiologic data (electrograms).

The situation depicted in Fig. 15–1B represents a later stage of the depolarization process, following epicardial breakthrough. Here, the EDL can be introduced in the same manner: For any exterior observation point, the potential generated by the UDL source(s) at the complete wave front(s) is the sum of the potentials generated by each of the subsections of the wave front. As before, the strength of the EDL is taken to be equal to the UDL strength (at the wave front) over any depolarized part of S_h, and to be zero elsewhere. The addition of the contributions of subsections is justified by the nature of the EDL. Just like that of the UDL, the nature of the EDL is that of a current source, specified by a current dipole surface distribution (see next section), for which the superposition (addition) principle holds true.

■ GENERALIZATION OF THE EDL

The EDL, just like the UDL, has the nature of an electric double layer. It differs from the UDL in that its strength is nonuniform over S_h. In the preceding introduction, the strength of the EDL is taken to be uniform over the depolarized parts of S_h and zero over the remaining parts. In this manner, the EDL may serve to explain the potential field during the depolarization phase only. At the end of this phase, the entire S_h borders depolarized tissue, and the EDL covers this closed surface. As a consequence, at this time, the contribution to the exterior potential field is zero because the solid angle subtended by any *closed* surface at any exterior observation point is zero.

In its generalization, the true electric source—the second-order spatial derivative of the transmembrane potential field *throughout ventricular mass*—is replaced by an equivalent source—an equivalent dipole surface density *at the surface* S_h bounding the myocardium. The time course of the local EDL strength is taken to be proportional to the local transmembrane potentials (TMP), $V_m(t)$, of the myocytes near S_h, with a proportionality constant set by the local values of the electric conductivity of the tissue. Its background can be found in the literature.[11] Its complete validity rests on an assumed spatial uniformity throughout the myocardium of the anisotropy ratio of intracellular and extracellular electric conductivities.[12] Although this assumption represents a so-called *first-order approximation* only, the EDL is currently the only model available with a direct link to cardiac electrophysiology that is able to describe the most prominent aspects of the genesis of the ECG. This applies in particular to the cardiac sources during the repolarization phase (ie, for describing the genesis of the T wave of the surface ECG).[13]

Prior to depolarization, all ventricular myocytes are polarized, with a resting potential $V_m(t) \approx -80$ mV. This creates a uniform EDL strength over S_h and, hence, a zero contribution to the external potential field and zero potential differences in all ECG leads. This is analogous to the situation of a single cell in its fully polarized state. By the time all myocytes have been activated, normally say 80 ms later, all values of the TMPs $V_m(t)$, which set the EDL strength at S_h, are close to a state having reversed polarity, $V_m(t) \approx +10$ mV, a state generally referred to as the depolarized state. If all $V_m(t)$ values were uniform over S_h, the external potential field would, once again, be zero. In fact, close to the parts of S_h where depolarization started, the $V_m(t)$ values will already have progressed more toward their resting value than at the parts activated last. This causes a nonuniform distribution of $V_m(t)$ values over S_h and, hence, produces a nonzero external field, causing nonzero values at the end of the QRS interval, with higher magnitudes the nonuniformity is greater. In the same manner, the nonuniformity in the $V_m(t)$ values over S_h values throughout the repolarization phase acts as the (EDL) source of the T wave voltages of the ECG. Significantly, if the time course during repolarization of $V_m(t)$ of all myocytes was the same, the T wave amplitudes in all ECG lead signals would be zero. Finally, if the myocardium is fully repolarized, and if all resting state values of $V_m(t)$ values are uniform, the external field is once more zero, accompanied by a return to zero baseline values of all ECG lead signals.

■ POTENTIALS GENERATED BY THE EDL

By using the EDL, the potential field in the external medium following the initiation of depolarization can be computed by splitting up S_h into numerous small patches. Individual source strengths proportional to the local value of $V_m(t)$ are assigned to each patch, weighted by the signed, individual solid angle that it subtends at the field point. Adding up the contributions of all patches (superposition theorem) then results in the value of the potential at the field point.

Any small membrane patch of a single cell acts as an elementary EDL that contributes to the extracellular field.[4,14] The most particular nature of this type of source is emphasized in the following example, illustrated in Fig. 15–2. Figure 15–2A shows the projection of a disk-shaped patch carrying a uniform strength situated at $x = 0$ along an x-axis in 3D space (line segment a). The surface normal of the patch (ie, the direction of the double layer) is directed along the x-axis. In Fig. 15–2B, the solid trace depicts the potential profile along the x-axis, which is proportional to the signed solid angle subtended by the disk at different positions of the observation point along the x-axis. Note the abrupt change in the sign of the potential and the accompanying jump (discontinuity) in the potential when crossing the double layer,[4] similar to the voltage jump observed when penetrating an active cellular membrane. The jump is the most characteristic feature of

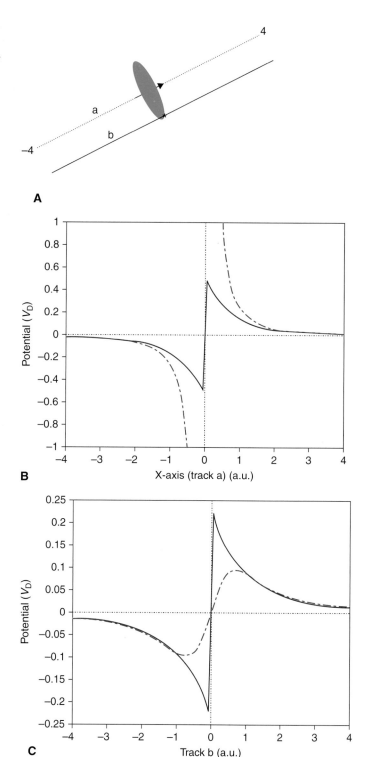

FIGURE 15–2. A. Projection in three-dimensional space of a circular disk with unit radius, carrying a double layer source with strength D (A/m) placed in an infinite medium with electric conductivity σ (siemens/m). The arrow marks the surface normal of the disk, as well as the single dipole approximation of the double layer source. **B.** Solid line indicates potential profile generated by the disk along line a, expressed in units $V_D = D/\sigma$ (V); dash-dot line indicates potential profile generated by a single (equivalent) dipole as represented by the arrow on the upper panel. **C.** Potential profiles similar to the ones on panel B, but now along line b. The scaling of the x-axis is in arbitrary units, with the value 1 being equal to the radius of the disk. Note that at distal observations points, for example at distances greater than 2, (the diameter of the disk) the potential profiles of the single dipole closely approximate those of the double layer.

the double layer source. It occurs, with identical magnitude, irrespective of the angle at which the patch is crossed and irrespective of the point of intersection. The magnitude of the generated voltage jump, V_D, can be used to specify the local double layer strength. When skimming the edge of the disk, as along line b on the upper panel, the discontinuity is still visible (Fig. 15–2C), but the magnitude is halved; potential profiles along lines that do not intersect the disk do not exhibit such discontinuities.

■ DIPOLAR APPROXIMATIONS OF THE EDL

At sufficiently large distances from the patch (as a rule of thumb, greater than twice the size of the patch), the potential field generated by the EDL is closely approximated by the field generated by a current dipole that is directed along the normal of the patch, as can be seen in Fig. 15–2. However, close to the patch, the potentials generated by the single dipole deviate greatly from the ones generated by the double layer. Note that in close proximity to the dipole location (track a; $x = 0$), the magnitude of the potential generated by the dipole tends to become infinite, which is a completely unphysiologic value.

The current dipole is probably the best known model of the cardiac electrical generator; it is the basis of vectorcardiography. In Einthoven's papers, as well as in his correspondence with Lewis and Wilson,[15] we see it appearing as an arrow drawn on a plane, representing the "electromotive force" of the heart. At the side of the head of the arrow (see Fig. 15–2), current is injected into the surrounding medium. The location is referred to as the source of the dipole; just below it (at the side of the tail of the arrow), exactly the same current is withdrawn from the medium; the location is referred to as the sink of the dipole. The nature of the current dipole can be likened to that of a circulation pump inside an aquarium.

The single current dipole as used in vectorcardiography can be viewed as the vector sum of the current dipoles, approximating the EDL of all patches of the heart surface S_h. It is a gross approximation of the full complexity of the cardiac electric activity (a so-called *equivalent generator*) that can be used during the entire QRST interval. In this application, a single dipole performs surprisingly well; it accounts for approximately 80% (representation power) of the potentials observed on the body surface. This holds true irrespective of whether a detailed volume conductor model is involved. However, the dipole cannot be interpreted directly in terms of the underlying electrophysiology. Some limited physiologic interpretability of the single dipole is present in situations where the electric activity is restricted to a small part of the myocardium. Examples are sources during the time interval directly following activation (eg, Wolff-Parkinson-White syndrome, ectopic beats) or during very late phases in depolarization.

THE THORAX MODEL

In Einthoven's papers, at first sight, the implied volume conductor model appears to be a large planar sheet of conductive paper. Inspected more closely, it is seen to relate to an infinite medium of homogeneous conductivity, at whose center the electric

sources are situated. Unrealistic as this volume conductor model may be, it proves to be highly valuable in the appreciation of the most significant characteristics of the potential fields generated by bioelectric sources.

For a spherical volume conductor with uniform internal electric conductivity and zero external conductivity (a somewhat more realistic volume conductor), a current dipole at its center produces potentials on the boundary of the sphere that are three-fold those in the infinite medium.

Since Einthoven's day, volume conductor models have grown increasingly more realistic. Initially, the relationship between source strength and the resulting potentials was derived from measurements taken from physical phantoms (torso tank models). Later, following the pioneering work by Gelernter and Swihart,[16] Lynn and Timlake,[17] Barnard et al,[18] and Barr et al,[19] the model-based analysis moved on to computations using digital computers. At present, after vast improvements in computing power and numerical algorithms, such computations can be performed easily. In the thorax model implemented in ECGSIM, the individual geometries of the relevant conductivity interfaces are used, measured by means of magnetic resonance methods. The model takes into account the relatively low conductivity of the lungs and the relatively high conductivity of blood in the cavities.[20,21]

The remaining main point of interest in the simulation of cardiac potentials is the selection of an appropriate source model for the particular application in hand.

MATRIX FORMULATION OF THE FORWARD PROBLEM

In ECGSIM, the simulation of the ECG is carried out by discretizing the EDL strength around N nodes of the numerical representation of the surface S_h at T subsequent time intervals of 1 ms. This is expressed by a matrix, **S**, having as its elements $S_{n,t}$, $n = 1 \ldots N$; $t = 1 \ldots T$. The temporal aspect of the source strength is described by a stylized version on a TMP wave form $V_m(t)$. Two examples of these wave forms are shown in Fig. 15–3.

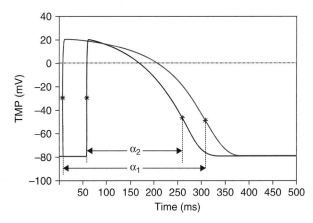

FIGURE 15–3. Two examples of stylized transmembrane potentials (TMP) at different patches of S_h, with activation recovery interval values α_1 and α_2, respectively. The asterisks mark the timing of the maximal slopes, in the upward slope taken as markers of local depolarization and in the downward slope as markers for the timing of local repolarization.

These are generated as the product of a number of S-shaped curves, known as the logistic functions.[22] Among the parameters involved in the specific variant of the wave forms, one is used for setting the local EDL strength at any node n, and two are used to specify the timing of local depolarization and repolarization, δ_n and ρ_n, respectively. The interval between these markers is the activation recovery interval (ARI), denoted here as $\alpha_n = \rho_n - \delta_n$. This interval reflects the absolute refractory period of the tissue.[23]

The transfer between sources and resulting potentials is described by a single, precomputed matrix $\mathbf{A}$, with elements $A_{l,n}$, $l = 1\ldots L$; $n = 1\ldots N$, with L being the number of field points of interest. The potentials Φ at the field points are computed from the matrix multiplication $\Phi = \mathbf{A}S$.

ABOUT ECGSIM

Upon installing the ECGSIM software (from http://www.ecgsim.org), a window comes into view on which four sections are marked, which will be referred to as the "panes" of the window

(Fig. 15–4). On the two panes on the left, the distribution over S_h of the EDL parameters may be displayed, such as the timing of local depolarization as shown on the Heart-pane and, on the TMP-pane, the TMP wave form assigned to the any of the nodes selected on the Heart-pane.

The two panes on the right display the results of the simulated surface potentials. The ECGs-pane in Fig. 15–4 displays a temporal image of the cardiac electric activity—that of the standard 12-lead ECG signals resulting from the default source parameter settings. On the Thorax-pane, an image of the corresponding body surface potential map (BSPM) is displayed, a snapshot taken at the time instant marked by the yellow bar drawn on the 12-lead signals shown on the ECGs-pane. This snapshot can be interpreted as a single frame of a movie animating the full spatiotemporal nature of the body surface potentials.

The ECGSIM software enables one to specify, or modify interactively, the timing of depolarization, $dep(n) = \delta_n$, and repolarization, $rep(n) = \rho_n$ of the TMPs at nodes n ($n = 1..N$), where $N = 257$ is the number of nodes at S_h. The difference $dur(n) = \alpha_n = rep(n) - dep(n)$ is the ARI taken as a measure of the local action potential duration. In addition, a value $str(n)$ ($0 \le str(n) \le 100\%$),

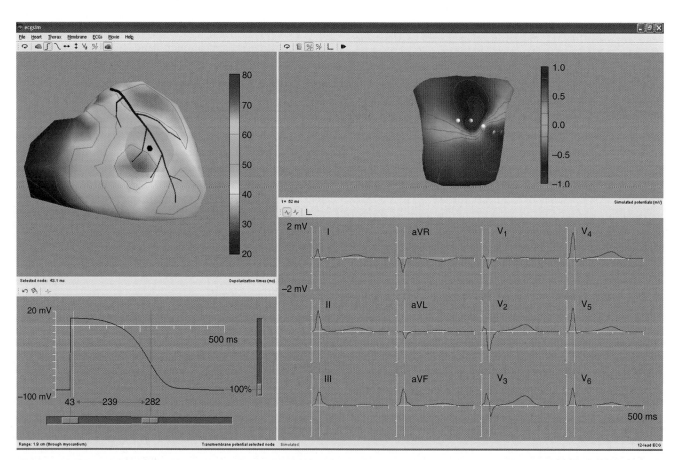

FIGURE 15–4. The main window of ECGSIM, comprising four panes. **Upper left.** The Heart-pane: the ventricular surface S_h composed of 510 small triangles (the equivalent double layer [EDL] patches) having $N = 257$ vertices–the nodes at which the EDL strength is specified. Note the single node highlighted and the shaded region around it, the significance of which is explained in examples to follow. **Lower left.** The TMP-pane: the transmembrane potentials (TMPs) assigned to the node highlighted on the Heart-pane. **Lower right.** The ECGs-pane: displaying the QRST signals of the standard 12-lead electrocardiogram (ECG) as simulated based on the TMPs assigned to the nodes. **Upper right.** The Thorax-pane: a frontal view of the thorax, on which the simulated body surface potential map (BSPM) is displayed corresponding to the time marked by the yellow vertical line in ECG traces shown on the ECGs-pane.

scaling the local magnitude of the TMP, can be set for each node. The effect of any such changes on the surface potentials (right panes) is shown instantaneously. An option is provided for viewing the animation (movie) of the sequence of BSPMs.

The potential field on S_h as generated by the EDL source may be displayed on the Heart-pane, the corresponding electrogram on the TMP-pane.

The interactive setting of any of the source parameters is mouse-controlled. The images desired to be displayed on the four panes may be selected from a toolbar, supported by pull-down menus. The two basic geometries shown on the upper panes may be rotated freely in space, thus providing different views of the total 3D aspects of the images. The boundaries of the panes may be shifted in order to increase the size of any pane of interest.

The ECGSIM package includes a full manual, specifying all of its options, as well as a brief introduction to its basic use. Specific options have been selected for creating the various images shown in the examples presented in the following sections.

THE ECG ACCORDING TO ECGSIM

In this section, we present several examples of how ECGSIM is able to provide a view on the link between electrophysiologic changes in the ventricles and the resulting changes in the body surface potentials. As an essential preliminary, we first describe the potentials resulting from the default parameter settings used to simulate the normal ECG. These potentials serve as a reference against which the effect of any implemented changes of the default parameters may be observed.

■ THE NORMAL ECG

The current version of ECGSIM deals with the simulation of the potential field outside the heart generated by the electric activity inside the ventricular myocardium. The potentials shown on the ECGs-pane of Fig. 15–4 depict the 12-lead ECG of a healthy, male subject. The Heart-pane presents an anterior view of the heart in its natural orientation as observed by magnetic resonance imaging. The color-coded function displayed is the timing of depolarization, $dep(n)$, on the surface S_h. The values of the factors scaling the TMP magnitude were given a (uniform) unit value. A slightly different view of the same data, exposing some parts of the septum and the endocardium, is shown in Fig. 15–5A. The timing of the local repolarization, $rep(n)$, used in the simulation is shown in Fig. 15–5B.

The realism of the potentials as based on these parameter settings can be judged from Fig. 15–6. In Fig. 15–6A, the simulated 12-lead ECG traces are shown in red, as on the ECGs-pane of Fig. 15–4. In addition, traces in blue are included, which represent the ECGs measured on the healthy subject studied. In Fig. 15–6B, another image of the cardiac electric activity is presented: the vectorcardiogram. Both panels are copied from the ECGs-pane after selecting the desired type of display.

The close correspondence between the measured data and those based on the data simulated by means of the EDL model (see Fig. 15–6) is a necessary, but not sufficient, indication of the general validity of the EDL in this particular application. It depends more critically on the realism of the major default parameters used—those setting the timing of local depolarization and repolarization. Their values, shown in Fig. 15–5, were obtained by means of dedicated inverse procedures,[13,24] the most recent upgraded version of which is described and evaluated in van Dam et al.[25]

The inversely computed depolarization sequence agrees qualitatively with the one observed in invasive procedures.[26] For the repolarization sequence, no such data are available. However, subsequent use of the EDL, examples of which are shown in the sequel, has fully corroborated the effectiveness of the EDL

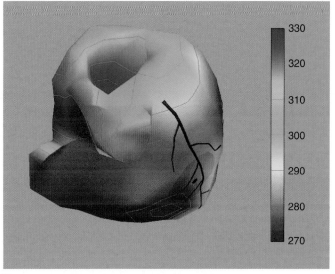

A   B

FIGURE 15–5. Images copied from the Heart-pane. **A.** The timing of depolarization $dep(n)$ on S_h used in simulating the normal electrocardiogram. The isochrones, supporting the color coding, are drawn at 10-ms steps. **B.** The distribution of the markers of the timing of local repolarization on S_h, $rep(n)$. The heavy dot highlights the location of the node n for which its transmembrane potential (TMP) is shown on the TMP-pane of Fig. 15–4. The geometry is shown in a slightly modified orientation compared with the one shown in Fig. 15–4, thus providing a view of parts of the endocardial and septal aspects of the ventricular myocardium.

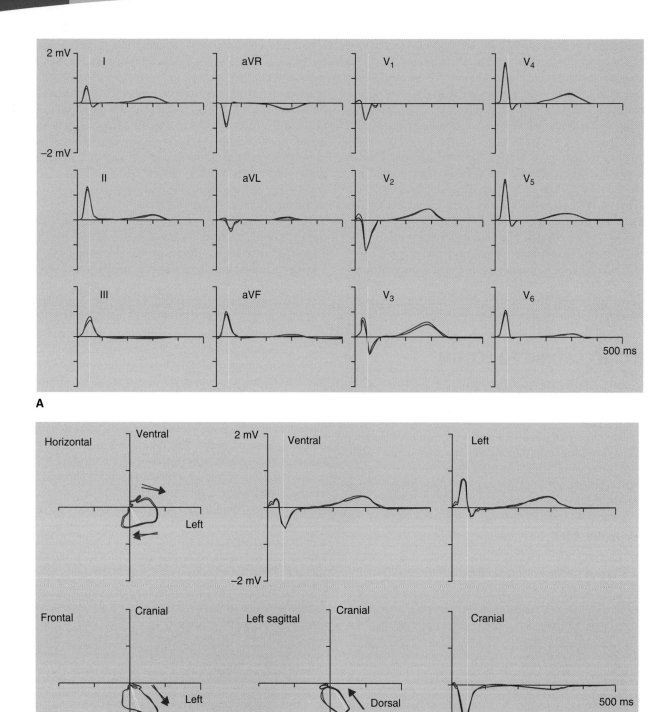

FIGURE 15–6. Images copied from the ECGs-pane. **A.** Red represents the 12-lead electrocardiogram (ECG) as simulated; blue represents the 12-lead reference ECG as measured on the healthy subject studied. The yellow vertical line at the zero crossing of the V_3 signal marks the timing of the snapshot of the body surface potential (BSP) map shown on the BSP-pane in Fig. 15–4. **B.** Vectorcardiographic representation of the same data; vector loops are projected on the horizontal, frontal, and left sagittal planes, as well as their projections on the three orthogonal axes, usually referred to as the X, Y, and Z lead signals.

in modeling for the signal components of the ECG during the ST-T interval.

As interesting as the close correspondence between the measured and the simulated data may be, the main significance of the interactive simulation tool lies in the opportunity that it provides for studying the effect of local changes in its default parameter settings as observed on the body surface potentials, as well as those on the surface S_h. All of the different parameter types can be varied interactively at a single node or in a region around the selected node, having a selectable size. The region affected may be restricted to the surface at which the node is situated (eg, the epicardium) or assigned to extend transmurally. In a basic variant, all parameters of a certain type [eg, the $dep(n)$ values] may be globally (ie, uniformly) shifted in time or scaled relative to their mean value.

A unique feature of the simulation is that it enables the study of the mean value over the body surface of the potential field generated by the cardiac electric activity. As is demonstrated in a later example, this is highly relevant in the understanding of the nature of the ST-T changes in the ECG observed during ischemia.

POTENTIAL FIELD AT S_h; ELECTROGRAMS

As mentioned previously, next to simulating body surface potentials, ECGSIM provides images of the potential fields generated on S_h, as well as their temporal representation in the form of electrograms.

Although the magnitude of the EDL is driven by the local TMPs (expressed in the unit V), its true nature is that of an electric current dipole source density (unit: A/m), feeding electric current into the tissues exterior to the ventricles. The potential field generated in the exterior medium close to S_h is distinct from that of the field of the local TMPs. A demonstration of this is shown in Fig. 15–7. The magnitude of the voltages shown in Fig. 15–7A is in agreement with those observed in electrophysiologic measurements. The timing of the fast upstrokes of the local TMP coincides with the fastest part in the down stroke of the local electrogram, as is demonstrated in Fig. 15–8. For a node at a local minimum in the timing of depolarization (wave front expanding from the node), the local electrogram has a characteristic rS morphology (Fig. 15–8A); for nodes at a local maximum in the timing of depolarization (the wave front closing in around the node), the morphology is of the Rs type

(Fig. 15–8B). For intermediate situations, the observed $(|S|-R)/(|S|+R)$ ratio depends on the local curvature of the local wave front,[27] in which R and $|S|$ denote the extreme values of the R and S wavelets.

BASIC STATISTICS OF THE TIMING PARAMETERS

One way of describing the genesis of the QRST wave forms is to attribute the sources to the dispersion of the timing of local depolarization and repolarization. Dispersion is a general term used for describing any inequality of the values of a set of parameters. Whatever the measure used for quantifying the dispersion, if the dispersion of the parameters specifying the wave forms of all TMPs were to be zero, a completely flat baseline in all ECG leads would be the result.

Crude, statistical measures for quantifying dispersion of any set of parameters are the standard deviation (SD) and their range (ie, the interval between their minimum and maximum values). Both measures are of interest when studying the way in which global changes in the TMPs affect the ECG wave forms. In Fig.15–9, a pop-up menu of ECGSIM is shown documenting these basic statistics for the default timing parameters (see Fig. 15–6). The sliders may be used to interactively change these global statistics and observe the effect on the body surface potentials (Thorax-pane and ECGs-pane). For the understanding of the origin of the morphology of the individual lead signals, the full distributions of the parameter values are required, such as the one shown in Fig. 15–5. Two examples of the effect of such global changes of the basic statistics are presented in the next paragraph.

In the first example (Fig. 15–10), the global dispersion of the apd values was reduced to zero, forcing their values over S_h to be uniform and, hence, the dispersion measures of dep and rep to be the same. The simulated T waves (red traces) in most of the

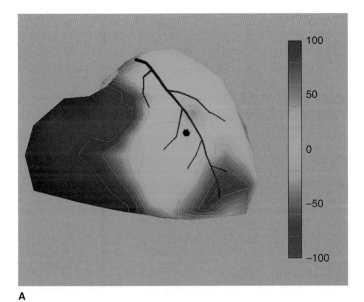

A

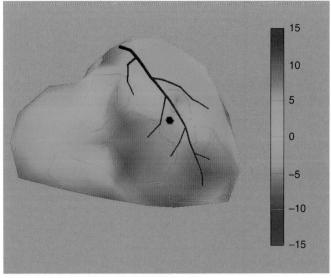

B

FIGURE 15–7. A. Color-coded image of the transmembrane potential field over the surface S_h, setting the strength of the equivalent double layer (EDL) at the time instant marked by the yellow bar in Fig. 15–6. Isopotential lines are drawn at 20-mV steps. **B.** The potential field just outside the surface S_h as generated by the EDL. Isopotential lines are drawn at 5-mV steps. Both potential fields are shown with reference to Wilson's central terminal.

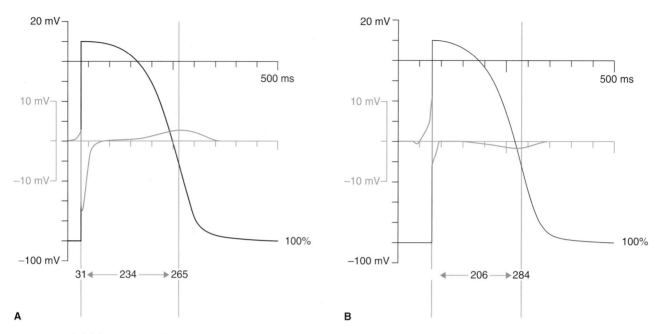

FIGURE 15–8. A. Black indicates transmembrane potential at a node overlaying a local minimum in the timing of depolarization. Light blue indicates electrogram at the same node. **B.** The same type of data for a node overlaying a local maximum in the timing of depolarization.

12-lead signals now show up with a polarity that is the reverse of the mean polarity of the simulated QRS complexes. These so-called *nonconcomitant polarities* are at odds with the ones observed on the measures data (blue traces), demonstrating that in reality the dispersion of *apd* values of the TMP is nonzero.

The second example (Fig. 15–11) demonstrates the effect of increasing the dispersion of the timing of repolarization *rep(n)*, while keeping its mean value and its pattern constant. Note the resulting increase of the magnitudes of the T waves. This effect is seen most clearly in the dominant T wave.[28]

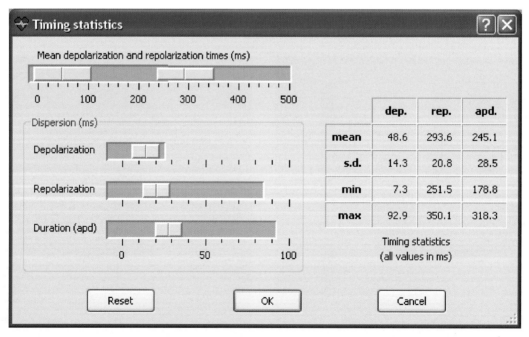

FIGURE 15–9. One of the pop-up menus of ECGSIM showing the basic statistics of the 257 parameters specifying the timing of local depolarization (*dep*) and repolarization (*rep*) and the measure of action potential duration (*apd* = *rep* − *dep*) of the distributions shown in Fig. 15–5. The sliders may be used to interactively vary any of the individual main statistics by shifting and scaling such that the pattern of the distribution over S_h remains the same, while observing the effects on the QRST wave forms as well as their effect on the other main statistics.

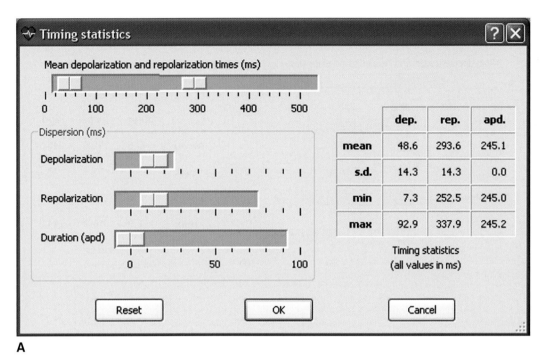

A

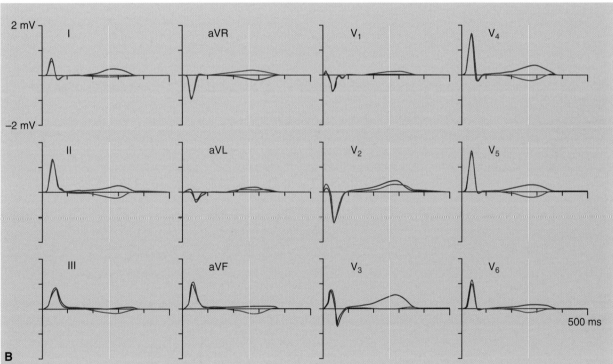

B

FIGURE 15–10. A. Basic statistics of the timing parameters after reducing the dispersion of the *apd* (action potential duration) values to zero. **B.** Red traces indicate simulation results for zero dispersion of *apd*. Blue traces indicate the measured 12-lead electrocardiogram (as on Fig. 15–5A). The yellow bar marks the time *t* = 293 ms, the mean value of the timing *rep*(*n*). Recall that *rep*(*n*) is the timing of the inflection point during the later part of repolarization (see Fig. 15–8). Full amplitude scale: 2 mV.

■ THE T WAVE

As with the QRS complexes, the genesis of the T wave is related to the spatial distribution of the TMPs. In contrast to those during the depolarization phase, the sources are of a much smaller strength and located throughout the myocardium rather than restricted to narrow, clearly defined wave fronts and active over a much longer period (eg, 100 ms for depolarization and 350 ms during normal repolarization). In healthy subjects, throughout the ST-T segment, the spatial pattern of the potential field generated over the thorax is much more sober and much more stable over time. A snapshot of the potential field with reference to Wilson's central terminal (WCT), *measured* over the thorax

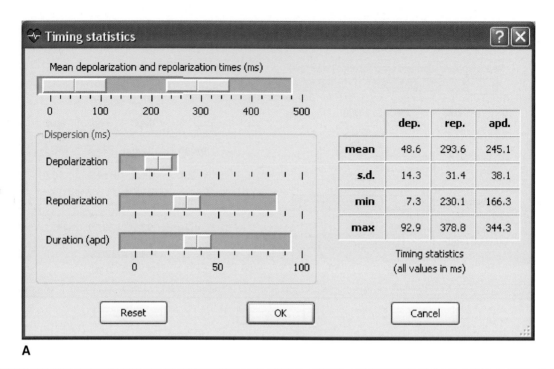

A

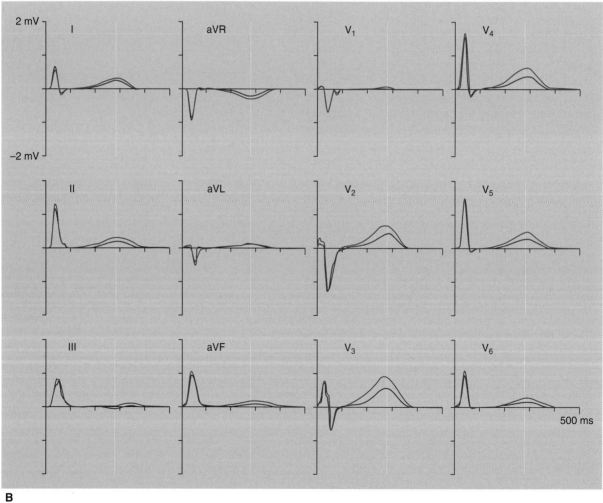

B

FIGURE 15–11. A. Basic statistics of the timing parameters after increasing the dispersion of the *rep* values by 50%. **B.** Red traces indicate simulation results after increasing the dispersion by 50%. Blue traces indicate measured 12-lead electrocardiogram (as on Fig. 15–5A). The yellow bar marks the time $t = 293$ ms, the mean value of the timing *rep(n)*. Recall that *rep(n)* represents the timing of the inflection points during the later part of repolarization (see Fig. 15–8).

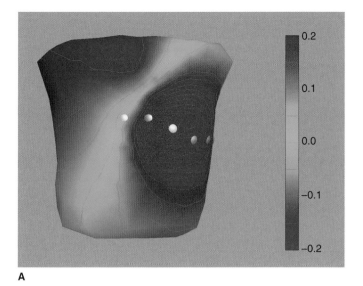
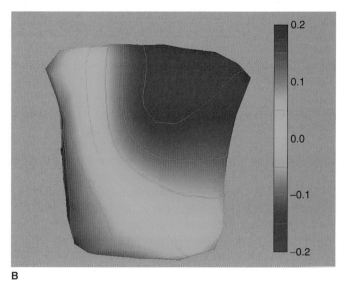

A   **B**

FIGURE 15–12. Measured body surface potential map at t = 293 ms as copied from the Thorax-pane. **A.** Anterior view. Silver-colored dots mark the positions of the six anterior sensing electrodes of the standard 12-lead system. **B.** Posterior view. Increments between subsequent isopotential lines = 50 μV. Potentials measured with respect to Wilson's central terminal.

at t = 293 ms after onset QRS is presented in Fig. 15–12. It demonstrates that in healthy subjects, most of the T waves in the standard 12-lead ECG are positive but, equally important, that vast areas are negative with respect to WCT. The pattern shown remains very stable over a period of more than 100 ms around the timing of apex T at t = 293 ms. This highly significant fact is illustrated in Fig. 15–13.

The dominant aspects of the normal BSPM pattern during the T wave are consistent with the distribution of the timing of repolarization found from the inverse procedure (see Fig. 15–5B). Following the complete depolarization of all myocytes, those that have depolarized early have progressed more toward their (negative) resting potential (repolarized) than those that depolarized later.[27] As a consequence, there is a consistent intracellular gradient of the intracellular potential

directed from the posterior basal part to the more anterior, apical part. The return current generated in the extracellular medium, demanded by the conservation of charge, sets up the pattern dominated by the local potential maximum commonly observed around the electrode sensing lead V_3 and the minimum near the right shoulder.

Besides this dominant factor, intracellular transmural gradients in the intracellular TMP values continuously set up transmural current sources directed from regions that have repolarized first to those repolarizing later. The dominant geometry of the left ventricle, a thick wall ellipsoidal-like structure with opposing electric forces in anterior and posterior wall segments, tends to cancel such transmural effects.

During repolarization, active electric sources are continuously present throughout the myocardium, extending over distances

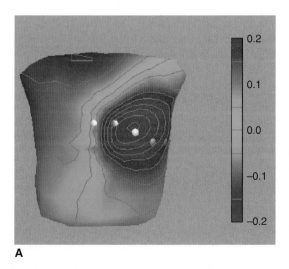
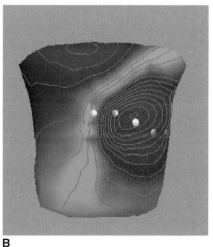
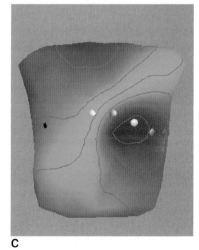

A   **B**   **C**

FIGURE 15–13. Anterior view of the thorax showing *measured* body surface potential maps at t = 243 ms (**A**), t = 293 ms (**B**), and t = 443 ms (**C**) from onset QRS, as copied from the Thorax-pane. Increments between subsequent isopotential lines = 50 μV. Potentials measured with respect to Wilson's central terminal. Note the stability of the patterns.

that are easily more than 8 cm. In view of this, the origin of the T wave can only be studied in a full-scale model of the ventricles.

In our opinion, any cause of T wave abnormality can only be fully understood against the background of a model of the T wave genesis in healthy subjects. The EDL model used in ECGSIM is such a model. Both the temporal (see Fig. 15–6) and the spatial aspects (not shown in this chapter) are replicated in the simulated data.

Examples of the use of the EDL model in the appreciation of basic notions of the genesis of the T wave are those illustrated in Figs. 15–10 and 15–11. The example presented in Fig. 15–11 indicates that the timing of the extremes in the T waves (apex-T magnitudes) reflects the dispersion of the timing of repolarization. If the dispersion were zero, no T waves would be visible on the ECG. The timing of the extremes reflects the mean value of the inflection points in the down slopes of the TMPs of the myocytes. A biophysical explanation of this property is described in van Oosterom.[28,29]

The examples shown in Figs. 15–10 and 15–11 relate to *global* changes in the timing of repolarization. The effect of *local* TMP changes is demonstrated in a number of the following subsections.

■ CHANGING THE TMP PARAMETERS LOCALLY

As mentioned before, all three major parameter types, $dep(n)$, $rep(n)$, and $str(n)$, specifying the $TMP(n)$ acting as the local strength of the EDL at node n can be varied interactively, either at any single node or in a region with a selectable size around it. In the example shown in Fig. 15–8A $dep(n) = 31$ ms, $rep(n) = 265$ ms, and $str(n) = 100\%$. The region affected may be restricted to the surface on which the node is situated (eg, the epicardium) or be assigned to extend transmurally. In addition, an option is included in ECGSIM referred to as "focus" in the pull-down menu that pops up from the item "membrane" on the menu bar. By selecting this option, an activation sequence is computed throughout the myocardium according to propagation at a uniform speed (Huygens principle). The resulting activation sequence may be studied as such or merged with a previously existing one. The merging is carried out based on the "first come first served principle" (ie, the smaller of the two activation times determined at the nodes is used in the computation of the potentials). Two examples of the effect of local changes in the timing parameters are presented first. Next, the effect of varying the scaling factor of the TMPs, $str(n)$, is shown in an application of the modeling of ECG changes during periods of acute ischemia.

The first example (Fig. 15–14) demonstrates the use of the "focus" option in simulating the wave forms in cases of the Wolff-Parkinson-White syndrome. In such cases, the depolarization sequence results from the fusion of an early activation along an anomalous pathway linking the atrial and ventricular myocardium and the normal activation initiated somewhat later via the bundle branches. The simulation first uses the "statistics" option (see Fig. 15–9) for delaying the normal, default activation sequence by 50 ms (using the mean slider for the *dep* values). Next, the result is merged with an activation initiated

at the location marked by the heavy dot shown on Fig. 15–14A. The propagation velocity starting from this "focus" at $t = 0$ was set at 0.8 m/s. Note the characteristic fast down slope of the QRS complexes.

The second example (Fig. 15–15) illustrates the effect of a local delay in the timing of repolarization. The default settings of $rep(n)$ on S_h, resulting in the close correspondence between measured and simulated data (see Fig. 15–6), were reduced on a segment of the epicardium of the right ventricle around the heavy dot shown in Fig. 15–15A. The reduction was set at 20 ms at the center of the region, tapering off linearly to zero at the edge. The resulting simulated QRST wave forms of the standard 12-lead ECG are shown (in red) on the lower panel, and the measured reference signals are shown in blue. The locations of the six anterior electrodes of leads V_1 to V_6 are included in the display, visualized by using one of the options of the Heartpane's menu bar. The electrode most proximal to the region of advanced timing of repolarization is the sensing electrode of lead V_2 (WCT being the reference). Correspondingly, the effect of this advanced repolarization timing can be observed most clearly on lead V_2: an increase of the apex-T value. Conversely, a local delay in the epicardial timing of this region gives rise to a reduced apex-T value (not shown here). By using ECGSIM, it can be easily demonstrated that a similarly advanced or delayed repolarization on the posteroinferior epicardium of the left ventricle having equal size gives rise to far smaller changes in the magnitudes of leads V_1 to V_6, with opposite polarity. The smaller magnitude reflects the larger distance between the affected region and the sensing electrodes.

The final example of the effect of changing the TMP parameters treats the topic of ECG changes during localized, acute ischemia. During such periods, the electric activity of the myocytes in the ischemic zone is abnormal; the magnitude of the TMP is smaller, the action potential duration (APD) is shorter, and the velocity of propagation in the ischemic zone is smaller than all of these factors compared with the nonischemic zone.[30,31] The expression of these effects on the ECG depends on the location and extent of the ischemic region. In the current version of ECGSIM, the direct modeling of ischemia is restricted to the most prominent of these effects—the reduction of the magnitude of the TMPs in the ischemic zone. This is effected by reducing the local values of the scaling factors $str(n)$ by means of the vertical slider in the TMP-pane (see Fig. 15–4). In this way, the resting potentials are set at smaller values (less negative values), as are the potentials following the upstroke (less positive values). The other two factors can be implemented by making the appropriate changes in the timing within the ischemic zone as well as in the surrounding nonischemic zone. This demands accurate information on how the timing might be affected, information that may not always be available. These two factors are indeed less prominently represented on the ECG.[32]

In the example shown in Fig. 15–16, an epicardial ischemic zone (shaded in Fig. 15–16A) has been modeled in this manner on the lateral free wall of the left ventricle. The value of $str(n)$ at the center of the ischemic region was set at 80%; toward its edge, it increased linearly to the default normal setting of 100%.

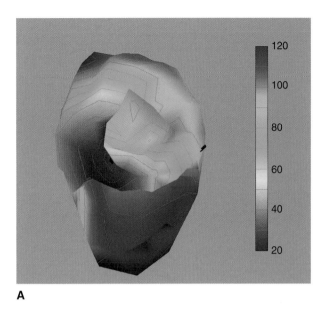

A

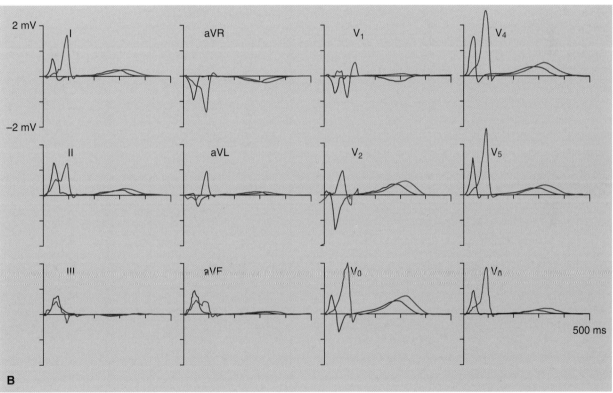

B

FIGURE 15–14. A. Simulated activation sequence of a Wolff-Parkinson-White case, a pattern resulting from the fusion of the activation along an anomalous pathway between atrial and ventricular myocardium, and the normal activation initiated via the bundle branches. Note the local minimum on the septum of the left ventricle, resulting from the normal activation. **B.** Simulated 12-lead electrocardiogram based on the activation sequence shown in panel A. Blue indicates the normal wave forms.

Figure 15–16A shows (in red) the simulated 12-lead ECG. The characteristic ST shifts observed during ischemia are brought out clearly through the comparison with normal (measured) reference data shown in blue. A BSPM at the middle of the ST-T segment (yellow time bar) is shown in Fig. 15–16B. Note that the ST-segment elevation is most pronounced in leads V_5 and V_6. The so-called reciprocal negativity (ST-segment depression above leads V_1 and V_2) can be seen to be poorly sampled

by these leads, the local extreme in this case being located well above the electrodes sensing V_1 and V_2. The direction of the shifts (elevation/depression) is difficult to understand without taking into account the volume conduction effects in the passive medium surrounding the heart. Moreover, the presence of the required high-pass filtering and the subsequent baseline definition tends to confuse the issue. This topic is addressed in the next subsection.

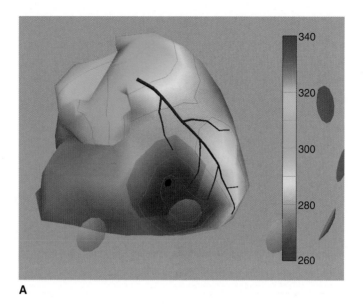

A

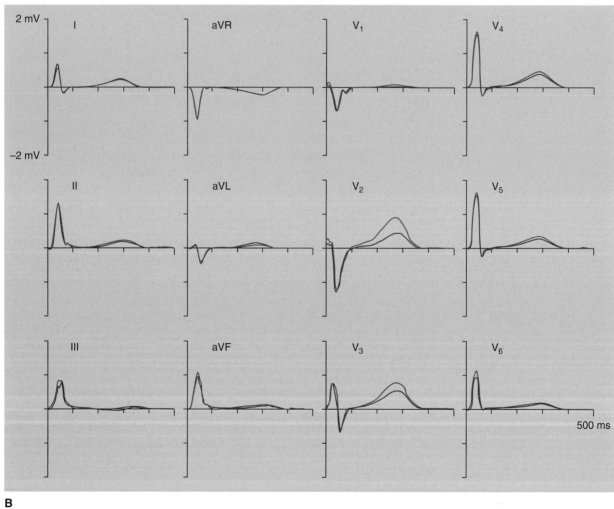

B

FIGURE 15–15. A. Distribution over S_h of the markers of the timing of local repolarization [$rep(n)$]. The values shown outside the shaded region depict the default setting used in Fig. 15–6. The values on the shaded region (epicardial only) were reduced relative to the default settings (by 20 ms at the center, tapering off linearly to a zero value at the edge). The transparent three-dimensional images of circular disks depict the positions of the precordial electrodes of the standard 12-lead system. **B.** Red indicates the resulting, simulated wave forms of the standard 12-lead electrocardiogram. Blue indicates the measured reference signals.

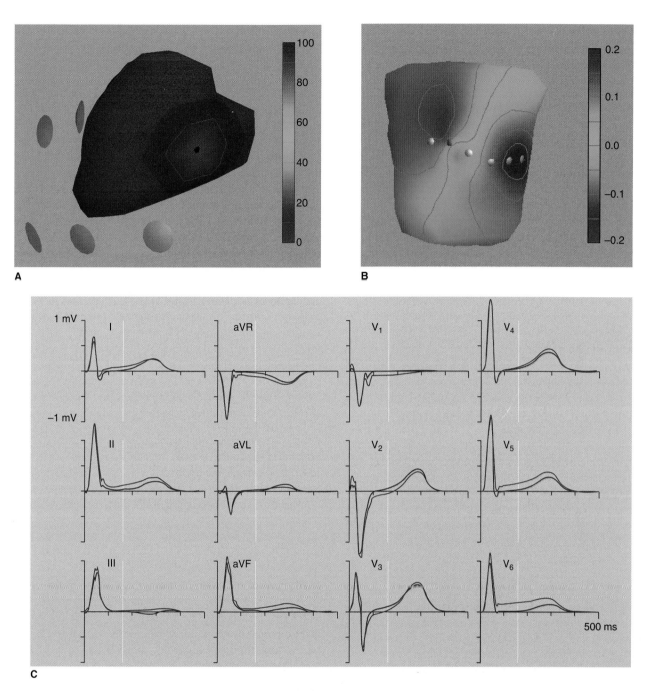

FIGURE 15–16. A. Left view of the ventricular surface S_h color coded by the function $str(n)$ scaling the local transmembrane potential. The values of $str(n)$ around the heavy black dot are set at 80%, whereas they increase linearly to 100% at the edge of the shaded region representing local epicardial ischemia. The lower two electrodes are the ones sensing V_5 and V_6. **B.** The body surface potential map at the time indicated by the yellow bar in the middle of the ST-T segment. **C.** Red indicates standard 12-lead signals; blue indicates the measured data for the nonischemic situation. All voltages are expressed in mV.

The ST-T changes illustrated here are the consequence of a nontransmural, epicardial ischemic zone. For transmural situations, the magnitudes tend to be smaller.

■ DIRECT CURRENT RECORDINGS; ST-T CHANGES

The recording of the ECG signals involves the measurement of electric potential differences generated at different locations on the body surface. Such bioelectric potentials commonly observed by means of electrodes placed on the body surface are always contaminated by contact potentials at the electrode-tissue interface. The magnitudes of these potentials are much larger than those of the ECG, are unknown, and may change slowly over time—the so-called baseline *wander* or *drift*. This problem is treated by including a high-pass filter in the first stage of the recording system. The resulting signal is referred to as an alternating current (AC) recording or high-pass filtering. This produces an output signal, which, when computed over a long time, has a zero mean value; the direct current (DC) component of the signal of a single beat is reduced to zero. If rapid perturbations of the contact potential occur, the baseline of the signal (ie, the time markers at which observed signals should be assigned a zero value) must be specified on a beat-to-beat basis. Even if the dynamic range of the input stage encompasses the full range of the sensor potentials (allowing a DC recording despite the presence of the contact potentials, a common feature in the most recent ECG recorders), the subsequent shift to a zero level remains to be *defined*.

The treatment of the problem is generally referred to as baseline *correction*. However, this is a somewhat misleading term because it assumes that the signal level that should be specified as zero is self-evident, which is not the case.

The problem of baseline definition is most pressing for recordings taken during periods of acute ischemia. As discussed in the previous subsection, during ischemia, the TMPs of the myocytes within the ischemic region differ from those in the nonischemic region; the resting potential decreases (tends to zero), and the upstroke is reduced. The size of these changes varies during the various stages of ischemia.[33] The intracellular coupling between myocytes in the ischemic region (I) and myocytes in the nonischemic region (NI) and the differences in the TMPs of the myocytes within these regions result in an electric current flow. During the time interval between the end of the T wave and the onset of the next QRS complex, the differences in the resting potentials in these regions result in a current flow in the intracellular myocardium directed from region I to region NI. In the extracellular domain, the direction of the current flow is in the opposite direction because charge is conserved. In the extracellular medium, this can be expressed by an equivalent current sink in the ischemic region, which lowers the nearby extracellular potentials.[33] During the activation of the tissue surrounding the ischemic zone, the potential difference between the regions is smaller, as is the loading effect.

The basic signals simulated by ECGSIM are (obviously) free of any of the problems created at the electrode-tissue interface. This permits the simulation of the true potential differences on the body surface. An illustration of this is shown in Fig. 15–17. The measured reference ECG (nonischemic, shown in blue) demanded a definition of the zero baseline. This was *defined* at the onset of the QRS and the end of the T wave, in fact at the onset of the next beat. In this manner, any influence of ongoing atrial electric activity (repolarization of the atria) is minimized.[34] The same procedure was applied to the (same) measured signals and the simulated ones shown in Fig. 15–16.

On the basis of the theory of the current flow between the ischemic and the nonischemic regions presented earlier, one would expect the potentials near leads V_5 and V_6 at the end of the T wave to be negative, whereas the potentials would be positive for the electrodes sensing V_1 and V_2. This is indeed observed in Fig. 15–17. The effect of the baseline correction applied to the ischemic signals shown in Fig. 15–16 is that the nonzero values at onset QRS and following the T wave show up in the baseline "corrected" signals as ST shifts having reversed polarity. This interpretation follows directly from the electrophysiologic studies by Janse et al.[33]

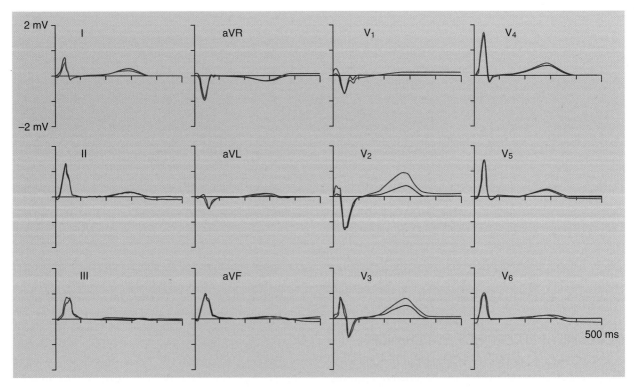

FIGURE 15–17. Red traces indicate simulated standard 12-lead signals under the ischemic conditions documented in Fig. 15–16, now shown in the direct current mode of "recording." Note the nonzero potential values at onset QRS and after the end of the T wave. Blue traces indicate the measured (nonischemic) signals.

CONCLUSION

As demonstrated in this chapter, the imaging of the basic spatiotemporal aspects of the genesis of the cardiac electric signals provides a powerful addition to the type of explanations commonly found in standard readers on the theory of the ECG.

The examples of the use of ECGSIM included in this chapter are by no means exhaustive. Topics left out to economize on space include the imaging of the properties of the transfer matrix that links sources and resulting potentials[35] and the animation of the spatiotemporal nature of the direction and magnitude of the dipole as used in vectorcardiography, linked to the geometry of ventricles and thorax.

In recent years, ECGSIM has attained world-wide application in different educational courses. Its major unique feature is the use of the EDL model, which is a source description that is far superior to that of the single current dipole. It has a direct link with the classic UDL model of cardiac activation and constitutes a source description of the electric sources during repolarization.

Next to its application in education, various papers have been published in which ECGSIM is applied as a research tool.[36-40] The ones listed have been based on version 1.3, which was restricted to the electric activity of the ventricles. In November 2010 an upgraded version (2.0) was released in which the electric activity of the atria was included.

REFERENCES

1. Einthoven W, de Lint K. Ueber das normale menschliche elektrokardiogram und uber die capillar-elektrometrische untersuchung einiger herzkranken. *Pflugers Arch Ges Physiol*. 1900;80:139-160.
2. Schalij MJ, Janse MJ, van Oosterom A, et al, eds. *Einthoven 2002; 100 Years of Electrocardiography*. Leiden, the Netherlands: The Einthoven Foundation; 2002:1-616.
3. van Oosterom A, Oostendorp TF. ECGSIM: an interactive tool for studying the genesis of QRST waveforms. *Heart*. 2004;90:165-168.
4. Wilson FN, Macleod AG, Barker PS. The distribution of action currents produced by the heart muscle and other excitable tissues immersed in conducting media. *J Gen Physiol*. 1933;16:423-456.
5. Holland RP, Arnsdorf MF. Solid angle theory and the electrocardiogram: physiologic and quantitative interpretations. *Progr Cardiovasc Dis*. 1977;19:431-457.
6. van Oosterom A. The equivalent double layer; source model for repolarization. In: Macfarlane PW, van Oosterom A, Pahlm O, et al, eds. *Comprehensive Electrocardiology*. Vol I. New York, NY: Springer-Verlag; 2009.
7. Plonsey R. *Bioelectric Phenomena*. New York, NY: McGraw-Hill; 1969.
8. van Oosterom A. Solidifying the solid angle. *J Electrocardiol*. 2002;35S:181-192.
9. Plonsey R, Barr RC. *Bioelectricity: A Quantitative Approach*. New York, NY: Springer; 2007.
10. van Oosterom A. Cell models: macroscopic source descriptions. In: Macfarlane PW, Lawrie TTV, eds. *Comprehensive Electrocardiology*. Vol 1. 1st ed. Oxford, United Kingdom: Pergamon Press; 1989:155-179.
11. Geselowitz DB. On the theory of the electrocardiogram. *Proc IEEE*. 1989;77/6:857-876.
12. Geselowitz DB. Description of cardiac sources in anisotropic cardiac muscle. Application of bidomain model. *J Electrocardiol*. 1992;25(Suppl):65-67.
13. van Oosterom A. Genesis of the T wave as based on an equivalent surface source model. *J Electrocardiogr*. 2001;34(Suppl):217-227.
14. Plonsey R. An extension of the solid angle formulation for an active cell. *Biophysical J*. 1965;5:663-666.
15. Snellen HA. *Selected Papers on Electrocardiography of Willem Einthoven*. Leiden, the Netherlands: Leiden University Press; 1977.
16. Gelernter HL, Swihart JC. A mathematical-physical model of the genesis of the electrocardiogram. *Biophys J*. 1964;4:285-301.
17. Lynn MS, Timlake WP. The numerical solution of singular equations of potential theory. *Numerische Mathematik*. 1968;11:77-98.
18. Barnard ACL, Duck IM, Lynn MS. The application of electromagnetic theory to electrocardiology. I. Derivation of the integral equations. *Biophys J*. 1967;7:443-462.
19. Barr RC, Ramsey M, Spach MS. Relating epicardial to body surface potentials by means of transfer coefficients based on geometry measurements. *IEEE Trans Biomed Eng*. 1977;24:1-11.
20. Brody DA. A theoretical analysis of intracavitary blood mass influence on the heart-lead relationship. *Circ Res*. 1956;IV:731-738.
21. van Oosterom A, Plonsey R. The Brody effect revisited. *J Electrocardiol*. 1991;24:339-348.
22. van Oosterom A, Jacquemet V. A parameterized description of transmembrane potentials used in forward and inverse procedures. Paper presented at the International Conference of Electrocardiology, Gdansk, Poland, June 1-4, 2005.
23. Haws CW, Lux RL. Correlation between in vivo transmambrane action potential durations and activation-recovery intervals from electrograms. *Circulation*. 1990;81:281-288.
24. Huiskamp GJM. *Noninvasive Determination of Human Ventricular Activation*. Nijmegen, the Netherlands: University of Nijmegen; 1989.
25. van Dam PM, Oostendorp TF, Linnenbank AC, et al. Non-invasive imaging of cardiac activation and recovery. *Ann Biomed Eng*. 2009;37:1739-1756.
26. Durrer D, van Dam RT, Freud GE, et al. Total excitation of the isolated human heart. *Circulation*. 1970;41:899-912.
27. van Oosterom A, Jacquemet V. The effect of tissue geometry on the activation recovery interval of atrial myocytes. *Physica D*. 2009;238:962-968.
28. van Oosterom A. The dominant T wave and its significance. *J Cardiovasc Electrophysiol*. 2003;14(Suppl 10):S180-S187.
29. van Oosterom A. The singular value decomposition of the T wave: its link with a biophysical model of repolarization. *Int J Bioelectromagnetism*. 2002;4:59-60.
30. Carmeliet E. Cardiac ionic currents and acute ischemia: from channels to arrhythmias. *Physiol Rev*. 1999;79:917-1017.
31. Kléber AG, Janse MJ, Wilms-Schopmann FJ, et al. Changes in conduction velocity during acute ischemia in ventricular myocardium of the isolated porcine heart. *Circulation*. 1986;73:189-198.
32. van Dam P, Oostendorp T, van Oosterom A. Application of the fastest route algorithm in the interactive simulation of the effect of local ischemia on the ECG. *Med Biol Eng Comput*. 2009;47:11-20.
33. Janse MJ, van Capelle FJL, Morsink H, et al. Flow of injury current and patterns of excitation during early ventricular arrhythmias in acute regional myocardial ischemia in isolated porcine and canaine hearts. Evidence for two different arrhythmogenic mechanisms. *Circ Res*. 1980;47:151-165.
34. Ihara Z, van Oosterom A, Hoekema R. Atrial repolarization as observable during the PQ interval. *J Electrocardiol*. 2006;39:290-297.
35. van Oosterom A, Huiskamp GJM. The effect of torso inhomogeneities on body surface potentials quantified by using tailored geometry. *J Electrocardiol*. 1989;22:53-72.
36. Pages A, Bonnet N, van Oosterom A, et al. What is ECGSIM able to do for ARVD. Paper presented at Cardiostim, Cannes, France, 2004.
37. Hooft van Huysduynen B, Swenne CA, Bax JJ, et al. Dispersion of repolarization in cardiac resynchronization therapy. *Heart Rhythm*. 2005;2:1286-1293.
38. Hooft van Huysduynen B, Swenne CA, Draaisma HHM, et al. Validation of ECG indices of ventricular repolarization heterogeneity. *J Cardiovasc Electrophysiol*. 2005;16:1097-1103.
39. Coronel R, Casini S, Koopmann TT, et al. Right ventricular fibrosis and conduction delay in a patient with clinical signs of brugada syndrome: a combined electrophysiological, genetic, histopathologic, and computational study. *Circulation*. 2005;112:2769-2777.
40. Svendsen MC, Oostendorp TF, Berbari EJ. Evaluation of auto-regressive modeling procedures for the detection of abnormal intra-QRS potentials using a boundary element electrocardiogram model. *Comput Cardiol*. 2007;34:289-292.

CHAPTER 16

GRAPHICAL ANALYSIS OF HEART RATE PATTERNS TO ASSESS CARDIAC AUTONOMIC FUNCTION

Phyllis K. Stein and Panagiotis Pantazopoulos

INTRODUCTION / 284

**INFORMATION FROM 5-MINUTE AVERAGED
HR PATTERNS / 284**

INFORMATION FROM POWER SPECTRAL ANALYSIS / 285
Bed and Wake Times / 286
Abnormalities in the HF Portion of the Power
    Spectral Plot / 288
Sleep-Disordered Breathing HR Patterns in the Power
    Spectral Plot / 288
Abnormal Organization of HRV Patterns on FFT / 288

INFORMATION FROM POINCARÉ PLOTS / 290

INFORMATION FROM BEAT-BY-BEAT HR TACHOGRAMS / 290
HR Tachograms to Identify Sleep Periods / 290
HR Tachograms to Identify Sleep-Disordered Breathing / 290
HR Tachograms to Identify Erratic Sinus Rhythm / 295
Other Patterns Potentially Visible on HR Tachograms / 296

**USING GRAPHICAL HRV TO SUPPLEMENT INTERPRETATION
OF HRV MEASURES / 296**

**INTEGRATING INFORMATION FROM MULTIPLE HRV
PLOTS / 296**

**COMBINING GRAPHIC HRV WITH OTHER IMAGING
MODALITIES / 297**

SUMMARY / 297

INTRODUCTION

A continuous electrocardiogram, whether from a Holter recording, an intensive care unit monitor, an overnight polysomnogram, or even a short-term recording, provides a signal that can yield information about the morphology and time of onset of each heartbeat. This information, exported as a "beat file" provides the basis for multiple ways of quantifying and categorizing heart rate variability (HRV), in most cases based on intervals between normal to normal (N-N) heartbeats only. The various methods for quantifying HRV (eg, time domain, frequency

domain, nonlinear) and their relationship to cardiac autonomic function have been described in multiple excellent reviews elsewhere.[1-3] Less appreciated is the power of using graphical images, also derived from beat files, to obtain information about normal and abnormal cardiac autonomic function, sinus node function, and sleep-disordered breathing.

The periods between successive heartbeats can be converted to a time series of instantaneous heart rates (60,000 milliseconds in a minute/time between beats in ms). Heart rate (HR) patterns can be examined on multiple scales, each providing both unique and overlapping information. HR itself can be plotted on a beat-by-beat basis, or HR averages and ranges over longer periods can be plotted. Power spectral analysis can mathematically deconstruct heartbeat patterns into their underlying rhythmic components using fast Fourier transforms (FFTs).[3] The structure of heartbeat patterns can be examined using Poincaré plots, which are plots of the interval between every pair of successive beats versus the next pair.

The current review will illustrate the types of information potentially available from these aspects of graphical HRV analysis (ie, 5-minute averaged HR patterns, hourly power spectral analysis, hourly Poincaré plots, and beat-by-beat HR tachograms). To accomplish this, we will primarily use representative plots from recordings selected from our database of subjects with and without known cardiovascular disease. From among the healthy subjects, we will examine graphical HRV in a younger adult with high HRV (the standard deviation of all normal-to-normal interbeat intervals [SDNN] = 198), an older adult with high HRV (SDNN = 167), and an older adult with low HRV (SDNN = 65). From among those with known cardiovascular disease, we will examine graphical HRV in a subject with very low HRV but normal HR patterns (SDNN = 63), a subject with periods of abnormal HR patterns (SDNN = 99), a subject with significant sleep-disordered breathing HR patterns (SDNN = 49), and a subject with atrial fibrillation (SDNN = 211).

INFORMATION FROM 5-MINUTE AVERAGED HR PATTERNS

Commercial Holter scanner reports often show plots of 5-minute averaged HR patterns. The presence or relative absence of a circadian rhythm of HR is clearly visible on these plots. Under normal circumstances, a clear decrease in HR during the night, a distinct rise in HR on awakening, and a relatively higher HR during the daytime are seen. Lack of circadian rhythm of HR is the primary determinant of low values for total HRV and suggests severe autonomic dysfunction and/or a complete lack of physical activity. In Fig. 16–1, the average HRs and their ranges for every 5 minutes are shown for four healthy subjects. The circadian rhythm of HR can be appreciated qualitatively by following the center line of the plots. A qualitatively normal circadian rhythm is clearly seen for the younger subject (see Fig. 16–1A) and the older subjects with high HRV (see Fig. 16–1B) and average HRV (see Fig. 16–1C), and approximate bed and wake times can be seen from the decrease in HR in the evening and the sharp increase in the morning, but in the older adult with low HRV

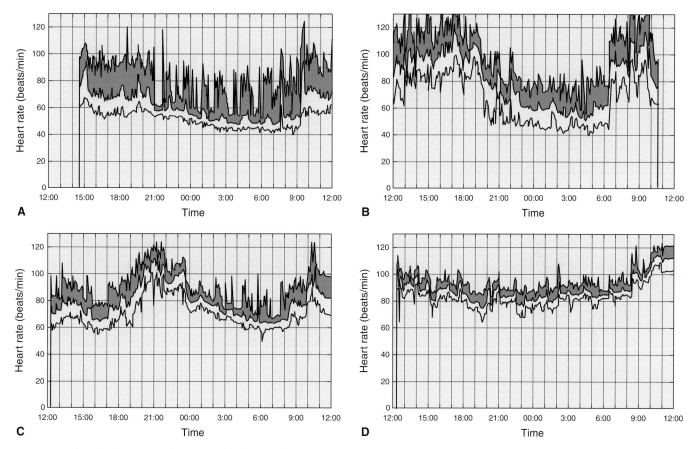

FIGURE 16–1. Plots of 5-minute average heart rate and maximum and minimum heart rate for each 5 minutes in (**A**) a young healthy man with high heart rate variability (HRV), (**B**) an older healthy man with high HRV, (**C**) an older healthy man with average HRV, and (**D**) an older man with low HRV. Green is heart rates above the average. Yellow is hearts below the average.

(see Fig. 16–1D), circadian rhythm is markedly attenuated and bed time is less clear.

Figure 16–2 shows 5-minute averaged HR plots for subjects with known cardiovascular disease. The patients in Fig. 16–2A,B have a diminished circadian rhythm, but a circadian rhythm is clearly visible in Fig. 16–2C. No circadian rhythm for HR is visible for the subject with atrial fibrillation (see Fig. 16–2D).

In Figs. 16–1 and 16–2, the top line of each plot shows the highest instantaneous HR in each 5-minute period, and the bottom line shows the lowest. The range of HRs within each period is a rough surrogate for the amount of HRV within each period. When the subjects with high HRV (see Fig. 16–1A,B) are compared with the subjects with lower HRV (see Fig. 16–1C,D), HR ranges are clearly less in subjects with lower HRV. HR ranges are still lower in the subject shown in Fig. 16–2A. Thus, examination of the range of HRs within each 5-minute period provides a qualitative sense of the amount of HRV present.

However, these HR ranges must be interpreted with caution, and examination of the HR ranges and circadian patterns of these ranges, as shown in these plots, could arouse suspicion of additional underlying problems beyond the lack of normal circadian rhythm. The clearest example is Fig. 16–2D (atrial fibrillation). Note the complete lack of a circadian rhythm and the extremely wide HR range. Abnormalities in cardiac rhythm may also be suspected in Fig. 16–2B,C, where there are periods of low HR range interspersed with periods of much higher HR ranges.

INFORMATION FROM POWER SPECTRAL ANALYSIS

Another way of displaying HR patterns is by frequency domain or power spectral analysis. This involves using FFTs or autoregressive methods to decompose the variations in HR into underlying frequencies that together constitute the whole HR pattern, roughly analogous to decomposing a single note in a symphony into the underlying sounds of the different instruments that are playing at once.[1,3] Normally, this process is performed on short segments of the signal (often 5 minutes) and then averaged over time. Only N-N interbeat intervals are used. If <80% of the time of segment is accounted from by N-N interbeat intervals (ie, >20% noise or ectopic beats), that segment is not usable for power spectral analysis. The reason for this is that the beat before and the beat after a nonnormal beat is excluded in power spectral analysis; thus, having >20% noise in a 5-minute segment means excluding >60% of the beats in that segment a priori. In a display of the results of power spectral analysis, the amount of variance (or amplitude, which is the square root of variance) at each underlying frequency is plotted on the y-axis, and the underlying frequency is plotted on the x-axis. Thus, the greater the HRV is, the greater the variance in HR and, therefore, the larger the area under the power spectral curve.

The various frequency domain HRV measures found in the literature are measures of the area under the FFT curve (or power) in groups of predefined underlying frequencies or "bands." These are usually reported as ultra low–frequency (ULF) power, very

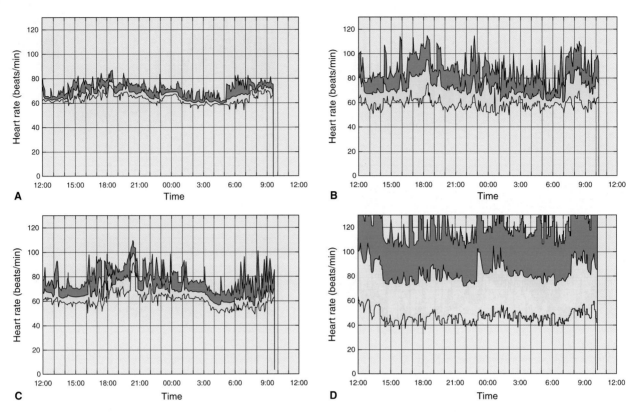

FIGURE 16–2. Plots of 5-minute average heart rate and maximum and minimum heart rate for each 5 minutes in (**A**) a cardiac patient with low heart rate variability (HRV), (**B**) a cardiac patient with abnormal HRV, (**C**) a cardiac patient with sleep-disorder breathing heart rate patterns, and (**D**) a cardiac patient with atrial fibrillation.

low–frequency (VLF) power, low-frequency (LF) power, and high-frequency (HF) power.[3] ULF power reflects variance in HR with a period of between 5 minutes and 24 hours and primarily reflects circadian HR patterns and long-term activity.[3] VLF power (variations from 20-second to 5-minute cycles) is believed to reflect the activity of the renin-angiotensin and parasympathetic systems, although it is exaggerated by periodic breathing patterns.[4] LF power (variations from 3-9 cycles/min) reflects the combined activity of the sympathetic and parasympathetic nervous systems and especially the activity of the baroreflex.[3] Beat-to-beat HR changes are quantified by HF power (variations at respiratory frequencies) and primarily reflect parasympathetic modulation of HR.[3] Differences in the amount of power in the different FFT bands are often used to compare cardiac autonomic function between subjects or within subjects after interventions, but as will be emphasized throughout this chapter, without graphical analysis of HR patterns, these numbers may prove to be misleading.[5]

Many commercial Holter scanning programs provide a single summarized plot of HRV power averaged over the entire recording. This plot is usually displayed as either amplitude versus frequency or ln amplitude versus ln frequency. The linear scale is more easily interpreted. Although 24-hour HRV plots are useful, more detailed information about changing autonomic function during the recording period can be obtained by plotting the HRV power spectral plot on an hourly basis. This, too, is available in some commercial Holter scanning systems. Notably, however, when hourly plots are used, information about the amount of ULF power is lost. Some of the information that can be gleaned by examining hourly FFTs is described in the following sections.

■ BED AND WAKE TIMES

Just as the circadian rhythm plots can suggest bed and wake times, examination of hourly power spectral plots can also identify these times in most people and sometimes even distinguish between quiet rest and sleep. The hour during which the subject became supine can often be identified as the hour when a distinct peak appears in the HF band. This peak appears because when people lie down, sympathetic activity declines and HR is under predominantly parasympathetic control, which leads to a large increase in respiratory sinus arrhythmia, which is vagally mediated.[6] Respiratory sinus arrhythmia, which is a speeding up of HR on inhalation and slowing down on exhalation, obviously occurs at the same frequency as respiration (ie, usually between 9 and 24 cycles/min). This frequency corresponds to the underlying oscillations of the HF power spectral HRV band (0.15-0.4 Hz). Moreover, the center frequency of this peak corresponds to the average breathing frequency during that period, and the magnitude of this peak reflects the degree of parasympathetic control of HR during that time. Often, supine rest can be distinguished from sleep because the center frequency of this peak declines at sleep onset compared with quiet rest and remains at that value during the night. Similarly, upon arising, this peak generally disappears. The reappearance of the HF peak during the middle of the day suggests a nap.

The 24 hourly power spectral amplitude plots for the healthy subjects originally shown in Fig. 16–1 are seen in Fig. 16–3. As indicated on the figure, hours with clearly visible HR peaks corresponding to times in bed and hours without such peaks

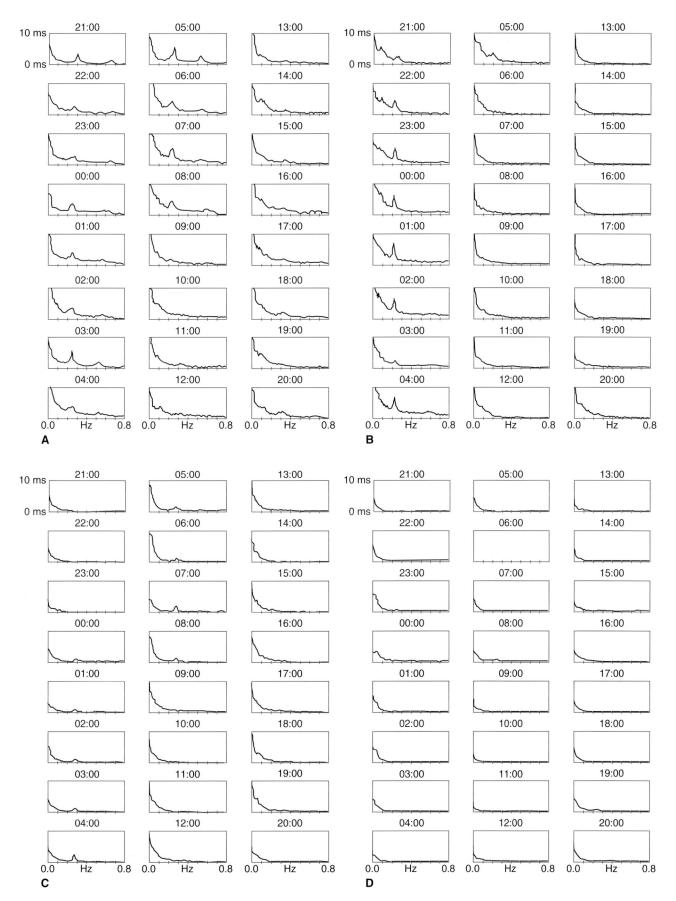

FIGURE 16–3. Plots of 5-minute averaged heart rate variability (HRV) spectral amplitudes for the same subjects shown in Fig. 16–1: (**A**) a young healthy man with high HRV, (**B**) an older healthy man with high HRV, (**C**) an older healthy man with average HRV, and (**D**) an older man with low HRV.

corresponding to times out of bed can clearly be identified for all but the subject with low HRV (see Fig. 16–3D).

Figure 16–4 shows 24 hourly spectral amplitude plots for the individuals with known cardiovascular disease originally shown in Fig. 16–2. Although the HF peak is extremely small for the subject with low HRV originally seen in Fig. 16–2A, close inspection can identify times in bed. In Fig. 16–4B, there are hours during the night with clear HF peaks that correspond to time in bed, but the HRV pattern is unclear in the hours immediately preceding and following them. The subject in Fig. 16–2C has clearly defined HF peaks during normal sleep hours, starting at 00:00, but additional HF peaks with a higher center frequency at 18:00 to 23:00 suggest that this subject was lying down for much of the time. Not surprisingly, no HF peak can be identified for the subject with atrial fibrillation.

ABNORMALITIES IN THE HF PORTION OF THE POWER SPECTRAL PLOT

Under normal circumstances, the HF peak of the power spectral plot, especially during sleep, is visible and distinct, as shown in most of the plots. As seen in Fig. 16–2A, even in patients with extremely low HRV, a clear, if small, HF peak can often be identified for the nighttime period, suggesting diminished but persevered vagal control of the heart. The absence of any such peak (as in Fig. 16–1D) suggests extreme parasympathetic dysfunction. Abnormalities in the shape of the HF peak suggest an underlying problem. For example, a disorganized peak in the HF band that has no clear center frequency (as in Fig. 16–2B) might suggest extremely irregular respiration or suggest the presence of either erratic sinus rhythm (ie, a high degree of sinus arrhythmia of nonrespiratory origin) or significant scanning error due to uneven detection of beat onsets.[5,7]

SLEEP-DISORDERED BREATHING HR PATTERNS IN THE POWER SPECTRAL PLOT

The association of sleep-disordered breathing with excessive sympathetic activation and the subsequent improvement in cardiac autonomic function with treatment have been well documented.[8] Clearly, sleep-disordered breathing is associated with multiple adverse outcomes, and just as clearly, it is very much underdiagnosed.[8-10] Graphical analyses of HRV offer a simple way to screen for this underlying condition. When sleep-disordered breathing is present, the patient experiences repeated episodes of loss of airflow and then abrupt awakenings to resume breathing. Unless autonomic dysfunction is extremely severe, each of these awakenings is accompanied by a sharp increase in HR, sometimes by as much as 25 to 30 beats per minute. Similarly, although generally briefer and more frequent, HR arousals can be caused by periodic limb movements (usually around every 20 seconds). Because sleep-disordered events occur at a frequency of between every 20 seconds to approximately every 90 seconds, this creates an oscillation in HR in the VLF band (which includes all HR oscillations at between every 20 seconds and every 5 minutes). This oscillation is also referred to as cyclic variation of HR (CVHR). Not surprisingly, this oscillation adds power at that underlying frequency in the HRV

power spectral plot, and the center frequency of that peak also indicates the underlying frequency of the CVHR. The plot from the older man with high HRV (see Fig. 16–3A) has considerable power in the VLF band during the night. In addition, there is a suggestion of a distinct VLF peak during different hours of the night. The plot from the older healthy man with average HRV (see Fig. 16–3C) shows considerably more VLF power in the 05:00, 06:00, and 08:00 hours than during the rest of the night, suggesting the presence of sleep-disordered breathing HR patterns during that period. The plots from the older healthy man with low HRV in Fig. 16–3D also suggest the presence of a peak in the VLF band between 00:00 and 03:00. In Fig. 16–4C, the plots from 01:00 and 02:00 show large VLF peaks corresponding to periods of sleep-disordered breathing that are not visible in the other examples but are relatively common in recordings from older adults and from cardiac patients. Although hourly power spectral plots are most useful for detecting CVHR peaks, often, if significant sleep-disordered breathing or periodic limb movements are present, this large VLF peak can be seen on the single averaged 24-hour FFT plot.

ABNORMAL ORGANIZATION OF HRV PATTERNS ON FFT

Not all FFT plots show a normal distribution of underlying rhythms in the different HRV bands. Aside from plots where there is little or no area under the curve, which indicate severely depressed autonomic function, other plots simply show an abnormal distribution of spectral power. Figure 16–4B,D shows examples of clearly abnormal plots. A side-by-side comparison of the normal and abnormal plots permits one to intuitively appreciate the differences. Abnormal plots are less organized. They have more area under the curve at frequencies above the HF band. They lack the characteristic HF peak or, in some cases, have a broad peak in the "wrong" place. This abnormal distribution of spectral power could be due to extremely inaccurate Holter scanning but more often indicates underlying irregularities in HR patterns that do not reflect normal cardiac autonomic function (erratic rhythm, as mentioned earlier) and may reflect higher risk of cardiovascular death. In both the Cardiovascular Health Study (CHS)[5] and the Cardiac Arrhythmia Suppression Trial (CAST),[11] we have reported that a higher prevalence of hours with erratic rhythm HR patterns is associated with increased risk of cardiovascular mortality. In the CAST study, a worsening of erratic rhythm HR patterns in association with antiarrhythmic therapy was also associated with increased risk of mortality.[11]

Although the precise origin of this abnormal rhythm has not been determined, it may reflect a form of sinus node dysfunction. However, from the perspective of using HRV to characterize cardiac autonomic function, as we have emphasized, these abnormal patterns are associated with higher HRV *numbers* that do not translate into "better" autonomic function.[5] Therefore, it is recommended that the underlying distribution of the HRV power spectrum be examined on an hourly basis and that clearly abnormal cases be excluded to avoid confounding HRV results. Because, as seen in this example, patients with periods

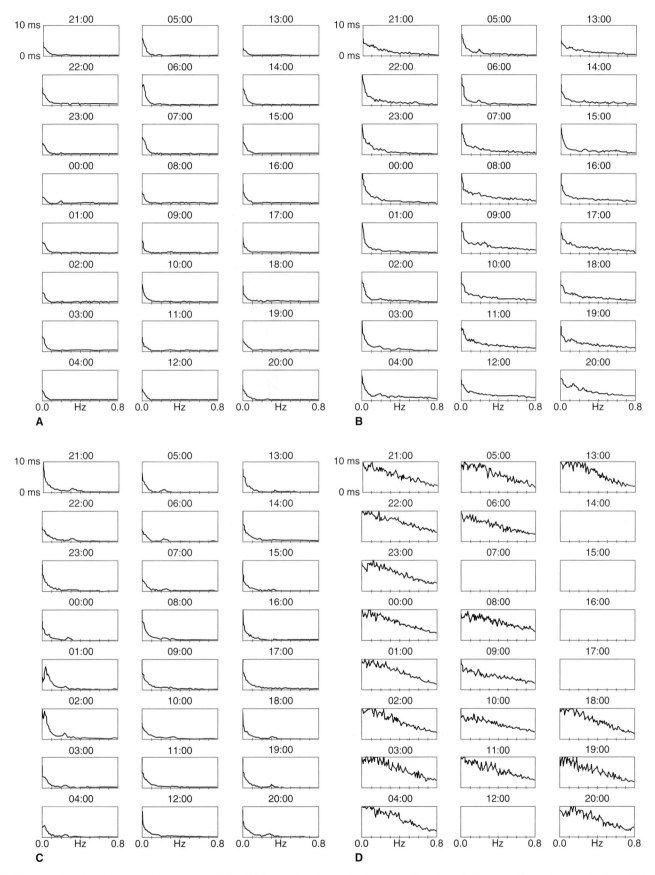

FIGURE 16–4. Plots of 5-minute averaged heart rate variability (HRV) spectral amplitudes for the same subjects shown in Fig. 16–2: (**A**) a cardiac patient with low HRV, (**B**) a cardiac patient with abnormal HRV, (**C**) a cardiac patient with sleep-disorder breathing HR patterns, and (**D**) a cardiac patient with atrial fibrillation.

of abnormal HR patterns do not necessarily have this rhythm throughout their entire recording, the question of how to adjust for this in determining HRV as a measure of autonomic function remains open. Clearly though, when this abnormal rhythm is prevalent during the recording, some HRV measures will not be meaningful. This topic will be discussed in greater detail at the end of this chapter.

INFORMATION FROM POINCARÉ PLOTS

A Poincaré plot is generated by plotting the time between two heartbeats versus the time between the next two for each pair of intervals on the recording. Although some investigators generate these plots from all R-R intervals, it can be more informative to use plots of N-N interbeat intervals only, because otherwise it is impossible to determine whether outliers are due to ectopy or erratic rhythm. Indeed, some investigators do deal with this by filtering or ignoring these beats, potentially measuring HRV only during the periods of normal sinus rhythm. This filtering, however, could result in the loss of potentially important information.

Just as with any other graphic display, *hourly* Poincaré plots show the amount of HRV, as seen in the area of the plots, in greater detail than a single 24-hour plot; more importantly, they provide a clear way to visualize the structure of the HR pattern at different times during the recording. Normal hourly plots are somewhat comet shaped or perhaps ellipsoid, although hours that contain both sleep and active periods might have two clusters. Abnormal plots are more disorganized, ranging from plots with a clearly visible central part and some outlier points to plots that seem splattered all over. Highly disorganized Poincaré plots have also been referred to as "complex" plots. Prior studies have supported the clinical importance of abnormal Poincaré plots generated from 24-hour R-R interval data.[12-14] These studies, have demonstrated an association between the presence of complex Poincaré plots and mortality among congestive heart failure patients. Abnormal Poincaré plots have also been associated with risk of ventricular tachycardia,[15] and in another study from the same group, in post–coronary artery bypass graft patients, more random HR patterns measured on postoperative day 1 predicted ischemic events.[16] Thus, Poincaré plots are also a sensitive way to identify recordings with an abnormal HR pattern in patients who could be at increased risk of cardiovascular events and in whom higher values for some HRV measures will be misleading.[7]

Figure 16–5 shows the hourly Poincaré plots for the subjects originally shown in Figs. 16–1 and 16–3. All of the plots are normally organized, although the young subject with high HRV (see Fig. 16–5A) clearly has more HRV during the daytime than the older subject with high HRV (see Fig. 16–5B). The decreased HRV in the older adult with average HRV (see Fig. 16–5C) and the even more depressed HRV in the older adult with low HRV are clearly visible as reduced area in the Poincaré plots.

Figure 16–6 shows the hourly Poincaré plots for the subjects with known cardiovascular disease originally shown in Figs. 16–2 and 16–4. Although the decreased HRV reflecting blunted

cardiac autonomic function is clearly visible, the *shapes* of the Poincaré plots in Fig. 16–6A,C are unremarkable. However, the plots in Fig. 16–6B reflect a combination of periods of essential normal sinus rhythm and periods of highly disorganized/erratic sinus rhythm. The plots for the patient with atrial fibrillation (see Fig. 16–6D) are, as would be expected, completely abnormal.

INFORMATION FROM BEAT-BY-BEAT HR TACHOGRAMS

A plot of instantaneous HR on a beat-to-beat basis and on an appropriate scale provides the most direct possible image of HRV. We have found that plotting HR on a series of 10-minute scales (0-100 beats/min) is excellent for these analyses. Only N-N interbeat intervals are used for this analysis. Figure 16–7 is an example of 1 hour's worth of data—six stacked 10-minute plots during quiet sleep. Respiratory sinus arrhythmia, seen as zig-zag HR patterns on the plots, and occasional arousals from sleep are clearly seen.

■ HR TACHOGRAMS TO IDENTIFY SLEEP PERIODS

Although the hour of lying down can usually be identified from hourly power spectral plots, a more precise estimate of lying down and getting up times can be made from beat-to-beat HR tachograms. The onset of lying down or sleep can be seen as the beginning of a period of lower and more regular HR and often the onset of a clearly seen HR pattern reflecting respiratory sinus arrhythmia. This clearly seen respiratory sinus arrhythmia pattern during sleep also provides information about breath-by-breath respiratory rate and a qualitative sense of the changing depth of respiration, which will be discussed in greater detail later. Figure 16–8 illustrates the difference in HR patterns between asleep and awake periods, 10 minutes apart, in the same subject (the older adult with average HRV). Note the higher mean HR (indicated by the average HR line) and the far greater irregularity of HR patterns during wake.

■ HR TACHOGRAMS TO IDENTIFY SLEEP-DISORDERED BREATHING

Although the presence of CVHR can often be identified from the hourly power spectral plot as described earlier, HR tachograms clearly identify the magnitude and duration of these cycles of regular arousals during sleep. The pattern of this CVHR often provides clues as to its origin. For example, especially during the early part of the night, repeated low-amplitude, relatively brief CVHR cycles at approximately 20-second intervals are often seen and suggest periodic limb movements. Higher amplitude, longer cycles suggest sleep-disordered breathing. A sharp increase in HR usually occurs when the patient arouses to breathe. HR returns to baseline when the patient falls back to sleep, at which point if there is sleep-disordered breathing, the airway collapses again. These events are associated with significant autonomic activation and have been shown, in some patients, to be association with spectacular surges in blood pressure. Although intuitively one might suspect that larger HR cycles are associated with more

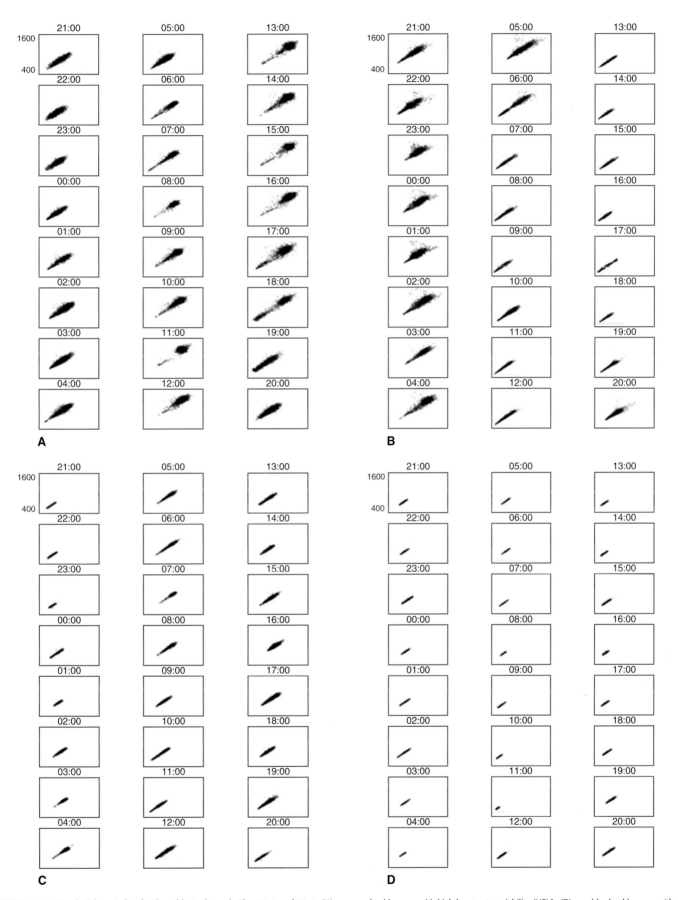

FIGURE 16–5. Hourly Poincaré plots for the subjects shown in Figs. 16–1 and 16–3: (**A**) a young healthy man with high heart rate variability (HRV), (**B**) an older healthy man with high HRV, (**C**) an older healthy man with average HRV, and (**D**) an older man with low HRV.

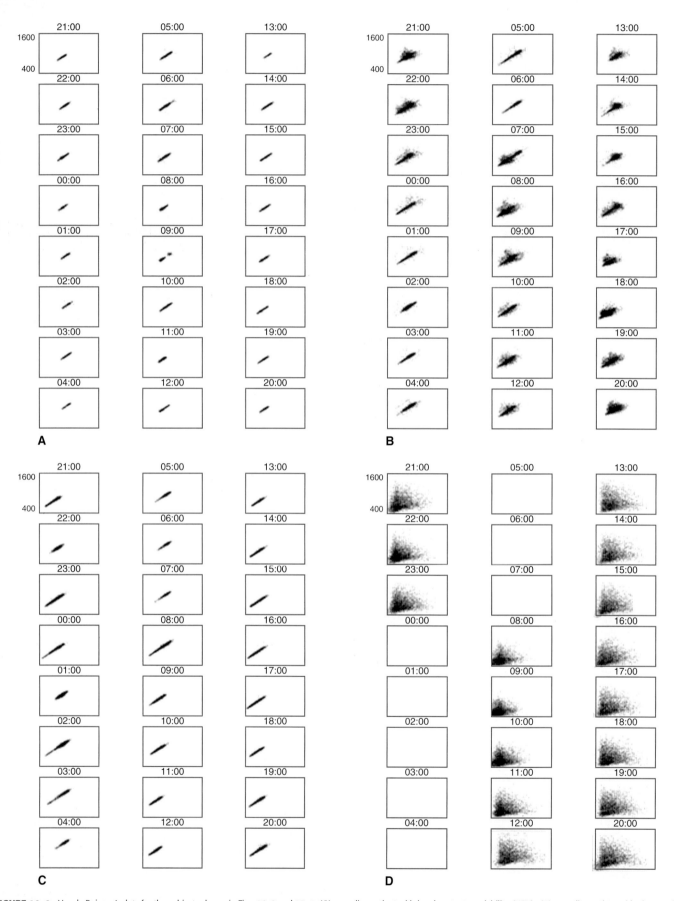

FIGURE 16–6. Hourly Poincaré plots for the subjects shown in Figs. 16–2 and 16–4: (**A**) a cardiac patient with low heart rate variability (HRV), (**B**) a cardiac patient with abnormal HRV, (**C**) a cardiac patient with sleep-disorder breathing HR patterns, and (**D**) a cardiac patient with atrial fibrillation.

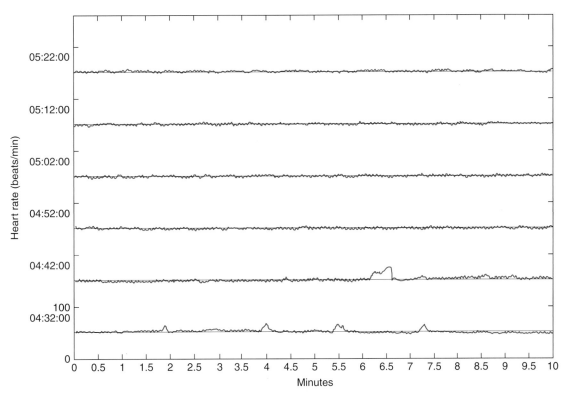

FIGURE 16–7. A 1-hour instantaneous heart rate tachogram during sleep. The tachogram is read from the bottom to the top. Each line is 10 minutes of beat-by-beat instantaneous heart rate for all normal heartbeats. The y-axis indicates 100 beats per minute between tick marks; the onset of each 10-minute segment is marked on the y-axis. The horizontal line for each plot represents the average heart rate during that 10-minute period.

severe sleep-disordered breathing, the magnitude of these cycles is also influenced by underlying autonomic function, and in the case of severely impaired autonomic function, severe sleep apnea HR changes might be barely visible on the tachogram. Note that respiratory sinus arrhythmia patterns can persist during the period of airflow obstruction, indicating a continuing respiratory effort. Although this pattern is often referred to as a *bradytachy* *pattern*, the commonly held view that obstruction of airflow is always associated with a significant bradycardia is not correct.[17] Such bradycardias do occur, especially in the presence of severe oxygen desaturations, but they are not a hallmark of the syndrome. Rather, the bradytachy pattern seen on electrocardiogram reflects the tachycardia of the HR arousal and the return to baseline HR after breathing is resumed.

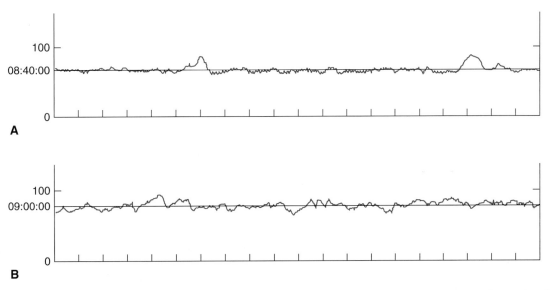

FIGURE 16–8. Heart rate tachograms (**A**) during sleep and (**B**) 10 minutes later in the same individual showing higher average heart rate and greater irregularity during wake compared with sleep.

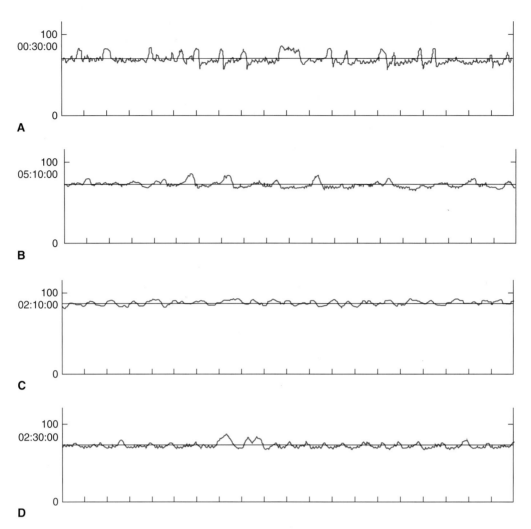

FIGURE 16–9. Samples of the heart rate (HR) tachogram for the subjects with suspected cyclic variation of HR based on Figs. 16–3 and 16–4: (**A**) the healthy older adult with high heart rate variability (HRV), (**B**) the older adult with average HRV, (**C**) the older adult with low HRV, and (**D**) the cardiac patient with a strong very low–frequency peak on the fast Fourier transform plot.

Figure 16–9 shows 10-minute sections of the HR tachograms from the subjects whose FFT plots in Figs. 16–3 and 16–4 previously suggested the presence of sleep-disordered breathing. In Fig. 16–9A, showing the older adult with high HRV, HR arousals are very sharp, and sleep is disrupted. This suggests either limb movements or perhaps what would be scored as "arousals for no apparent reason." The older adult with average HRV shown in Fig. 16–9B did not have CVHR until the morning hours. This is a typical pattern consistent with the greater amount of rapid eye movement (REM) sleep (with more intense CVHR) toward morning and the possibility that the patient is lying on his back, which increases the likelihood of sleep-disordered breathing. In Fig. 16–9C, the sleep-disordered breathing HR pattern of the older adult with average HRV is seen. The mixture of longer and short HR arousals suggests the possibility of a mixture of sleep-disordered breathing events of varied severity. Finally, Fig. 16–9D shows CVHR from the cardiac patient originally seen in Fig. 16–2C. This CVHR pattern of relatively short HR arousals suggests the presence of hypopneas (periods of decreased airflow) rather than obstructive apneas (full cessation of airflow).

None of the patients selected to illustrate various aspects of HR pattern analysis proved to have either severe obstructive sleep apnea HR patterns or central sleep apnea HR patterns. Therefore, these patterns are illustrated in Fig. 16–10. Figure 16–10A shows typical HR patterns for severe obstructive sleep apnea. Note the sharp increase in HR at the beginning of the CVHR and the relative abrupt decrease in HR at the termination of the event. Although the examples shown in Fig. 16–10 have regular cycles of CVHR, regularity is not always present.[18] Of special clinical interest is the identification of central sleep apnea (lack of airflow due to failure to breathe) and Cheyne-Stokes respiration (a combination of central hypopnea or apnea and then periodic respiration) from HR tachograms. CVHR due to central sleep apnea is typically of lower amplitude and flatter shape than that due to apneas or hypopneas, because the resumption of respiration is not associated with a sharp HR arousal. Patients with central sleep apnea tend to have relatively low HRV on the tachogram; however, respiratory sinus arrhythmia is usually visible, and therefore, the lack of respiratory effort or the periodic respiration can usually be identified. Figure 16–10B shows a tachogram with a central sleep apnea HR

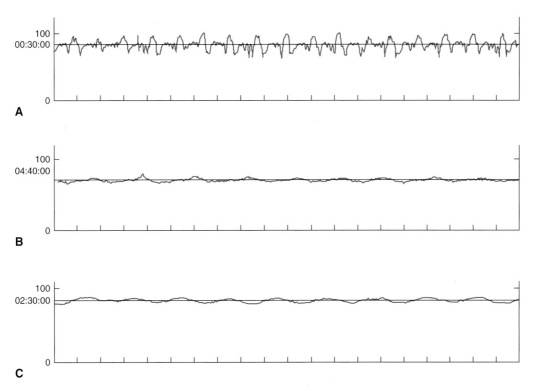

FIGURE 16–10. Examples of sleep-disordered breathing from other subjects: (**A**) severe obstructive sleep apnea, (**B**) central sleep apnea, and (**C**) Cheyne-Stokes respiration.

pattern. Figure 16–10C shows clearly identifiable Cheyne-Stokes respiration HR patterns.

■ HR TACHOGRAMS TO IDENTIFY ERRATIC SINUS RHYTHM

Beat-to-beat HR tachograms can also reveal arrhythmias that are not apparent on ordinary Holter scanning. Respiratory sinus arrhythmia, as has been seen in the previous examples, is seen as a saw-tooth pattern on the HR tachogram and is especially visible during supine rest. However, there is another form of sinus arrhythmia that is highly irregular even though

there is no visible difference in the P waves or PR intervals on Holter scanning. As previously mentioned, the presence of this erratic sinus rhythm can be identified from both FFT plots and from Poincaré plots. However, HR tachograms provide the most direct evidence for its presence.[5] Figures 16–11A (from the subject originally shown in Figs. 16–2B, 16–4B, and 16–6B) and 16–11B (from a different subject) show examples of HR tachograms with erratic HR patterns. As mentioned, time and frequency domain HRV measures are confounded by erratic rhythm. However, many of the newer, nonlinear measures (eg, the short-term fractal scaling exponent) actually capture this increased randomness in HR patterns, which

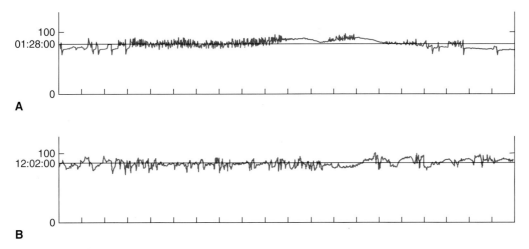

FIGURE 16–11. Heart rate tachograms during periods of erratic rhythm (**A**) in the cardiac patient whose data are shown in Figs. 16–2C, 16–4C, and 16–6C and (**B**) in a different individual.

is likely the reason they perform so well as predictors of cardiovascular outcomes.[18-20]

■ OTHER PATTERNS POTENTIALLY VISIBLE ON HR TACHOGRAMS

Extremely abnormal HR tachograms can suggest severe scanning error, and investigation of the original recording is advised before any conclusions are drawn. Additional patterns are also seen on HR tachograms, although their clinical significance is unknown. Tachograms reveal episodes of "sinus bigeminy," an alternating pattern of slightly faster and slower HRs that is often not noticed on Holter scanning and that is remarkably common. Tachograms also reveal various oscillating HR patterns, including one with an oscillation at approximately 6 cycles/min that we have observed in a small number of high-risk patients and others where the HR cycles up and down for long periods of time, as if the system cannot find a stable state. Although generation of numbers for statistical comparison is the goal of HRV research, it cannot be emphasized enough that looking at the primary data, the actual beat-to-beat HR patterns, is essential for results to be meaningful.

USING GRAPHICAL HRV TO SUPPLEMENT INTERPRETATION OF HRV MEASURES

Graphical analysis of HR patterns can potentially permit more accurate measurement of HRV. To apply this, it is important to qualitatively understand the scope of different HRV measures. Certain measures primarily reflect total HRV and therefore mostly circadian rhythms. These measures include SDNN, the standard deviation of the averages of N-N intervals for every 5 minutes (SDANN), total power, and ULF power. Because the largest contribution to HRV is circadian rhythm, these measures are less affected by erratic rhythm, sleep-disordered HR patterns, or even scanning error unless it is really severe.[5] Of the circadian HRV measures, SDANN and ULF power, which are roughly equivalent,[21] are the least affected and can, arguably, even be used to measure HRV in cases of atrial fibrillation.[22] Thus, results of a 24-hour recording can generally categorize subjects as having low or high HRV even in the presence of very abnormal rhythms. Average HR is also unaffected by these abnormal rhythms, although it could be elevated by the arousals of severe sleep apnea. However, a high SDNN due to a monotonically increasing HR through the entire recording (which we have seen) is clearly not comparable to an SDNN that reflects circadian rhythm. This supports the importance of examining plots of HR patterns or, at the very least, examining hourly average HRs.

The second group of HRV measures is "intermediate" and reflects HRV on a scale of approximately 5 minutes or less. These measures include the average standard deviation of 5-minute N-N intervals (SDNNIDX), VLF power (which reflects variations in HR at cycles of 20 seconds to 5 minutes), and LF power (which reflects variations in HR at 3-9 cycles/min). VLF power is especially unaffected by erratic rhythm,

sinus bigeminy, and subtle scanning error because it does not include cycles below every 20 seconds, but it is exaggerated by sleep apnea (although only for part of the 24-hour period) and by oscillating HR patterns. LF power reflects underlying oscillations of HR at about 3 to 9 cycles/min and is exaggerated by abnormal HR patterns.

The third class of HRV measures reflects beat-to-beat changes. This group includes the percentage of N-Ns >50 ms different from the prior one (pNN50), root mean square of the average difference in N-N interval between successive pairs of beats (rMSSD), HF power, and various ratio measures such as the LF/HF ratio, normalized LF power, and normalized HF power. It is often assumed that these measures reflect parasympathetic control of HR or, in the case of the ratio measures, some sort of balance between the two arms of the autonomic nervous system.[1] These measures, however, are totally confounded by erratic rhythm, scanning error, and sinus bigeminy, which significantly exaggerate them.[5] Putting them into the denominator, as is done with the ratio measures, simply adds to the problem.

Thus, examination of graphical HR patterns is essential before deciding to include subjects in a standard HRV analysis. When graphical plots seem normal, HRV can meaningfully be calculated. When they are clearly abnormal, it is likely that only the circadian measures and VLF power will be meaningful. Short-term HRV measures are meaningless when erratic rhythm is present, and erratic rhythm is common among both cardiac patients and older adults in whom HRV may be useful for risk stratification.

INTEGRATING INFORMATION FROM MULTIPLE HRV PLOTS

Scanning of all of the Holter recordings shown in the figures was carefully verified. Revisiting the series of plots shown for the different subjects, it becomes clear that some subjects have normally configured plots by every test. In those subjects, traditional time or frequency domain HRV, whether high or low, can be calculated and should reflect cardiac autonomic function. Although, with experience, direct visualization of the HR tachogram provides an excellent starting point, a set of 24 hourly Poincaré plots and FFTs, each printed on a single page, provide a rapid way to assess each continuous electrocardiogram recording, and those that are normally organized by FFT and Poincaré plot criteria can generally be accepted for HRV analysis. The question of what to do with abnormal plots is complex and is the subject of ongoing investigations. At a minimum, the Holter scanning should be verified to ensure that the irregular rhythm is not due to undetected ectopy or nonuniform detection of beat onsets. If, however, this rhythm is truly present, as mentioned, circadian HRV measures, calculation of VLF power, and nonlinear methods can still be applied to characterize HRV for research studies. Short-term measures are meaningless in these cases, expect that when they appear to be unusually high relative to total HRV or to the population being studied, they are a red flag for erratic rhythm.

Clinically, each of these plots, including hourly HR tachograms plotted on a 10-minute scale, is available from at least one commercial Holter system, but no system, to our knowledge, provides all of them. Some clinical scanners attempt to detect CVHR that indicates sleep-disordered breathing. Measures like the short-term fractal scaling exponent and other novel nonlinear HRV measures are not yet commercially available. These require high-quality Holter scanning and further validation of their potential clinical utility.

COMBINING GRAPHIC HRV WITH OTHER IMAGING MODALITIES

The relationship of autonomic assessments from imaging and HRV analysis has been explored in numerous prior studies. For example, HRV has been studied in relation to cardiac iodine 123 (^{123}I)-meta-iodobenzylguanidine (MIBG) uptake, a direct measure of sympathetic nerve innervation of the ventricles of the heart. Not surprisingly, although sympathetic innervation of the ventricles and sympathetic innervation of the sinoatrial node are not the same thing, post–myocardial infarction patients with globally impaired cardiac ^{123}I-MIBG were also found to have impaired HRV.[23] The relationship between HRV and cardiac ^{123}I-MIBG parameters was confirmed in a group of implantable cardioverter-defibrillator (ICD) recipients by Koutelou et al[24] and among diabetic patients by Freeman et al.[25] Furthermore, baroreceptor sensitivity, LF power, rMSSD, and MIBG wash-out were independent predictors of fast ventricular arrhythmia episodes over an average of 32 months of follow-up among the ICD recipients.[24] The relationship of HRV to ventricular function during exercise as assessed by radionuclide imaging has also been explored. For example, Nagaoka et al[26] reported a relationship between depressed ventricular response to exercise and decreased HRV during different time periods in patients with idiopathic cardiomyopathy. However, these investigations have been limited by the assumption that low HRV is the only marker for abnormalities in cardiac autonomic function and high values for HRV reflect greater health. Moreover, the nature of the underlying HR patterns was never taken into account. As has been illustrated earlier, low HRV is only one form of abnormal HRV. Thus, future studies incorporating both numeric and graphical methods for analysis of HRV promise to enhance the combined power imaging and HRV for risk stratification and understanding of the underlying physiology of different cardiac pathologies.

SUMMARY

Use of graphical plots of HR patterns provides additional clinically relevant information that would be missed by the numeric measurements; in addition, visualization of HR patterns by some graphical method is absolutely essential before many of the numerical measurements can be said to have any true meaning. With current computer technology, generation of graphical plots of HR patterns is neither difficult nor time consuming. Potentially, therefore, the future of ambulatory ECG analysis, whether from Holter recordings or some other form of inpatient or outpatient telemetry, will incorporate such plots, thereby markedly adding to the utility of HRV-type analysis for both research and clinical practice.

REFERENCES

1. Acharya UR, Joseph KP, Kannathal N, et al. Heart rate variability: a review. *Med Bio Eng Comput.* 2006;44:1031-1051.
2. Thayer JF, Yamamoto SS, Brosschot JF. The relationship of autonomic imbalance, heart rate variability and cardiovascular disease risk factors. *Int J Cardiol.* 2010;141:122-131.
3. Kleiger RE, Stein PK, Bigger JT Jr. Heart rate variability: measurement and clinical utility. *Ann Noninvasive Electocardiol.* 2005;10:88-101.
4. Taylor JA, Carr DL, Myers CW, et al. Mechanisms underlying very-low-frequency RR interval oscillations in humans. *Circulation.* 1998;98:547-555.
5. Stein PK, Domitrovich PP, Hui N, et al. Sometimes higher heart rate variability is not better heart rate variability: results of graphical and non linear analyses. *J Cardiovasc Electrophysiol.* 2005;16:954-959.
6. Grossman P, Taylor EW. Toward understanding respiratory sinus arrhythmia: relations to cardiac vagal tone, evolution and biobehavioral functions. *Biol Psychol.* 2007;74:263-285.
7. Wiklund U, Hörnsten R, Karlsson M, et al. Abnormal heart rate variability and subtle atrial arrhythmia in patients with familial amyloidotic polyneuropathy. *Ann Noninvasive Electrocardiol.* 2008;13:249-256.
8. Somers VK, White DP, Amin R, et al. Sleep apnea and cardiovascular disease: an American Heart Association/American College of Cardiology Foundation Scientific Statement from the American Heart Association Council for High Blood Pressure Research Professional Education Committee, Council on Clinical Cardiology, Stroke Council, and Council on Cardiovascular Nursing. *J Am Coll Cardiol.* 2008;19:686-717.
9. Friedman O, Logan AG. The price of obstructive sleep apnea-hypopnea: hypertension and other ill effects. *Am J Hypertens.* 2009;22:474-483.
10. Pack AI, Gislason T. Obstructive sleep apnea and cardiovascular disease: a perspective and future directions. *Prog Cardiovasc Dis.* 2009;51:434-452.
11. Stein PK, Le QC, Domitrovich PP; Cast Investigators. Development of more erratic heart rate patterns is associated with mortality post-myocardial infarction. *J Electrocardiol.* 2008;41:110-115.
12. Woo MA, Stevenson WG, Moser DK, et al. Patterns of beat-to-beat heart rate variability in advanced heart failure. *Am Heart J.* 1992;123:704-710.
13. Brouwer J, van Veldhuisen DJ, Man in 't Veld AJ, et al; the Dutch Ibopamine Multicenter Trial Study Group. Prognostic value of heart rate variability during long-term follow-up in patients with mild to moderate heart failure. *J Am Coll Cardiol.* 1996;28:1183-1189.
14. Bonaduce D, Petretta M, Marciano M, et al. Independent and incremental prognostic value of heart rate variability in patients with chronic heart failure. *Am Heart J.* 1999;138:273-284.
15. Mäkikallio TH, Seppänen T, Airaksinen KEJ, et al. Dynamic analysis of heart rate may predict subsequent ventricular tachycardia after myocardial infarction. *Am J Cardiol.* 1997;80:779-783.
16. Laitio TT, Mäkikallio T, Huikuri H, et al. Relation of heart rate dynamics to the occurrence of myocardial ischemia after coronary artery bypass grafting. *Am J Cardiol.* 2002;89:1176-1181.
17. Stein PK, Duntley SP, Domitrovich PP, et al. A simple method for detecting sleep-disordered breathing using Holter monitoring. *J Cardiovasc Electrophysiol.* 2003;14:467-473.
18. Stein PK, Reddy A. Non-linear heart rate variability and risk stratification in cardiovascular disease. *Indian Pacing Electrophysiol J.* 2005;1:210-220.
19. Stein PK, Sanghavi D, Sotoodehnia N, et al. Association of Holter-based measures including T-wave alternans with risk of sudden cardiac death in the community-dwelling elderly: the Cardiovascular Health Study. *J Electrocardiol.* 2010;43:251-259.

20. Huikuri HV, Perkiömäki JS, Maestri R, et al. Clinical impact of evaluation of cardiovascular control by novel methods of heart rate dynamics. *Philos Transact A Math Phys Eng Sci.* 2009;13:1223-1238.

21. Bilge AR, Stein PK, Domitrovich PP, et al. Assessment of ultra low frequency band power of heart rate variability: validation of alternative methods. *Int J Cardiol.* 1999;71:1-6.

22. Frey B, Heinz G, Binder T, et al. Diurnal variation of ventricular response to atrial fibrillation in patients with advanced heart failure. *Am Heart J.* 1995;129:58-65.

23. Yoshida N, Nozawa T, Igawa A, et al. Modulation of ventricular repolarization and R-R interval is altered in patients with globally impaired cardiac 123I-MIBG uptake. *Ann Noninvasive Electrocardiol.* 2001;6:55-63.

24. Koutelou M, Katsikis A, Flevari P, et al. Predictive value of cardiac autonomic indexes and MIBG washout in ICD recipients with mild to moderate heart failure. *Ann Nucl Med.* 2009;23:677-684.

25. Freeman MR, Newman D, Dorian P, Barr A, Langer A. Relation of direct assessment of cardiac autonomic function with metaiodobenzylguanidine imaging to heart rate variability in diabetes mellitus. *Am J Cardiol.* 1991;80:247-250.

26. Nagaoka H, Kubota S, Iizuka T, Imai S, Nagai R. Relation between depressed cardiac response to exercise and autonomic nervous activity in mildly symptomatic patients with idiopathic dilated cardiomyopathy. *Chest.* 1996;109:925-932.

CHAPTER 17

DEVELOPMENT OF THE HEART, WITH PARTICULAR REFERENCE TO THE CARDIAC CONDUCTION TISSUES

Robert H. Anderson, Aleksander Sizarov, and Antoon F. M. Moorman

INTRODUCTION / 299

THE BASIC CARDIAC BUILDING PLAN / 299

MORPHOLOGIC RECOGNITION OF THE POSTNATAL
    CONDUCTION TISSUES / 300

FORMATION OF THE DEFINITIVE ATRIAL CHAMBERS / 302

DEVELOPMENT OF THE CONDUCTION TISSUES / 305
    The Sinus Node / 306
    The Atrioventricular Node / 306
    The Nature of the Interatrial Myocardium / 308
    The Atrioventricular Conduction Axis / 308
    The Ventricular Conducting Tissues / 308
    The Atrioventricular Ring Tissues / 309
    The Atrioventricular Insulating Planes / 310
    The Pulmonary Venous Myocardial Sleeves / 310
    The Myocardium of the Outflow Tracts / 310

CONCLUSION / 310

INTRODUCTION

It is, perhaps, unfortunate that the myocytes that generate and dissipate the cardiac impulse throughout the myocardial body are known as the cardiac conduction tissues, because all myocytes within the heart possess the capacity to conduct. The alternative title, the "specialized tissues," is equally unfortunate, because from a developmental stance, as we will show, the so-called *conducting tissues*, in particular the nodal components, share important features with the myocytes of the primary heart tube. It is their so-called "working" partners that show more evidence of developmental specialization. In this chapter, therefore, we will describe the processes whereby the initial heart tube grows by addition of myocardium at both its venous and arterial pole, how it loops, and how eventually it becomes converted into the four-chambered organ. In this definitive structure, it is the sinus node that generates the cardiac impulse, this being propagated within the atrial musculature, delayed in the atrioventricular node, and

then conducted rapidly to the ventricular myocardium through the atrioventricular bundle, its branches, and the ventricular ramifications known as Purkinje fibers. We will also discuss the fate of the more widespread areas of primary myocardium found in the developing heart because it is almost certainly the remnants of these areas in the postnatal heart that are the substrates for many cardiac arrhythmias. In contrast, with regard to perhaps the most important arrhythmia in the ageing population, namely atrial fibrillation, we will show how the pulmonary myocardial sleeves, known now to be the substrate for many forms of atrial fibrillation, are derived from so-called working rather than specialized conducting tissues.

THE BASIC CARDIAC BUILDING PLAN

The overall structure of the developing heart and the basic arrangement of the definitive heart are preserved across the vertebrates, from fish to man. When first seen during development, the heart is laid down as a linear myocardial tube, with venous and arterial poles (Fig. 17–1A). Conduction through this linear tube begins at the venous pole and proceeds toward the arterial pole. With ongoing development, cavities balloon from the tube, to which additional material is rapidly added at both poles. In the most basic plan, the myocardium that will form the atrial chambers balloons from the primary tube into the dorsal direction, whereas the myocardium of the developing ventricles balloons in ventral fashion (Fig. 17–1B). Concomitant with the ballooning of these pouches from the linear, or primary, tube, it becomes possible to record an electrocardiogram.[1] At these early stages, it is not possible to recognize any "conduction tissues" when assessing the cardiac structure histologically. It is possible, however, to distinguish the characteristics of the myocytes in the different parts of the developing heart according to their molecular signatures. Thus, the myocytes of the primary heart tube do not express the connexin proteins responsible for the formation of fast-conducting gap junctions.[2] As a consequence, at this early stage, the blood is propelled through the developing heart in a sluggish, peristaltic fashion. In contrast, the myocytes forming the walls of the developing atrial and ventricular chambers express the molecules that ensure rapid conduction and synchronous contraction, such as the gap-junctional proteins connexin 40 and 43.[3] This myocardium making up the walls of the developing chambers is called *working*, or *secondary, myocardium*. It is possible to distinguish subtypes within the working myocardium.[4] The myocytes making up the atrial working myocardium conduct faster and express the rapidly contracting atrial myosin isoform, whereas the myocytes within the developing ventricles express the slow myosin isoform,[5] which is also expressed in slow-twitch skeletal muscle. Whereas myocytes within both the atrial and ventricular working myocardial walls express atrial natriuretic factor, the atrial myocytes that are added via the so-called *dorsal mesocardium*, the area that will eventually form the myocardial sleeves of the pulmonary veins, do not express this gene (Fig. 17–2).

We now know that, in the mammalian heart, the initial component of the linear heart tube forms little more than the embryonic

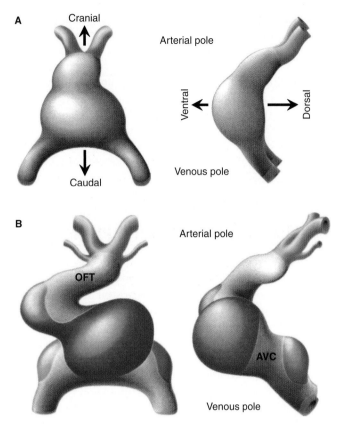

FIGURE 17–1. Morphogenesis of the early heart tube in mammals. **A.** The prototypic linear heart tube as seen in ventral (left) and right lateral (right) views. **B.** The prototypic looping and chamber-forming heart tube in similar views. The primary myocardium is gray, the myocardium of the atrial chambers ballooning dorsally in parallel at the venous pole is blue, and the myocardium of the ventricular chambers growing ventrally in sequence along the heart tube is red. At the linear tube stage in human, there is no secondary myocardium present. The chamber myocardium is first seen locally at the stage of looping and does not involve the entire circumference of the tube. Note that the primary myocardium of the venous pole, the atrioventricular canal (AVC), and the outflow tract (OFT) is continuous, with no formation of rings.

atrioventricular canal.[6] Additional material remains to be added to the developing heart at both the venous and arterial poles from the so-called *second heart field*, although it is debated whether this is derived from a separate field or rather from ongoing temporal migrations of cells from a single source.[7,8] Regardless, the end result is that the heart tube elongates and bends concomitant with the addition of the new material at its venous and arterial poles.[9] As it bends, the cavities of the atrial and ventricular chambers balloon from the linear tube,[10] with the atrial appendages in the mammalian heart ballooning in parallel from the atrial component of the primary tube, but with the apical components of the ventricles ballooning in series from the ventricular part of the developing heart (Fig. 17–3A). The molecular signatures of the developing myocardial components are well seen in the mouse heart on the 12th day of development, albeit the apical trabecular component of the right ventricle is only just beginning to balloon at this stage (Fig. 17–3B,C). The evidence in the mouse heart, now known to be replicated during development of the human heart, shows that the areas of primary myocardium are extensive. It is from these areas that, with time, there will be formation of the components of the so-called *conduction system* as recognized in the definitive heart.[11]

MORPHOLOGIC RECOGNITION OF THE POSTNATAL CONDUCTION TISSUES

As we will discuss, our studies on the developing heart, as yet unpublished, showed the location of the remnants of the initial primary myocardium, now providing insights into the location of arrhythmic substrates in the postnatal heart. The parts of the primary myocardium, including those of the sinus venosus persisting as the components of the so-called *cardiac conduction tissues* in the definitive postnatal heart, can be recognized morphologically based on the criteria established by Aschoff[12] and Mönckeberg[13] at the beginning of the twentieth century.[12,13] The conduction tissues, according to these criteria, should be histologically distinguishable from surrounding myocardium, should be traceable from one section of the specimen to another, and, if forming tracts, should be insulated from the other myocardium by connective tissue. Thus, all different components of the cardiac conduction tissues in the definitive

left ventricle and atrioventricular canal. Recent evidence from the mouse heart shows that, from the stance of lineage, the ventricular septum is derived from this embryonic left ventricle, whereas the entire mural component of the left ventricle is derived from the

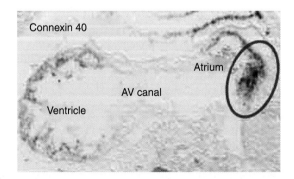
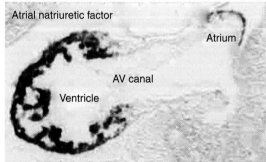

FIGURE 17–2. The domains of the atrial musculature are distinguished based on their expression of the different molecular markers. In the left panel, we show of the pattern of expression of mRNA for the gap-junctional protein connexin 40, whereas the right panel shows the pattern of expression of mRNA for atrial natriuretic factor (ANF). Both sections are taken sagittally through the mouse embryonic heart at embryonic day 9½. At the dorsal aspect of the atrium, there is a special part of the muscle, which is positive only for connexin 40 (red circle in left panel). We called this part the mediastinal myocardium. Note the absence of both connexin 40 and ANF in the musculature bordering the atrioventricular (AV) canal.

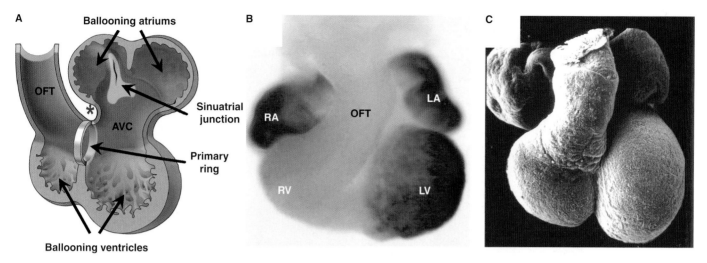

FIGURE 17-3. The basic plan of the chamber-forming heart in the mammalian embryo. **A.** We show schematically the arrangement of the locally differentiating atrial and ventricular chambers (shown in blue) and the primary myocardium (shown in gray). In this scheme, the outflow tract (OFT) is tilted away to show the relationships of the atrial pouches, the primary interventricular ring, and the atrioventricular canal (AVC). Note the continuity of the primary myocardium of the sinuatrial junction, the atrioventricular canal, and outflow tract at the inner curvature (asterisk). **B.** We show the mouse embryonic heart at embryonic day 11½, stained as a whole mount following in situ hybridization for the atrial natriuretic factor (ANF). This marks the differentiating chamber myocardium of the right atrial (RA) and left atrial (LA) appendages and the right ventricle (RV) and left ventricle (LV). At the stage shown, the expression of ANF in the right ventricle is seen only dorsally. **C.** We show a scanning electron micrograph of the human embryonic heart at a comparable stage of development. Note the essential similarity in the arrangement of the ballooning chambers and the location of the atrial appendages to either side of the outflow tract.

postnatal heart (Fig. 17–4) can be recognized morphologically using histologic stainings and the fulfillment of the criteria, established by Mönckeberg[13] and Aschoff.[12] The exemplar of such a conduction tract, as shown by Tawara,[14] is the atrioventricular conduction axis (Fig. 17–5A). The sinus and atrioventricular nodes, in contrast, are not insulated from the atrial musculature, thus fulfilling only two of the three criteria (Fig. 17–5B,C). The morphologic features that permit recognition of the regular cardiac nodes also permit additional areas of atrial myocardium to be recognized as being histologically specialized. However, use of these same criteria shows that the pulmonary venous myocardial sleeves and the internodal atrial myocardium, at least in terms of gross histology, are made up of working myocytes.[15]

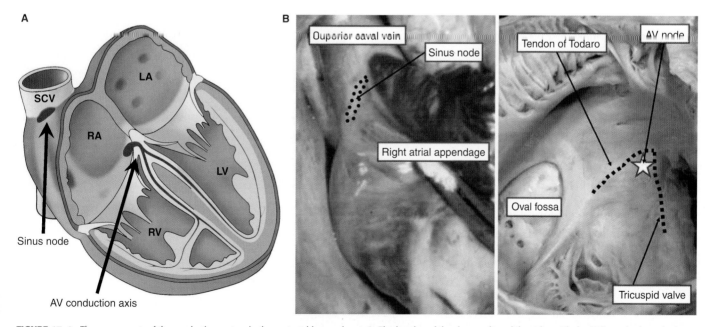

FIGURE 17-4. The components of the conduction system in the postnatal human heart. **A.** The location of the sinus node and the atrioventricular (AV) conduction axis shown in a schematic fashion. **B.** The gross anatomy of the human heart as related to the cardiac nodes. The sinus node is located at the right side of the junction between the superior caval vein (SCV) and the right atrial appendage. The AV node (star in right side of pane B) is located normally at the apex of the triangle of Koch (dotted line). LA, left atrium; LV, left ventricle; RA, right atrium; RV, right ventricle; SCV, superior caval vein.

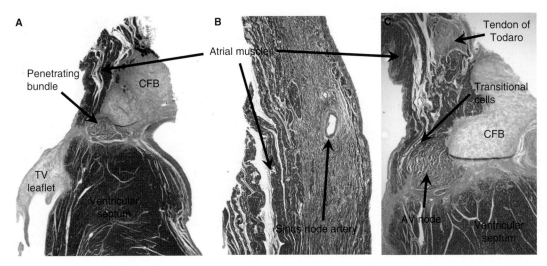

FIGURE 17–5. Histologic characteristics of the conduction system in the postnatal human heart. Serial sections through the atrioventricular (AV) conduction axis (**A** and **C**) and the sinus node (**B**) were stained with the Masson's trichrome, which colors muscle tissues in red and collagen in blue. The penetrating bundle (A), sinus node (B), and AV node (C) are all made up of histologically distinct cells, which can be traced through serial sections. The penetrating bundle is also isolated by the connective tissue from the adjacent working myocardium, which is not the case for the nodes. Note the presence of extensive zones of transitional cells between the working atrial myocardium and the compact part of the AV node in panel C. CFB, central fibrous body. TV, tricuspid valve.

FORMATION OF THE DEFINITIVE ATRIAL CHAMBERS

The sinus and atrioventricular nodes and the pulmonary myocardial sleeves are all components of the definitive atrial chambers.[16] Knowledge of the development of these components, therefore, requires an appreciation of the morphologic stages involved in formation and separation of the morphologically right and left atrial chambers. It requires, in particular, an understanding of the formation of the atrial septum. Therefore, prior to considering the steps involved in formation of the cardiac nodes themselves, we will review our own understanding of the developmental heritage of the left and right atrial chamber myocardium.

The entire linear heart tube, including the venous pole and the part from which the atrial appendages will balloon, is made up of primary myocardium. The appendages, with walls made of chamber myocardium, balloon in parallel fashion from the primary myocardium. Subsequent to looping of the heart tube, they are positioned rightward and leftward relative to the developing outlet component of the heart (see Fig. 17–3B,C). At the stage at which the systemic venous tributaries enter the atrial component of the tube, which they do in relatively symmetrical fashion, there has been no formation of the lungs. However, it is important to appreciate that the atrial component of the tube remains connected dorsally to the mediastinal mesenchyme through the so-called *dorsal mesocardium*, where the pulmonary vein will develop (Fig. 17–6). With ongoing development, there is a shift in the relationship of the systemic venous tributaries so that, eventually, they open to the right side of the developing atrial component. In the mouse heart, anatomic boundaries of a discrete intrapericardial systemic venous sinus possessing myocardial walls do not become recognizable until after the tributaries have come to open to the prospective right atrium.[4]

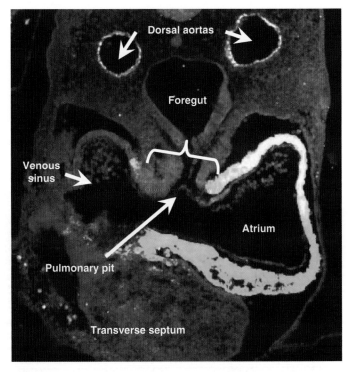

FIGURE 17–6. This transverse section is from a young human embryonic heart at Carnegie stage 12 and shows ballooning of the atrial and ventricular chambers. The atrial component of the heart tube is connected to the mediastinal mesenchyme at the ventral surface of the foregut by the so-called dorsal mesocardium (bracket). The section was stained immunofluorescently for myocardial marker SERCA-2a protein, which is revealed by the light green color.

In the human heart, in contrast, the venous sinus is recognizable morphologically, as a compartment within the pericardial cavity, albeit its walls initially are not myocardial. In both mouse and man, nonetheless, the left-sided venous tributary, which will

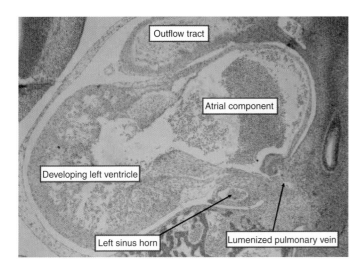

FIGURE 17–7. This sagittal section is through a human embryonic heart at Carnegie stage 14, when atrial and ventricular septation is beginning. Note the solitary opening of the newly lumenized pulmonary vein to the atrial component of the heart. The opening is adjacent to the developing left atrioventricular junction, which contains the left sinus horn. Note that the horn, which will become the coronary sinus, possesses its own muscular wall and has no connection with the pulmonary vein. Stained using hematoxylin and eosin.

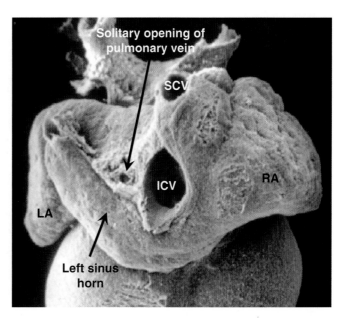

FIGURE 17–8. This scanning electron micrograph showing the dorsal aspect of a human heart is from an embryo at the same stage as the section shown in Fig. 17–7. It shows the opening of the pulmonary vein through the persisting dorsal mesocardial connection (dorsal mesenchyme) above the left sinus horn (future coronary sinus) and left of the joining of the superior caval vein (SCV) and inferior caval vein (ICV). LA, left atrium; RA, right atrium.

become the coronary sinus in man, retains its own myocardial walls, passing inferior to the dorsal mesocardial connection as it extends to open in the right atrium (Fig. 17–7). Concomitant with this rightward shift of the atrial connections of the systemic venous tributaries, the dorsal mesocardium itself also undergoes significant remodeling.

When first seen, the internal atrial location of the mesocardial connection is marked by the so-called *pulmonary ridges*, which flank an imperforate pit in the dorsal wall of the undivided atrium.[17] With further development, it is possible to trace from this pit an endocardial strand through the mediastinal mesenchyme to the ventral surface of the foregut, where lung buds will eventually develop. With ongoing development, this strand lumenizes to form the pulmonary vein (see Fig. 17–7), which enters the atrium through the dorsal mesocardial connection (Fig. 17–8). At later stages of development, the walls of the newly formed pulmonary vein become myocardial, and neither in mouse nor man do they have any direct connection with the myocardial walls clothing the tributaries of the systemic venous sinus.[4,17]

Concomitant with the rightward shift of the tributaries of the systemic venous sinus, septation of the atrial component of the developing heart commences. This is achieved initially by growth toward the atrioventricular canal of a crescentic muscular shelf, the primary atrial septum, or "septum primum." As it grows toward the atrioventricular canal, which undergoes division by formation of two atrioventricular endocardial cushions, there is a space between the leading edge of the developing septum, which carries a mesenchymal cap, and the atrial surfaces of the cushions. This space is the primary atrial foramen, or "foramen primum" (Fig. 17–9). The foramen is closed by union of the mesenchymal cap on the leading edge of the primary septum and the extracardiac dorsal mesenchyme, or

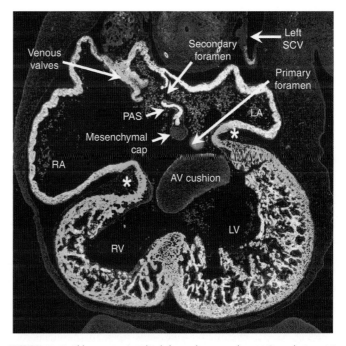

FIGURE 17–9. This transverse section is from a human embryo at Carnegie stage 16, when atrial septation is being completed. The section was stained immunofluorescently for myocardial marker troponin I, which is shown by the light green color. The primary atrial septum (PAS) is well seen, with the mesenchymal cap on its leading edge, just prior to closure of the primary atrial foramen. The secondary foramen has already appeared at the atrial roof. Note the location of the venous valves, which mark the boundaries of the systemic venous sinus, now exclusively committed to the developing right atrium (RA). There is a muscular continuity between atriums and ventricles via the atrioventricular (AV) canal musculature (asterisks). The AV cushions have already separated the lumen of the AV canal into separate streams. LA, left atrium; LV, left ventricle; RV, right ventricle; SCV, superior caval vein.

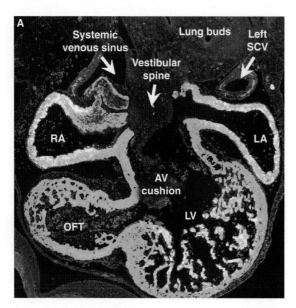
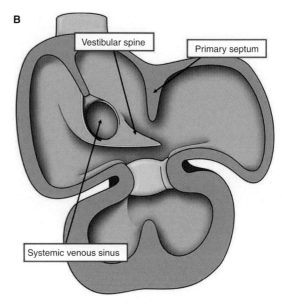

FIGURE 17–10. The transverse section shown in panel **A** is from a slightly younger human embryo compared with the one shown in Fig. 17–9, namely at Carnegie stage 15. It was also stained for troponin I, which is depicted by the light green color. The section shows how additional tissue, contiguous with the mesenchyme around the lung buds, is protruding into the atrial lumen. This tissue is the vestibular spine, or dorsal mesenchymal protrusion. Its location is shown schematically in panel **B**, which is a cartoon based on the original illustration made by Wilhelm His the Elder.[19] AV, atrioventricular; LA, left atrium; LV, left ventricle; OFT, outflow tract; RA, right atrium; SCV, superior caval vein.

vestibular spine, with the endocardial cushions.[18] By the time of fusion, the upper edge of the septum has already broken down to form the secondary atrial foramen, or "foramen secundum" (see Fig. 17–9). As the primary septum fuses with the cushions to close the primary foramen, it completes the confinement of the pulmonary venous return to the left atrium. During this period, the right pulmonary ridge becomes very pronounced and now is recognizable as the vestibular spine, or "spina vestibuli,"[19] also known as the dorsal mesenchymal protrusion[20] (Fig. 17–10). The area occupied initially by the spine and the mesenchymal cap most probably becomes the extensive muscular anteroinferior rim of the oval foramen. This process of formation of the anteroinferior rim of the oval fossa, as we will see, is particularly important in forming the atrial septal connections of the atrioventricular node, albeit the mechanisms of formation have yet to be established.

During and after division of the atrial chambers and formation of the definitive anteroinferior border of the oval foramen, marked changes have also occurred in the location of the pulmonary veins. The initially solitary venous opening is first seen adjacent to the developing left atrioventricular junction (see Fig. 17–7). Eventually, four veins open to the atrial roof (Fig. 17–11).[21] Only after the venous openings have become translocated to the atrial roof does it become possible to recognize the infolded superior atrial fold that eventually separates the opening of the superior caval vein to the right atrium from the right-sided pulmonary venoatrial junctions. This area, although usually known as the "septum secundum," is no more than a fold in the superior atrial roof, a feature made more obvious in the postnatal heart by the fat that accumulates within the groove.[22]

Concomitant with the rightward shift of the systemic venous tributaries and their incorporation into the right atrium, its

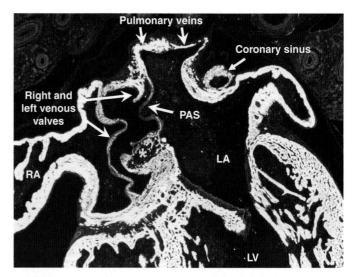

FIGURE 17–11. The transverse section through the heart of the human embryo at the end of the embryonic period, specifically at Carnegie stage 23, has been stained for troponin I, depicted by light green, and shows two of the four pulmonary veins opening to the roof of the left atrium (LA). Note the mesenchymal tissue between the primary atrial septum (PAS) and the musculature of the atrioventricular junction, with small islands of cardiomyocytes (asterisk) showing impending muscularization of the future inferoanterior rim of the oval foramen. Note also that, although the right venous valve remains prominent at this stage, the left valve has almost disappeared. LV, left ventricle; RA, right atrium.

floor, composed of primary myocardium, becomes an integral part of the morphologically right atrium. The boundary between the floor of the venous sinus and the appendage becomes particularly prominent and is recognizable in the formed heart as the terminal crest.[16] During fetal life, the entirety of the boundary between the systemic venous sinus and the remainder of the right atrium is marked by extensive muscular folds known as the venous valves. These structures usually regress to greater or lesser extent in the postnatal heart, with parts of the right valve persisting as the Eustachian and Thebesian valves, guarding the orifices of the inferior caval vein and coronary sinus, respectively. The left venous valve usually disappears in its entirety in the human heart. By the time of birth, the musculature forming the floor of the systemic venous sinus has become indistinguishable in terms of gross histology from the remaining atrial musculature, but its initial location within the sinus is indicative of its primary myocardial heritage. Further myocardium of primary origin, but converted into working myocardium at birth, is also found within the vestibules of both atria just above the atrioventricular valves. This is the atrioventricular canal musculature, which is sequestrated within the atrial component concomitant with formation of the fibroadipose plane of atrioventricular insulation.[23] Apart from this vestibular myocardium, the remainder of the left atrial musculature is derived either from chamber or dorsal mediastinal myocardium and has never possessed a primary myocardial phenotype.[4,24] As we will discuss, these differences in developmental heritage are crucial in determining the potential anatomic substrates for atrial arrhythmias.

DEVELOPMENT OF THE CONDUCTION TISSUES

As we have emphasized already, it is possible to record an electrocardiogram from the developing embryo long before the final appearance of all components of the conduction system can be recognized histologically in the postnatal heart.[1] This is because, again as already emphasized, all myocardial cells within the heart have the ability to conduct the cardiac impulse, albeit to a different extent.[25] The ability to record an adult type of electrocardiogram from the embryonic heart without a definitive conduction system coincides with the initiation of the local ballooning and differentiation of the fast-conducting chambers from the slow-conducting primary heart tube.[26] The rapid conduction between the myocytes making up the secondary myocardium of the chambers is due to their linkage by large and fast-conducting gap junctional complexes,[27] which are absent from the slowly conducting primary myocardium.[28] Subsequent to the ballooning of the atrial appendages and the growth of the ventricles, the remaining primary myocardium becomes recognizable as the outflow tract, atrioventricular canal, and the corridor of myocardium, which extends from the atrioventricular canal to incorporate the orifices of the systemic venous tributaries. Our knowledge of the subsequent changes to this primary myocardium, which for the most part becomes converted in terms of its histologic appearance to so-called *working myocardium*, has accrued from experiments carried out largely in the mouse. Thus, in the developing mouse heart, the primary myocardium that will not develop into chamber myocardium is distinguished by the expression of the gene encoding Tbx3, a T-box transcription factor, which represses the chamber program of gene expression (Fig. 17–12).[29] By tracing the location of this transcription factor and related factors such as Tbx18[24,30] in the myocardial walls of the systemic venous sinus, it has been possible, in the mouse heart, to chart with accuracy the location of those areas of primary myocardium that persist as the definitive postnatal conduction tissues. Recent expressional analyses in the developing human heart from our own laboratory, as yet unpublished, largely confirm the findings in the mouse, taking account of the morphologic differences in the arrangement of the postnatal conduction tissues between the two species.

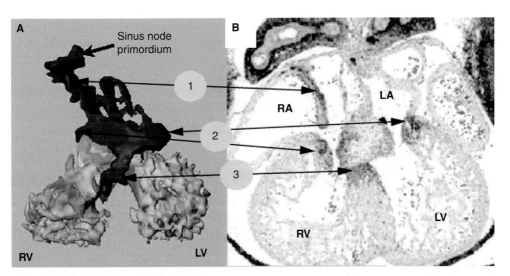

FIGURE 17–12. The section in panel **B** shows the pattern of expression of the Tbx3 gene in the embryonic mouse heart at day 12½ of development, whereas panel **A** shows the three-dimensional (3D) reconstruction of the domain of expression of the gene (shown in red). Note how the Tbx3-positive cells, shown by the dark blue color in panel B, mark the developing conduction system, as can be appreciated from the 3D reconstruction. Already at this relatively early stage of development, it is possible to appreciate the position of the future atrioventricular (AV) bundle on the crest of the ventricular septum (3), the atrioventricular AV ring tissues (2), the internodal myocardium along the right venous valve (1), and the future sinus node.[29] LA, left atrium; LV, left ventricle; RA, right atrium; RV, right ventricle.

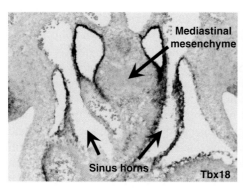
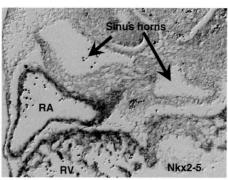
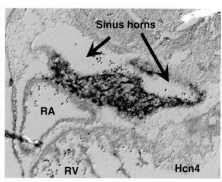

FIGURE 17–13. The gene expression profile of the inflow region in the mouse embryonic heart at day 10½ of development, as assessed by in situ hybridization of mRNA for transcription factors Tbx18 (left), Nkx2-5 (middle), and pacemaker channel Hcn4 (right). Note that in the heart, Tbx18 and Hcn4 are expressed only in the cells making up the walls of the sinus horns, whereas Nkx2-5 specifically is not expressed in these structures. RA, right atrium; RV, right ventricle.

THE SINUS NODE

From the outset of the formation of the cardiac tube, pacemaker activity always originates at the intake of the heart.[31] Recent molecular experiments have revealed the molecular mechanism whereby this is achieved.[30,32] With ongoing development, the systemic venous sinus and its tributaries, or left and right common cardinal veins, become incorporated into the pericardial cavity and acquire myocardial sleeves. The myocardium of the systemic venous tributaries is characterized by the expression of the T-box transcription factor Tbx18, by the expression of the important pacemaker channel Hcn4, and by the absence of expression of the cardiac transcription factor Nkx2-5 (Fig. 17–13).[24,32] Under direction of the transcription factor Pitx2c, the pacemaker phenotype becomes restricted to the right sinuatrial junction and is recognizable as the sinus node (Fig. 17–14).[32] The remaining areas become working myocardium when assessed both histologically and molecularly. Within 6 weeks of development in the human embryo, the primordium of the sinus node can be recognized in sections processed in standard histologic fashion, which coincides with positivity for the pacemaker channel Hcn4 (Fig. 17–15). If the findings in the mouse are, indeed, paralleled in the human heart, then the location of the primary myocardium around the mouth of the coronary sinus and along the terminal crest offers some explanation for the origins of abnormal electrical activity in patients with atrial arrhythmias.

THE ATRIOVENTRICULAR NODE

As with the sinus node, most of our knowledge concerning the genetic regulation of the development of the atrioventricular node has emerged over the past decade subsequent to multiple investigations of the mouse heart. There are known important differences in the function of the atrioventricular node between mouse and man, most probably related to the size of the heart.[33] There are also significant differences in the architectural arrangement of the myocytes making up the compact node and its transitional zones in human[34] as compared with the mouse.[35,36] There are also differences in the relationship of the atrioventricular muscular sandwich relative to the aortic root. Because of the marked off setting of the leaflets of the mitral and tricuspid valves in man, the compact node is a half-oval set against the central fibrous body, with transitional cells forming a marked overlay not seen in the mouse. The penetrating atrioventricular bundle is also appreciably shorter in man compared with mouse. It is important, therefore, to remember interspecies diversity when considering the developmental aspects.

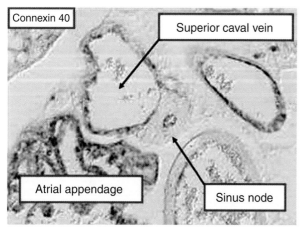
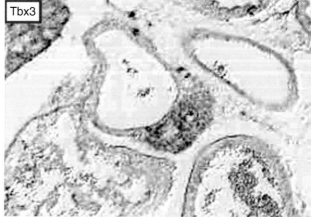

FIGURE 17–14. Molecular characterization of the sinus node at the late fetal stage in the mouse, as assessed by in situ hybridization of mRNA for connexin 40 (left) and Tbx3 (right). The cells of the sinus node are specifically positive for Tbx3, which is not expressed in the atrial musculature, and lacking connexin 40. Connexin 40 is expressed in the myocardium of atrial chambers, the sleeve of the superior caval vein, and the endothelium of the sinus node artery.

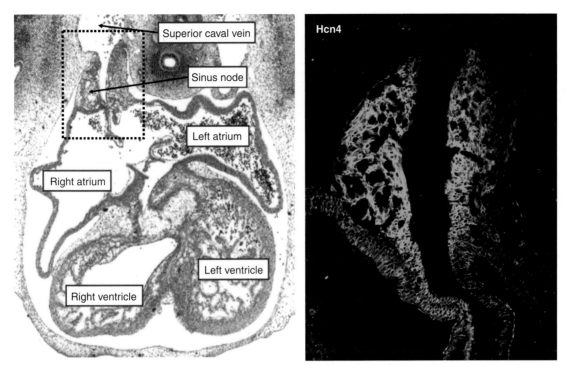

FIGURE 17–15. Morphologic and molecular recognition of the sinus node primordium in the human embryonic heart at Carnegie stage 16. Appreciate the characteristic appearance of the sinus node as a thickened manchette at the junction of the superior caval vein with the right atrium (left panel, hematoxylin and eosin). The right panel shows the enlargement of the region boxed in the left panel from another human embryo of the same developmental stage showing strong expression of the pacemaker channel Hcn4 in the cells making up the sinus node primordium.

In the mouse, recent lineage studies have shown that the compact part of the node is derived from the atrioventricular canal musculature, with its primary phenotype.[6] This part of the atrioventricular node, therefore, as with the sinus node, is distinguished by its content of Tbx3.[29] During further development, it acquires a highly specific transcriptional profile that is distinct from both the working myocardium and the original primary myocardium.[37] The atrioventricular canal musculature can also be recognized histologically in the human heart at 6 weeks of development (Fig. 17–16). Initially, after the primary foramen

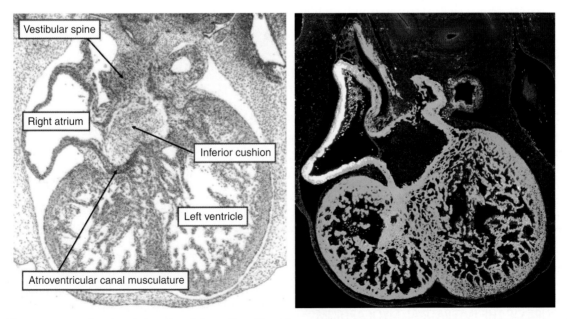

FIGURE 17–16. These transverse sections through the embryonic heart of two different human embryos at Carnegie stage 16 are taken through the dorsal aspect of the atrioventricular canal. The left panel (stained with hematoxylin and eosin) illustrates how the histologic characteristics of the more densely situated cells of the atrioventricular canal musculature make it possible to distinguish them as a part of the developing atrioventricular node. The right panel (immunofluorescence staining for troponin I) serves as a reference for discerning the myocardial tissues from mesenchymal tissues.

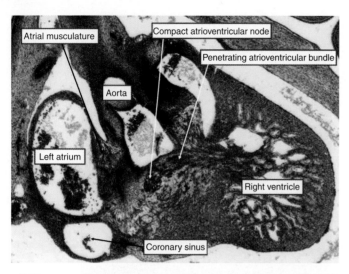

FIGURE 17–17. This sagittal section, from a human embryo at Carnegie stage 18, is prepared in a plane comparable with the subcostal oblique echocardiographic plane. It shows how the developing central fibrous body initially interposes between the atrioventricular conduction axis and the atrial musculature. Note the histologic characteristics of more densely packed cells of the atrioventricular node and penetrating bundle, which are surrounded by more loose tissue, as discernable already at this embryonic stage of human development.

has been closed, the mesenchymal tissues that eventually form the central fibrous body interpose between the atrioventricular canal musculature, which will form the compact part of the atrioventricular node and its inferior extensions, and the musculature of the atrial septum (Fig. 17–17). The connection of the definitive node, via transitional cells, with the musculature of the atrial septum requires subsequent muscularization of the tissues contributed via the vestibular spine and the mesenchymal cap. As discussed earlier, an extensive array of transitional cells interpose between the working atrial myocytes and the cells of the compact atrioventricular node in man.[34] It remains to be established with certainty whether it is these transitional cells or the nodal inferior extensions that form the clinically important slow and fast pathways for atrioventricular nodal conduction. In terms of development, nonetheless, the slow pathway represents the continuation of the atrioventricular canal musculature into the vestibule of the tricuspid valve. The larger part of this ring, in histologic terms, becomes transformed into working myocardium, but its origin as primary myocardium probably accounts for its role as the slow nodal pathway.[38] The fast pathway, in contrast, extends from the anterosuperior rim of the atrial septum to make contact with the atrioventricular nodal myocytes. This connection cannot be formed developmentally until after the muscularization of the vestibular spine and the mesenchymal cap. The precise origin of this pathway remains to be established.

■ THE NATURE OF THE INTERATRIAL MYOCARDIUM

The criteria for histologic recognition of conducting tracts were established to defuse a suggestion that "specialized" pathways exist to preferentially conduct the sinus impulse through the atrial myocardium into the atrioventricular node. These sensible criteria were ignored by investigators who subsequently suggested that such "specialized" tracts did exist within the atrial musculature. In terms of gross histology, there are no insulated tracts extending between the cardiac nodes.[39] The preferential conduction that does exist within the muscular pathways is the consequence of the packing of the individual atrial myocytes.[40] In developmental terms, there is a corridor of primary myocardium extending from the sites of formation of the sinus and atrioventricular nodes.[4] In the formed heart, the terminal crest is the boundary between the floor of the atrial component of the primary heart tube and the right atrial appendage. Remnants of this primary myocardium could serve as substrates for abnormal automaticity in the right atrium. In terms of gross histology in the postnatal heart, however, these areas are indistinguishable from the remainder of the working atrial myocardium.[39]

■ THE ATRIOVENTRICULAR CONDUCTION AXIS

It was the monumental monograph of Sunao Tawara,[14] now also available in an excellent English translation,[41] that clarified the arrangement of the atrioventricular conduction axis. He showed that the atrioventricular node was but the commencement of a tract of histologically distinct myocytes that could be traced eventually into the ventricular Purkinje cells. The proximal ventricular part of this axis is directly continuous with the compact atrioventricular node, which, in turn, is part of a larger developmental entity, recognized in the human heart by the expression of the GlN2 antigen[42] and that can be traced round the vestibule of the tricuspid valve and the aortic root, eventually returning to the atrioventricular axis itself as a "dead-end tract." The entirety of the axis is initially part of a ring of primary myocardium that surrounds the embryonic interventricular foramen (Fig. 17–18). In the mouse heart, when taking the border between node and penetrating bundle as the site at which the axis becomes insulated by the fibrous tissue of the central fibrous body,[14] a tongue of the ventricular component can be traced as the inferior part of the compact atrioventricular node. Such a dual origin of the proximal atrioventricular conduction axis is also supported circumstantially in human hearts by evidence from the arrangements seen in patients with rare forms of congenitally complete atrioventricular dissociation.[43] Whether the arrangement seen in the mouse also exists in the developing human heart remains to be established.

■ THE VENTRICULAR CONDUCTING TISSUES

In the normal situation, it is the atrioventricular conduction axis that provides the only muscular continuity between the atrial and ventricular muscles masses. There have also been discussions as to whether the myocardial cells making up this axis, including the so-called *Purkinje myocytes*, are derived by recruitment of working myocardial cells or differentiate directly from primary myocardium.[44,45] Lineage studies, as yet unpublished, suggest that the myocytes making up the proximal part of the ventricular component of the axis are derived from the initial primary myocardium of the heart tube. The primary myocardium, however, is slowly conducting. The purpose of the ventricular bundle branches and their peripheral ramifications, in contrast, is to

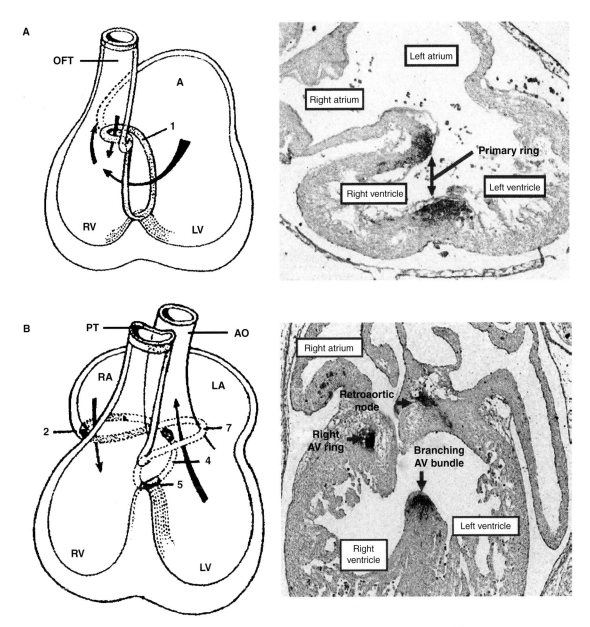

FIGURE 17–18. Morphologic changes in the arrangement of the tissues of the initial primary ring. The left side of the panels shows schematic representations of the primary ring and its derived tissues, as was reconstructed by Wessels et al[42] from the serial sections of human embryos at Carnegie stage 15 (**A**) and stage 18 to 19 (**B**) immunohistochemically stained using antibody to the chick nodose ganglion (GlN2), as shown in the right side of the panels (with brown color). Although the function of the antigen to which GlN2 antibody binds is still unknown, it was helpful by enabling one to follow the changes that occur in the atrioventricular canal and developing conduction system during septation of the human heart. At the earlier stage (A), GlN2 expression marks the location of the primary ring, which is the precursor to the atrioventricular conduction system, as can be appreciated from section of the older embryo (B), where it is possible to see how the ring has now expanded to encircle the right atrioventricular (AV) junction, forming the right AV ring bundle, and also passes behind the aortic root, forming a retroaortic node. Numbers pointing to different parts of the primary ring tissues in the left side of the panels indicate the following: 1, initial position of the primary ring; 2, right AV ring bundle; 4, penetrating AV bundle; 5, branching portion of AV bundle; and 7, retroaortic root branch. A, atrium; AO, aorta; LA, left atrium; LV, left ventricle; OFT, outflow tract; PT, pulmonary trunk; RA, right atrium; RV, right ventricle.

ensure rapid activation of the working ventricular myocardium, with the activation commencing at the ventricular apexes so as to ensure systolic ejection of the blood into the arterial trunks. The bundle branches and the ventricular Purkinje myocytes, therefore, are derived from the initial trabeculated component of the ventricular walls,[46] with their myocytes joined together by rapidly conducting connexins.

■ THE ATRIOVENTRICULAR RING TISSUES

Another debate relating to cardiac conduction concerned the presence of recognizable node-like structures in the right atrial vestibular myocardium. These entities were recognized by Kent[47] at the turn of the nineteenth century, albeit erroneously interpreted by him as providing multiple muscular connections across the atrioventricular junctions of the normal heart. The structures are the remnants of the ring of primary atrioventricular canal myocardium that forms the vestibule of the tricuspid valve (see Fig. 17–18). The T-box transcription factor Tbx3, which represses the chamber program of gene expression, is expressed in the entirety of the initial ring (see Fig. 17–12). In very rare circumstances, the remnants can persist as histologically recognizable structures that function as substrates for ventricular preexcitation in otherwise normally structured hearts.[48] They can also form anomalous atrioventricular nodes in the setting of congenital malformations such as congenitally corrected transposition and double inlet left ventricle.[49,50] In the developing heart, the ring of atrioventricular canal musculature crosses over the atrioventricular conduction axis, forming a mass of histologically recognizable tissue in the atrial musculature directly dorsal to the aortic root (see Fig. 17–18B). This so-called retroaortic node is separated from the atrioventricular node itself by the insulating tissues of the central fibrous body. It does not become an integral part of the normal atrioventricular node.

■ THE ATRIOVENTRICULAR INSULATING PLANES

In the postnatal heart, it is only the atrioventricular conduction axis that provides a muscular pathway between the atrial and ventricular myocardial masses. As we have discussed, it is possible to record an adult-type electrocardiogram long before specialized conducting tracts can be recognized.[1] At these initial stages, muscular continuity is found throughout both atrioventricular junctions, with the muscular continuity being provided by the primary atrioventricular canal myocardium (see Fig. 17–9). Recent experiments using lineage data have shown that the atrioventricular canal region contributes significant material to the left ventricular inlet component.[6] Part of the initial canal musculature, nonetheless, becomes sequestered in the atrial tissues subsequent to the formation of the fibrous insulating planes.[23] The separating planes themselves are often considered part of an extensive fibrous skeleton. In reality, this is far from the case. In the right atrioventricular junction of the postnatal human heart, it is rare to find a well-formed fibrous annulus supporting the hinges of the leaflets of the tricuspid valve. Instead, it is the fibroadipose tissue of the atrioventricular groove that separates the atrial from the ventricular myocytes. On the left side, the fibrous annulus is better formed, supporting the mural leaflet of the mitral valve. In relation to the anterior, or aortic, leaflet of the mitral valve, it is initially possible to see the musculature of the inner heart curve. With ongoing development, this muscle disappears, leaving aortic-to-mitral fibrous continuity. The precise timing of the disruption of the extensive areas of initial myocardial continuity around the atrioventricular junctions has still to be established for the human heart, as does the mechanism permitting retention of those muscular bridges[51] known to be the substrates for ventricular preexcitation.[52]

■ THE PULMONARY VENOUS MYOCARDIAL SLEEVES

With the recognition that atrial fibrillation in many patients can be cured by creating electrical discontinuity between the pulmonary venous myocardial sleeves and the remainder of the left atrial musculature,[53] suggestions have been made that this myocardium is itself histologically specialized. Some have argued that the myocytes making up the sleeves are "Purkinje-like" and hence histologically specialized.[54] Rigorous examination of the sleeves in the human heart shows this not to be the case.[55] The pulmonary sleeves are made up of aggregated working myocytes, and there is no evidence that the sleeves are histologically distinct or specialized. An alternative explanation for the "specialization" is that the myocardium itself is initially derived from the systemic venous sinus.[56] There is no evidence to support this notion either, with a wealth of evidence showing that the myocytes within the sleeves have never had a primary myocardial heritage.[57]

■ THE MYOCARDIUM OF THE OUTFLOW TRACTS

In contrast to the pulmonary venous myocardial sleeves, which have no relationship to the embryonic primary myocardium, the myocardium making up the ventricular outflow tracts had the primary myocardial phenotype during the embryonic phase of development. Much interest has been focused on this myocardium as the substrate for ventricular tachycardias, the more so because some such tachycardias can be cured by ablation, placing the lesions distal to the anatomic ventriculoarterial junction.[58] There is no question that the entirety of the myocardium of the common ventricular outflow tract is initially of the primary variant or that this myocardium initially extends to the margins of the pericardial cavity (Fig. 17–19A).[59] During development, the distal part of the outflow tract rapidly changes to an arterial phenotype,[60] albeit the mechanisms of the transformation have yet to be established. Subsequent to the formation of the intrapericardial arterial trunks, a sleeve of primary myocardium encloses the entirety of the developing aortic and pulmonary roots (Fig. 17–19B).[60] Eventually this myocardium also regresses in a proximal direction, but even in the postnatal heart, it is possible to recognize crescents of ventricular myocardium at the bases of all the pulmonary valvar sinuses and in two of the aortic valvar sinuses.[61] These crescentic areas were initially made up of primary myocardium. In the postnatal heart, they cannot be distinguished histologically from the remainder of the ventricular myocardium. Parts of the muscular sleeve could persist on the epicardial aspect of the arterial valves, even extending into the walls of the arterial trunks. The dead-end tract of the primary interventricular ring also persists on the crest of the ventricular septum in the aortic root.[62] It remains to be established which, if any, of these muscular structures are the substrates for ventricular tachycardias.

CONCLUSION

Much has been learned over the last two decades concerning the development of the heart and the formation of the specialized conducting tissues. The majority of this evidence has come from the study of the murine heart. We have sought to summarize this evidence in our chapter, showing its relevance to the understanding of normal cardiac conduction and the understanding of clinical cardiac arrhythmias. At present, the majority of the evidence concerning development is derived from study of

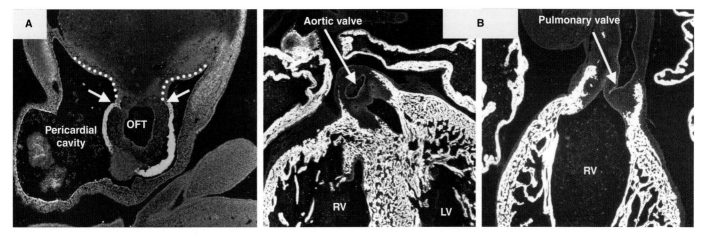

FIGURE 17–19. Muscular phenotype of the outflow tract in the human embryonic heart. **A.** Troponin I staining of the transverse section through the undivided outflow tract (OFT) of the human embryo at Carnegie stage 14. Note the presence of the myocardium (depicted by green color) at this high level, where cardiac outflow tract is bordered (arrows) by pericardial wall (dotted lines). At the end of the human embryonic period, at Carnegie stage 23, after completion of the septation of the heart and division of the outflow into aortic and pulmonary arterial parts, the myocardial tissue (depicted by white color) is still present at the level of both aortic and pulmonary valves (**B**). LV, left ventricle; RV, right ventricle.

the mouse heart. Furthermore, as yet, it has not been possible to achieve consensus as to how the time-honored criteria of Aschoff and Mönckeberg can best be modified to take note of the huge advances made in the understanding of the molecular signatures of the cardiac specialized tissues.[15] Within the next few years, we should be able to extend these investigations to the developing human heart. In particular, comparable advances in imaging should permit studies to be made of the developing human heart, ideally correlating these findings with electrocardiographic changes. Comparisons of these changes in the development of the normally structured heart, for example, with the morphology seen in the setting of common atrioventricular junction[63] should permit clarification of the roles played by the atrial septal inputs to the atrioventricular node. We anticipate that these future investigations will confirm the hypotheses advanced in this chapter.

REFERENCES

1. Paff GH, Boucek RJ, Harrell TC. Observations on the development of the electrocardiogram. *Anat Rec.* 1968;160:575-582.
2. Delorme B, Dahl E, Jarry-Guichard T, et al. Expression pattern of connexin gene products at the early developmental stages of the mouse cardiovascular system. *Circ Res.* 1997;81:423-437.
3. Van Kempen MJA, Vermeulen JLM, Moorman AFM, Gros DB, Paul DL, Lamers WH. Developmental changes of connexin40 and connexin43 mRNA-distribution patterns in the rat heart. *Cardiovasc Res.* 1996;32:886-900.
4. Soufan AT, van den Hoff MJ, Ruijter JM, et al. Reconstruction of the patterns of gene expression in the developing mouse heart reveals an architectural arrangement that facilitates the understanding of atrial malformations and arrhythmias. *Circ Res.* 2004;95:1207-1215.
5. Wessels A, Vermeulen JL, Virágh S, Kálmán F, Lamers WH, Moorman AF. Spatial distribution of "tissue-specific" antigens in the developing human heart and skeletal muscle. II. An immunohistochemical analysis of myosin heavy chain isoform expression patterns in the embryonic heart. *Anat Rec.* 1991;229:355-368.
6. Aanhaanen WT, Brons JF, Domínguez JN, et al. The Tbx2+ primary myocardium of the atrioventricular canal forms the atrioventricular node and the base of the left ventricle. *Circ Res.* 2009;104:1267-1274.
7. Buckingham M, Meilhac S, Zaffran S. Building the mammalian heart from two sources of myocardial cells. *Nat Rev Genet.* 2005;6:826-835.
8. Moorman AF, Christoffels VM, Anderson RH, van den Hoff MJ. The heart-forming fields: one or multiple? *Philos Trans R Soc Lond B Biol Sci.* 2007;362:1257-1265.
9. van den Berg G, Abu-Issa R, de Boer BA, et al. A caudal proliferating growth center contributes to both poles of the forming heart tube. *Circ Res.* 2009;104:179-188.
10. Moorman AFM, Christoffels VM. Cardiac chamber formation: development, genes and evolution. *Physiol Rev.* 2003;83:1223-1267.
11. Christoffels VM, Burch JB, Moorman AF. Architectural plan for the heart: early patterning and delineation of the chambers and the nodes. *Trends Cardiovasc Med.* 2004;14:301-307.
12. Aschoff L. Referat über die herzstörungen in ihren beziehungen zu den spezifischen muskelsystemen des herzens. *Verh Deutsch Pathol Ges.* 1910;14:3-35.
13. Mönckeberg JG. Beiträge zur normalen und pathologischen anatomie des herzens. *Verh Deutsch Pathol Ges.* 1910;14:64-71.
14. Tawara S. *Das Reizleitungssystem des Säugetierherzens. Eine Anatomisch-Histologische Studie über des Atrioventricular Bundel und die Purkinjescher Folden.* Jena, Germany: G. Fischer; 1906.
15. Moorman AFM, Christoffels VM, Anderson RH. Anatomic substrates for cardiac conduction. *Heart Rhythm.* 2005;2:875-886.
16. Anderson RH, Cook AC. The structure and components of the atrial chambers. *Europace.* 2007;9(Suppl 6):vi3-vi9.
17. Webb S, Brown NA, Wessels A, Anderson RH. Development of the murine pulmonary vein and its relationship to the embryonic venous sinus. *Anat Rec.* 1998,250:325-334.
18. Mommersteeg MT, Soufan AT, de Lange FJ, et al. Two distinct pools of mesenchyme contribute to the development of the atrial septum. *Circ Res.* 2006;99:351-353.
19. His W. Die area interposita, die Eustachische klappe und die apina vestibuli. In: His W, ed. *Anatomie Menschlicher Embryonen. Zur Geschichte der Organe.* Vol. 3. Jena, Germany: Verlag von FCW Vogel; 1885:149-152.
20. Wessels A, Anderson RH, Markwald RR, et al. Atrial development in the human heart: an immunohistochemical study with emphasis on the role of mesenchymal tissues. *Anat Rec.* 2000;259:288-300.
21. Webb S, Kanani M, Anderson RH, Richardson MK, Brown NA. Development of the human pulmonary vein and its incorporation in the morphologically left atrium. *Cardiol Young.* 2001;11:632-642.
22. Anderson RH, Webb S, Brown NA. Clinical anatomy of the atrial septum with reference to its developmental components. *Clin Anat.* 1999;12:362-374.
23. Wessels A, Markman MW, Vermeulen JL, Anderson RH, Moorman AF, Lamers WH. The development of the atrioventricular junction in the human heart. *Circ Res.* 1996;78:110-117.

24. Christoffels VM, Mommersteeg MTM, Trowe MO, et al. Formation of the venous pole of the heart from an Nkx2-5-negative precursor population requires Tbx18. *Circ Res.* 2006;98:1555-1563.

25. de Jong F, Opthof T, Wilde AA, et al. Persisting zones of slow impulse conduction in developing chicken hearts. *Circ Res.* 1992;71:240-250.

26. Moorman AF, Christoffels VM. Development of the cardiac conduction system: a matter of chamber development. *Novartis Found Symp.* 2003;250:25-34.

27. Severs NJ. Cardiac muscle cell interaction: from microanatomy to the molecular make-up of the gap junction. *Histol Histopathol.* 1995;10:481-501.

28. Miquerol L, Dupays L, Théveniau-Ruissy M, et al. Gap junctional connexins in the developing mouse cardiac conduction system. *Novartis Found Symp.* 2003;250:80-98.

29. Hoogaars WM, Tessari A, Moorman AF, et al. The transcriptional repressor Tbx3 delineates the developing central conduction system of the heart. *Cardiovasc Res.* 2004;62:489-499.

30. Wiese C, Grieskamp T, Airik R, et al. Formation of the sinus node head and differentiation of sinus node myocardium are independently regulated by Tbx18 and Tbx3. *Circ Res.* 2009;104:388-397.

31. van Mierop LHS. Localization of pacemaker in chick embryo heart at the time of initiation of heartbeat. *Am J Physiol.* 1967;212:407-415.

32. Mommersteeg MT, Hoogaars WM, Prall OW, et al. Molecular pathway for the localized formation of the sinoatrial node. *Circ Res.* 2007;100:354-362.

33. Meijler FL, Billette J, Jalife J, et al. Atrioventricular conduction in mammalian species: hemodynamic and electrical scaling. *Heart Rhythm.* 2005;2:188-196.

34. Becker AE, Anderson RH. Morphology of the human atrioventricular junctional area. In: Wellens HJJ, Lie KI, Janse MJ, eds. *The Conduction System of the Heart. Structure, Function and Clinical Implications.* Leiden, the Netherlands: Stenfert Kroese BV; 1976:263-286.

35. Viragh Sz, Challice CE. The development of the conduction system in the mouse heart. IV. Differentiation of the atrioventricular conduction system. *Dev Biol.* 1982;89:25-40.

36. Thaemert JC. Fine structure of the atrioventricular node as viewed in serial sections. *Am J Anat.* 1973;136:43-66.

37. Horsthuis T, Buermans HP, Brons JF, et al. Gene expression profiling of the forming atrioventricular node using a novel Tbx3-based node-specific transgenic reporter. *Circ Res.* 2009;105:61-69.

38. McGuire MA, de Bakker JM, Vermeulen JT, et al. Atrioventricular junctional tissue. Discrepancy between histological and electrophysiological characteristics. *Circulation.* 1996;94:571-577.

39. Janse MJ, Anderson RH. Specialized internodal atrial pathways: fact or fiction? *Eur J Cardiol.* 1974;2:117-136.

40. Spach MS, Kootsey JM. The nature of electrical propagation in cardiac muscle. *Am J Physiol.* 1983;244:H3-H22.

41. Tawara S. *The Conduction System of the Mammalian Heart. An Anatomico-Histological Study of the Atrioventricular Bundle and the Purkinje Fibers.* Translation by Shimada M, Suma K. London, United Kingdom: Imperial College Press; 2000.

42. Wessels A, Vermeulen JL, Verbeek FJ, et al. Spatial distribution of "tissue-specific" antigens in the developing human heart and skeletal muscle. III. An immunohistochemical analysis of the distribution of the neural tissue antigen G1N2 in the embryonic heart; implications for the development of the atrioventricular conduction system. *Anat Rec.* 1992;232:97-111.

43. Anderson RH, Wenink ACG, Losekoot TG, Becker AE. Congenitally complete heart block. Developmental aspects. *Circulation.* 1977;56:90-101.

44. Christoffels VM, Moorman AF. Development of the cardiac conduction system: why are some regions of the heart more arrhythmogenic than others? *Circ Arrhythm Electrophysiol.* 2009;2:195-207.

45. Gourdie RG, Harris BS, Bond J, et al. Development of the cardiac pacemaking and conduction system. *Birth Defects Res C Embryo Today.* 2003;69:46-57.

46. Mikawa T, Fischman DA. The polyclonal origin of myocyte lineages. *Annu Rev Physiol.* 1996;58:509-521.

47. Kent AFS. Researches on the structure and function of the mammalian heart. *J Anat Physiol.* 1893;14:233-254.

48. Anderson RH, Ho SY, Gillette PC, Becker AE. Mahaim, Kent and abnormal atrioventricular conduction. *Cardiovasc Res.* 1996;31:480-491.

49. Anderson RH, Becker AE, Arnold R, Wilkinson JL. The conducting tissues in congenitally corrected transposition. *Circulation.* 1974;50:911-923.

50. Anderson RH, Arnold R, Thaper MK, Jones RS, Hamilton DI. Cardiac specialized tissues in hearts with an apparently single ventricular chamber (double inlet left ventricle). *Am J Cardiol.* 1974;33:95-106.

51. Hahurij ND, Gittenberger-De Groot AC, Kolditz DP, et al. Accessory atrioventricular myocardial connections in the developing human heart: relevance for perinatal supraventricular tachycardias. *Circulation.* 2008;117:2850-2858.

52. Becker AE, Anderson RH. The Wolff-Parkinson-White syndrome and its anatomical substrates. *Anat Rec.* 1981;201:169-177.

53. Haissaguerre M, Jais P, Shah DC, et al. Electrophysiological end point for catheter ablation of atrial fibrillation initiated from multiple pulmonary venous foci. *Circulation.* 2000;101:1409-1417.

54. Perez-Lugones A, McMahon JT, Ratliff NB, et al. Evidence of specialized conduction cells in human pulmonary veins of patients with atrial fibrillation. *J Cardiovasc Electrophysiol.* 2003;14:803-809.

55. Ho SY, Cabrera JA, Tran VH, Farre J, Anderson RH, Sanchez-Quintana D. Architecture of the pulmonary veins: relevance to radiofrequency ablation. *Heart.* 2001;86:265-270.

56. Blom NA, Gittenberger-de Groot AC, Jongeneel TH, de Ruiter MC, Poelmann RE, Ottenkamp J. Normal development of the pulmonary veins in human embryos and formulation of a morphogenetic concept for sinus venosus defects. *Am J Cardiol.* 2001;87:305-309.

57. Mommersteeg MTM, Brown NA, Prall OWJ, et al. Pitx2c and Nkx2-5 are required for the formation and identity of the pulmonary myocardium. *Circ Res.* 2007;101:902-909.

58. Gonska BD, Brune S, Bethge KP, Kreuzer H. Radiofrequency catheter ablation in recurrent ventricular tachycardia. *Eur Heart J.* 1991;12:1257-1265.

59. Boukens BJ, Christoffels VM, Coronel R, Moorman AF. Developmental basis for electrophysiological heterogeneity in the ventricular and outflow tract myocardium as a substrate for life-threatening ventricular arrhythmias. *Circ Res.* 2009;104:19-31.

60. Ya J, van den Hoff MJ, de Boer PA, et al. Normal development of the outflow tract in the rat. *Circ Res.* 1998;82:464-472.

61. Sutton JP III, Ho SY, Anderson RH. The forgotten interleaflet triangles: a review of the surgical anatomy of the aortic valve. *Ann Thorac Surg.* 1995;59:419-427.

62. Kurosawa H, Becker AE. Dead-end tract of the conduction axis. *Int J Cardiol.* 1985;7:13-20.

63. Thiene G, Wenink AC, Frescura C, et al. Surgical anatomy and pathology of the conduction tissues in atrioventricular defects. *J Thorac Cardiovasc Surg.* 1981;82:928-937.

SECTION III

Cardiovascular Multimodal Imaging in Key Clinical Problems

18. Congenital Heart Disease: Atrioventricular Septal Defect. . . 315

19. Right Ventricular Cardiomyopathies 322

20. Ischemic Heart Disease 354

21. Acute Myocardial Infarction 360

22. Diseases of the Aorta 368

23. Peripheral Vascular Disease 392

24. Pulmonary Vascular Disease. 402

25. Atrial Fibrillation. 420

CHAPTER 18

CONGENITAL HEART DISEASE: ATRIOVENTRICULAR SEPTAL DEFECT

Nina Hakačova

INTRODUCTION / 315

CHALLENGES OF AVSD / 315

ANATOMY OF AVSD / 315

IMAGING OF AVSD: ANATOMY / 315
  Echocardiography / 315
  Imaging of the Atrioventricular Valve Function / 317
  Electrophysiology of the AVSD / 318

MECHANISMS UNDERLYING THE ELECTROPHYSIOLOGIC FEATURES IN AVSD / 320
  Conduction System / 320
  Conduction System and Atrioventricular Valve Complex / 320

SIGNIFICANCE OF UNDERSTANDING ELECTROANATOMIC RELATIONSHIPS / 320

CONCLUSION / 320

INTRODUCTION

Major advances in the field of pediatric cardiology and cardiac surgery over the last several decades have led to an improvement in survival rates of the patients with congenital heart disease. During this period, improvements in surgical and medical treatments have been accompanied by developments in a spectrum of diagnostic modalities. Integration of different modalities in clinical and research environments is being used for better understanding and better managing of complex cardiac conditions.

Ideally, few noninvasive imaging modalities should be able to delineate all aspects of the anatomy and evaluate physiologic consequences of the lesion(s) in patients with congenital heart disease. Moreover, the imaging modalities used should be cost effective and portable, not cause excessive discomfort and morbidity, and not expose patients to harmful effects of ionizing radiation. To limit the number of imaging modalities used in diagnosis and therapy, research is being performed to evaluate and validate techniques that could potentially serve as noninvasive or minimally invasive imaging modalities that would replace those which are invasive and less available.

The aim of this chapter is to present a model of how noninvasive multimodal imaging can improve the understanding of pathophysiology and increase the accuracy of the diagnosis of the specific congenital heart disease. The focus is on the heart with atrioventricular septal defect (AVSD).

CHALLENGES OF AVSD

Appropriate diagnosis and detailed assessment of the anatomic and functional features of AVSD presents challenges. Particularly, accurate preoperative assessment of the atrioventricular valve component is crucial since long-term outcomes for surgical repairs of AVSDs depend on the successful repair of the left atrioventricular valve. Moreover, surgical destruction of the conduction system may occur in cases of inappropriate diagnosis because AVSDs have different conduction pathways compared with defects that have separate atrioventricular valves.[1]

Understanding the electroanatomic and functional relationships in hearts with AVSDs is suggested to permit differentiation of atrioventricular defects from other similar abnormalities.

ANATOMY OF AVSD

AVSD is anatomically characterized by abnormal development of the atrioventricular valve junction.[2-6] In addition, the overall atrioventricular valve complex including valve leaflets and papillary muscles is abnormally developed. Figure 18–1 schematically depicts main differences in the normal (Fig. 18–1A) and primum AVSD heart (Fig. 18–1B) anatomy. Atrioventricular valve leaflets are different from normal mitral and tricuspidal leaflets because atrioventricular valve leaflets guard a common atrioventricular junction and are displaced. In addition, valve leaflets may be asymmetric, the mural leaflet may be abnormally small. Displacement and sometimes even dysfunction of the papillary muscles is present. Those changes are often associated with pre- and postoperative regurgitation of the valve.[1-9] Left ventricular papillary muscles are positioned further from the septum compared with normal, with the posterior papillary muscle more so than the anterior papillary muscle.[1] Thus, specifically, the posterior papillary muscle is a marker of distinction between AVSDs and other similar defects such as defects with mitral clefts.[1]

AVSD is further characterized by inflow tract shortening and by outflow tract lengthening. Left ventricular outflow tract is transformed into a longer channel, and therefore, the ratio between the inflow and outflow is smaller than that in healthy controls.[10,11]

IMAGING OF AVSD: ANATOMY

■ ECHOCARDIOGRAPHY

Two-dimensional (2D) echocardiography (ECHO) is the current standard noninvasive imaging tool used for the morphologic and functional assessment of the AVSD and provides global preoperative data in the majority of cases.[12] Figure 18–2 and

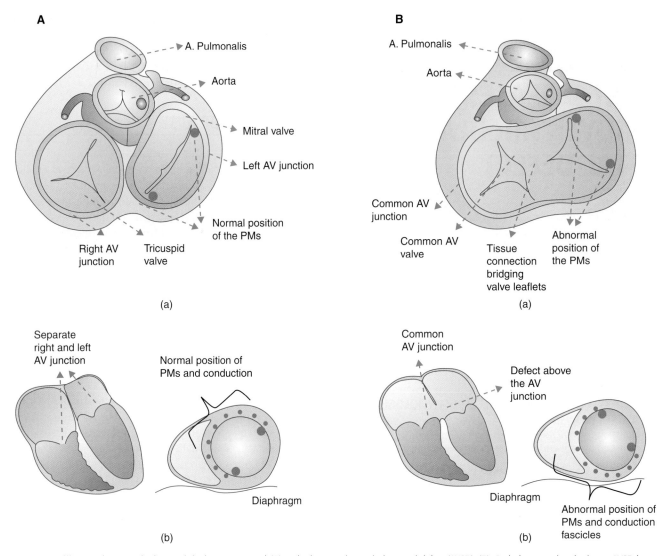

FIGURE 18–1. Differences in anatomic characteristics between normal (**A**) and primum atrioventricular septal defect (AVSD) (**B**). Both the normal and primum AVSD hearts are first shown from modified left anterior oblique view at the level of the valves (a). The apical four-chamber view and short axis view of the heart at the level of papillary muscles are also presented (b). A, arteria; AV, atrioventricular; PMs, papillary muscles. The image was modified from Adachi I, Uemura H, McCarthy KP, et al. Surgical anatomy of atrioventricular septal defect. *Asian Cardiovasc Thorac Ann.* 2008;16:497-502.

the related Moving Image show the 2D image of the primum AVSD. The morphology of the defect and atrioventricular valve is presented.

With advances in imaging technology, three-dimensional (3D) ECHO has been shown to primarily facilitate the accurate anatomic and functional assessment of complex spatial anatomic features and relationships of the anatomic and functional abnormalities involved in AVSD.[12] 3D ECHO provides more detailed information about anatomic and functional assessment of the atrioventricular valve, the relationships between the leaflets of the valves, with each other and with other heart structures.[13] Figure 18–3 and the related Moving Image show an example of the assessment of the anatomy of the atrioventricular valve by using 3D ECHO imaging. Relationships between the leaflets and dynamics of the valve leaflet motion can be seen on the cine image. This anatomic information is of value for the clinician in planning surgical treatment because it provides

a more detailed anatomic definition of interrelations between structures.[14]

The atrioventricular valve apparatus consists of the annulus, leaflets, chordae, and papillary muscles. Because the atrioventricular valve apparatus is complex, 2D ECHO is often not sufficient to provide full information of the atrioventricular valve relationships. Real-time 3D imaging permits display of the entire circumference of the atrioventricular annulus. This is important information in surgical repair of the valves (eg, annuloplasty). Whereas 2D imaging shows the edges of the leaflets in multiple different views, real-time 3D imaging shows the entire surface of the leaflet in a single display. Leaflets can be inspected from either the atrial side or the ventricular side, depicting, for example, buckling, cleft, or deficiencies. The advantage is that all of the information can be obtained from a single data set without the need to scan and sweep from different windows, as is required in 2D imaging.[15] 3D ECHO

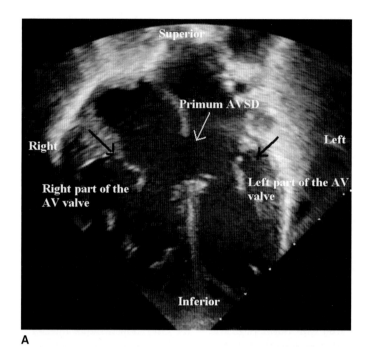

A

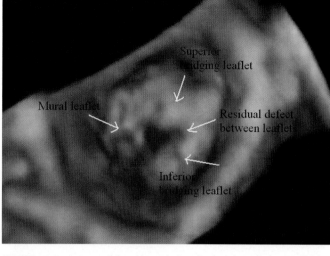

FIGURE 18–3. Anatomy of the atrioventricular valve in atrioventricular septal defect (AVSD) imaged using three-dimensional echocardiography. Mural and anterior and posterior bridging leaflets are visualized. The picture is taken after suturing of the bridging leaflets. Residual defect is seen between the bridging leaflets. See also Moving Image 18–3.

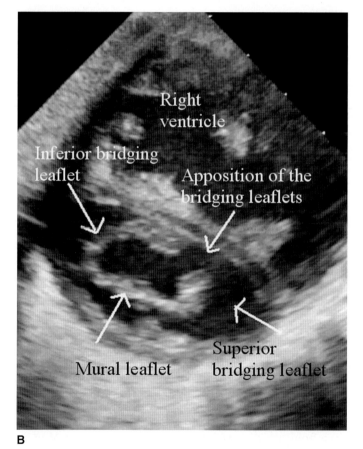

B

FIGURE 18–2. A. Anatomy of the atrioventricular septal defect (AVSD) imaged using two-dimensional echocardiographic imaging. Apical four-chamber view shows the premium AVSD defect between the atria and the common atrioventricular (AV) junction with left and right parts of the common AV valve. See also Moving Image 18–2A. **B.** Subcostal short axis view shows the anatomy of the left part of the atrioventricular valve. Bridging leaflets and mural leaflet are depicted. Moving Image 18–2B shows the function of the left atrioventricular valve with insufficiency through the apposition of the bridging leaflets.

provides new insight into the dynamic morphology of the left-sided atrioventricular valve and left ventricular outflow tract anatomy.[16,17] In the clinical scenario, it clarifies the pathology, particularly in complex lesions where the incremental information has an impact on therapeutic decision making.

■ IMAGING OF THE ATRIOVENTRICULAR VALVE FUNCTION

Morbidity of the left atrioventricular valve remains an important concern.[18-20] Reoperation of valve failure is complex and involves annular reduction, commissurotomy, closure of the residual defect in the apposition of the bridging leaflets, and patch enlargement of the atrioventricular valve. Although the surgeon has the opportunity to inspect the atrioventricular valve and test its competency with saline, this latter technique is nonphysiologic and might provide an incomplete evaluation of the true nature of the valve failure. 2D ECHO with color Doppler scanning is the current standard for both preoperative and postoperative assessment of patients with AVSD. Figure 18–4 and the related Moving Image show the color Doppler ECHO used for assessment of the function of the atrioventricular valve. The limitation of the 2D perspective is its difficulty to provide details regarding the status of the commissures, the precise location of the regurgitant jets, sites of poor coaptation, and the presence of clefts. Color Doppler scanning is a helpful adjunct, but the true extent and location of the regurgitant jets might be difficult to appreciate in a 2D image, particularly in cases with multiple jets caused by the phenomena of jet entrainment.

3D color-flow ECHO is a complementary technique with potential to assess the more precise mechanism of the valve dynamics and valve insufficiency. Figure 18–5 and the related Moving Image show the 3D flow through the atrioventricular

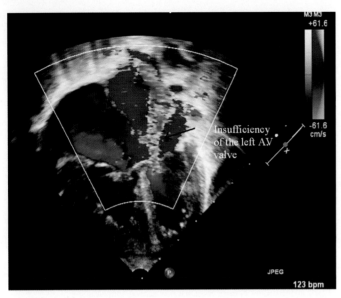

FIGURE 18–4. Two-dimensional echocardiography image of the insufficiency of the atrioventricular (AV) valve. Image is presented from the apical long axis view. See also Moving Image 18–4.

valve. 3D color Doppler images can identify regurgitation jets in three dimensions and in a more precise relationship to the leaflets of the atrioventricular valve. This facilitates the identification of anatomic details and mechanism of the valve failure. Redundancy of the valve leaflets and/or defective coaptation can be demonstrated during real-time 3D imaging of the motion of the leaflets. The contribution of poor coaptation and/or dysplastic leaflets to the degree of valve regurgitation can be documented with the 3D geometry of the regurgitant jet.

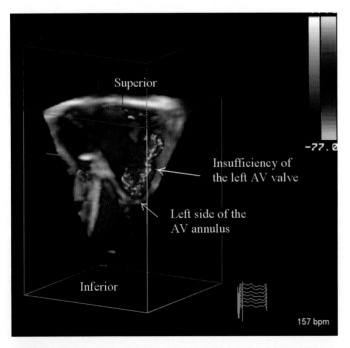

FIGURE 18–5. Three-dimensional flow of the insufficiency of the left-sided atrioventricular (AV) valve. See also Moving Image 18–5.

■ ELECTROPHYSIOLOGY OF THE AVSD

Left axis deviation is considered a "hallmark" of AVSD.[21] Superior orientation of the QRS loop in the frontal and sagittal planes was even suggested as a sign that differentiates AVSD from other cardiac abnormalities.[22] By gaining insight into the developmental relationships between the conduction system and heart structures, improvement in diagnosis can be achieved.

Electrophysiologic abnormalities were studied by using several different techniques including vectorcardiogram, body surface potential maps, and epicardial mapping, with the aim of describing the abnormality of electrical activation in detail and to use the activation patterns to differentiate AVSD from other similar lesions.[21,22]

Vectorcardiogram

As shown in Fig. 18–6, the major portion of the QRS loop in the frontal plane is superiorly oriented in AVSD patients compared with normals, in whom the QRS loop is rather inferiorly and horizontally placed.[21] This displacement, also known as *counterclockwise rotation*, of the QRS loop in the frontal plane is a very common vectorcardiographic finding in patients with AVSD.[21,22]

Body Surface Maps

Spach et al[23] used body surface maps to study electrophysiologic abnormalities in AVSD. The distribution of cardiac potentials on the body surface in patients with AVSD differed in a characteristic pattern from the normal group. Figure 18–6 shows an example of data from a child with AVSD (Fig. 18–7B) and a child with a normal heart (Fig. 18–7A).

Using Fig. 18–7 as reference, the initial phase of ventricular depolarization in the AVSD patient (a*) started more inferiorly and more leftward, compared with the normal child (a). The depolarization wave then migrated more superiorly (b*) and after that shifted to the right (c*). During the second half of the heart cycle, depolarization was shifted superiorly and to the left (d*, e*) and finished by depolarization of the right ventricle (f*). Depolarization followed then an inferosuperior direction in the AVSD patient (2f*, 2g*) and finished by depolarization of the right ventricle (2h*, 2j*). In summary, the main difference compared with the normal group was the late depolarization of the superior part of the left ventricle.

An interesting finding in f* is the emergence of nondipolar content on the surface of the child with AVSD. This means that within the heart, there was a presence of more than one overall wave front, which caused the simultaneous presence of more than one maximum or minimum. This finding is characteristic for patients with AVSD. It was suggested that the transient absence of a null zone suggests the marked predominance of active wave fronts within the heart progressing in an endocardial-to-epicardial direction. Durrer et al[24] demonstrated that the diaphragmatic surface of the left ventricle activates abnormally early in AVSD patients. Wave fronts in the ventricular free walls are spreading in an endocardial-to-epicardial direction as the

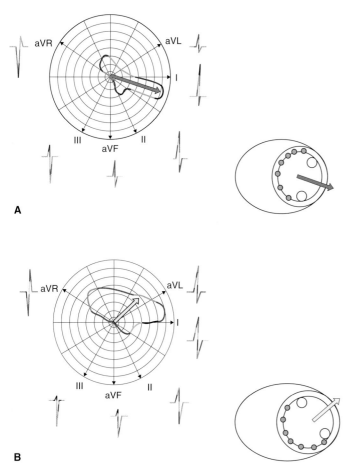

A

B

FIGURE 18–6. Differences in electrophysiologic characteristics presented by vector-cardiogram in a child with normal heart (**A**) and a child with primum atrioventricular septal defect (AVSD) (**B**). The vectorcardiogram is projected in the frontal plane and supplemented with the corresponding QRS complexes in limb leads (I, II, III, aVF, aVR, and aVL). Different colors in the vectorcardiogram represent time intervals of 10 ms. The thick arrow represents direction of the average QRS vector in the frontal plane. Corresponding displacement of the papillary muscles and bundle branch fascicles is shown besides both vectorcardiograms.

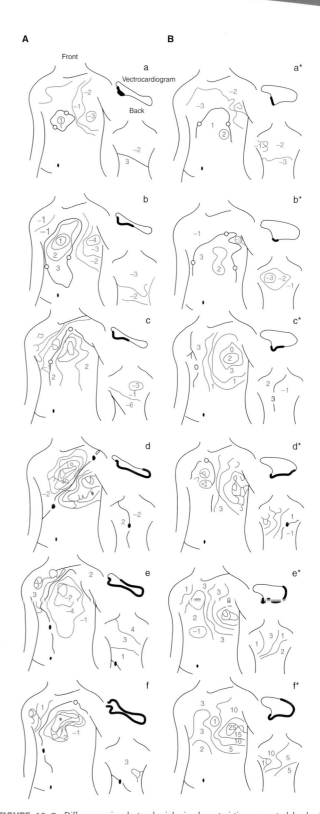

FIGURE 18–7. Differences in electrophysiologic characteristics presented by body surface maps in a child with normal heart (**A**) and a child with primum atrioventricular septal defect (AVSD) (**B**). The electrophysiologic event of one cardiac cycle is divided into time intervals of 10 ms labeled by letters "a-f" in normal heart and "a*-i*" in primum AVSD. The pictures of the body surface maps are acquired each 10 ms. That represents 10 ms interval of the cardiac cycle. The numbers shown within the maps indicate voltage in millivolts. Red color indicates positive zone; blue color indicates negative zone; black line indicates null zone. The figure was modified from Spach et al.[23]

diaphragmatic surface of the left ventricle completes its activation with epicardial breakthrough.

Epicardial Mapping

Durrer et al[24] examined the epicardial excitation in four patients with AVSD. An intramural electrode was used for recordings. The greatest differences in left ventricular excitation, as compared with normal, were present at the basal region of the posterior wall. In patients with normal hearts, the earliest epicardial activation time found was 70 ms after the beginning of the left ventricular cavity potential, whereas in patients with AVSD, values of 28 to 34 ms were found. Therefore, Durrer at al[24] considered the finding to be suggestive of the existence of a relatively large posterobasal area activated at least 30 ms earlier than normal.

After epicardial breakthrough at the basal part of the posterior wall, however, the excitatory forces moved to the anterior and posterolateral parts of the left ventricle and progressed in a more superior direction.

MECHANISMS UNDERLYING THE ELECTROPHYSIOLOGIC FEATURES IN AVSD

■ CONDUCTION SYSTEM

It was recently proposed that abnormal development of the conduction system follows the development of the heart anatomy.[25] The effort to understand and explain the reason for the previously described abnormalities of left ventricular depolarization with left QRS axis deviation as a result led to studies concerning electroanatomic aspects of the AVSD.

It was proposed that differences in atrioventricular valve relationships to the septum affect not only the shunting level but also the location of the atrioventricular node.[7,26-28] The bundle of His was found to also be displaced.[23] By performing iodine staining of the peripheral conduction system of the left ventricle, it was shown that the bundle of His entered the ventricular muscle area in a position that was located inferiorly compared with the normal entrance of the left bundle branch.[29] From the bundle of His, multiple branches extended over the diaphragmatic surface of the left ventricle. No discrete organized pattern, as present in the normal heart with an anterior and posterior division, was visible in the AVSD hearts. There was general dispersion of multiple arborizations emanating over the inferior septal border out over the left ventricular free wall. A large septal area superior to the defect in the outflow tract of the left ventricle was completely void of conduction system. The arrangement of the conduction system in AVSD with inferior displacement of the bundle of His was suggested to result in different order of depolarization sequences in the heart and thus left axis deviation.[30]

■ CONDUCTION SYSTEM AND ATRIOVENTRICULAR VALVE COMPLEX

From developmental studies, it is known that the conduction system develops from the trabecular system of the ventricle.[31] The location of the papillary muscles was recently suggested to predict the location of the conduction system and thus the sequences of electrical activation in the heart.[32]

As stressed earlier, papillary muscles belong to the atrioventricular valve complex and are abnormally positioned in AVSD patients.[1] The relationship between papillary muscles and conduction system may be key to understanding some electrophysiologic abnormalities.[33] Recently, the association between QRS axis deviation and position of papillary muscles has been suggested in AVSD patients.[34] The main finding was that in AVSD patients, the left deviation of the QRS axis correlated with the anatomic imbalance of the positions of the mitral papillary muscles.

SIGNIFICANCE OF UNDERSTANDING ELECTROANATOMIC RELATIONSHIPS

Abnormalities associated with the AVSD are complex. Diagnostic confusions of AVSD with other heart defects have been reported.[35,36] The ability to distinguish AVSD from other congenital heart defects early and precisely is important because

AVSD patients may present with severe hemodynamic complications early in the course and require different surgical management with the awareness that the displacement of the atrioventricular conduction tissues varies markedly between AVSD and other lesions.[1,36]

Left atrioventricular valve regurgitation remains the most common residual defect.[37] Deterioration of the atrioventricular valve can be progressive and rapid and can lead to congestive heart failure early in infancy.[38] Prediction of the functional outcomes of left atrioventricular valves following the repair of AVSDs is of interest.[38-40] It was shown previously that mitral valve regurgitation correlates with changes in the 3D geometry of the subvalvular apparatus and the annulus. Abnormal anatomic and electrical constellation leads to abnormal dynamics of the atrioventricular valve function. Important practical implications can be drawn from this information regarding approaches to restore a more favorable geometry and might explain why, in some cases, a simple annuloplasty ring might fail to improve mitral valve regurgitation.

Detailed understanding of the atrioventricular valve complex in association with electrophysiologic abnormalities may be beneficial in predicting the atrioventricular valve abnormalities and outcome of patients with AVSD according to the papillary muscle positions and abnormalities of the conduction system. Association between the papillary muscle positions, conduction system, and function of the left ventricle and atrioventricular valve may be of interest in designing surgical procedures dealing with anatomic and electrophysiologic relationships and may predict their effects on the restoration of the ventricular performance.

CONCLUSION

The major determinants of ventricular contraction and thus ventricular function are anatomic arrangements and the sequence of ventricular electrical activation. The ventricular activation sequence changes during heart development concomitantly with its anatomy.[1] In patients with congenital heart disease, abnormal electrical activation reflects abnormal development of anatomic arrangements, and they both may influence heart performance and function.

This chapter highlights the main anatomic, functional, and electrophysiologic abnormalities associated with AVSD. The use of multimodal imaging modalities is suggested in the assessment of the electroanatomic and functional relationships.

Moving Images

All moving images are located on the complementary DVD.

REFERENCES

1. Kohl T, Silverman NH. Comparison of cleft and papillary muscle position in cleft mitral valve and atrioventricular septal defect. *Am J Cardiol.* 1996;77:164-169.
2. Anderson RH, Ho SY, Becker AE. Anatomy of the human atrioventricular junctions revisited. *Anat Rec.* 2000;260:81-91.

3. Anderson RH, Ho SY, Falcao S, et al. The diagnostic features of atrioventricular septal defect with common atrioventricular junction. *Cardiol Young*. 1998;8:33-49.

4. Silverman NH, Zuberbuhler JR, Anderson RH. Atrioventricular septal defects: cross-sectional echocardiographic and morphologic comparisons. *Int J Cardiol*. 1986;13:309-331.

5. Baron MG, Wolf BS, Steinfeld L, et al. Endocardial cushion defects. Specific diagnosis by angiocardiography. *Am J Cardiol*. 1964;13:162-175.

6. Falcao S, Daliento L, Ho SY, et al. Cross sectional echocardiographic assessment of the extent of the atrial septum relative to the atrioventricular junction in atrioventricular septal defect. *Heart*. 1999;81:199-205.

7. Thiene G, Wenink AC, Frescura C, et al. Surgical anatomy and pathology of the conduction tissues in atrioventricular defects. *J Thorac Cardiovasc Surg*. 1981;82:928-937.

8. Meijboom EJ, Wyse RK, Ebels T, et al. Doppler mapping of postoperative left atrioventricular valve regurgitation. *Circulation*. 1988;77:311-315.

9. Kanani M, Elliott M, Cook A, et al. Late incompetence of the left atrioventricular valve after repair of atrioventricular septal defects: the morphologic perspective. *J Thorac Cardiovasc Surg*. 2006;132:640-646.

10. Gallo P, Formigari R, Hokayem NJ, et al. Left ventricular outflow tract obstruction in atrioventricular septal defects: a pathologic and morphometric evaluation. *Clin Cardiol*. 1991;14:513-521.

11. Piccoli GP, Gerlis LM, Wilkinson JL, et al. Morphology and classification of atrioventricular defects. *Br Heart J*. 1979;42:621-632.

12. Chen GZ, Huang GY, Liang XC, et al. Methodological study on real-time three-dimensional echo-cardiography and its application in the diagnosis of complex congenital heart disease. *Chin Med J (Engl)*. 2006;119:1190-1194.

13. Espinola-Zavaleta N, Munoz-Castellanos L, Kuri-Nivon M, et al. Understanding atrioventricular septal defect: anatomoechocardiographic correlation. *Cardiovasc Ultrasound*. 2008;6:33.

14. Del Pasqua A, Sanders SP, de Zorzi A, et al. Impact of three-dimensional echocardiography in complex congenital heart defect cases: the surgical view. *Pediatr Cardiol*. 2009;30:293-300.

15. Uno K, Takenaka K, Ebihara A, et al. Value of live 3D transoesophageal echocardiography in the diagnosis of mitral valve lesions. *Eur J Echocardiogr*. 2009;10:350-351.

16. van den Bosch AE, Ten Harkel DJ, McGhie JS, et al. Surgical validation of real-time transthoracic 3D echocardiographic assessment of atrioventricular septal defects. *Int J Cardiol*. 2006;112:213-218.

17. van den Bosch AE, van Dijk VF, McGhie JS, et al. Real-time transthoracic three-dimensional echocardiography provides additional information of left-sided AV valve morphology after AVSD repair. *Int J Cardiol*. 2006;106:360-364.

18. El-Najdawi EK, Driscoll DJ, Puga FJ, et al. Operation for partial atrioventricular septal defect: a forty-year review. *J Thorac Cardiovasc Surg*. 2000;119:880-889; discussion 889-890.

19. Abbruzzese PA, Napoleone A, Bini RM, et al. Late left atrioventricular valve insufficiency after repair of partial atrioventricular septal defects: anatomical and surgical determinants. *Ann Thorac Surg*. 1990;49:111-114.

20. Poirier NC, Williams WG, Van Arsdell GS, et al. A novel repair for patients with atrioventricular septal defect requiring reoperation for left atrioventricular valve regurgitation. *Eur J Cardiothorac Surg*. 2000;18:54-61.

21. Beregovich J, Bleifer S, Donoso E, et al. The vectorcardiogram and electrocardiogram in persistent common atrioventricular canal. *Circulation*. 1960;21:63-76.

22. Liebman J, Nadas AS. The vectorcardiogram in the differential diagnosis of atrial septal defect in children. *Circulation*. 1960;22:956-975.

23. Spach MS, Boineau JP, Long EC, et al. Genesis of the vectorcardiogram in endocardial cushion defects. *Proceedings of the Long Island Jewish Hospital Symposium*. Amsterdam, the Netherlands: North-Holland Publishing Co; 1965:307-326.

24. Durrer D, Roos JP, van Dam RT. The genesis of the electrocardiogram of patients with ostium primum defects (ventral atrial septal defects). *Am Heart J*. 1966;71:642-650.

25. Sedmera D, Reckova M, Bigelow MR, et al. Developmental transitions in electrical activation patterns in chick embryonic heart. *Anat Rec A Discov Mol Cell Evol Biol*. 2004;280:1001-1009.

26. Brandenburg RO, Burchell HB, Toscano-Barbosa E. Electrocardiographic studies of cases with intracardiac malformations of the atrioventricular canal. *Proc Staff Meet Mayo Clin*. 1956;31:513-523.

27. Anderson RH, Ho SY. The morphology of the specialized atrioventricular junctional area: the evolution of understanding. *Pacing Clin Electrophysiol*. 2002;25:957-966.

28. Khairy P, Mercier LA, Dore A, et al. Partial atrioventricular canal defect with inverted atrioventricular nodal input into an inferiorly displaced atrioventricular node. *Heart Rhythm*. 2007;4:355-358.

29. Lev M. The architecture of the conduction system in congenital heart disease. I. Common atrioventricular orifice. *AMA Arch Pathol*. 1958;65:174-191.

30. Borkon AM, Pieroni DR, Varghese PJ, et al. The superior QRS axis in ostium primum ASD: a proposed mechanism. *Am Heart J*. 1975;90:215-221.

31. James TN. Cardiac conduction system: fetal and postnatal development. *Am J Cardiol*. 1970;25:213-226.

32. Nakaya Y, Hiraga T, Mori H. Histopathologic studies of the conduction system in marked left-axis deviation. *Am J Cardiol*. 1987;60:95-98.

33. Hakacova N, Robinson AM, Olson CW, et al. The relationship between mitral papillary muscles positions and characteristics of the QRS complex. *J Electrocardiol*. 2008;41:487-490.

34. Hakacova N, Wagner GS, Idriss SF. Electroanatomic relationships in patients with primum atrioventricular septal defect. *JACC Cardiovasc Imaging*. 2009;2:1357-1365.

35. Smallhorn JF, de Leval M, Stark J, et al. Isolated anterior mitral cleft. Two dimensional echocardiographic assessment and differentiation from "clefts" associated with atrioventricular septal defect. *Br Heart J*. 1982;48:109-116.

36. Sigfusson G, Ettedgui JA, Silverman NH, et al. Is a cleft in the anterior leaflet of an otherwise normal mitral valve an atrioventricular canal malformation? *J Am Coll Cardiol*. 1995;26:508-515.

37. Minich LL, Atz AM, Colan SD, et al. Partial and transitional atrioventricular septal defect outcomes. *Ann Thorac Surg*. 2010;89:530-536.

38. Manning PB, Mayer JE Jr, Sanders SP, et al. Unique features and prognosis of primum ASD presenting in the first year of life. *Circulation*. 1994;90:II30-II35.

39. Bharucha T, Sivaprakasam MC, Haw MP, et al. The angle of the components of the common atrioventricular valve predicts the outcome of surgical correction in patients with atrioventricular septal defect and common atrioventricular junction. *J Am Soc Echocardiogr*. 2008;21:1099-1104.

40. Anderson RH, Zuberbuhler JR, Penkoske PA, et al. Of clefts, commissures, and things. *J Thorac Cardiovasc Surg*. 1985;90:605-610.

CHAPTER 19

RIGHT VENTRICULAR CARDIOMYOPATHIES

Vincent L. Sorrell, Julia H. Indik, Nishant Kalra, and Frank I. Marcus

INTRODUCTION / 322

**GENERAL CONCEPTS OF RV ANATOMY
    AND PHYSIOLOGY / 322**

SELECTED NONINVASIVE RV IMAGING TECHNIQUES / 325
    Echocardiography / 325
    Nuclear Cardiology / 335
    CMR Imaging / 336
    Multidetector Cardiac Computed Tomography / 338

SELECTED INVASIVE IMAGING TECHNIQUES / 338
    Cine Angiography of the RV / 338
    Intracardiac Echocardiography / 340

SPECIFIC RV CARDIOMYOPATHIES / 340
    General Approach (Algorithm) / 340
    RV Dysfunction Secondary to LV Dysfunction / 340
    RV Infarction / 340
    RV Volume Overload / 342
    Congenital Heart Disease / 342
    RV Pressure Overload / 343
    Pericardial Constriction / 345
    Arrhythmogenic RV Cardiomyopathy/Dysplasia / 346
    UHL Anomaly / 350

FUTURE ASPECTS OF RV MULTIMODAL IMAGING / 350

INTRODUCTION

The evaluation of right ventricular (RV) size and function in normal and pathologic conditions is challenging due to its complex shape and nonsymmetrical contraction. Unlike the left ventricle (LV), the RV is crescent shaped and truncated, with separate inflow and outflow portions. The normal RV is triangular (curved) when viewed sagittally, crescent shaped when viewed axially, and similar to a teapot when viewed coronally (Fig. 19–1). It is thin walled, highly trabeculated, and devoid of the LV's extensive circumferential myofibrillar architecture. The RV apex may be dominated by the shape and function of the LV apex or may be entirely separate and independent ("butterfly" apex) (Fig. 19–2).[1] The RV is strongly influenced by the normally concave interventricular septum, and its shape is influenced by acute and chronic pathologic pressure and volume changes. Whereas the normal LV has the shape of a prolate ellipse (and becomes a sphere in many disease states), there is no convenient model that accurately approximates normal or pathologic RV geometry.

This chapter describes the unique characteristics of the RV and offers a comprehensive, multimodal imaging approach to the investigation of the normal and pathologic RV.

GENERAL CONCEPTS OF RV ANATOMY AND PHYSIOLOGY

The RV is notable for its distinctive shape, heavy trabeculation, prominent moderator band, and lack of fibrous continuity between the tricuspid and pulmonic valves. The RV can be considered to be composed of three components: the inflow (or inlet), the outflow (outlet, conus, or infundibulum), and the apex. The RV inflow tract and outflow tract are separated by the thick crista supraventricularis band of muscle fibers. The apex is virtually immobile and usually tethered to the LV apex. These three parts develop separately, are independently subjected to congenital malformations, and have unique responses to pathology and pharmacologic interventions. The RV myocardium is usually 2- to 3-mm thick with subepicardial myofibers arranged in a circumferential network parallel to the atrioventricular groove, encircling the RV outflow tract (RVOT), and then becoming more spirally orientated near the RV apex.[2,3] The inflow is mainly composed of circumferential fibers in the subepicardium and longitudinal fibers in the subendocardium. At the outflow tract, both subendocardial and subepicardial fibers run longitudinally. The majority of the RV myocardium is devoid of the middle circumferential myofiber array that is dominant in the LV and is much more dependent on longitudinal shortening for ejection than the LV.[4] During systole, at the inflow tract, there is longitudinal shortening from base to apex and circumferential motion toward the common septum. Thus, simple global measures of RV function are difficult due to the two portions contracting perpendicular to each other.

The global RV performance is determined by the following regional contraction patterns: (1) movement of the basal free wall toward the apex (the "bellows effect"); (2) the contraction of the RVOT; (3) the contribution of the LV (tethering) at the interventricular insertion sites; and (4) the influence of the ventricular septum (interventricular dependence). Interventricular dependence is illustrated by impairment of RV function due to the adjacent diseased LV, but not necessarily due to a myopathic process itself.[5] This should be considered when assessing RV performance. The evaluation of regional RV wall motion must take into consideration the variable contraction patterns near the moderator, parietal, and septomarginal bands because the muscle bundles may alter the symmetric contraction of the RV free wall (Table 19–1).

These features of RV contraction are important in understanding and estimating RV function. Because the predominant RV fractional shortening is significantly greater longitudinally than circumferentially, an evaluation of longitudinal shortening provides a relatively simple and reliable estimate of global RV function. RV function is also influenced by volume shifts that occur with normal respiration. During inspiration, venous return increases, causing an increased RV preload, with a slight but detectable increase in RV stroke volume. Therefore, when

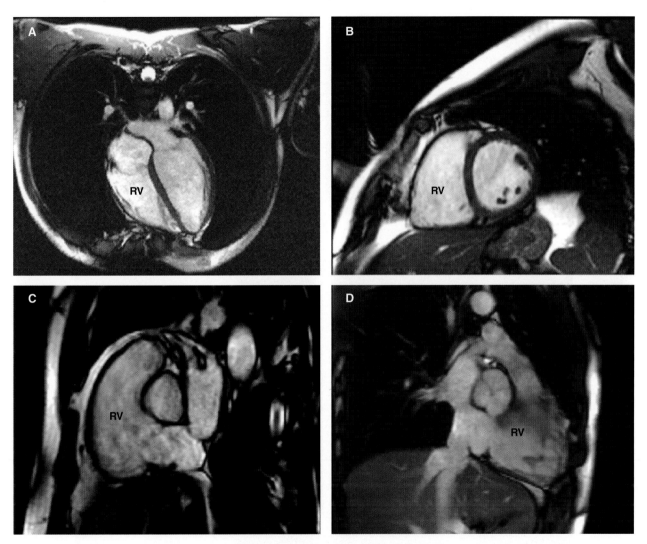

FIGURE 19–1. Representative cardiac magnetic resonance (CMR) white blood images. The normal right ventricle (RV) is crescent shaped when viewed axially (**A**), triangular (curved) when viewed sagittally (**B** and **C**), and similar to a teapot when viewed coronally (**D**).

TABLE 19–1. Incidence of Right Ventricular Wall Motion Abnormalities in the Various Planes According to the Segment Involved, Type, and Relation to the Insertion of the Moderator Band/Trabeculae

Findings n = 29 (100%)	Axial n (%)	SAX n (%)	LAX n (%)
Segment affected			
Apicolateral	23 (79.3)	-	10 (34.5)
Mediolateral	10 (34.5)	-	5 (17.2)
Basolateral	-	-	-
Inferolateral	-	4 (13.8)	-
Wall motion abnormality	*25 (86.2)*	*4 (13.8)*	*12 (41.4)*
Dyskinesia	19 (79.3)	-	9 (31.0)
Hypokinesia	9 (31.0)	-	3 (10.3)
Bulging	2 (6.9)	4 (13.8)	3 (10.3)
Relation to insertion MB			
To right	14 (48.3)	-	4 (13.8)
To left	6 (20.7)	2 (6.9)	3 (10.3)

Modified from: Sievers B, et al. Right ventricular wall motion abnormalities in healthy subjects imaged with cardiovascular magnetic resonance imaging and characterized with a new segmental model. *J Cardiovasc Magn Res*. 2004;6:601-608.

carefully measuring RV performance, one should consider whether data were acquired during inspiration, expiration, or apnea (preferred). Lastly, a regional difference in response to inotropic stimulation has been observed, with the RVOT being more reactive than the RV inflow tract.[6] This may be important when evaluating response to treatment with inotropic drugs.

The LV and RV have the same stroke volume, but the upper limit of normal RV volume is greater than the LV. This explains why the normal RV ejection fraction (EF) is lower than the LVEF (example: RV in diastole, 100 mL; RV in systole, 55 mL; RV stroke volume, 45 mL; RVEF = 45/100 = 45%; LV in diastole, 90 mL; LV in systole, 45 mL; LV stroke volume, 45 mL; LVEF = 45/90 = 50%).

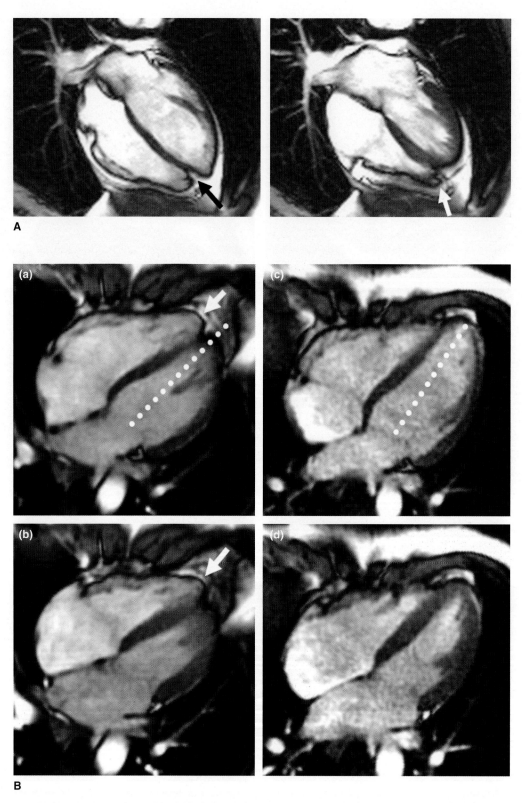

FIGURE 19–2. A. Cardiac magnetic resonance imaging white blood (steady-state free precession) cine image. The right ventricular (RV) apex is entirely separate and independent from the left ventricular (LV) apex ("butterfly" apex; black arrow). **Left.** Diastole. **Right.** Systole. Note the thin hypokinetic RV apex in this normal patient (white arrow). **B.** Importance of foreshortening. This is a normal volunteer without heart disease. Note the left panel images (**a** = diastole; **b** = systole) that were obtained within minutes of the right panel images (**c** = diastole; **d** = systole). The image on the left was obtained with a slightly inferior angulation relative to the truly aligned four-chamber view on the right creating a foreshortened LV long axis diameter (dotted lines equal length). Due to the pyramidal RV shape, this inferior angulation creates an elongated RV cavity relative to the LV. This creates a falsely dilated RV cavity and also accentuates the RV apex, which appears separated from the LV ("butterfly") and hypokinetic (arrows). See Moving Image 19–2B.

The pulmonary circulation normally has a low vascular resistance, and consequently, the RV has short isovolumic contraction time (ICT) and isovolumic relaxation time (IRT). The superficial circumferential fibers contract during the ICT, but during the ejection period, the deeper longitudinal fibers contract and are responsible for the longitudinal shortening. During the phase of isovolumic contraction, the longitudinal shortening of the RV occurs mainly during the ejection phase of the cardiac cycle controlled by the subendocardial fibers. Onset of RV ejection at the outflow tract is delayed approximately 25 to 50 ms after the onset of contraction of the inflow tract. These anatomic considerations provide the potential for specific regional markers of RV contractility.

In summary, RV function is difficult to assess due to its complex anatomy and physiology. Various noninvasive and invasive techniques have been used to evaluate RV function and their strengths and limitations will be discussed.

SELECTED NONINVASIVE RV IMAGING TECHNIQUES

■ ECHOCARDIOGRAPHY

Echocardiography is and will likely remain a first-line diagnostic imaging modality for evaluating the RV structure and function because of its availability and because it is a noninvasive, rapid, portable, and comprehensive approach to assess patients with suspected right heart disease. Accurate evaluation of RV morphology and function requires integration of multiple echocardiographic views, including parasternal long and short axis, RV inflow, apical four-chamber, and subcostal views.[7] Although multiple quantitative methods for RV assessment are listed, assessment of RV structure and function remains mostly qualitative in clinical practice. Methods commonly used to calculate the LV volume may be used to calculate RV volumes but are less accurate due to the complex geometry. Due to these inherent limitations, a number of geometry-independent parameters have been proposed.

One-Dimensional Echocardiography (M-Mode)

The commonly reported RV internal diameter obtained with M-mode in the parasternal long axis view is an unreliable marker of RV dilation because the anterior RV wall is often poorly seen. The irregular RV shape may result in the M-mode cursor transecting either the wider central plane or a narrower peripheral site because the cursor may transect the RV in an oblique manner.

The total tricuspid annular descent or tricuspid annular plane systolic excursion (TAPSE) is an important marker of RV global systolic function (normal, 20 mm). The TAPSE can be derived from M-mode analysis of the lateral tricuspid annular ring or Doppler tissue imaging (DTI) color display (Fig. 19–3). Interestingly, for such a simple marker of RV function, the correlation between TAPSE and RVEF by cardiac magnetic resonance (CMR) was superior to radionuclide techniques and three-dimensional estimates of RVEF.[8]

Two-Dimensional Echocardiography

Normally, the LV appears larger than the RV in the parasternal long and short axis and the apical four-chamber view. To use this evaluation of RV size, care must be taken not to foreshorten the LV and overestimate the relative RV size (see Fig. 19–2B). For volume calculations, additional problems are encountered. During RV dilation, the already complex geometry undergoes significant and variable shape changes. Therefore, geometric formulas used for normal RV shapes are not likely to be valid in pathologic conditions. Despite attempts to obtain orthogonal RV images necessary for volume calculations, most commonly using the apical four-chamber and subcostal views, it remains difficult to validate that they are orthogonal.[9]

Because the RVOT is composed of a preponderance of circumferential myofibers, this region is an estimate of global RV function. The RVOT fractional shortening can be calculated as the percentage of the RVOT diastolic diameter minus the systolic diameter divided by the diastolic diameter. Either two-dimensional (2D) or M-mode echocardiography of the basal parasternal short axis view at the level of the aortic root can be used to measure this value, and this value has been shown to correlate with TAPSE. Importantly, it closely correlates with other physiologic events, such as the shortened pulmonary acceleration time recorded at the cusp level in patients with pulmonary hypertension.[10]

The RVEF can be determined using the area-length method applied to the apical four-chamber view or an adequate subcostal view.[11] Similar to its proven value in the assessment of LV diseases, contrast echocardiography has recently been shown to be of value in evaluating the presence of RV pathology.[12] Occasionally, agitated saline contrast alone may improve the visualization of the RV borders. If ineffective, a contrast agent (activated perflutren) can be administered to improve the echocardiographic assessment of the RV size and global and regional function (Fig. 19–4). When image quality is suboptimal, contrast should be administered and has been demonstrated to be safe and cost effective.[13]

Global, systolic RV function can be assessed quantitatively using 2D echocardiography analysis as percentage of change in the RV cavity area from end-diastole to end-systole in the apical four-chamber view. End-diastole is identified by the onset of the R wave, whereas end-systole is regarded as the smallest RV cavity size just before the tricuspid valve opening. Endocardial borders of the RV free wall and septum are traced from base to apex, and the RV fractional area change (RV FAC) is defined using the following formula: (end-diastolic area – end-systolic area)/(end-diastolic area) × 100 (Fig. 19–5). Heavy RV trabeculation makes endocardial tracing difficult and requires an adequate quality image for accuracy of this parameter. This technique incorporates the RV inflow tract and the apex but excludes the RVOT and may overestimate RV function if focal regional dysfunction exists in this region. The percentage of RV FAC is a relatively simple parameter that is a surrogate marker of the RVEF and correlates well with CMR-derived RVEF ($r = 0.80$).[14]

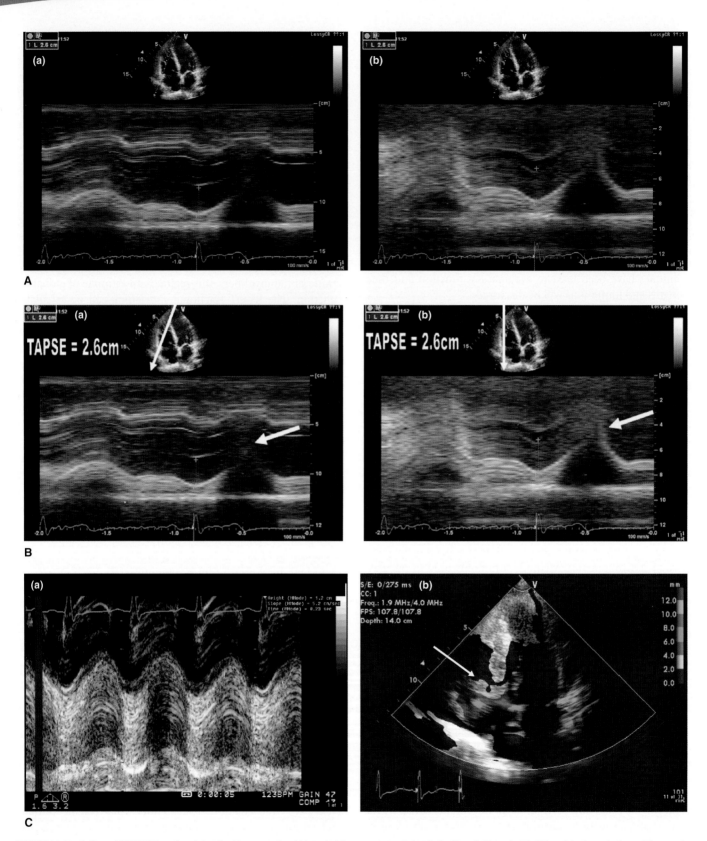

FIGURE 19–3. A. Normal TAPSE (26 mm) as determined by conventional M-mode (**a**) versus anatomic (vertically aligned) M-mode (**b**). Although both methods provide reproducible values, the conventional M-mode that includes the RV cavity is easier to measure with higher signal-to-noise ratio at end-systole (arrows). **B.** The TAPSE can be derived from M-mode analysis (**a**) of the lateral tricuspid annular ring or Doppler tissue imaging color display (**b**). This patient has normal global RV function with TAPSE >20 mm and "purple" basal RV (white arrow). **C.** Markedly reduced global RV systolic function and a TAPSE of 12 mm. Note the red and yellow color at the base of the RV instead of the normal purple display (white arrow).

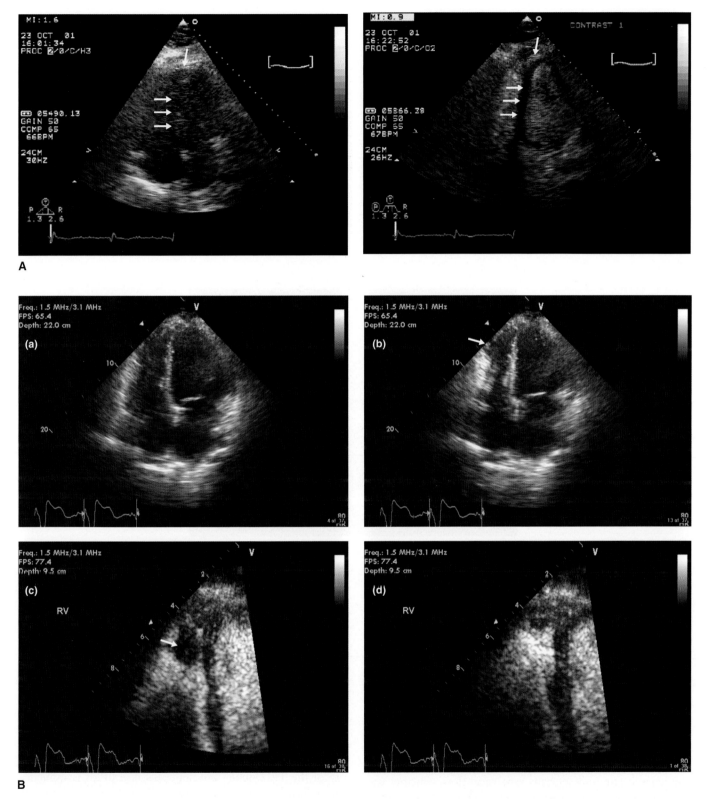

FIGURE 19–4. A. Contrast echocardiography. A second-generation contrast agent (activated Perflutren) can be administered to improve the echocardiographic assessment of the right ventricular (RV) size and global and regional function. **Left** (unenhanced image). RV apex and septal border (arrows) cannot be seen. **Right** (contrast enhanced). Both the RV endocardial border and the RV apex are seen (arrows). The RV apex occupies the cardiac apex, which is abnormal and consistent with RV dilation. **B.** Contrast echocardiography. Unenhanced apical 4-chamber view in diastole (a) and systole (b). A wall motion abnormality is suggested at end-systole (arrow). Contrast-enhanced images in diastole (c) and systole (d) reveal a large filling defect consistent with a thrombus not previously suspected (arrow). A large filling defect (arrow) is seen in the RV apex of this patient with a dilated cardiomyopathy (normal coronary arteries). See Moving Image 19–4B.

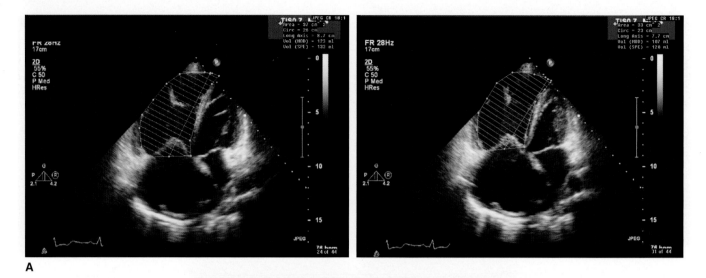

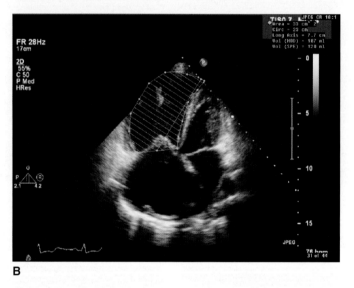

FIGURE 19–5. A. B. Transthoracic 2D echocardiographic images in diastole (left) and systole (right). Endocardial borders of the right ventricular free wall and septum are traced from base to apex, and the RV FAC% is defined using the following formula: (end-diastolic area – end-systolic area)/(end-diastolic area) × 100 (%). In this patient, there is severely reduced RV systolic function. See Moving Image 19–5B.

Conventional Doppler Techniques

Pulsed wave Doppler tricuspid flow velocity helps evaluate RV filling and, indirectly, RV diastolic function. Peak flow velocity in early diastole (E wave), peak velocity at atrial contraction (A wave), tricuspid deceleration time, and tricuspid A wave duration are variables that can be compared with their mitral counterparts to assess for unilateral or bilateral heart disease. The hepatic vein and superior vena caval flow velocities can be obtained with pulsed wave Doppler and analyzed during apnea or in response to volume changes that occur with normal respiration. Increased flow reversals in the hepatic vein (>20%) or superior vena cava (>10%) during apnea suggest increased right-sided heart filling pressures. Increased flow reversals in response to inspiration or expiration can be seen in patients with restrictive or constrictive cardiomyopathies, respectively.[15-17]

Because tricuspid regurgitation (TR) is common, the rate of RV pressure increase can be obtained from the continuous-wave spectral Doppler TR signal. The time interval (dt) necessary to increase the TR velocity from 0 to 2 m/s is measured (Fig. 19–6). This represents a pressure change (dP) of 16 mm Hg. The dP/dt value is considered normal if it is greater than 400 mm Hg/s.[18] The accuracy of this method is directly dependent on the quality of the TR Doppler envelope. Because dP/dt is influenced by preload, adding the maximal TR velocity (P_{max}) into the equation as dP/dt/P_{max} compensates for changes in preload.[19] In patients with dominant RV failure, TR-derived dP/dt/P_{max}, but not dP/dt alone, has been identified as a clinically useful index of RV contractility.

The RV index of myocardial performance (RIMP; or Tei index) is defined as the sum of the ICT and IRT divided by the ejection time and is increased in either systolic or diastolic RV

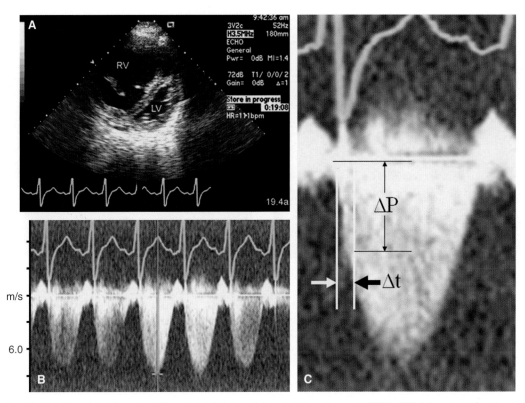

FIGURE 19–6. Two-dimensional (2D) and Doppler echocardiography. Calculation of time derivative of pressure (dP/dt; $\Delta P/\Delta t$) from the tricuspid regurgitation (TR) spectral Doppler envelope. **A.** 2D echocardiography demonstrating dilated right ventricle (RV) with "compressed" left ventricle (LV) from severe pulmonary hypertension. **B.** Estimated pulmonary artery systolic pressure >5 m/s (>100 mm Hg). **C.** Zoom TR spectral Doppler image. The time interval (Δt) necessary to increase the TR velocity from 0 to 2 m/s (or from 1 to 3 m/s if marked pulmonary hypertension is present, as in this case example) is measured. ΔP, change in pressure.

dysfunction (Fig. 19–7).[20] An elevated RIMP has been shown to be an early sign of RV dysfunction in cardiac amyloidosis.[21] Patients with hypertrophic cardiomyopathy and exertional dyspnea have an increased global RIMP compared to those without dyspnea.[22] A value ≥0.40 has a sensitivity of 81% and a specificity of 85% to diagnose RVEF <35%. A value <0.25 has a sensitivity of 70% and a specificity of 89% to identify patients with RVEF ≥0.50.[23] Doppler-derived RIMP measurement correlates with the CMR-derived RVEF and is a simple and reliable method for the evaluation of RV function in adults with repaired tetralogy of Fallot. This index is a marker of prognosis in patients with heart failure and primary pulmonary hypertension and has been used for risk stratification.[24,25]

Tissue Doppler Imaging

Tissue Doppler imaging of the RV is a useful and readily applicable adjunct to the comprehensive echocardiography Doppler assessment of the RV by transthoracic echocardiography. Tissue Doppler imaging permits analysis of the RV longitudinal myocardial velocity. Because the RV is composed of a network of clockwise and counter-clockwise endocardial and epicardial longitudinal myofibers, the RV myocardial velocity reflects RV systolic function. Similar to the LV, five major deflections are visualized on tissue Doppler imaging of the RV tricuspid

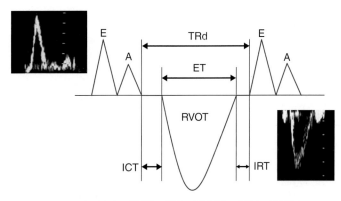

Tei index (IMP) = ICT + IRT/ET or TRd – ET/ET

FIGURE 19–7. The Tei index (of myocardial performance) is measured using conventional pulsed wave Doppler. The tricuspid inflow (E and A waves) and the right ventricular outflow tract (RVOT) spectral Doppler analysis is all that is required. Because this requires two different ultrasound windows (and different cardiac cycles), care must be given to minimize time lag between image acquisition (and thereby minimize changes in HR). To obtain the Tei index from one ultrasound window and reduce chance for HR difference errors, the duration of the tricuspid regurgitation (TRd) can be used if tricuspid regurgitation is present. A, tricuspid inflow late (atrial) wave; E, tricuspid inflow early wave; ET, ejection time; IMP, index of myocardial performance; IVCT, isovolumic contraction time; IVRT, isovolumic relaxation time.

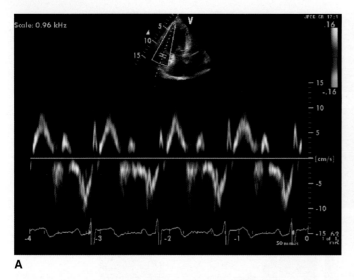 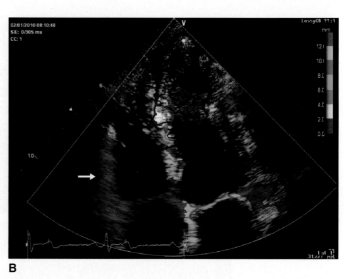

A   **B**

FIGURE 19–8. A. Five major deflections are visualized on tissue Doppler imaging of the right ventricular (RV) tricuspid annulus: the isovolumic contraction time wave (ICT), systolic velocity (Sa), isovolumic relaxation time wave (IRT), early diastolic velocity (Ea), and late diastolic velocity (Aa). **B.** Tissue Doppler evaluation of the RV myocardium allows for color coding of the derivative of tissue velocity (displacement). Note the normal visually estimated tricuspid annular plane systolic excursion (TAPSE) where the basal half of the RV myocardial wall moves >12 mm at end-systole (purple color of the basal RV; arrow).

annulus: ICT wave, systolic velocity, IRT wave, early diastolic velocity, and late diastolic velocity (Fig. 19–8). Timing of the RV events can be measured using a high frame rate, leading to an alternative calculation of RIMP (Fig. 19–9A). Because short time measurements are analyzed to derive this value, it is imperative that high-quality tissue Doppler imaging tracings are obtained with satisfactory temporal resolution.

Tissue Doppler can also be used to record the peak systolic velocity of the tricuspid annulus (s'). In healthy individuals, the lower normal limit at the basal RV lateral wall is ≥14 ± 2 cm/s for DTI spectral displays and ≥10 ± 2 cm/s for DTI color displays. This velocity has been shown to correlate more closely with CMR-derived RVEF than the fractional area change (FAC), DTI-derived tissue displacement, systolic strain, and strain rate.[26] An s' <9.5 cm/s identifies patients with an RVEF <40%.[27] Thresholds of >12, 12 to 9, and <9 cm/s allow differentiation between normal (>55%), moderately reduced (30%-55%), and severely reduced (<30%) RVEF, respectively.[28]

Myocardial velocity of the RV free wall as measured by DTI during the ICT phase has also been used to estimate RV contractility. However, this parameter is more sensitive to loading conditions than the other listed markers. Myocardial acceleration during the earliest phase of ICT is a novel index for the assessment of RV contractile function that is less affected by preload and afterload changes.[29] This index is calculated by dividing myocardial velocity during ICT by the time interval from the onset of this wave to the time at peak velocity (Fig. 19–9).

Tissue Doppler measures are dependent on the Doppler cursor angle. This limitation is overcome with 2D strain measures (speckle tracking) and, being angle independent, allows the evaluation of regional function in all myocardial segments, including the ventricular apex (Fig. 19–10). Ultrasound "speckles" in the RV wall are tracked and allow the determination of the global

and regional, frame-to-frame measure of myocardial velocities, 2D strain, and strain rate. Peak systolic strain and strain rate, particularly of the basal RV free wall, are significantly impaired in patients with pulmonary arterial hypertension and have been used as an index of RV function.[30]

The quantification of regional myocardial function remains a challenge. One main limitation of conventional DTI is that an akinetic segment may still possess measurable myocardial velocities due to being tethered to a normal adjacent myocardial segment. Strain and strain rate are indices of myocardial deformation that largely overcome this limitation. Strain rate (velocity of deformation) can be calculated from the spatial gradient

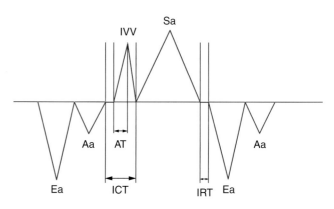

FIGURE 19–9. A. The Tei index (of myocardial performance) may also be measured using myocardial tissue Doppler echocardiography (TDE) instead of conventional Doppler. The tricuspid annular TDE spectral analysis is all that is required. This method only uses one ultrasound window and reduces the chance for heart rate difference errors. The acceleration time (AT) of the isovolumic contraction time (ICT) may also be obtained (see text for details). Aa, tricuspid TDE annular late (atrial) wave; AT, acceleration time; Ea, tricuspid TDE annular early wave; IRT, isovolumic relaxation time; IVV, (isovolumic velocity); Sa, tricuspid TDE annular systolic wave.

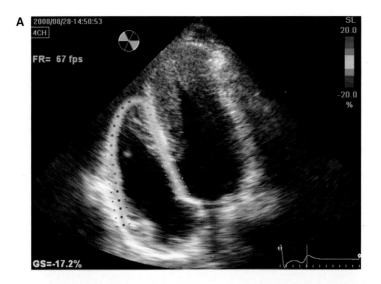

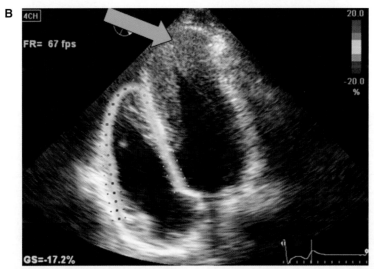

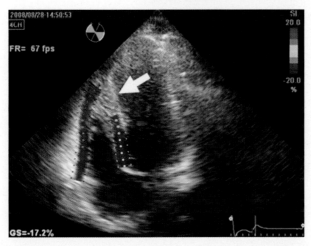
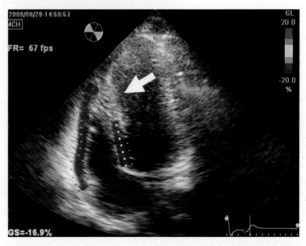

FIGURE 19–10. RV speckle tracking allows for color coding of normal two-dimensional strain that is not dependent on cursor angle limitations, which is a limitation of tissue Doppler echocardiography. **A.** End-diastole. **B.** End-systole. Images in **B** were acquired at different times demonstrating the reproducibility of results. Red = normal. Note the mildly abnormal distal septal and apical region on both data sets (pink; white arrow). Although this may be an artifact from using a technique designed for the left ventricle (LV), in this patient with an apical hypertrophic cardiomyopathy (note LV apex; green arrow), abnormal apical strain of the RV would be expected.

in velocities recorded between two neighboring points in the tissue (Fig. 19–11).[31] The longitudinal RV strain and strain rate values are higher and more inhomogeneous than those in the LV. Mean values for longitudinal strain and strain rate are lowest in the basal RV segments and increase toward the apical segments. Strain rate imaging is independent of overall motion.

The quantification of regional RV function using either 2D or DTI strain values is feasible and reproducible.[32] This technique has a potential role in the initial and serial assessment of patients with primary or secondary RV disease and correlates with invasive and CMR findings of RV performance.[33]

Three-Dimensional Echocardiography

Three-dimensional (3D) echocardiographic analysis of the RV has recently been reported to eliminate the geometric intricacies of the RV. Due to the nongeometric 3D shape of the RV, the measurement of RV volume is challenging, resulting in numerous qualitative, but limited quantitative, measures. Recently, real-time 3D echocardiography (RT3DE) has become available and can provide reliable, reproducible measures of RV volumes

independent of geometric assumptions.[34] By manually tracing the endocardial borders during systole and diastole, the RV volumes are determined, and RVEF is calculated. Because an image of the entire RV is acquired in a single pyramidal data set, any acoustic window will increase the likelihood that adequate quality data are obtained (Fig. 19–12). For measuring RV volume and RVEF, RT3DE is more accurate and reproducible than 2D echocardiography and has less variation and higher correlation to CMR.[35] Normal RT3DE values of the RV size and function are listed in Table 19–2.[36]

In a study of 200 patients, including normal controls and patients with valvular heart disease, pulmonary hypertension, and dilated cardiomyopathies, RT3DE results were compared with results from conventional 2D and RV Doppler flow and showed a positive correlation of 3D RVEF with TAPSE, FAC, and peak s′ tissue Doppler echocardiography (TDE) velocity and a negative correlation with pulmonary artery pressure.[37] Adequate, good-quality 3D acquisition was obtained in nearly all patients with a mean time of 3 ± 1 minutes. The technique of RT3DE has been validated in phantoms, animals

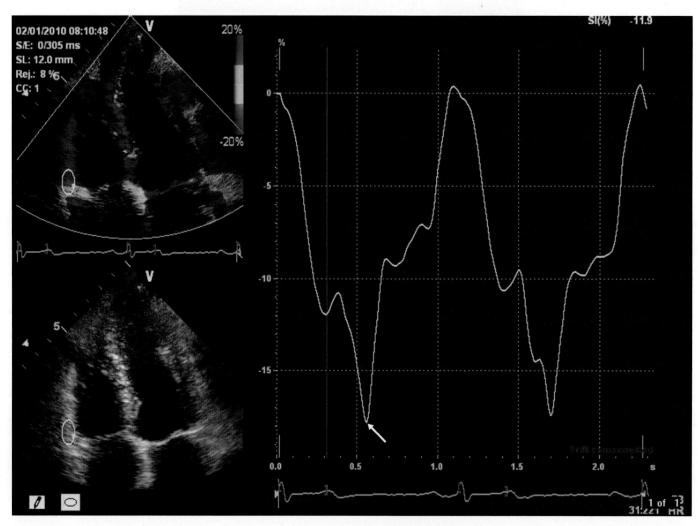

FIGURE 19–11. Tissue Doppler echocardiography quantitative strain assessment of basal right ventricular deformation. The peak systolic strain is normal at −18% (arrow).

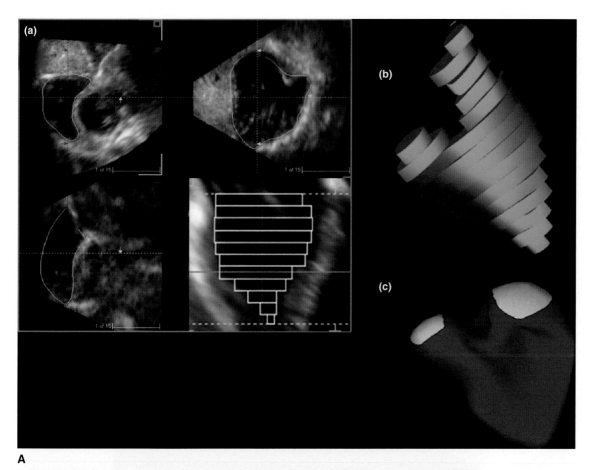

A

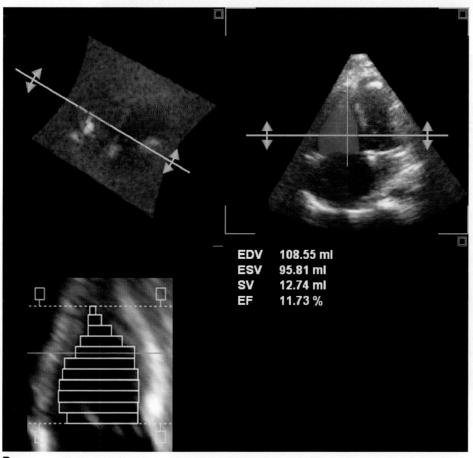

EDV	108.55 ml
ESV	95.81 ml
SV	12.74 ml
EF	11.73 %

B

FIGURE 19–12. A. Three-dimensional (3D) echocardiography. **a.** Right ventricular (RV) triplane series with stacked right ventricular slices. Manual traced RV endocardial borders from the sagittal, coronal, and axial orientations provide a disk summation method (Simpson's rule) of volume and ejection fraction (EF) (**b**) and creation of a dynamic, smoothed 3D surface model (**c**). This method incorporates the longitudinal motion (tricuspid annular plane systolic excursion), the RV outflow tract contraction (fractional area change), and the interventricular dependence (septal contour). **B.** 3D echocardiography. This patient has a markedly dilated RV and severely reduced RVEF (see normal values in Table 19–2). EDV, end-diastolic volume; ESV, end-systolic volume; SV, stroke volume. See Moving Image 19–12B. **C.** Color-coded, regional surface maps of the RV provide assessment of regional contraction patterns and segmental time-volume curves. Red = apex; green = RV inflow; yellow = RV outflow. **D.** 3D echocardiogram. Because the entire RV is acquired in a single pyramidal data set, any available acoustic window will increase the likelihood that adequate quality data are obtained. This is the same patient as in Fig. 19–5 (note the similarity of the calculated RVEF demonstrating severe global RV dysfunction).

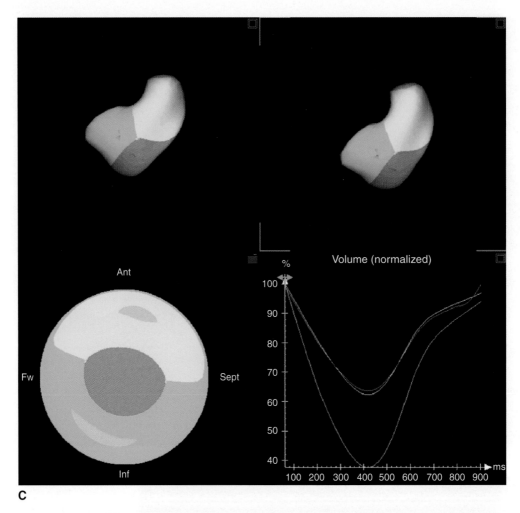

C

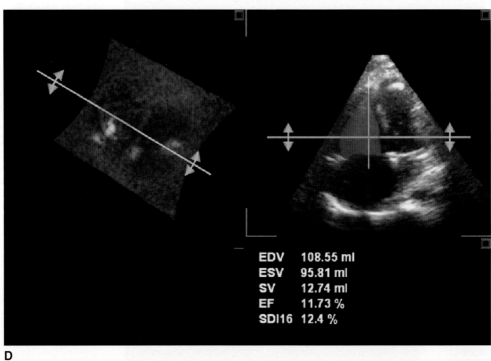

EDV	108.55 ml
ESV	95.81 ml
SV	12.74 ml
EF	11.73 %
SDI16	12.4 %

D

FIGURE 9–12. *(continued)*

TABLE 19–2. Normal Right Ventricular Volume/Body Surface Area Using CMR and RT3DE

Volume	n	CMR (mL/m²) Mean (SD)	RT3DE (mL/m²) Mean (SD)
EDV			
All	71	71.3 (12.9)	70.0 (12.9)
Men	36	67.1 (12.1)	65.4 (13.4)
Women	35	75.6 (12.4)	74.7 (13.0)
ESV			
All		33.5 (9.9)	33.4 (10.3)
Men		28.6 (8.1)	29.2 (10.7)
Women		38.4 (9.1)	37.8 (7.4)
FF			
All		53.3 (8.7)	52.6 (9.9)
Men		57.5 (7.0)	56.2 (9.1)
Women		49.0 (8.8)	48.9 (9.5)

Note the consistent findings that female right ventricular (RV) cavities are larger and the RV ejection fraction is lower than male RV cavities.

CMR, cardiac magnetic resonance; EDV, end-diastolic volume; EF, ejection fraction; ESV, end-systolic volume; RT3DE, real-time three-dimensional echocardiography; SD, standard deviation.

Modified from: Gopal AS, et al. Normal values of right ventricular size and function by real-time three-dimensional echocardiography: comparison to cardiac magnetic resonance imaging. *J Am Soc Echocardiogr.* 2007;20:445-455.

studies, adult patients with RV cardiomyopathies, and children with congenital heart diseases.[38] Excellent correlation exists with magnetic resonance imaging (MRI) reference standards, although there is a common underestimation of RV volumes. Although additional data from RT3DE studies including a wider variety of RV pathologies are needed, this option appears to be the most cost-effective reference standard for quantitative RV volume and EF determination.

Transesophageal Echocardiography

In patients with suboptimal transthoracic echocardiographic windows, transesophageal echocardiography (TEE) may be considered because the esophageal window is frequently adequate for cardiac assessment. There are few studies reported on the use of this method for assessment of the RV. Most reports are from intraoperative studies where inotropic medications and rapid fluid shifts limit the interpretation of reported findings. In a study of 25 children with atrial septal defects undergoing surgical correction, 90% had adequate 3D TEE studies.[39] RV volumes had an excellent correlation with direct surgical measures ($r^2 = 0.99$), obtained at the end of surgery by injecting saline solution through the tricuspid valve using a graduated syringe, but had a slight, consistent overestimation.

If tricuspid or pulmonic valve disease is suspected, this is a valuable complementary diagnostic tool. This approach is also useful for the assessment of the atrial septum for congenital defects or to determine whether RVOT obstruction is a cause

of RV dilation or dysfunction. In general, TEE is reserved for patients in whom the transthoracic echocardiogram is suboptimal, despite the use of contrast, and when CMR is unavailable.

■ NUCLEAR CARDIOLOGY

First-Pass Radionuclide Angiography

Radionuclide angiography (RNA) is the historical reference standard for RVEF and has been used to measure global and regional RV abnormalities.[40] A significant advantage of this technique is its reliance on a count-based method that is independent of geometry. This technique relies on separation of the radioactivity within the RV from adjacent structures, especially the right atrium. The RVEF is calculated by tracing the RV cavity in an end-diastolic and end-systolic frame. The most accurate method to achieve this is a gated first-pass RNA. This ensures that the radioisotope remains within the RV cavity and allows acquisition of RV functional data prior to the isotope crossing the pulmonary vasculature and contaminating the field of interest with left atrial and LV radioactivity. Although nuclear scans are widely available, first-pass RNA studies are not commonly performed.

Equilibrium-Gated RNA

Multigated acquisition (MUGA) equilibrium scans are used for analysis of functional LV data but are not optimal for RV assessment and result in underestimation of the RVEF. We have found that first-pass RNA correlates better with CMR determined RVEF, as compared with gated equilibrium RNA.[41]

Myocardial Perfusion Imaging Single Photon Emission Computed Tomography

Myocardial perfusion imaging (MPI) using electrocardiogram (ECG)-gated single photon emission computed tomography (SPECT) is commonly performed for evaluation of myocardial ischemia. It is not used primarily to evaluate LV (or RV) function, but this information is obtained and is valuable when an ischemia assessment is performed. Its specific role in evaluating RV pathology is limited. Indirect evidence of RV dilation and RV hypertrophy may be seen as increased RV radiotracer uptake, but SPECT cannot clarify whether this is due to valvular or congenital heart disease, pulmonary arterial hypertension, or a primary RV cardiomyopathy.[42] MPI is most valuable to assess LV myocardial ischemia or scar and may assist in the indirect assessment of the patient with RV cardiomyopathy.

Radiolabeled Meta-Iodobenzylguanidine Imaging

Radiolabeled iodine 123–meta-iodobenzylguanidine (^{123}I-mIBG), also known as iobenguane, an analog of the false neurotransmitter guanethidine, is used to scintigraphically map the adrenergic system in the myocardium. This agent localizes in adrenergic nerve terminals primarily by the norepinephrine transporter and is decreased in heart failure patients with the poorest prognosis.[43,44] Because sympathetic innervation of the heart participates in the regulation of myocardial contractility and because there is a link between catecholamine hypersensitivity and ventricular arrhythmias, there may be diagnostic value for predicting arrhythmic substrate in cardiomyopathies. Abnormalities of myocardial ^{123}I-mIBG uptake have been reported to be predictive of ventricular arrhythmias and sudden cardiac death in patients with idiopathic ventricular fibrillation.[45] The RV myocardium cannot be adequately studied with this agent, but coexistent LV involvement may be identified earlier than with other diagnostic modalities.

■ CMR IMAGING

Black Blood, Static Imaging

High spatial resolution images can be obtained using spin-echo CMR sequences and ECG and respiratory gating optimized to minimize cardiac motion artifacts.[46] This provides high image detail of the RV myocardium to assess cavity shape, wall thickness, and intracavitary structures such as the papillary muscles and moderator band. A fat saturation pulse can confirm the presence and extent of fat. Cardiac valves, being thinner

and highly mobile, are less well visualized than they are with echocardiography (Fig. 19–13A).

White Blood, Cine Imaging

It is possible to accurately calculate both LV and RV volumes simultaneously by CMR.[35,47] Both ventricles are imaged in the same acquisition, and multiple short axis slices are obtained. From each short axis slice of known thickness, the area is calculated, and the summed volumes are determined using Simpson's rule (Fig. 19–13B). This method is not dependent on acoustic windows, is not limited by geometric assumptions, and rarely has poor-quality results. CMR has excellent interstudy reproducibility in healthy subjects, patients with heart failure, and patients with hypertrophy. Quantitative RV volume and function have been validated in a large, multiethnic study.[48]

CMR is considered the reference standard for research investigations and for serial measures in patients with chronic heart diseases, especially involving the RV. Rarely, assessment of the RV volume may be challenging due to poor delineation of the

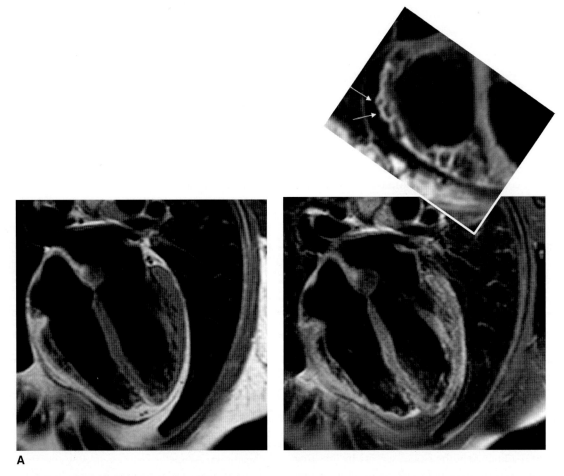

FIGURE 19–13. **A.** Cardiac magnetic resonance imaging. Black blood spin-echo sequence (left) with fat saturation demonstrated (right) and a zoom image (top) confirming extensive fatty myocardial replacement (arrows) in the patient with confirmed arrhythmogenic right ventricular cardiomyopathy/dysplasia (ARVC/D). **B.** Cardiac MRI using a white blood steady-state free precession (SSFP) cine image sequence. Simpson's rule is used to obtain 10 short axis slices for comprehensive assessment of the entire heart from base (1) to apex (10). The endocardium of the right ventricle (RV) and left ventricle (LV) is manually traced. **C.** Cardiac MRI image in patient with ARVC/D. Myocardial delayed contrast enhancement sequence. **Left.** Short axis. **Right.** Long axis. Note the black LV myocardium (normal; white arrows) compared with extensive fibrosis of the white RV myocardium (black arrows).

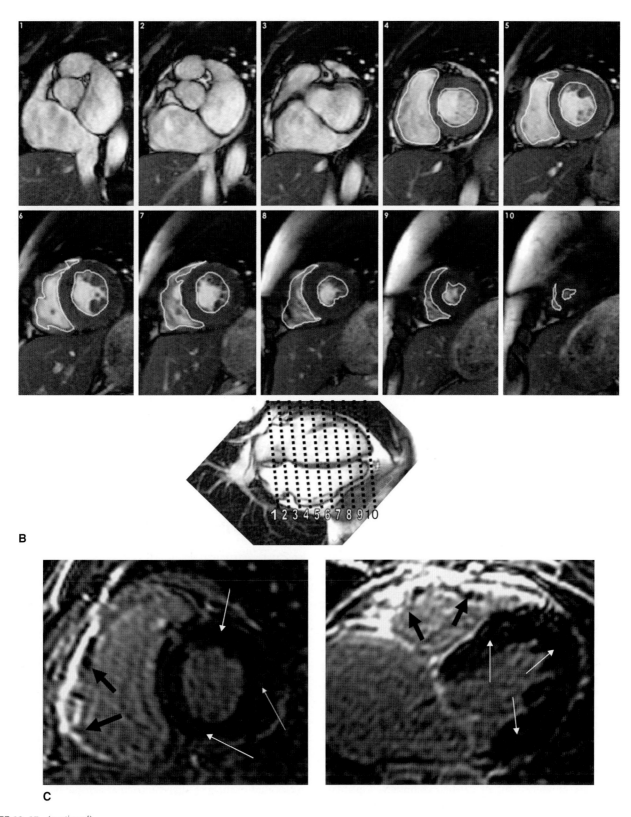

FIGURE 19–13. (*continued*)

endocardial border, especially in end-systole due to elimination of blood from intertrabecular spaces. Partial volume artifacts may occasionally reduce the quality of the RV apex. Also, the inability to visualize the pulmonic valve may overestimate RV volume by including PA volume as well. CMR is relatively contraindicated in patients with pacemakers, implantable defibrillators, cerebral aneurysm clips, and other non–CMR-compatible metallic devices. Presently, CMR is considered to be an appropriate test for evaluation of RV volume, mass, and function.[49]

Tagging Sequences

Although global RV volume and function are reliably measured using cine CMR, abnormalities in these parameters occur relatively late in the course of the disease. Earlier markers of RV dysfunction, frequently regional, would be valuable. There are numerous reports on the value of quantitative regional strain assessment as an early marker of many cardiac diseases. Myocardial tagging using modern CMR imaging sequences allows quantitative assessment of subtle regions of cardiac dysfunction.[50] This method of regional RV wall assessment will eventually become the diagnostic reference tool of choice for subtle and/or early RV pathology.

Myocardial Delayed Contrast Enhancement

A valuable component of CMR imaging is the ability to characterize myocardial tissue using the previously mentioned sequences coupled with the infusion of gadolinium contrast. The normal and pathologic wash-out kinetics of contrast have been well validated and provide evidence of normal or abnormal myocardial tissues. Although initially established for LV myocardial diseases, this technique can also be used for the thinner walled RV myocardium, although its reliability is less well established (Fig. 19–13C).[51]

■ MULTIDETECTOR CARDIAC COMPUTED TOMOGRAPHY

Cardiac computed tomography (CCT) provides high-quality 3D data sets for postprocessing that can be used to obtain both global and regional RV function parameters and anatomic volume with high spatial and adequate temporal resolution within a breath-hold using ECG synchronization (Fig. 19–14). The ability to assess functional information of the RV represents another important application of CCT, especially in patients with acute pulmonary emboli and congenital cardiovascular disease commonly referred for CCT. The accuracy of volume and regional functional measurements depends on the spatial and temporal resolution as well as the timing of the contrast enhancement of cardiac chambers. Optimal contrast timing requires a priori determination to maximize visualization of either the RV or LV or both ventricles equally. Reconstruction of thin myocardial slices reduces partial volume effect and provides a sharper definition of endocardial borders. Retrospective cardiac gating has the advantage of enabling image reconstructions at any point throughout the cardiac cycle and is essential for functional analysis. Few studies have been published on RV global function assessment

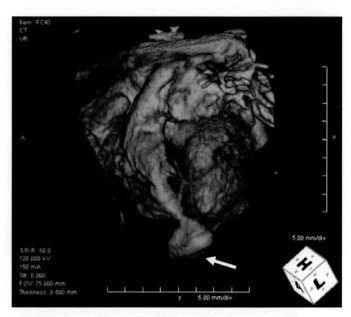

FIGURE 19–14. Cardiac computed tomography angiography, three-dimensional, volume-rendered image, end-systolic phase, with contrast timed to fill both the right ventricular (RV) and left ventricular chambers. A large, focal diverticulum (arrow) is seen in the RV apex in a newborn infant with congenital heart disease. See Moving Image 19–14.

in comparison with standard modalities. Due to the current lower temporal resolution of CCT compared with echocardiography or CMR, a slight overestimation of the ventricular volumes may be expected.[52]

SELECTED INVASIVE IMAGING TECHNIQUES

■ CINE ANGIOGRAPHY OF THE RV

To perform an angiogram of the RV that is suitable for both qualitative and quantitative analysis, there must be good opacification during contrast injection. Either a pigtail catheter (5-French) or Berman catheter (6- or 7-French) can be used. RV angiograms are performed in several views: (1) anterior-posterior; (2) lateral; (3) right anterior oblique (RAO) 30°; and (4) left anterior oblique (LAO) 60°. The catheter should be positioned within the chamber but not touching the walls because this can create artifact wall motion abnormalities as well as ectopic ventricular complexes. A high frame rate of 30 frames per second is preferred, with 40 to 50 mL of contrast injected at a rate of 12 to 15 mL/s.[53] The patient should be instructed to hold his or her breath, and the table should not be moved. Cardiac cycles that occur just after ventricular ectopic beats should not be analyzed.

The interpretation of the RV angiogram is complex because the RV is an asymmetric chamber with nonuniform contraction. In normal subjects, the most vigorous contraction occurs in the tricuspid inflow region, which can also be measured as the TAPSE. Less vigorous contraction occurs in the inferior wall and apex, whereas the anterior wall, outflow tract, and septum have minimal contraction. A quantitative assessment of wall motion compared with normal subjects is helpful to assess the significance of segments that have a visual impression of hypokinesis.[54] The RAO 30° image display is commonly used to assess RV contraction.

RV volumes and EFs can be computed from angiographic views of end-diastole and end-systole. Volume formulae based on calculation of the projected area and length in one or two fluoroscopic views have been derived based on various geometric models such as the hemi-ellipse model and pyramids incorporating projected areas from the RAO 30° and LAO 60° views or the RAO 30° view alone or in combination with area and length from anterior-posterior and lateral fluoroscopic views.[55-58] For instance, the formula for volume proposed by Ferlinz[57] and validated with volumes measured by water displacement of an RV cast is given as follows: Volume = $0.6*A_{RAO}*A_{LAO}/L_{RAO}$ +

3.9 (mL), where A_{RAO} and A_{LAO} are the projected areas in the RAO 30° and LAO 60° views and L_{RAO} is the projected distance in the RAO 30° view from the pulmonic valve to the point that bisects the inferior wall (Fig. 19–15). Commercial software is also available to compute volumes (PIE Medical Imaging, Maastricht, the Netherlands).[59]

Volume measurements require a calibration to a standard-sized object in the fluoroscopic view. This can be achieved with a metal ball or ruler placed on the chest or by measurement of the projected diameter of the known size of the intracardiac catheter used for injection of dye. A magnified high-resolution image of the catheter is needed because a small measurement error will translate to a large error in volume as the calibration constant is proportional to the third power of the catheter diameter. Calculation of the EF does not require image calibration. In a

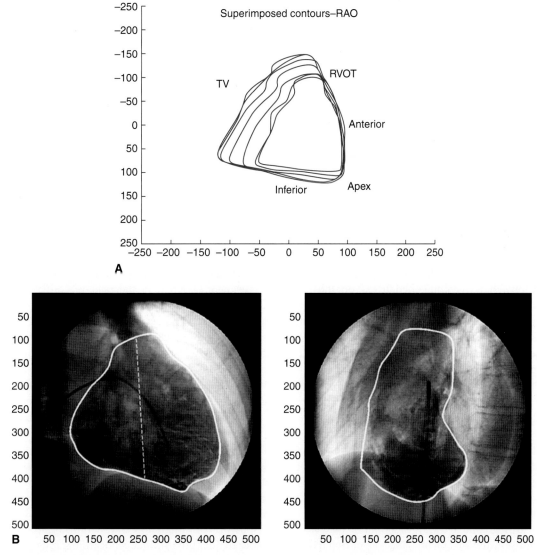

FIGURE 19–15. A. A series of superimposed contours of the right ventricle (RV) imaged in the right anterior oblique (RAO) 30° view is shown in a normal subject. Wall motion is greatest in the tricuspid valve (TV) region and least in the RV outflow tract (RVOT) and anterior wall. **B.** Contours drawn in the RAO 30° (left) and left anterior oblique 60° (right) views. To compute the RV volume using the two-view formula by Ferlinz,[57] the projected area in each view is measured, as well as the length (dashed line in left panel) from the pulmonic valve to the bisected base in the RAO 30° view.

small series of pediatric and adult patients, there was good correlation between angiographically derived volumes and those computed from CMR imaging.[59]

Angiographically derived RV volume and EF have been studied in certain patient populations. In arrhythmogenic right ventricular cardiomyopathy/dysplasia (ARVC/D) subjects, angiographically derived RVEF is reduced compared with normal subjects.[53,60] RV end-diastolic volumes are increased in athletes compared with nonathletes.[61] In athletes with ventricular arrhythmias, the RV end-systolic volume is increased compared with athletes without ventricular arrhythmias, raising the concern that high-performance exercise may trigger arrhythmias and structural changes in the RV or unmask an early stage of ARVC/D.

■ INTRACARDIAC ECHOCARDIOGRAPHY

Intracardiac echocardiography (ICE) can be used to measure the RV volumes and function using a 10-MHz ICE catheter and acquiring sequential cross-sectional images from RV apex to base during a calibrated pullback.[62] Volumes were calculated in an in vitro model by applying Simpson's algorithm, and these correlated well with actual volumes (standard error of estimate [SEE] = 2.3 mL, $r = 0.98$). Also, a beating-heart canine model was used, and findings were compared with actual volumes measured by an intracavitary balloon connected to an external column. Good correlations were observed between ICE and actual values for diastolic (SEE = 4.1 mL, $r = 0.97$), systolic (SEE = 3.4 mL, $r = 0.96$), and EF (SEE = 3.1%, $r = 0.87$) values. This technique has been demonstrated to accurately assess quantitative RV parameters and provides the researcher and clinician with an additional diagnostic tool.

SPECIFIC RV CARDIOMYOPATHIES

■ GENERAL APPROACH (ALGORITHM)

The proposed approach is recommended based on the data presented in this review, although no imaging protocol has been proven to be superior. Initially, conventional echocardiography is used to establish a rapid assessment of the RV size and function (Fig. 19–16). Additional echocardiographic techniques are added for serial investigations or when RV size and function remain in question after the conventional approach.[63] Due to the limited data on normal RV dimensions adjusted for body size and gender, the majority of these findings are qualitative, and quantitative findings are currently not sufficient to determine mild or early concealed disease. One such parameter is the estimation of RV size and function using the conventional apical four-chamber view and tracing the RV endocardium in diastole and systole to obtain the FAC. The RV image should be optimized to maximize the diameter of the tricuspid annulus and the RV length.

Complex echocardiographic techniques should be used selectively. Contrast infusion and/or TEE imaging is an option if there are suboptimal transthoracic windows. Nuclear first-pass RNA may be of value when echocardiography images are suboptimal or clinical questions remain. If CMR is available, this should be used as the reference standard for research and as an alternative

to first-pass RNA when echocardiographic images are not diagnostic. When gating artifacts or MRI contraindications require an alternative reference standard, invasive RV angiography or ICE should be considered. If noninvasive coronary artery imaging is performed using multidetector CT scan, the RV can be assessed using a multiphasic reconstruction technique.

Finally, when evaluating the patient with heart failure who has a dilated RV, color flow Doppler should be performed to look for features characteristic of ASD, Ebstein anomaly, or severe TR. Conventional Doppler can establish the diagnosis of pulmonary hypertension or pulmonic stenosis. In the absence of these findings, RV infarction, ARVC/D, and cardiac contusion should be considered. Uhl anomaly is a diagnosis of exclusion. The discussion of disease-specific pathologic examples follow.

■ RV DYSFUNCTION SECONDARY TO LV DYSFUNCTION

The most common cause of RV dysfunction is passive influence due to LV dysfunction. Therefore, any diagnostic tool for RV assessment must also be capable of adequate LV assessment. This is a significant limitation of first-pass RNA. Comprehensive biventricular imaging is possible with 2D and 3D echocardiography as well as CMR. Echocardiography Doppler has a distinct advantage of being able to evaluate the anatomy and function of the cardiac valves and indirectly assess cardiac hemodynamics.

In patients with chronic systolic heart failure (LVEF ≤45%) and moderate to severe mitral regurgitation, TAPSE is highly discriminating.[64] Survival was 45% in those with the worst TAPSE, whereas it was 82% in those with TAPSE >14 mm. The RVEF is also an independent predictor of survival in patients with moderate heart failure.[65]

■ RV INFARCTION

The clinical triad of hypotension, elevated right atrial pressure, and clear lung fields may be due to pericardial effusion, tamponade, or acute pulmonary emboli. In addition to a specific search for ST-segment elevation in the right precordial ECG leads, global RV size and regional RV function should be assessed. This can be accomplished with portable 2D echocardiography. In addition to evaluating the RV regional contraction pattern, the presence of pericardial fluid, tamponade, and severity of tricuspid regurgitation can be observed. The parasternal short axis view shows inferior RV wall continuity and has the highest reported sensitivity (82%) for detecting a hemodynamically important RV infarction.[66]

RV infarction is relatively commonly associated with an ECG pattern of inferior myocardial infarction, and these patients have a poor prognosis.[67] Furthermore, the diagnostic clinical constellation and the ECG findings of RV infarction are not as accurate compared with more advanced imaging techniques. Recently, it was demonstrated that delayed myocardial contrast was present in the inferior RV myocardial wall in patients with RV myocardial infarction and that this finding was significantly more frequent than either echocardiography or ECG abnormalities.[68] Interestingly, these authors also found RV wall motion abnormalities in patients without RV infarction confirming that segmental RV contraction alone is not specific for RV pathology and occurs in normal controls.

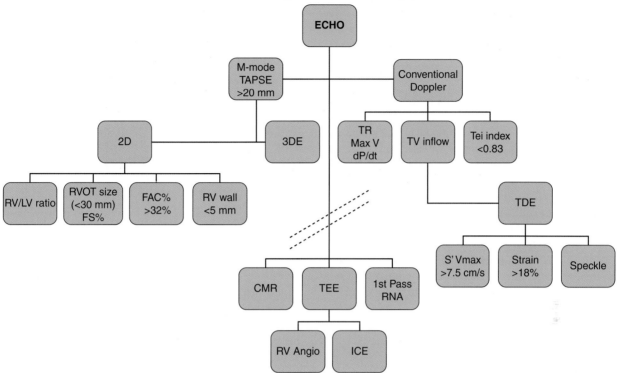

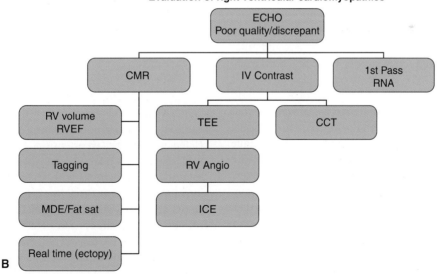

FIGURE 19–16. A. Proposed algorithm for a multimodal imaging approach to the evaluation of right ventricular (RV) cardiomyopathies. A careful evaluation starting with qualitative and quantitative, one-dimensional (M-mode), two-dimensional (2D), three-dimensional (3D), and Doppler echocardiography is recommended. When the echocardiography (ECHO) exam is suboptimal or the results are discrepant with suspected findings or other clinical evidence, additional imaging tools are required (double dashed-line). Confirming abnormal ECHO findings with abnormal findings from images below the dashed lines will increase the accuracy of rare pathologic findings (such as arrhythmogenic right ventricular cardiomyopathy/dysplasia [ARVC/D]). 3DE, three-dimensional echocardiography; Angio, angiography; CMR, cardiac magnetic resonance; FAC%, fractional area change; ICE, intracardiac echocardiography; LV, left ventricle; RNA, radionuclide angiography; RVOT, right ventricular outflow tract; TAPSE, tricuspid annular plane systolic excursion; TDE, tissue Doppler echocardiography; TEE, transesophageal echocardiography; TR, tricuspid regurgitation; TV, tricuspid valve. **B.** Proposed algorithm for a multimodal imaging approach to the evaluation of RV cardiomyopathies when the ECHO exam is suboptimal or the results are discrepant (or suspicion for rare pathology such as ARVC/D). Administration of intravenous (IV) contrast is simple but often inadequate to optimally image the RV. CMR is the reference standard and should be considered the next most important imaging tool when available. First-pass RNA may be used in place of CMR for RV volume and function assessment. TEE and cardiac computed tomography (CCT) are additional next-line options. RV angiography and/or ICE are invasive and reserved for continued suboptimal testing/discrepant results or when subsequent management decisions remain in doubt. Fat sat, fat saturation; MDE, myocardial delayed enhancement.

Decreased RV systolic function is a major risk factor for death, sudden death, heart failure, and stroke after myocardial infarction. For every 5% reduction in FAC%, there was a 1.53 increased risk of fatal and nonfatal cardiovascular outcomes.[69]

■ RV VOLUME OVERLOAD

The RV can accept large volume changes acutely with minimal decrease in RV performance. Chronic RV volume overload may cause RV failure. RV volume overload in the absence of pulmonary hypertension is common in valvular and congenital heart diseases. The RV function is usually preserved because the RV initially accommodates volume overload better than an increase in pressure. It is difficult to image large RV cavities by 3D echocardiography and TEE imaging because the entire cardiac data set may be too large to be included in the imaging field. Invasive RV angiography also must adjust image acquisition (higher contrast volume, higher rate of infusion) to maintain adequate images. Regardless of the RV size or function, CMR and first-pass RNA images are usually adequate for analysis.

■ CONGENITAL HEART DISEASE

General Overview

Although quantitative estimates of RV size and function are less accurate than the methods used for LV assessment, they are superior to the most commonly used visual, or "eyeball," assessment. In a study of 22 patients with right-sided congenital heart disease who underwent both echocardiography and reference CMR, investigators compared the interpretations of four echocardiographers. The ability of the echocardiographer to correctly classify the RV into one of four CMR-defined categories of size and function was only 50% and 41%, respectively. There was both over- and underestimation.[70] RT3DE data were obtained in 28 patients with congenital heart disease and a wide range of RV size and function. The investigators used a modified apical window that enabled visualization of the RVOT and compared conventional manual measures (19 minutes) to a rapid automated technique (5 minutes). They found an excellent overall correlation of RVEF and size ($r = 0.83$-0.92; depending on method and parameter) but a consistent underestimation (~20 mL) of RV volumes (especially in the largest RV cavities) with CMR-derived data obtained within 2 hours of the RT3DE study.[71] Although only half the study patients had adequate images for RT3DE analysis, this study lends further hope that a more accurate, automated, and rapid echo method may be available to assess the size and function of complex congenital malformations of the RV.

Atrial Septal Defect

Left to right cardiac shunting is a common cause of RV dilation. The right atrium and pulmonary artery are also dilated in atrial septal defect (ASD). If the pulmonary artery is normal, it is highly unlikely that a significant right-to-left cardiac shunt exists. In addition to diagnostic imaging modalities capable of assessing RV volume overload, there are incremental advantages of 2D and 3D echocardiography because they can assess the anatomy, size, and significance of cardiac shunting. When clini-

cal or imaging suspicion for an ASD exists but is not confirmed, one should search for an anomalous pulmonary vein that may mimic all of the features of an ASD.

Tetralogy of Fallot With Pulmonary Regurgitation

Pulmonary regurgitation is anticipated after repair of tetralogy of Fallot, and valve replacement is recommended if the RV function begins to fail (Fig. 19–17). Complete RV recovery is less likely after significant RV dilation and dysfunction occurs. Therefore, early identification of severe RV dysfunction is important. The rate of acceleration of the RV lateral wall s′ wave by TDE has been used for this purpose.[72] This index was found to be valuable in patients with tetralogy of Fallot who had variable amounts of pulmonary regurgitation (preload). Myocardial tagging with CMR should also provide an early marker of RV dysfunction but has yet to be adequately studied in this population.

Ebstein Anomaly

Apical displacement of the tricuspid valve septal leaflet insertion >8 mm/m^2 is diagnostic of this entity.[73] The tricuspid valve leaflet is redundant and elongated. Unlike many congenital heart diseases, Ebstein anomaly may first be diagnosed in the adult. These patients may present with exertional dyspnea and a diagnosis of cor pulmonale or similar incorrect diagnosis. Numerous masqueraders of Ebstein anomaly exist (eg, tricuspid valve dysplasia, prolapse or traumatic flail leaflet, ARVC/D), and they can be diagnosed with adequate 2D echocardiography or CMR. Endocarditis may also mimic this disease and either transthoracic echocardiography or TEE should confirm this pathology. Ebstein anomaly should be considered in the differential diagnosis of all patients with right heart dilatation.

Patent Ductus Arteriosus

A patent arterial duct in the adult is usually small and clinically silent. A moderate-sized patent ductus arteriosus is usually manifest by a continuous murmur, LV dilation, and shunt-related pulmonary hypertension. Echocardiography using 2D and Doppler flow analysis is most commonly used to make this diagnosis. In all patients with secondary pulmonary hypertension and RV dysfunction, the possible presence of a patent ductus arteriosus should be carefully evaluated by color flow Doppler.[74] These shunts can be readily closed percutaneously, and this should be considered even with pulmonary arterial hypertension (pulmonary artery pressure greater than two thirds of the systemic arterial pressure; or pulmonary vascular resistance exceeds two thirds of the systemic vascular resistance) if the left to right shunt is at least 1.5:1. Cardiac MRI and CCT can provide clear 3D volume-rendered images to assist with operative interventions. Cardiac MRI can also accurately assess the degree of cardiac shunting.

Congenital Absence of the Pericardium

RV dilation is common in this entity and may mimic RV volume overload.[75] Cardiac MRI and CT are excellent modalities to distinguish this cause of RV dilation due to their ability to obtain excellent pericardial images.[76] It is critical to distinguish

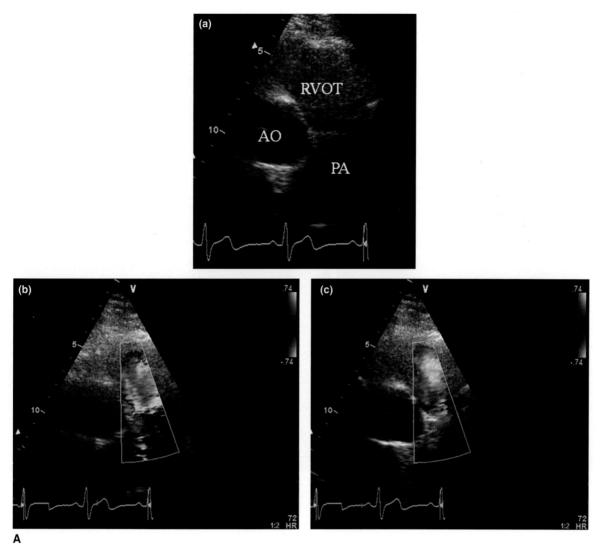

FIGURE 19–17. A. Basal short axis two-dimensional (2D) (**a**) and color flow Doppler (**b**, systole; **c**, diastole) echocardiogram. Dilated right ventricular outflow tract (RVOT) and pulmonary artery (PA) in a patient after tetralogy of Fallot repair with residual severe (free) pulmonic regurgitation (PR). **b.** Blue = flow away from transducer (from RVOT to PA). **c.** Red = PR flow toward transducer (from PA to RVOT). AO, aorta; See Moving Image 19–17A. **B.** Transthoracic 2D echocardiogram in a patient with Ebstein anomaly. The right side is markedly dilated in all views (**a**, parasternal long axis; **b**, parasternal short axis; **c**, apical four-chamber view; **d**, subcostal view). See Moving Image 19–17B.

complete pericardial absence from partial absence because the latter entity places the patient at risk for cardiac herniation and fatal myocardial strangulation. Again, CMR and CCT can usually confirm the diagnosis.[77]

Carcinoid Heart Disease

This is a relatively rare disease that often presents with tricuspid and pulmonic valve pathology (mixed stenosis/regurgitation), with RV dilation and dysfunction. It is commonly diagnosed with transthoracic echocardiography and Doppler flow analysis. Occasionally, the valves are spared and the primary involvement is a metastatic tumor mass of the RV (or LV) myocardium.[78] Diagnostic tools that can characterize the myocardium are valuable. Nuclear SPECT imaging (using the radioisotope technetium 99m and routine MPI sequencing) and CMR (T2 short tau inversion recovery) have been reported to clearly distinguish the tumor mass from the adjacent myocardium.[79]

■ RV PRESSURE OVERLOAD

Unlike RV volume overload, RV pressure overload (RVPO) is most commonly associated with RV dysfunction and with right ventricular hypertrophy (RVH), if chronic. The RV is unable to adequately adjust to acute pressure overload, such as due to pulmonary emboli, and acute regional RV failure, commonly with apical sparing (McConnell sign), ensues (Fig. 19–18).[80] The reason for apical "sparing" may be partly related to the fact that the RV apical contraction is primarily due to LV contraction and the RV apex is pulled toward the LV, creating the illusion of normal RV contraction. The free wall of the RV, lacking the apical interventricular continuity (no "LV tethering"), is more notably dysfunctional. Gradual RV pressure overload creates less acute changes in RV size and function and provides time for some degree of RV compensation.

Both TAPSE and RIMP have been reported to correlate well with clinical, biochemical, and echocardiographic parameters of poor clinical outcomes after acute pulmonary emboli.[81]

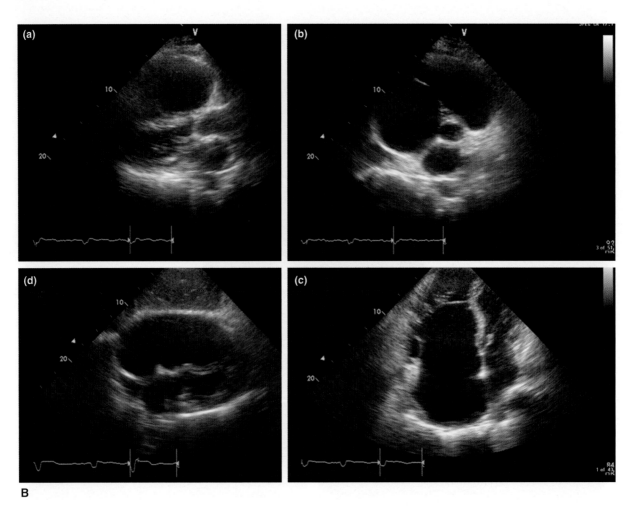

FIGURE 19–17. (*continued*)

Echocardiography is again the first-line diagnostic approach to assess these patients. Normal wall thickness of the RV is 2 to 3 mm and can be measured using 2D echocardiography or, less commonly, M-mode. Up to 5-mm wall thickness is usually considered normal due to difficulties in distinguishing myocardium from epicardium and confirming a perpendicular alignment. The subcostal view is the most reliable for assessment of RVH, whereas the apical four-chamber view is the least reliable. Using M-mode echocardiography in the subcostal view, a wall thickness ≥5 mm was abnormal with a 90% sensitivity and 94% specificity.[82] In addition to RV volume and function assessment, continuous wave spectral Doppler of the TR jet is able to accurately assess the degree of RVPO that is not possible with other imaging tools. CCT is becoming the initial diagnostic imaging test to assess pulmonary emboli. RV enlargement identified with CT predicts early death and adverse clinical events in patients with acute pulmonary emboli.[83,84]

Pulmonary Hypertension due to Left Heart Disease (Group 2)

It is difficult to differentiate pulmonary arterial hypertension (PAH; group 1) from pulmonary hypertension secondary to left heart disease (group 2), especially in patients with normal LV global systolic function. Comprehensive transthoracic echocardiographic imaging

with TDE is uniquely able to provide relatively accurate, noninvasive estimates of left atrial pressure in these patients. However, if severe PAH is present and associated with RV dysfunction, then LV filling is reduced, and the accuracy of echocardiography/Doppler to differentiate primary from secondary PAH is diminished.[85] Volume loading, or performing exercise TDE, may assist in this distinction. Because treatment algorithms vary based on the type of PAH, further studies are required to determine the optimal diagnostic method to confirm group 2 PAH secondary to diastolic dysfunction.

In patients with congenital heart disease (group 1 PAH) or chronic obstructive pulmonary disease (group 3 PAH) and pulmonary hypertension, DTI-derived RV strain is a sensitive index of segmental contractile function and correlates with invasively derived RV stroke volume index.[86-89]

Pulmonary Arterial Hypertension (Group 1)

The echocardiographic findings in idiopathic PAH are similar to those in patients with cor pulmonale. However, patients with group 1 PAH often have greater RVH and septal flattening (even concavity toward the LV), and this may precede inferior vena cava plethora.[90] Doppler echocardiography can estimate the pulmonary artery systolic pressure, evaluate the right atrial

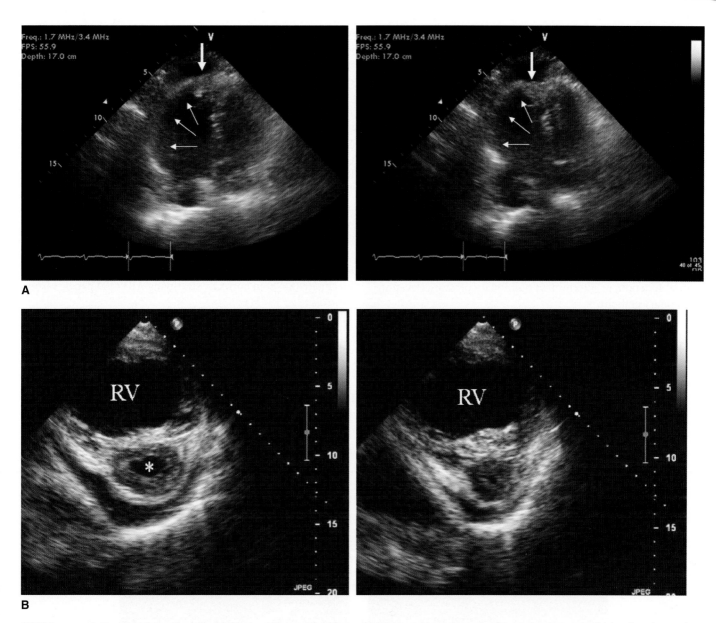

FIGURE 19–18. A. Transthoracic two-dimensional (2D) echocardiogram. The right ventricle (RV) is unable to adequately adjust to acute pressure overload, such as due to pulmonary emboli, and acute regional RV failure, commonly with apical sparing (McConnell sign), ensues. See text for details. **B.** Transthoracic 2D echocardiography (diastole [left]; systole [right]) in a patient with severe pulmonary artery hypertension. The RV is severely dilated and the left ventricle (*) is small and underfilled. Also see Fig. 19–6.

and RV size and function, and evaluate the atrial and ventricular septum for cardiac shunting. Cardiac CT (direct) and nuclear ventilation-perfusion scan (indirect) can exclude the presence of significant pulmonary emboli.

The RIMP (Tei index) is an important risk-stratifying parameter in patients with PAH. The survival rate of patients with PAH and a Tei index ≥0.83 is worse after 1 year than in those with a Tei index <0.83.[91] In a multivariate model, this was the only echocardiographic parameter that was an independent predictor of an adverse outcome.

■ PERICARDIAL CONSTRICTION

The clinical presentation of patients with pericardial constriction may be similar to that of patients with an RV cardiomyopathy. Doppler echocardiography can be used for this assessment. Mitral, aortic, tricuspid valve flow; hepatic, pulmonary, and superior vein flow; and the respiratory variation provide the physiologic clues to this diagnosis.[92] TDE has been found to have consistent and predictable findings in patients with pericardial constriction.[93] The longitudinal velocity of the basal interventricular septum is increased and may exceed the normally higher basal LV lateral wall longitudinal velocity. This is thought to be due to a compensatory effect of the longitudinal myofibers in the setting of impaired circumferential and radial contraction from the constriction process. The reversal of the relation between the lateral and medial e′ velocities (ie, annulus reversus) is an important diagnostic clue to the presence of constriction. It is likely that this variable myofiber response to pathology occurs in other

LV and RV settings but has yet to be identified. In addition to these Doppler-detected physiologic alterations that result from increased pericardial pressures, the pericardium can readily be visualized with CMR or CTA.

■ ARRHYTHMOGENIC RV CARDIOMYOPATHY/ DYSPLASIA

ARVC/D, clinically described nearly 30 years ago, represents the prototypical RV cardiomyopathy.[54] It has been extensively studied and reported in a large international registry. In ARVC/D, the RV has an abnormal structure and function; in the late stage, there can be RV failure due to fibrofatty replacement of the RV myocardium with normal pulmonary pressures. Because 5 mm Hg is adequate to maintain a pressure difference from the RVOT to the pulmonary vasculature, right heart failure usually requires concomitant LV dysfunction (systolic or diastolic), loss of atrial function, or intermittent pulmonary pressure elevation (pulmonary emboli).[94]

There is no single specific diagnostic finding in patients with ARVC/D. Therefore, the diagnosis requires using a combination of clinical, ECG, genetic, and multimodal imaging findings. However, some morphologic features are consistently seen in patients meeting ARVC/D task force criteria.[95]

A normal FAC ≥32% was present in nearly all controls, and an FAC <32% was found in 65% of ARVC/D newly diagnosed probands but only 3% of controls.[95] Additional markers of more subtle RV dysfunction can be used when the RV FAC is normal

and include tissue Doppler imaging, TAPSE, and the RIMP (Fig. 19–19).[96] Peak RV systolic velocity <7.5 cm/s and peak RV strain <18% were shown to best identify patients with phenotypically mild ARVC/D and an apparently normal RV.[97]

In an effort to quantify the RV size, Nava et al[98] studied 132 patients with ARVC/D and categorized RV dilation having an end-diastolic volume of <75 mL/m^2, 75 to 120 mL/m^2, and >120 mL/m^2 as mild, moderate, and severe, respectively (Fig. 19–20).[98] These authors also noted patterns of regional RV dysfunction. Milder forms of the disease affect the RV apex. The RV inflow was impaired at all disease stages, and enlargement of the RVOT correlated with disease severity because it was dilated in 100% of those with severe disease, 50% of those with moderate disease, and only 29% of those mild disease. Others have shown the diagnostic importance of dilation of the RVOT. A cutoff value of 30 mm has a high sensitivity (89%) and specificity (86%) in correctly stratifying ARVC/D patients from controls (Fig. 19–21).

Because the hallmark of fibrofatty infiltration of the RV myocardium is regional dysfunction, careful assessment of tissue deformation using tissue Doppler imaging seems logical and was recently confirmed as a viable option for this purpose. In a small subset of 34 patients confirmed to have ARVC/D by task force criteria, a cutoff value of –18.2% had a 97% sensitivity and a 91% specificity for the diagnosis of this disease.[99] The ability of this method to differentiate ARVC/D from other RV diseases has yet to be substantiated.

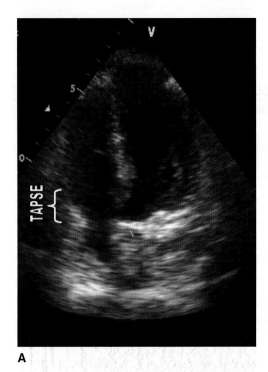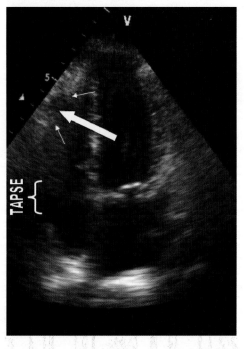

A

FIGURE 19–19. A. Regional right ventricular (RV) dysfunction in arrhythmogenic RV cardiomyopathy/dysplasia (ARVC/D). Transthoracic two-dimensional (2D) echocardiographic image, in apical four-chamber orientation in diastole (left) and systole (right). There is a focal regional RV wall motion abnormality (large arrow = aneurysm; small arrows = edge of aneurysm) in this patient with suspected ARVC/D. Despite the moderate-sized aneurysm, the tricuspid annular plane systolic excursion (TAPSE) was normal (24 mm). **B.** Same patient as in **A.** Note the normal TAPSE (arrow). **C.** Global RV systolic dysfunction. Transthoracic 2D echocardiographic image, in apical four-chamber orientation in diastole (right) and systole (left). There is global RV wall hypokinesis. Consistent with marked RV systolic dysfunction, the TAPSE was very abnormal (12 mm).

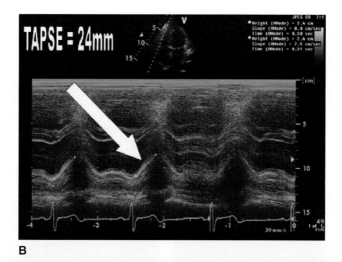

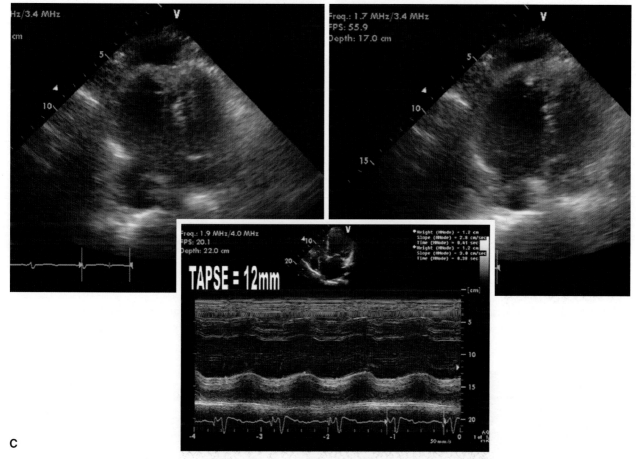

FIGURE 19–19. (continued)

Despite the potential for CMR to be the reference standard for ARVC/D due to its ability to quantify RV size, evaluate global and regional function, and image fat (fat suppression sequence) and fibrosis (delayed contrast sequence), assessment of this disease entity remains a challenge. This is likely due to the variation of CMR image acquisition, the variable distribution and extent of fatty infiltration depending on disease severity, and the knowledge that some degree of fatty infiltration and regional outward systolic motion abnormalities are commonly seen in normal controls.[100] Reliance on the finding of RV fat or subtle regional wall motion abnormality (especially near the moderator band and RV apex) may result in overdiagnosis of ARVC/D.[101] In normal individuals, epicardial fat overlies the RV (often with a clear line of demarcation) and is most noted in

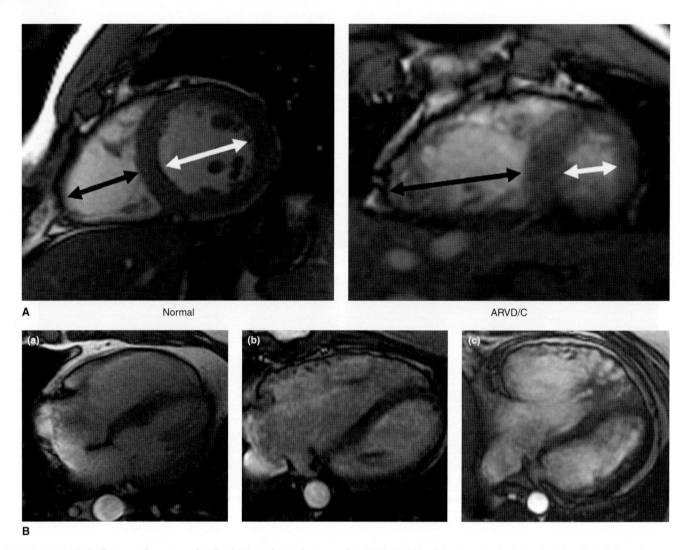

FIGURE 19–20. A. Cardiac magnetic resonance imaging (MRI) steady-state free precession (SSFP) white blood cine image in short axis orientation. Diastolic image in a normal volunteer (left) and in a patient with documented arrhythmogenic right ventricular (RV) cardiomyopathy/dysplasia (ARVC/D; right). Note the dilated RV cavity (black arrows) relative to the left ventricular (LV) cavity (white arrows). **B.** Cardiac MRI SSFP images from three different patients with ARVC/D demonstrating the variation in phenotypic expression; straight axial orientation. **a.** Mild RV dilation (EDVi <75 mL/m²; RV similar in size to LV). **b.** Moderate RV dilation (end-diastolic volume index [EDVi] 75-120 mL/m²; RV larger than LV); **c.** Severe RV dilation (EDVi >120 mL/m²; RV markedly larger than the LV).

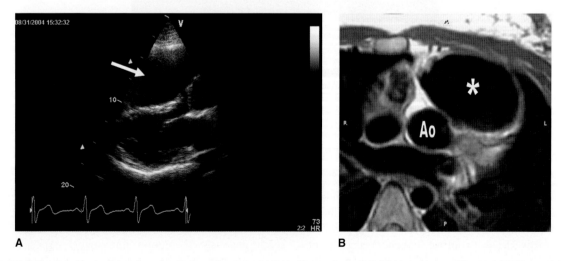

FIGURE 19–21. A. Parasternal long-axis two-dimensional echocardiogram in a patient with a markedly dilated right ventricular outflow tract (RVOT; arrow). **B.** Cardiac magnetic resonance imaging black blood spin-echo sequence, in basal short axis orientation. Severe RVOT dilation (*) in a patient with suspected arrhythmogenic right ventricular cardiomyopathy/dysplasia. AO, aorta.

the atrioventricular groove and near the apex. In patients with ARVC/D, the hyperintense fat signal extends through this line of demarcation indicating infiltration into the RV epicardium (usually in the RV inflow or outflow regions).[102] To minimize the variability of image acquisition, standard CMR protocols have been published and deviations should be minimized.[103]

The presence of fibrosis in the RV is not normal and provides an important diagnostic clue to the presence of ARVC/D (Fig. 19–22). Delayed contrast enhancement with CMR correlates with histopathologic changes and regions of wall motion

abnormalities, inversely correlates with RV global function, and predicts sustained ventricular tachycardia during electrophysiologic testing.[104] CMR provides an excellent method for the assessment of ARVC/D when there is a high-quality, expertly interpreted examination. If the CMR is completely normal, it may eliminate the need for subsequent invasive testing.

CT imaging in ARVC/D is usually reserved for patients with contraindications to CMR. The advantages of CT are quick scan time, minimal operator dependence, and consistent image quality, and it can be used in patients with pacemakers and

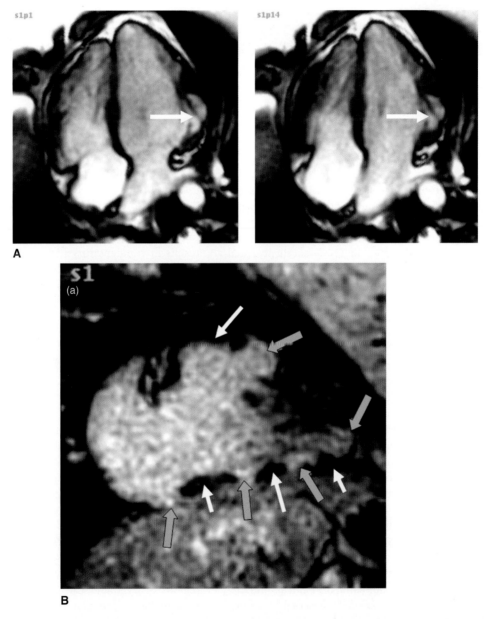

FIGURE 19–22. A. Cardiac magnetic resonance imaging steady-state free precession image (left, diastole; right, systole) in apical four-chamber orientation in a patient with a plakophilin genetic mutation (arrhythmogenic right ventricular cardiomyopathy/dysplasia). There is biventricular dilation and both global and regional dysfunction. Arrow = large lateral left ventricle aneurysm. See Moving Image 19–22A. **B.** Cardiac magnetic resonance. Myocardial delayed contrast enhancement sequence in the same patient as in **a.** Right ventricular (RV) two-chamber view orientation. Note the multiple segments of contrast enhancement (white myocardium; green arrows) interspersed within regions of normal RV myocardium (black myocardium; white arrows).

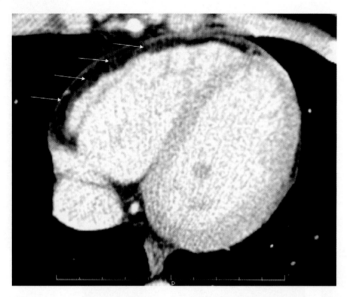

FIGURE 19–23. Cardiac computed tomography. Extensive fat is seen adjacent to the right ventricular (RV) myocardium. This has a value of –50 Hounsfield units (HU), which is consistent with epicardial fat and not intramyocardial fat (usually 5 to –17 HU) This patient had normal RV size and function and no evidence for arrhythmogenic right ventricular cardiomyopathy/dysplasia.

implantable cardioverter-defibrillator devices. Attenuation of intramyocardial fat (5 to –17 Hounsfield units; HU) is significantly less than attenuation of normal myocardium (73 ± 14 HU) and greater than epicardial fat (–65 ± 10 HU) (Fig. 19–23).[105] Another advantage of CT is excellent visualization of the mediastinum to assess for lymphadenopathy, a marker of sarcoidosis, which is known to mimic ARVC/D.[106] Disadvantages include low temporal resolution and registration artifacts limiting wall motion assessment, image deterioration from lead artifacts, and the requirement for retrospective gating, which increases radiation exposure making this procedure less optimal for the young or for serial investigations.

Angiography remains a reference imaging standard of the RV for the diagnosis of ARVC/D. The well-known regions of abnormal function, termed the "triangle of dysplasia," consisting of the RVOT, apex, and subtricuspid valve regions, can be examined in multiple angiographic views for hypokinesis, akinesis, or dyskinesis (aneurysmal segments). In addition to wall motion abnormalities, angiography can delineate other abnormalities, such as prolonged persistence of dye in aneurysmal segments.[107] Angiography may also reveal a polycyclic contour, or cauliflower-like appearance, a specific but nonsensitive finding for ARVC/D, because this occurs in advanced stages of the disease. Thick trabeculation (>4 mm) with deep horizontal fissuring, referred to as "pile d'assiettes," is characteristic in ARVC/D, particularly if it involves the moderator band, the papillary muscles, and the apex and superior-apical region.[108] Nonetheless, marked trabeculation can also occur in normal subjects and needs to be evaluated in conjunction with other RV abnormalities.

In a cohort of ARVC/D patients, wall motion was decreased by more than 30% at the tricuspid valve region and by 50% in the subtricuspid region compared to normal individuals.[109]

Furthermore, a poor TAPSE excursion correlated with decreased RVEF.[110] However, because there is minimal contraction of the RVOT and anterior wall in normal subjects, the wall motion in these regions is not significantly different in ARVC/D patients.

The fact that ARVC/D is rare only compounds the difficulty of diagnosing it. Combining a rare disease with the difficulty in interpretation of the irregular shaped RV leads to over- and underdiagnosis of ARVC/D.[101] When the imaging abnormality is documented by at least two imaging modalities, it increases the accuracy of the finding. If present on only one imaging test, RV angiography should be considered, or the tests should be referred to experts for re-evaluation. In 89 patients with an initial diagnosis of ARVC/D (34% who received an implantable cardioverter-defibrillator device) who were sent for expert re-evaluation, only 24 (27%) met task force criteria for ARVC/D. Importantly, none of the 46 patients diagnosed solely by CMR criteria of wall thinning and RV myocardial fat fulfilled ARVC/D criteria.[111]

■ UHL ANOMALY

This unusual RV cardiomyopathy is typified by an extremely thin ("paper-thin") RV wall with essentially endocardial apposition to the epicardium, sparing the normal mid-myocardial layer. If the majority of the RV is involved, ineffective RV contraction results in the RV acting as a conduit for blood, rather than a pumping chamber. Lack of myocardial contraction should be recognized with any diagnostic tool capable of critically evaluating myocardial segments. Lack of RV contraction results in compensatory hyperdynamic septal contraction and hypertrophied RA wall. Although displaying many characteristics of ARVC/D, this anomaly is rarely seen in adults, has not been found to be congenital, and does not have significant fatty replacement.[112]

FUTURE ASPECTS OF RV MULTIMODAL IMAGING

With modern echocardiographic imaging probes, one can see a well-defined separation of the interventricular septum into RV and LV myofibers.[113] It is not known if this feature will eventually improve our understanding of RV performance and, specifically, how the interventricular septum influences the RV. This warrants additional investigation.

One particularly interesting imaging technique with direct application to ARVC/D is radiolabeled ^{123}I-mIBG, also known as iobenguane, an analog of the false neurotransmitter guanethidine. Japanese investigators have demonstrated LV myocardial ^{123}I-mIBG defects in ARVC/D patients that correspond to regions of CCT and CMR fatty infiltration.[114] None of these patients had ventricular tachycardia originating from the LV on electrophysiologic testing. It was previously shown that ^{123}I-mIBG LV defects commonly localize in the ventricular septum and regions contiguous to the RV.[115] These regions are anatomically and sympathetically related. A subepicardial, primarily RV, dysplastic cardiomyopathy would likely impair the

LV in this region early in its disease progression. Further investigation is required to fully evaluate the potential of advanced radiopharmaceuticals for the investigation of these patients. It is likely that additional specific molecular agents will become available and provide incremental diagnostic and managerial roles in this and other rare cardiomyopathies.

Multigated RNA is still considered the reference standard for ventricular volume and function assessment, although CMR has become more accurate and does not expose the patient to irradiation. Time-volume activity curves generated with RNA can accurately assess global and regional RV motion with adequate temporal resolution. Using offline software and novel processing techniques to reduce noise and focusing on regions of dyskinesia, this method effectively distinguishes normal controls from ARVC/D patients with regional or diffuse hypokinesia.[116] Nonetheless, it is not specific for ARVC/D, but rather demonstrates any RV pathologic, dyssynchronous motion. It is not known whether this will provide incremental value to the previously listed alternative techniques.

Genetic markers aimed at reclassifying specific cardiomyopathies and assisting in treatment development are rapidly being identified. For example, ARVC/D shows autosomal dominant inheritance and has been mapped to eight chromosomal loci, with mutations identified thus far in seven genes. One gene mutation shares an arrhythmic profile with familial catecholaminergic polymorphic ventricular tachycardia. Furthermore, two recessive forms are caused by mutations in junctional plakoglobin (Naxos disease) and desmoplakin (Carvajal syndrome).[117] A link with ion channel disorders (channelopathies) has been described beyond the primary structural pathologic findings. Given the subtlety of early morphologic changes in this disease and the inherent difficulties in evaluating early RV impairment from any pathology, the ability to detect genotypic impairment will influence the future assessment of phenotypic expression using multimodal imaging.

Moving Images

All moving images are located on the complementary DVD.

REFERENCES

1. Sorrell VL, Altbach MI, Kudithipudi V, Squire SW, Goldberg SJ, Klewer SE. Cardiac MRI is an important complementary tool to Doppler echocardiography in the management of patients with pulmonary regurgitation. *Echocardiogr J.* 2007;24: 316-328.
2. Haddad F, Hunt SA, Rosenthal DN, et al. Right ventricular function in cardiovascular disease. Part I. Anatomy, physiology, aging, and functional assessment of the right ventricle. *Circulation.* 2008;117:1436-1448.
3. Sheehan F, Redington A. The right ventricle: anatomy, physiology and clinical imaging. *Heart.* 2008;94:1510-1515.
4. Sanchez-Guintana D, Anderson RH, Ho SY. Ventricular myoarchitecture in tetralogy of Fallot. *Heart.* 1996;76:280-286.
5. Santamore WP, Dell'Italia LJ. Ventricular interdependence: significant left ventricular contributions to right ventricular systolic function. *Prog Cardiovasc Dis.* 1998;40:289-308.
6. Denault AY, Chaput M, Couture P, Hebert Y, Haddad F, Tardif JC. Dynamic right ventricular outflow tract obstruction in cardiac surgery. *J Thorac Cardiovasc Surg.* 2006;132:43-49.
7. Horton KD, Meece RW, Hill JC. Assessment of the right ventricle by echocardiography: a primer for cardiac sonographers. *J Am Soc Echocardiogr.* 2009;22:776-792.
8. Kjaergaard J, Petersen CL, Kjaer A, Schaadt BK, Oh JK, Hassager C. Evaluation of right ventricular volume and function by 2D and 3D echocardiography compared to MRI. *Eur J Echocardiogr.* 2006;7:430-438.
9. Levine RA, Gibson TC, Aretz T, et al. Echocardiographic measurement of right ventricular volume. *Circulation.* 1984;69:497-505.
10. Lindqvist P, Henein M, Kazzam E. Right ventricular outflow-tract fractional shortening: an applicable measure of right ventricular systolic function. *Eur J Echocardiogr.* 2003;4:29-35.
11. Silverman NH, Hudson S. Evaluation of right ventricular volume and ejection fraction in children by two-dimensional echocardiography. *Pediatr Cardiol.* 1983;4:197-203.
12. Arora H, Virani SS, Simpson L, Stainback RF. Contrast echocardiography for right-sided heart conditions. Case reports and literature review. *Tex Heart Inst J.* 2008;35:38-41.
13. Wei K, Mulvagh SL, Carson L, et al. The safety of Derfinity and Optison for ultrasound image enhancement: a retrospective analysis of 78,383 administered contrast doses. *J Am Soc Echocardiogr.* 2008;21:1202-1206.
14. Anavekar NS, Gerson D, Skali H, Kwong RY, Yurcel K, Solomon SD. Two-dimensional assessment of right ventricular function: an echocardiographic-MRI correlate study. *Echocardiography.* 2007;24:452-456.
15. Appleton CP, Hatle LK, Popp RL. Superior vena cava and hepatic vein Doppler echocardiography in healthy adults. *J Am Coll Cardiol.* 1987;10:1032-1039.
16. Klein AL, Hatle LK, Burstow DJ, et al. Comprehensive Doppler assessment of right ventricular diastolic function in cardiac amyloidosis. *J Am Coll Cardiol.* 1990;15:99-108.
17. Appleton CP, Jensen JL, Hatle LK, Oh JK. Doppler evaluation of left and right ventricular diastolic function: a technical guide for obtaining optimal flow velocity recordings. *J Am Soc Echocardiogr.* 1997;10:271-292.
18. Anconina J, Danchin N, Selton-Suty C, et al. Noninvasive estimation of right ventricular dP/dt in patients with tricuspid valve regurgitation. *Am J Cardiol.* 1993;71:1495-1497.
19. Selton-Suty C, Juilliere Y. Non-invasive investigations of the right heart: how and why? *Arch Cardiovasc Dis.* 2009;102:219-232.
20. Kanzaki H, Nakatani S, Kawada T, Yamagishi M, Sunagawa K, Miyatake K. Right ventricular dP/dt/P(max), not dP/dt(max), noninvasively derived from tricuspid regurgitation velocity is a useful index of right ventricular contractility. *J Am Soc Echocardiogr.* 2002;15:136-142.
21. Kim WH, Otsuji Y, Yuasa T, Minagoe S, Seward JB, Tei C. Evaluation of right ventricular dysfunction in patients with cardiac amyloidosis using Tei index. *J Am Soc Echocardiogr.* 2004;17:45-49.
22. Morner S, Lindqvist P, Waldenstrom A, Kazzam E. Right ventricular dysfunction in hypertrophic cardiomyopathy as evidenced by the myocardial performance index. *Int J Cardiol.* 2008;124:57-63.
23. Schwerzmann M, Samman AM, Salehian O, et al. Comparison of echocardiographic and cardiac magnetic resonance imaging for assessing right ventricular function in adults with repaired tetralogy of Fallot. *Am J Cardiol.* 2007;99:1593-1597.
24. Meluzin J, Spinarova L, Hude P, et al. Prognostic importance of various echocardiographic right ventricular functional parameters in patients with symptomatic heart failure. *J Am Soc Echocardiogr.* 2005;18:435-444.
25. Yeo TC, Dujardin KS, Tei C, Mahoney DW, McGoon MD, Seward JB. Value of a Doppler-derived index combining systolic and diastolic time intervals in predicting outcome in primary pulmonary hypertension. *Am J Cardiol.* 1998;81:1157-1161.
26. Wang J, Prakasa K, Bomma C, et al. Comparison of novel echocardiographic parameters of right ventricular function with ejection fraction by cardiac magnetic resonance. *J Am Soc Echocardiogr.* 2007;20:1058-1064.
27. De Castro S, Cavarretta E, Milan A, et al. Usefulness of tricuspid annular velocity in identifying global RV dysfunction in patients with primary pulmonary hypertension: a comparison with 3D echo-derived right ventricular ejection fraction. *Echocardiography.* 2008;25:289-293.
28. Tuller D, Steiner M, Wahl A, Kabok M, Seiler C. Systolic right ventricular function assessment by pulsed wave tissue Doppler imaging of the tricuspid annulus. *Swiss Med Weekly.* 2005;135:461-468.
29. Vogel M, Schmidt MR, Kristiansen SB, et al. Validation of myocardial acceleration during isovolumic contraction as a novel noninvasive index of right ventricular contractility. Comparison with ventricular pressure-volume relations in an animal model. *Circulation.* 2002;105:1693-1699.

30. Pirat B, McCulloch ML, Zoghbi WA. Evaluation of global and regional right ventricular systolic function in patients with pulmonary hypertension using a novel speckle tracking method. *Am J Cardiol.* 2006;98:699-704.

31. Kowalski M, Kukulski T, Jamal F, et al. Can natural strain and strain rate quantify regional myocardial deformation? A study in healthy subjects. *Ultra Med Biol.* 2001;27:1087-1097.

32. Teske AJ, De Boeck BWL, Olimulder M, Prakken NH, Doevendans PA, Cramer MJM. Echocardiographic assessment of regional right ventricular function. A head to head comparison between 2D-strain and tissue Doppler derived strain analysis. *J Am Soc Echocardiogr.* 2007;21: 275-282.

33. Rajagopalan N, Simon MA, Shah H, Mathier MA, Lopez-Candales A. Utility of right ventricular tissue Doppler imaging: correlation with right heart catheterization. *Echocardiography.* 2008;25:706-711.

34. Jenkins C, Chan J, Bricknell K, Strudwick M, Marwick TH. Reproducibility of right ventricular volumes and ejection fraction using real-time three-dimensional echocardiography: comparison with cardiac MRI. *Chest.* 2007;131:1844-1851.

35. Grothues F, Moon JC, Bellenger NG, Smith GS, Klein HU, Pennell DJ. Interstudy reproducibility of right ventricular volumes, function, and mass with cardiovascular magnetic resonance. *Am Heart J.* 2004;147:218-223.

36. Gopal AS, Chukwu EO, Iwuchukwu CF, et al. Normal values of right ventricular size and function by real-time three-dimensional echocardiography: comparison to cardiac magnetic resonance imaging. *J Am Soc Echocardiogr.* 2007;20:445-455.

37. Tamborini G, Brusoni D, Torres Molina JE, et al. Feasibility of a new generation three-dimensional echocardiography for right ventricular volumetric and functional measurements. *Am J Cardiol.* 2008;102:499-505.

38. Shiota T. 2D echocardiography: evaluation of the right ventricle. *Curr Opin Cardiol.* 2009;24:410-414.

39. Grison A, Maschietto N, Reffo E, et al. Three-dimensional echocardiographic evaluation of right ventricular volume and function in pediatric patients: validation of the technique. *J Am Soc Echocardiogr.* 2007;20: 921-929.

40. Steele P, Kirch D, LeFree M, Battock D. Measurement of right and left ventricular ejection fractions by radionuclide angiocardiography in coronary artery disease. *Chest.* 1976;70:51-56.

41. Johnson LL, Lawson MA, Blackwell GG, Tauxe EL, Russell K, Dell'Italia LJ. Optimizing the method to calculate right ventricular ejection fraction from first-pass data acquired with a multicrystal camera. *J Nucl Cardiol.* 1995;2:372-379.

42. Movahed MR, Hepner A, Lizotte P, Milne N. Flattening of the interventricular septum (D-shaped left ventricle) in addition to high right ventricular tracer uptake and increased right ventricular volume found on gated SPECT studies strongly correlates with right ventricular overload. *J Nucl Cardiol.* 2005;12:428-434.

43. Sisson JC, Shapiro B, Meyers L, et al. Metaiodobenzylguanidine to map scintigraphically the adrenergic nervous system in man. *J Nucl Med.* 1987;28:1625-1636.

44. Agostini D, Verberne HJ, Burchert W, et al. I-123-mIBG myocardial imaging for assessment of risk for a major cardiac event in heart failure patients: insights from a retrospective European multicenter study. *Eur J Nucl Med Mol Imaging.* 2008;35:535-546.

45. Paul M, Schafers M, Kies P, et al. Impact of sympathetic innervation on recurrent life-threatening arrhythmias in the follow-up of patients with idiopathic ventricular fibrillation. *Eur J Nucl Med Mol Imaging.* 2006;33:866-870.

46. Pennell DJ, Sechtem UP, Higgins CB, et al. Clinical indications for cardiovascular magnetic resonance (CMR): Consensus Panel report. *Eur Heart J.* 2004;25:1940-1965.

47. Mooij CF, de Wit CJ, Graham DA, Powell AJ, Geva R. Reproducibility of MRI measurements of right ventricular size and function in patients with normal and dilated ventricles. *J Magn Reson Imaging.* 2008;28:67-73.

48. Tandri H, Daya SK, Nasir K, et al. Normal reference values for the adult right ventricle by magnetic resonance imaging. *Am J Cardiol.* 2006;98: 1660-1664.

49. Hendel RC, Patel MR, Kramer CM, et al. ACCF/ACR/SCCT/SCMR/ASNC/ NASCI/SCAI/SIR 2006 appropriateness criteria for cardiac computed tomography and cardiac magnetic resonance imaging: a report of the American College of Cardiology Foundation Quality Strategic Directions Committee Appropriateness Criteria Working Group, American College of Radiology, Society of Cardiovascular Computed Tomography, Society for Cardiovascular Angiography and Interventions, and Society of Interventional Radiology. *J Am Coll Cardiol.* 2006;48:1475-1497.

50. Youssef A, Ibrahim ESH, Korosoglou G, Abraham MR, Weiss RG, Osman NF. Strain-encoding cardiovascular magnetic resonance for assessment of right-ventricular regional function. *J Cardiovasc Magn Reson.* 2008;10:33.

51. Grosse-Wortmann L, Macgowan CK, Vidarsson L, Yoo SJ. Late gadolinium enhancement of the right ventricular myocardium: is it really different from the left? *J Cardiovasc Magn Res.* 2008;10:20.

52. Plumhans C, Muhlenbruch G, Rapaee A, et al Assessment of global right ventricular function on 64-MDCT compared with MRI. *Am J Roent.* 2008;190:1358-1361.

53. Wichter T, Indik J, Daliento L. Diagnostic role of angiography. In: Marcus FI, Nava A, Thiene G, ed. *Arrhythmogenic Right Ventricular Cardiomyopathy/ Dysplasia: Recent Advances.* Milan, Italy: Springer Verlag; 207:147-158.

54. Marcus FI, Fontaine GH, Guiraudon G, et al. Right ventricular dysplasia: a report of 24 adult cases. *Circulation.* 1982;65:384-398.

55. Boak JG, Bove AA, Kreulen T, Spann JF. A geometric basis for calculation of right ventricular volume in man. *Cathet Cardiovasc Diagn.* 1977;3:217-230.

56. Ferlinz J, Gorlin R, Cohn PF, Herman MV. Right ventricular performance in patients with coronary artery disease. *Circulation.* 1975;52:608-615.

57. Ferlinz J. Measurements of right ventricular volumes in man from single plane cine angiograms. A comparison to the biplane approach. *Am Heart J.* 1977;94:87-90.

58. Arcilla RA, Tsai P, Thilenius O, Ranniger K. Angiographic method for volume estimation of right and left ventricles. *Chest.* 1971;60:446-454.

59. Wellnhofer E, Ewert P, Hug J, et al. Evaluation of new software for angiographic determination of right ventricular volumes. *Int J Cardiovasc Imaging.* 2005;21:575-585.

60. Daliento L, Rizzoli G, Thiene G, et al. Diagnostic accuracy of right ventriculography in arrhythmogenic right ventricular cardiomyopathy. *Am J Cardiol.* 1990;66:741-745.

61. Ector J, Ganame J, van der Merwe N, et al. Reduced right ventricular ejection fraction in endurance athletes presenting with ventricular arrhythmias: a quantitative angiographic assessment. *Eur Heart J.* 2007;28:345-353.

62. Vazquez de Prada JA, Chen MH, Guerrero JL, et al. Intracardiac echocardiography: in vitro and in vivo validation for right ventricular volume and function. *Am Heart J.* 1996;131:320-328.

63. Rudski LG, Wyman WL, Afilalo J, Hua L, Handschumacher MD, et al. *J Am Soc Echocardiogr* 2010; 23: 685-713.

64. Lloyd Dini F, Conti U, Fontanive P, et al. Right ventricular dysfunction is a major predictor of outcome in patients with moderate to severe mitral regurgitation and left ventricular dysfunction. *Am Heart J.* 2007;154:172-179.

65. de Groote P, Milliare A, Hossein C, et al. Right ventricular ejection fraction is an independent predictor of survival in patients with moderate heart failure. *J Am Coll Cardiol.* 1998;32:948-954.

66. Lopez-Sendon J, Garcia-Fernandez MA, Coma-Canella I, Yanguela MM, Banuelos F. Segmental right ventricular function after acute myocardial infarction: two-dimensional echocardiographic study in 63 patients. *Am J Cardiol.* 1983;51:390-396.

67. Mehta SR, Eikelboom JW, Natarajan MK, et al. Impact of right ventricular involvement on mortality and morbidity in patients with inferior myocardial infarction. *J Am Coll Cardiol.* 2001;37:37-43.

68. Kumar A, Abdel-Aty H, Kriedemann I, et al. Contrast-enhanced cardiovascular magnetic resonance imaging of right ventricular infarction. *J Am Coll Cardiol.* 2006;48:1969-1976.

69. Anavekar NS, Skali H, Bourgoun M, et al. Usefulness of right ventricular fractional area change to predict death, heart failure, and stroke following myocardial infarction (from the VALIANT ECHO Study). *Am J Cardiol.* 2008;101:607-612.

70. Puchalski MD, Williams RV, Askovich B, Minich LL, Mart C, Tani LY. Assessment of right ventricular size and function: echo versus magnetic resonance imaging. *Congenit Heart Dis.* 2007;2:27-31.

71. Khoo NS, Young A, Occleshaw C, Cowan B, Zeng ISL, Gentles TL. Assessments of right ventricular volume and function using three-dimensional echocardiography in older children and adults with congenital heart disease: comparison with cardiac magnetic resonance imaging. *J Am Soc Echocardiogr.* 2009;22:1279-1288.

72. Toyono M, Harada K, Tamura M, Yamamoto F, Takada G. Myocardial acceleration during isovolumic contraction as a new index of right ventricular contractile function and its relation to pulmonary regurgitation in patients after repair of tetralogy of Fallot. *J Am Soc Echocardiogr.* 2004;17:332-337.

73. Edwards WD. Embryology and pathologic features of Ebstein's anomaly. *Progr Pediatr Cardiol.* 1993;2:5-15.

74. Therrien J, Connelly MS, Webb GD. Patent ductus arteriosus. *Curr Treat Options Cardiovasc Med.* 1999;4:341-346.

75. Payvandi MN, Kerber RE. Echocardiography in congenital and acquired absence of the pericardium: an echocardiographic mimic of right ventricular volume overload. *Circulation.* 1976;53:86-92.

76. Murat A, Artas H, Yilmaz E, Ogur E. Isolated congenital absence of the pericardium. *Pediatr Cardiol.* 2008;29:862-864.

77. Wang ZJ, Reddy GP, Gotway MB, Yeh BM, Hetts SW, Higgins CB. CT and MR imaging of pericardial disease. *Radiographics.* 2003;23:167-180.

78. Kasi VJ, Ahsanudin AN, Gilbert C, Orr L, Moran J, Sorrell VL. Isolated metastatic myocardial carcinoid tumor in a 48-year old man. *Mayo Clin Proc.* 2002;77:591-594.

79. Schiavone WA, Baker C, Prasad SK. Imaging myocardial carcinoid with t2-STIR CMR. *J Cardiovasc Magn Res.* 2008;10:10-14.

80. McConnell MV, Solomon SD, Rayan ME, Come PC, Goldhaber SZ, Lee RT. Regional right ventricular dysfunction detected by echocardiography in acute pulmonary embolism. *Am J Cardiol.* 1996;78:469-473.

81. Holley AB, Cheatham JG, Jackson JL, Moores LK, Villines TC. Novel quantitative echocardiographic parameters in acute PE. *J Thromb Thrombolysis.* 2009;28:506-512.

82. Prakash R, Matsukubo H. Usefulness of echocardiographic right ventricular measurements in estimating right ventricular hypertrophy and right ventricular systolic pressure. *Am J Cardiol.* 1983;51:1036-1040.

83. Schoepf UJ, Kucher N, Kipfmueller F, Quiroz R, Costello P, Goldhaber SZ. Right ventricular enlargement on chest computed tomography: a predictor of early death in acute pulmonary embolism. *Circulation.* 2004;110:3276-3280.

84. Quiroz R, Kucher N, Schoepf UJ, et al. Right ventricular enlargement on chest computed tomography: prognostic role in acute pulmonary embolism. *Circulation.* 2004;109:2401-2404.

85. Gurudevan SV, Malouf PJ, Auger WR, et al. Abnormal left ventricular diastolic filling in chronic thromboembolic pulmonary hypertension. True diastolic dysfunction or left ventricular underfilling. *J Am Coll Cardiol.* 2007;49:1334-1339.

86. Urheim S, Cauduro S, Frantz R, et al. Relation of tissue displacement and strain to invasively determined right ventricular stroke volume. *Am J Cardiol.* 2005;96:1173-1178.

87. Rajagopalan N, Simon MA, Mathier MA, Lopez-Candales A. Identifying right ventricular dysfunction with tissue Doppler imaging in pulmonary hypertension. *Int J Cardiol.* 2008;128:359-363.

88. Weidemann F, Eyskens B, Mertens L, et al. Quantification of regional right and left ventricular function by ultrasonic strain rate and strain indexes after surgical repair of tetralogy of Fallot. *Am J Cardiol.* 2002;90:133-138.

89. Vitarelli A, Conde Y, Cimino E, et al. Assessment of right ventricular function by strain rate imaging in chronic obstructive pulmonary disease. *Eur Respir J.* 2006;27:268-275.

90. Simonneau G, Robbins, IM, Beghetti M, et al. Updated clinical classification of pulmonary hypertension. *J Am Coll Cardiol.* 2009;54:S43-S54.

91. Yeo TC, Dujardin KS, Tei C, et al. Value of a Doppler-derived index combining systolic and diastolic time intervals in predicting outcome in primary pulmonary hypertension. *Am J Cardiol.* 1998;81:1157-1161.

92. Hatle HK, Appleton CP, Popp RL. Differentiation of constrictive pericarditis and restrictive cardiomyopathy by Doppler echocardiography. *Circulation.* 1989;79:357-370.

93. Reuss CS, Wilansky SM, Lester SJ, et al. Using mitral 'annulus reversus' to diagnose constrictive pericarditis. *Eur J Echocardiogr.* 2009;10:372-375.

94. Marcus FI, Nava A, Thiene G, eds. *Arrhythmogenic RV Cardiomyopathy/Dysplasia: Recent Advances.* New York, NY: Springer; 2007.

95. Yoeger DM, Marcus FI, Sherrill D, et al. Echocardiographic findings in patients meeting task force criteria for ARVD: new insights from the multidisciplinary study of ARVD. *J Am Coll Cardiol.* 2005;45:860-865.

96. Yoeger DM, Marcus FI, Sherrill D, et al. Right ventricular myocardial performance index in probands from the multicenter study of ARVD. *J Am Coll Cardiol.* 2005;45:147A.

97. Prakasa KR, Wang J, Tandri H, et al. Utility of tissue Doppler and strain echocardiography in arrhythmogenic right ventricular dysplasia/cardiomyopathy. *Am J Cardiol.* 2007;100:507-512.

98. Nava A, Batice B, Basso C, et al. Clinical profile and long term follow up of 37 families with ARVC. *J Am Coll Cardiol.* 2000;36:2226-2233.

99. Teske AJ, Cox MG, De Boeck BW, et al. Echocardiographic Tissue deformation imaging quantifies abnormal regional right ventricular function in arrhythmogenic right ventricular dysplasia/cardiomyopathy. *J Am Soc Echcoardiogr.* 2009;22:920-927.

100. Sievers B, Addo M, Franken U, et al. Right ventricular wall motion abnormalities in healthy subjects by cardiovascular magnetic resonance imaging and characterized with a new segmental model. *J Cardiovasc Magn Res.* 2004;6:601-608.

101. Bomma C, Rutberg J, Tandri H, et al. Misdiagnosis of ARVD/C. *J Cardiovasc Electrophysiol.* 2004;15:300-306.

102. Tandri H, Bomma C, Calkins H, Bluemke DA. Magnetic resonance and computed tomography imaging in arrhythmogenic right ventricular dysplasia. *J Magn Reson Imaging.* 2004;19:848-858.

103. Jain A, Tandri H, Calkins H, Bluemke DA. Role of cardiovascular magnetic resonance imaging in arrhythmogenic right ventricular dysplasia. *J Cardiovasc Magn Reson.* 2008;10:32.

104. Tandri H, Saranthan M, Rodriquez ER, et al. Noninvasive detection of myocardial fibrosis in ARVC using delayed-enhancement magnetic resonance imaging. *J Am Coll Cardiol.* 2005;4:98-103.

105. Bomma C, Tandri H, Nasir K, et al. Role of helical CT in qualitative and quantitative evaluation of ARVD. *Pacing Clin Electrophysiol.* 2003;1:965.

106. Ott P, Marcus FI, Sobonya RE, et al. Cardiac sarcoidosis masquerading as right ventricular dysplasia. *Pacing Clin Electrophysiol.* 2003;26:1498-1503.

107. Wichter T, Indik J, Daliento L. Diagnostic role of angiography. In: Marcus FI, Nava A, Thiene G, ed. *Arrhythmogenic Right Ventricular Cardiomyopathy/Dysplasia: Recent Advances.* Milan, Italy: Springer Verlag; 2007:147-158.

108. Daliento L, Rizzoli G, Thiene G, et al. Diagnostic accuracy of right ventriculography in arrhythmogenic right ventricular cardiomyopathy. *Am J Cardiol.* 1990;66:741-745.

109. Indik JH, Wichter T, Gear K, Dallas WJ, Marcus FI. Quantitative assessment of angiographic right ventricular wall motion in arrhythmogenic right ventricular dysplasia/cardiomyopathy (ARVD/C). *J Cardiovasc Electrophysiol.* 2008;19:39-45.

110. Hebert J-L, Chemla D, Gerard O, et al. Angiographic right and left ventricular function in arrhythmogenic right ventricular dysplasia. *Am J Cardiol.* 2004;93:728-733.

111. Marcus FI, Zareba W, Calkins H, et al. Arrhythmogenic right ventricular cardiomyopathy/dysplasia clinical presentation and diagnostic evaluation: results from the North American Multidisciplinary Study. *Heart Rhythm.* 2009;6:984-992.

112. Greer ML, McDonald C, Adatia I. MRI of Uhl's anomaly. *Circulation.* 2000;101:E230-E232.

113. Boettler P, Claus P, Herbots L, et al. New aspects of the ventricular septum and its function: an echocardiographic study. *Heart.* 2005;91:1343-1348.

114. Takahashi N, Ishida Y, Maeno M, et al. Noninvasive identification of left ventricular involvements in arrhythmogenic right ventricular dysplasia: comparison of 123I-MIBG, 201TlCl, magnetic resonance imaging and ultrafast computed tomography. *Ann Nucl Med.* 1997;11:233-241.

115. Wichter T, Hindricks G, Lerch H, et al. Regional myocardial sympathetic dysinnervation in arrhythmogenic right ventricular cardiomyopathy: an analysis using 123I-meta-iodobenzylguanidine scintigraphy. *Circulation.* 1994;89:667-683.

116. Mariano-Goulart D, Déchaux L, Rouzet F, et al. Diagnosis of diffuse and localized arrhythmogenic right ventricular dysplasia by gated blood-pool SPECT. *J Nucl Med.* 2007;48:1416-1423.

117. Maron BJ, Towbin JA, Thiene G, et al. Contemporary definitions and classification of the cardiomyopathies: An American Heart Association Scientific Statement from the Council on Clinical Cardiology, Heart Failure and Transplantation Committee; Quality of Care and Outcomes Research and Functional Genomics and Translational Biology Interdisciplinary Working Groups; and Council on Epidemiology and Prevention. *Circulation.* 2006;113:1807-1816.

CHAPTER 20
ISCHEMIC HEART DISEASE

Brian B. Ghoshhajra, Ricardo C. Cury,
and Richard D. White

INTRODUCTION / 354

THE ISCHEMIC CASCADE: A FRAMEWORK FOR
   CATEGORIZATION / 354

RADIOGRAPHY/FLUOROSCOPY / 354

ULTRASOUND / 354

STRESS ECHOCARDIOGRAPHY / 355

COMPUTED TOMOGRAPHY / 355

MAGNETIC RESONANCE IMAGING / 358

NUCLEAR CARDIOLOGY / 358

INVASIVE IMAGING METHODS / 359

INTRODUCTION

The available imaging arsenal for the detection and management of ischemic heart disease has never been larger. Many new noninvasive imaging techniques have obviated the need for many invasive diagnostic procedures and offer risk stratification of patients with known and newly detected disease. Imaging allows the stratification of patients with preclinical disease, beyond that of clinical risk factors. Finally, in cases of invasive diagnostic workups, new imaging modalities now offer highly accurate quantification and adjunctive information that was previously not possible.

THE ISCHEMIC CASCADE: A FRAMEWORK FOR CATEGORIZATION

Given the often overwhelming array of imaging modalities and potential findings from each given imaging test, a framework with which to categorize imaging findings is useful. The "ischemic cascade" that follows coronary artery occlusion (Fig. 20–1), as first described by Nesto and Kowalchuk,[1] provides such a framework. By establishing the progression from clinically unrecognized parameters to myocardial infarction, the concept of the ischemic cascade allows the physician to recognize and categorize the potential findings from a given imaging study and interpret them along a clinically meaningful spectrum.

The progression along the continuum of detectable abnormalities of the myocardium is preceded by detectable precursors

affecting the coronary arteries, namely atherosclerotic changes, although simple coronary arterial disease may not lead to ischemic consequences. In the presence of a discrete coronary artery stenosis or generalized arteriopathy significant enough to cause significantly decreased myocardial blood flow at rest or during stress (exercise or pharmacologically induced), perfusion defects can be initially detected. Diastolic myocardial dysfunction follows and then systolic dysfunction. Eventually, electrocardiogram (ECG) changes and infarction can be detected. Various imaging tests can detect or infer the presence of myocardial ischemia or infarct. These findings are summarized in Table 20–1.

Therefore, in this chapter, we discuss each imaging modality and outline the potential findings offered by each modality along the preclinical and clinical sequence of the ischemic cascade. When selecting the appropriate test for a given patient, the multisociety appropriateness criteria can serve as guidelines, allowing evidence-based expert consensus to guide the clinician in evaluating complex imaging decisions in an efficient manner.[2-5] In many cases, the complementary information provided by multiple tests is essential to patient management.[6] In certain instances, hybrid imaging allows simultaneous acquisition of this information (ie, positron emission tomography [PET]/computed tomography angiography [CTA] or single photon emission computed tomography [SPECT]/computed tomography [CT]).[7]

RADIOGRAPHY/FLUOROSCOPY

Chest radiography is a universally available, relatively inexpensive test that allows reliable assessment of cardiac size and of the sequelae of ischemic heart disease such as pulmonary venous hypertension, pulmonary edema from cardiogenic origin, and focal edema from ischemic valve disease (such as mitral regurgitation). Although normal radiographs cannot exclude ischemic heart disease, this easily performed test can reliably detect changes over time in patients with known heart disease.[8] X-ray fluoroscopy has historically been used to detect coronary calcification and cardiac size but is no longer used due to the availability of more reliable methods.

ULTRASOUND

Cardiac ultrasound, or echocardiography, is a widely available, radiation-free modality that is routinely used in the diagnosis and management of all forms of heart disease. Transthoracic echocardiography is the most commonly performed imaging examination in the United States.[9] Although limited by operator-dependent techniques, acoustic windows, and body habitus in obese patients, echocardiography plays a key role, offering robust information without the use of iodinated contrast or ionizing radiation. Transesophageal echocardiography, an invasive test, allows more reliable acoustic windows and imaging planes at the expense of time and invasiveness. Echocardiography allows the assessment of ventricular and

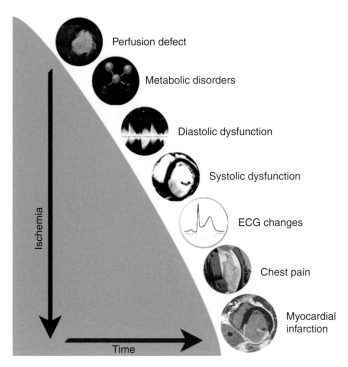

FIGURE 20–1. Following coronary stenosis or occlusion, a progression of detectable abnormalities of the myocardium begins with decreased myocardial blood flow (perfusion defects) at rest or during stress (exercise or pharmacologically induced). Diastolic myocardial dysfunction then follows, with later systolic dysfunction. Eventually, electrocardiogram (ECG) changes and progression to infarction occur. Various imaging tests can detect or infer these abnormalities.

atria size, global and regional left ventricular function, diastolic function (tissue relaxation/ventricular filling), myocardial wall thickness, and assessment for valvular disease. Doppler ultrasound also allows measurement of flow and calculation of gradients, such as in cases of valve dysfunction.[3] New techniques in echocardiography such as deformation (tissue tracking imaging), application of contrast, and three-dimensional imaging can expand the potential role of echocardiography and aid in selected cases.

TABLE 20–1. Complementary Imaging Modalities: Each Imaging Modality Demonstrates Unique Strengths and Weaknesses

Modality	Echo	CT	MRI	SPECT	PET	SCA
Plaque	–	+++	+	–	–	++
Perfusion defect	–	+	+++	++	+++	–
Diastolic dysfunction	+++	+	+++	–	–	–
Systolic dysfunction	+++	++	+++	+	+	+
Infarction	+	++	+++	++	++	+
Other findings	+++	+++	+++	+	+	+

CT, computed tomography; Echo, echocardiography; MRI, magnetic resonance imaging; PET, positron emission tomography; SCA, selective coronary angiography; SPECT, single photon emission computed tomography.

STRESS ECHOCARDIOGRAPHY

Stress echocardiography, performed with dobutamine (pharmacologic stress) and/or low-level exercise, allows the detection of induced wall motion abnormalities, a key finding along the ischemic cascade. This finding alone results in a high diagnostic accuracy for the detection of significant coronary artery disease (CAD).[2] Two different meta-analyses have been performed comparing the performance of stress echocardiography to conventional coronary angiography. The first included patients with an intermediate pretest likelihood of CAD (25%-75%), and the angiographic definition of significant coronary heart disease was either ≥50% or ≥70%. Stress echocardiography had a sensitivity and specificity of 76% and 88%, respectively, in six studies of 510 patients.[10]

The second meta analysis compared exercise echocardiography and exercise SPECT myocardial perfusion imaging with coronary angiography, with extent of stenosis varying between ≥50% and 75%. The two tests had similar sensitivity (85% for echocardiography and 87% for SPECT), but the specificity for stress echocardiography was significantly higher (77% for echocardiography vs 64% for SPECT).[11]

COMPUTED TOMOGRAPHY

CT of the heart has been performed for decades, but the challenges of cardiac motion and ECG gating have until recently been daunting. Early success with electron-beam CT allowed reliable quantification of calcium scores, which highly correlate with (preclinical) CAD burden.[12] However, this expensive technology has not become widely available.

With the advent of multidetector CT (MDCT), routine assessment of the coronary arteries became widely available. MDCT offers reliable calcium scoring. The use of calcium scoring can be used to lower the likelihood of CAD, but numerous recent studies have shown that a significant proportion of patients have only noncalcified plaque, which will be missed by calcium scoring CT.[13] Calcium scoring can help manage asymptomatic patients at intermediate risk for CAD by providing additional information compared with traditional risk factors alone,[14] which may help assess for preclinical manifestations of ischemic heart disease.

ECG-gated cardiac CT with intravenous bolus contrast enhancement has allowed the collection of a dynamic, three- or four-dimensional data set. Case 1 (illustrated in Fig. 20–2) demonstrates three-dimensional coregistration of CTA data in the multimodality workup of a patient for ischemic heart disease. Combined with advanced multiplanar reconstruction workstations, MDCT offers reliable coronary angiography by using 64-slice MDCT technology or higher. The direct visualization of coronary arteries and their lumen has been proven to be highly accurate in patients with satisfactory low and regular heart rates (often requiring β-blockade to achieve the necessary heart rate for scanning).[15] New scanner technologies such as increasing z-axis detector length, dual-source scanners, and prospective ECG triggering have allowed continual improvements in image quality, temporal resolution, and radiation doses.[16]

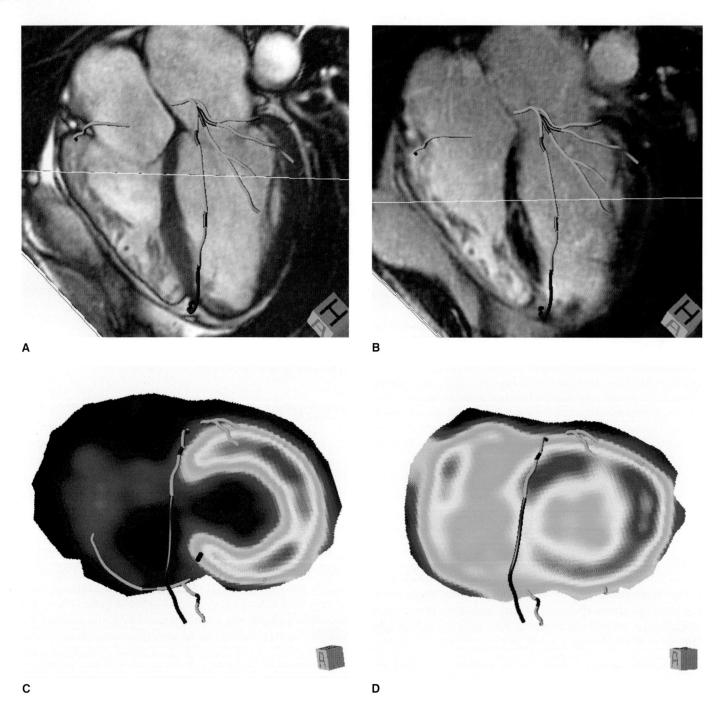

FIGURE 20–2. Case 1: Multimodality imaging for ischemic heart disease. Coregistration of computed tomography (CT), magnetic resonance imaging (MRI), fluorodeoxyglucose (FDG) positron emission tomography (PET) viability, and rubidium PET perfusion imaging allows the complementary roles of each modality to guide appropriate management. Fusions of multidetector CT (MDCT) and cine/delayed enhancement MRI images (**A** and **B**), MDCT and rubidium-PET perfusion images (**C**), and MDCT and FDG-PET images (**D**) demonstrate stenosis in the left anterior descending artery territory (red arterial map), corresponding to apical thinning and late gadolinium enhancement consistent with infarct on the MRI images (**A** and **B**), septal perfusion defect (**C**), and viability on FDG-PET images (**D**).

ECG-gated cardiac multidetector CTA can be used to reliably assess for CAD and can reliably exclude significant CAD, particularly in patients with low to intermediate probability of CAD.[5] One growing application of coronary CTA is the assessment of low- to intermediate-risk patents presenting to the emergency department with acute chest pain. Several trials demonstrated that a strategy using coronary CTA can decrease time for diagnosis, length of stay, and hospital costs, with zero major adverse cardiac events 30 days after discharge with a negative coronary CTA.[17-19]

Other established applications are assessment of coronary anomalies; patients presenting with atypical angina and low to intermediate likelihood of CAD; patients presenting with non-diagnostic or inconclusive stress tests; patients with new onset of heart failure and low to intermediate probability of CAD; and patients before valvular surgery to rule out CAD. Three recent multicenter trials confirmed prior observations of single-center studies demonstrating that 64-slice MDCT has a high sensitivity and specificity with a moderate positive predictive value and an excellent negative predictive value.[20-22]

More recent publications have validated the use of ECG-gated cardiac CT for complications of ischemic disease, such as coronary and ventricular aneurysms, myocardial thinning, and global and regional dysfunction. Case 2 (illustrated in Fig. 20–3) demonstrates CT of a left ventricular aneurysm. Preliminary research has demonstrated potential use for other manifestations of ischemic heart disease, such as myocardial characterization, and rest or stress perfusion defects.[23,24] Contrast CT can be contraindicated in cases of severe renal dysfunction, contrast allergy, and severe congestive heart failure.

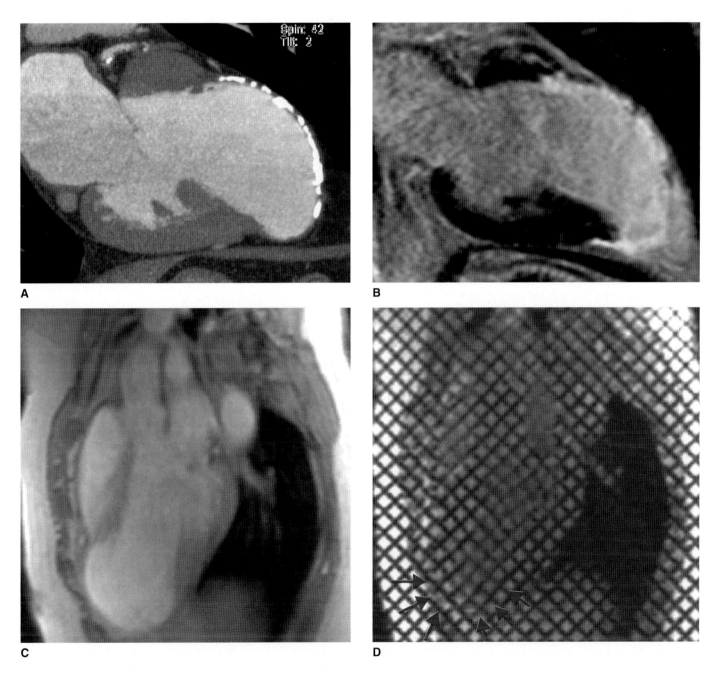

FIGURE 20–3. Case 2: Complementary roles of imaging modalities before and after intervention. **A.** Preoperative gated cardiac computed tomography demonstrates calcification, thinning, and thin mural thrombus in the mid to distal anterior wall and apex, consistent with aneurysm. **B.** Delayed-enhancement magnetic resonance imaging (MRI) with nulling of the normal myocardium demonstrates late gadolinium enhancement consistent with scar, while at the same time confirming viability of the remainder of the noninfarcted myocardium. Cine-MRI allows assessment of the ventricular size and function (**C**), while myocardial wall dynamics are demonstrated by the cine-tagged images (**D**). The tagged images shown in (D) are reconstructed in systole, demonstrating slight outward deformation of the tag lines (arrows), indicating dyskinesis. The patient underwent ventricular restoration with the Dor procedure, and MRI subsequently was performed for assessment of the myocardium. **E.** and **F.** Postsurgical MRI demonstrated restored ejection fraction and improved dynamic myocardial function. Cine images (E) now demonstrate restored postoperative configuration of the ventricle, and tagged images (F) appropriate systolic thickening (arrows) of the restored ventricle.

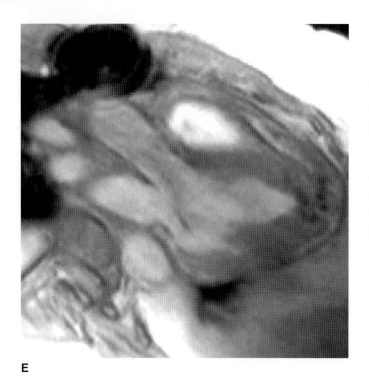

E

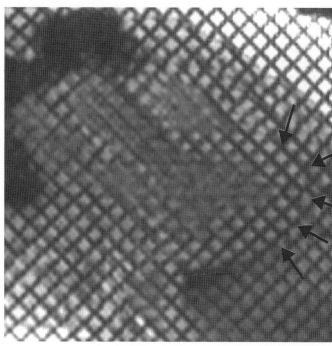

F

FIGURE 20–3. *(continued)*

MAGNETIC RESONANCE IMAGING

The use of cardiac magnetic resonance imaging (MRI) for ischemic heart disease is promising and still in its early stages. This modality allows accurate assessment of myocardial function (see Fig. 20–2, Case 1, for an example of ventricular thinning consistent with infarction), as well as first-pass myocardial perfusion (bolus of gadolinium agent during pharmacologic stress) and delayed enhancement (myocardial necrosis and scar). Because of the exquisite contrast resolution and excellent temporal resolution, MRI can identify subendocardial and transmural perfusion defects and characterize the transmyocardial perfusion gradient.[25] Use of cardiac MRI to assess the late manifestations of ischemic heart disease is well established.[26] The use of MRI to identify delayed enhancement allows reliable assessment of myocardial necrosis and scar and the identification of patterns of scar consistent with ischemic myocardial infarction. Case 2 (see Fig. 20–3) demonstrates findings of scar in a left ventricular aneurysm. In cases of cardiomyopathy of unknown origin, MRI allows excellent differentiation of ischemic cardiomyopathy from other causes of nonischemic cardiomyopathy.[27] MRI can also offer unmatched ability for tissue characterization, which can be useful in differentiating true aneurysm from pseudoaneurysm, evaluating for pericardial adhesions, and imaging in cases where echocardiography windows are limited. Phase-contrast MRI can evaluate and quantify flow in cases of shunting or valvular dysfunction. Limitations of MRI include safety issues relating to implantable hardware, such as automatic implantable cardioverter-defibrillators/pacemakers, and issues with contrast-enhanced MRI, such as gadolinium-induced nephrogenic systemic fibrosis (particularly in patients with severe renal dysfunction).[5]

NUCLEAR CARDIOLOGY

The use of radionuclide imaging is often a vital part of the imaging of ischemic heart disease. Stress myocardial perfusion imaging can be performed to detect relative perfusion defects, a sign of unbalanced coronary blood flow from significant stenosis. This test is frequently used and can identify ischemic territories, infer the distribution of coronary lesions, demonstrate fixed defects (infarcts), and quantify systolic function, each of which carries independent prognostic value beyond or in addition to the simple presence of ischemic myocardium. In certain situations, the test is limited, such as in cases of balanced ischemic lesions, obesity, and breast attenuation and diaphragmatic artifacts.[4] Myocardial perfusion imaging can be performed with SPECT or PET. SPECT and PET can be used with radiotracers targeted at perfusion (eg, technetium-based and rubidium agents, respectively) and myocardial viability (eg, thallium and fluorine 18 fluorodeoxyglucose, respectively). Myocardial perfusion can be especially helpful in cases of known ischemic heart disease, a situation where quantitation of ischemic burden can be essential to guide management. Newer hybrid scanners (PET/CT and SPECT/CT) can offer simultaneous acquisition of nuclear and CT data, offering the benefits of calcium scoring, attenuation correction, and even anatomic CTA in conjunction with myocardial perfusion data.[28] Case 1 (see Fig. 20–2) demonstrates rubidium PET and fluorodeoxyglucose PET in the workup for myocardial ischemia and viability, respectively. Advances in nuclear cardiology can include evaluation of ischemic memory with iodine 123–15-(p-iodophenyl)-3-(R,S)-methylpentadecanoic acid (BMIPP) in which an area at risk of acute myocardial infarction can be detected as a defect even a couple of weeks after the myocardial insult.

INVASIVE IMAGING METHODS

The multimodality imaging workup of ischemic heart disease often ends in selective coronary angiography (SCA), which offers the ability to both diagnose and treat CAD in a single setting. Imaging options at SCA include contrast angiography and intravascular ultrasound, which can characterize the luminal wall and allow evaluation of stents.[29] Invasive coronary angiography also allows simultaneous functional measurements by assessing the functional flow reserve (ie, pressure measurements).[30]

REFERENCES

1. Nesto RW, Kowalchuk GJ. The ischemic cascade: temporal sequence of hemodynamic, electrocardiographic and symptomatic expressions of ischemia. *Am J Cardiol*. 1987;59:23C-30C.
2. Douglas P, Khandheria B, Stainback R, Weissman N. ACCF/ASE/ACEP/AHA/ASNC/SCAI/SCCT/SCMR 2008 appropriateness criteria for stress echocardiography: a report of the American College of Cardiology Foundation Appropriateness Criteria Task Force, American Society of Echocardiography, American College of Emergency Physicians, American Heart Association, American Society of Nuclear Cardiology, Society for Cardiovascular Angiography and Interventions, Society of Cardiovascular Computed Tomography, and Society for Cardiovascular Magnetic Resonance endorsed by the Heart Rhythm Society and the Society of Critical Care Medicine. *J Am Coll Cardiol*. 2008;51:1127-1147.
3. Douglas PS, Khandheria B, Stainback RF, et al. ACCF/ASE/ACEP/ASNC/SCAI/SCCT/SCMR 2007 appropriateness criteria for transthoracic and transesophageal echocardiography: a report of the American College of Cardiology Foundation Quality Strategic Directions Committee Appropriateness Criteria Working Group, American Society of Echocardiography, American College of Emergency Physicians, American Society of Nuclear Cardiology, Society for Cardiovascular Angiography and Interventions, Society of Cardiovascular Computed Tomography, and the Society for Cardiovascular Magnetic Resonance endorsed by the American College of Chest Physicians and the Society of Critical Care Medicine. *J Am Coll Cardiol*. 2007;50:187-204.
4. Hendel RC, Berman DS, Di Carli MF, et al. ACCF/ASNC/ACR/AHA/ASE/SCCT/SCMR/SNM 2009 appropriate use criteria for cardiac radionuclide imaging: a report of the American College of Cardiology Foundation Appropriate Use Criteria Task Force, the American Society of Nuclear Cardiology, the American College of Radiology, the American Heart Association, the American Society of Echocardiography, the Society of Cardiovascular Computed Tomography, the Society for Cardiovascular Magnetic Resonance, and the Society of Nuclear Medicine: endorsed by the American College of Emergency Physicians. *Circulation*. 2009;119:e561-e587.
5. Hendel RC, Patel MR, Kramer CM, et al. ACCF/ACR/SCCT/SCMR/ASNC/NASCI/SCAI/SIR 2006 appropriateness criteria for cardiac computed tomography and cardiac magnetic resonance imaging: a report of the American College of Cardiology Foundation Quality Strategic Directions Committee Appropriateness Criteria Working Group, American College of Radiology, Society of Cardiovascular Computed Tomography, Society for Cardiovascular Magnetic Resonance, American Society of Nuclear Cardiology, North American Society for Cardiac Imaging, Society for Cardiovascular Angiography and Interventions, and Society of Interventional Radiology. *J Am Coll Cardiol*. 2006;48:1475-1497.
6. Shaw L, Narula J. Bridging the detection gap chasm of risk: where can computed tomography angiography take us? *JACC Cardiovasc Imaging*. 2009;2:524-526.
7. Kaufmann P. Cardiac hybrid imaging: state-of-the-art. *Ann Nucl Med*. 2009;23:325-331.
8. Chakko S, Woska D, Martinez H, et al. Clinical, radiographic, and hemodynamic correlations in chronic congestive heart failure: conflicting results may lead to inappropriate care. *Am J Med*. 1991;90:353-359.
9. Martin NM, Picard MH. Two years of appropriateness criteria for echocardiography: what have we learned and what else do we need to do? *J Am Soc Echocardiogr*. 2009;22:800-802.
10. Garber AM, Solomon NA. Cost-effectiveness of alternative test strategies for the diagnosis of coronary artery disease. *Ann Intern Med*. 1999;130:719-728.
11. Fleischmann KE, Hunink MG, Kuntz KM, Douglas PS. Exercise echocardiography or exercise SPECT imaging? A meta-analysis of diagnostic test performance. *JAMA*. 1998;280:913-920.
12. Rumberger JA, Simons DB, Fitzpatrick LA, Sheedy PF, Schwartz RS. Coronary artery calcium area by electron-beam computed tomography and coronary atherosclerotic plaque area. A histopathologic correlative study. *Circulation*. 1995;92:2157-2162.
13. Hausleiter J, Meyer T, Hadamitzky M, Kastrati A, Martinoff S, Schömig A. Prevalence of noncalcified coronary plaques by 64-slice computed tomography in patients with an intermediate risk for significant coronary artery disease. *J Am Coll Cardiol*. 2006;48:312-318.
14. Greenland P, Bonow RO, Brundage BH, et al. ACCF/AHA 2007 clinical expert consensus document on coronary artery calcium scoring by computed tomography in global cardiovascular risk assessment and in evaluation of patients with chest pain: a report of the American College of Cardiology Foundation Clinical Expert Consensus Task Force (ACCF/AHA Writing Committee to Update the 2000 Expert Consensus Document on Electron Beam Computed Tomography) developed in collaboration with the Society of Atherosclerosis Imaging and Prevention and the Society of Cardiovascular Computed Tomography. *J Am Coll Cardiol*. 2007;49:378-402.
15. Hendel RC, Budoff MJ, Cardella JF, et al. ACC/AHA/ACR/ASE/ASNC/HRS/NASCI/RSNA/SAIP/SCAI/SCCT/SCMR/SIR 2008 key data elements and definitions for cardiac imaging: a report of the American College of Cardiology/American Heart Association Task Force on Clinical Data Standards (Writing Committee to Develop Clinical Data Standards for Cardiac Imaging). *J Am Coll Cardiol*. 2009;53:91-124.
16. Brodoefel H, Burgstahler C, Tsiflikas I, et al. Dual-source CT: effect of heart rate, heart rate variability, and calcification on image quality and diagnostic accuracy. *Radiology*. 2008;247:346-355.
17. Goldstein JA, Gallagher MJ, O'Neill WW, Ross MA, O'Neil BJ, Raff GL. A randomized controlled trial of multi-slice coronary computed tomography for evaluation of acute chest pain. *J Am Coll Cardiol*. 2007;49:863-871.
18. Hoffmann U, Nagurney JT, Moselewski F, et al. Coronary multidetector computed tomography in the assessment of patients with acute chest pain. *Circulation*. 2006;114:2251-2260.
19. Hollander JE, Chang AM, Shofer FS, McCusker CM, Baxt WG, Litt HI. Coronary computed tomographic angiography for rapid discharge of low-risk patients with potential acute coronary syndromes. *Ann Emerg Med*. 2009;53:295-304.
20. Miller JM, Rochitte CE, Dewey M, et al. Diagnostic performance of coronary angiography by 64-row CT. *N Engl J Med*. 2008;359:2324-2336.
21. Meijboom WB, Meijs MFL, Schuijf JD, et al. Diagnostic accuracy of 64-slice computed tomography coronary angiography: a prospective, multicenter, multivendor study. *J Am Coll Cardiol*. 2008;52:2135-2144.
22. Budoff M, Dowe D, Jollis J, et al. Diagnostic performance of 64-multidetector row coronary computed tomographic angiography for evaluation of coronary artery stenosis in individuals without known coronary artery disease: results from the prospective multicenter ACCURACY (Assessment by Coronary Computed Tomographic Angiography of Individuals Undergoing Invasive Coronary Angiography) trial. *J Am Coll Cardiol*. 2008;52: 1724-1732.
23. Blankstein R, Shturman LD, Rogers IS, et al. Adenosine-induced stress myocardial perfusion imaging using dual-source cardiac computed tomography. *J Am Coll Cardiol*. 2009;54:1072-1084.
24. Cury RC, Nieman K, Shapiro M, Butler J, Nomura C. Comprehensive assessment of myocardial perfusion defects, regional wall motion, and left ventricular function by using 64-section multidetector CT. *Radiology*. 2008;248:466-475.
25. Klem I, Heitner JF, Shah DJ, et al. Improved detection of coronary artery disease by stress perfusion cardiovascular magnetic resonance with the use of delayed enhancement infarction imaging. *J Am Coll Cardiol*. 2006;47: 1630-1638.
26. Kim RJ, Fieno DS, Parrish TB, et al. Relationship of MRI delayed contrast enhancement to irreversible injury, infarct age, and contractile function. *Circulation*. 1999;100:1992-2002.
27. Calore C, Cacciavillani L, Boffa GM, et al. Contrast-enhanced cardiovascular magnetic resonance in primary and ischemic dilated cardiomyopathy. *J Cardiovasc Med (Hagerstown)*. 2007;8:821-829.
28. Dicarli M. Hybrid PET/CT is greater than the sum of its parts. *J Nucl Cardiol*. 2008;15:118-122.
29. Kim S-H, Hong M-K, Park D-W, et al. Impact of plaque characteristics analyzed by intravascular ultrasound on long-term clinical outcomes. *Am J Cardiol*. 2009;103:1221-1226.
30. Tonino PAL, De Bruyne B, Pijls NHJ, et al. Fractional flow reserve versus angiography for guiding percutaneous coronary intervention. *N Engl J Med*. 2009;360:213-224.

CHAPTER 21

ACUTE MYOCARDIAL INFARCTION

Joey F. A. Ubachs, Lia E. Bang, Jacob T. Lønborg, Philip Hasbak, Nina Hakačova, and Galen S. Wagner

INTRODUCTION / 360

ELECTROCARDIOGRAM / 360
    Anderson-Wilkins Acuteness Score / 360
    Sclarovsky-Birnbaum Ischemia Grading System / 361
    Localizing Myocardial Ischemia / 361

MYOCARDIAL PERFUSION SPECT / 362

CARDIAC MAGNETIC RESONANCE IMAGING / 362

POSITRON EMISSION TOMOGRAPHY / 362

MYOCARDIAL SALVAGE / 362

PATIENTS / 362
    Patient 1: Complete Myocardial Salvage—Aborted
        Infarction / 363
    Patient 2: Partial Myocardial Salvage / 364
    Patient 3: No Myocardial Salvage Because of Low
        Protection / 364
    Patient 4: No Myocardial Salvage Because of Late Presentation
        and Low Protection / 365
    Patient 5: Extension of Infarction Because of Interventional
        Embolization / 365

CLINICAL RELEVANCE / 366

INTRODUCTION

When a patient is presented at the emergency department or to a mobile emergency system with acute chest pain, the first assessment includes a standard 12-lead electrocardiogram (ECG). When chest pain is caused by an acute coronary occlusion, the initial ECG can show ST-segment elevation, which meets the criteria that indicate an ST-segment elevation myocardial infarction (STEMI). All five patients included in this chapter presented with first-time STEMI due to an occluded left anterior descending coronary artery as documented by emergency coronary angiography (Fig. 21–1).

The ECG is the initial modality used in the evaluation of patients with suspected acute myocardial infarction. It provides general information about presence and location of the acute ischemia/infarction process. Several ECG scoring systems are being used for assessment of the extent of the initially ischemic myocardium and also the extent of the final infarction. There are, however, limitations in using the ECG as a modality for sizing either the ischemic or infarcted region. In its current form, the ECG does not provide an image of the electrical activation or recovery. New methods are currently in development to transform the ECG waveforms into cardiac images, with algorithms to quantify key aspects of the ischemia/infarction process such as extent, acuteness, and severity.[1-3]

The five patients included in this chapter represent the varied outcomes that can result from acute percutaneous coronary intervention (PCI) that is intended to provide maximal salvage of ischemic myocardium. The ECG was used to assess the Anderson-Wilkins Acuteness Score and the Sclarovsky-Birnbaum Severity Ischemia Grade on the initial ECG to indicate the patient's potential for recovery of the involved region of myocardium.[4,5] Cardiovascular magnetic resonance (CMR) imaging was performed on all patients. Two patients received myocardial perfusion single photon emission computed tomography (SPECT) with the radioactive tracer injected prior to opening of the occluded vessel, and the other three patients received SPECT imaging with injection of the radioactive tracer only after the occluded vessel was opened. Positron emission tomography (PET) was performed on these three patients.

In this chapter, the methods used for analysis will be described briefly, followed by description and visualization of the five presented patients. The category of outcome for each of the patients is also considered.

ELECTROCARDIOGRAM

■ ANDERSON-WILKINS ACUTENESS SCORE

The ECG Anderson-Wilkins Acuteness Score indicates the acuteness of an episode of acute myocardial infarction on a continuous scale from 4.0 to 1.0; 4.0 represents a hyperacute process, while 1.0 indicates a late, subacute process. The score is based on the comparative T wave amplitudes versus abnormal Q wave durations in each of the leads with ST-segment elevation or tall T waves. The *acuteness phase* is designated for each of these leads based on the presence (A) or absence (B) of a tall T wave and the absence (1) or presence (2) of an abnormal Q wave, with 1A being the most acute (tall T waves without abnormal Q waves) and 2B being the least acute (positive but not tall T waves with abnormal Q waves).[4]

The Anderson-Wilkins Acuteness Score is then calculated from the following formula:

$$\frac{4(\#\,leads\,1A)+3(\#\,leads\,1B)+2(\#\,leads\,2A)+(\#\,leads\,2B)}{Total\,leads\,with\,1A,1B,2A,or\,2B}$$

In Fig. 21–2, representing the example ECG of patient 1, an ST-segment elevation or tall T wave can be seen in leads I and aVL and in leads V_1 to V_6. All leads except V_1 show a tall T wave and no abnormal Q wave. Lead V_1 has a Q wave but no tall T wave. The final Anderson-Wilkins Acuteness Score is 3.6, indicating the presence of a highly acute myocardial infarction.

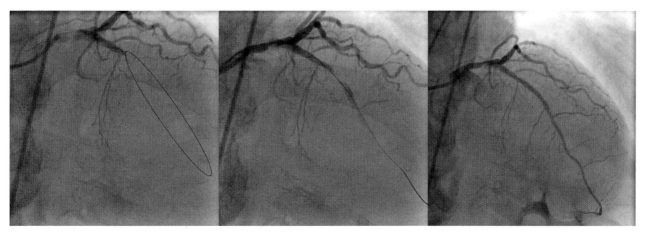

FIGURE 21–1. Angiography. Coronary angiogram during percutaneous coronary intervention of patient 4 are shown. The left panel shows an occlusion within the left anterior descending coronary artery (LAD). The red ellipse shows the actual location of the LAD. The middle panel shows the coronary artery with the transducer placed in the LAD. The right panel shows the LAD after percutaneous coronary intervention resulting in TIMI (thrombolysis in myocardial infarction) 3 flow.

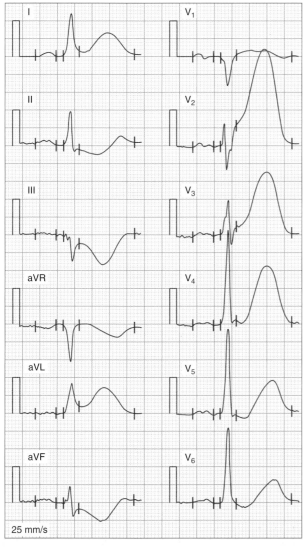

FIGURE 21–2. Initial electrocardiogram for patient 1 showing ST-segment elevation in leads I, aVL, and V_1 to V_3. In addition, tall T waves can be seen in leads I, aVL, and V_2 to V_6. The red vertical lines represent from left to right: P wave onset, P wave offset, QRS onset, QRS offset, and T wave offset.

SCLAROVSKY-BIRNBAUM ISCHEMIA GRADING SYSTEM

The Sclarovsky-Birnbaum Ischemia grading system is based on assessment of changes in the T wave, ST segment, and terminal part of the QRS complex, as a method for estimating the severity of ischemia as influenced by protection by either collateral vessels or metabolic preconditioning.[5] The grading system consists of three grades representing increasing severity: grade I—tall upright T waves without ST-segment elevation; grade II—ST-segment elevation in at least two adjacent leads without terminal QRS distortion; and grade III—ST-segment elevation with terminal QRS distortion in two or more adjacent leads. Figure 21–2 shows an example of grade II ischemia when assessed by the grading system.

LOCALIZING MYOCARDIAL ISCHEMIA

The clinical management of patients with acute coronary occlusion involves a complex assessment of the extent and severity of changes of both ischemia and infarction within the left ventricle. Often, the assessed methods are presented in different formats, and within each method, the orientation of the heart, angle selection for cardiac planes, nomenclature for segments, and assignment of segments to coronary arterial territories have evolved independently. This evolution has been based on the inherent strengths and weaknesses of the technique and the practical clinical application of these modalities as they are used for patient management. This independent evolution has resulted in a lack of standardization and has made accurate intra- and cross-modality comparisons difficult. A uniform method for display that allows for side-by-side comparison would therefore simplify data interpretation. Cerquiera et al[6] proposed a 17-segment standardized polar plot representation for the left ventricle, where the outer boundaries of the polar plot represent the base of the left ventricle and where the center of the polar plot represents the apex of the left ventricle. The 17-segment model facilitates multimodal imaging approaches.

Cain et al[7] used the polar plot representation for comparing myocardial perfusion SPECT, regional function by CMR, and viability by CMR. More recently, Ubachs et al[3] and Bacharova et al[1] developed ECG methods to visualize the ST-segment deviation on a polar plot representation (see Chapters 7 and 11). Ubachs et al[3] used the presence of ST-segment elevation on the standard 12-lead ECG to locate the ischemic myocardium based on the infarct distribution method described by Strauss and Selvester.[8] Bacharova et al[1] used the dipolar electrocardiotopography (DECARTO) method, where the center of the location is provided by the spatial orientation of the resultant ST vector.

MYOCARDIAL PERFUSION SPECT

Perfusion defect size by myocardial perfusion SPECT has been shown to correlate well with ex vivo measures of myocardial ischemia when the perfusion tracer is injected prior to PCI.[9] Its evolution and use over the last decades has made myocardial perfusion SPECT the gold standard for quantification of myocardial ischemia (see Chapter 3). However, it has been shown that the perfusion defect size has a strong correlation with the myocardial infarct size when the myocardial perfusion SPECT is performed a few days after opening of the coronary artery.[10]

CARDIAC MAGNETIC RESONANCE IMAGING

Along with recent technical advances, CMR imaging has become a powerful tool for the evaluation of irreversible myocardial injury. During acute myocardial infarction, cell membranes lose integrity and rupture, which increases the extracellular volume. By using an extracellular contrast medium, this region of irreversibly damaged myocardium can be accurately identified.[11] CMR imaging is usually undertaken 10 to 30 minutes after injection of an extracellular contrast medium.

Therefore, CMR imaging can be considered the reference method for in vivo visualization of myocardial infarction (see Chapter 6).

More recently, CMR has been introduced as a method for quantification of the myocardium at risk by using a T2-weighted sequence that visualizes myocardial edema. This method has been validated in both animals[12] and humans.[13] In the patients presented in this chapter, there is a difference in imaging parameters. Patients 1 and 2 were imaged using an 8-mm slice thickness, whereas patients 3, 4, and 5 were imaged using a 15-mm slice thickness. This probably results in a slight overestimation of the myocardium at risk in patients 3, 4, and 5 due to partial volume effect in the most basal slices.

POSITRON EMISSION TOMOGRAPHY

Unlike myocardial perfusion SPECT imaging, which detects single photons, PET imaging detects paired simultaneous annihilation photons. This coincidence detection leads to least an increase in the sensitivity of PET compared with myocardial perfusion SPECT, with improved image quality.

Flow reserve (hyperemic flow/baseline flow) and absolute quantification of regional, baseline, and maximal myocardial perfusion (in mL/min/g tissue) are feasible and well validated using dynamic PET image acquisition. These quantitative data can support visual and semiquantitative image interpretation and improve detection of preclinical and multivessel coronary artery disease. PET provides a sensitivity of 91% and a specificity of 89% for the diagnosis of obstructive coronary artery disease.[14] Just as in myocardial perfusion SPECT, PET imaging uses ionizing radiation that can result in late adverse biologic effects. But positron-emitting tracers typically provide less radiation burden when compared with myocardial perfusion SPECT tracers due to their short half-lives.

The most widely used tracers for evaluating myocardial perfusion with PET in clinical practice are generator produced rubidum-82, cyclotron produced nitrogen-13 ammonia, and to some degree oxygen-15 water. Another commonly used PET tracer is fluorine-18 fluoro-2-deoxy-D-glucose (^{18}F-FDG). The uptake and retention of ^{18}F-FDG reflects the activity of the various glucose transporters and hexokinase-mediated phosphorylation in a matter similar to unlabeled glucose. In the setting of ischemic heart disease, viable myocardium often exhibits a shift in substrate utilization from aerobic to anaerobic metabolism. Therefore, ^{18}F-FDG imaging can be used to assess glycolytic activity of the myocardium during ischemia.

More information on positron emission tomography can be found in Chapter 3

MYOCARDIAL SALVAGE

The myocardium at risk, defined as the hypoperfused myocardium during acute coronary occlusion, is an important measure because a variable amount of this area will become infarcted. Therefore, to assess the efficacy of reperfusion therapy, it is necessary to determine how much myocardium is salvaged by measuring the final infarct size in relation to the initial myocardium at risk. The initial myocardium at risk is determined by myocardial perfusion SPECT and the finally infarcted myocardium is determined by CMR for the two patients in whom the radioactive tracer was injected prior to reperfusion. For the other three patients, T2-weighted CMR was used to assess myocardium at risk.

Myocardial salvage is defined as:

$$\frac{100 \times (\text{Initial myocardium at risk} - \text{Finally infarcted myocardium})}{\text{Initial myocardium at risk}}$$

PATIENTS

The five patients included in this chapter are from two study sites; patients 1 and 2 are from Skåne University Hospital in Lund, Sweden; and patients 3, 4, and 5 are from Copenhagen University Hospital in Copenhagen, Denmark. All five patients received standard and DECARTO ECG studies to estimate the location of the ischemic myocardium and CMR imaging with late gadolinium enhancement to measure infarct size.

All patients also received CMR imaging with a T2-weighted sequence to measure the myocardium at risk. The three patients from Copenhagen University Hospital received ^{18}F-FDG PET imaging to estimate the infarcted myocardium and the potentially viable myocardium with sufficient metabolic abnormality to appear abnormal by this method.

In patients with acute coronary occlusion, reperfusion before loss of myocardial viability can potentially salvage some portion of the ischemic cells so that they return to their normal contractile function. However, because there is a limited amount of time that non-blood-perfused myocardial cells can rely on anaerobic metabolism for preservation of their anatomy and physiology, the time to reperfusion is critical.[15] This can also be called the *salvagability time window.*

There are several specific etiologies for failure to achieve salvage. One is an excessive delay between time of acute coronary occlusion and time of reperfusion, as illustrated by patient 2.

There is also the variable level of "ischemic protection" provided by preexisting collateral vessels and/or ischemic preconditioning. Prior episodes of ischemia facilitate both of these protective mechanisms. Patients without prior ischemia may have a much shorter salvagability time window, as illustrated by patient 3.

Even when the patient receives reperfusion within their salvagability time window, the therapeutic intervention could be complicated by distal embolization of a portion of the thrombus. The embolic material could occlude native or collateral vessels, producing ischemia and potentially infarction of additional myocardium. An example is presented by patient 5.

Even when the ischemic myocardium is salvaged, there is physiologic delay in its resumption of contractile function by the metabolic process termed *stunning.*[16] The oxygen and glucose provided by the reperfusing blood is used to restore both cellular physiologic function and biochemical substrate. There may be further delay in resumption of contractile function caused my many pathologic processes, and this has been termed *hibernation.* For patient 2, significant myocardial salvage has been achieved, and for patient 1, total salvage has been achieved. However, this salvaged myocardium requires time before providing its contribution to the global left ventricular contractile function.

PATIENT 1: COMPLETE MYOCARDIAL SALVAGE–ABORTED INFARCTION

A 71-year-old man with no history of myocardial infarction was admitted to the emergency department with a complaint of increasing chest pain while warming up for a game of tennis. Since then, approximately 90 minutes had passed. The admitting ECG showed sinus rhythm and ST-segment elevation in leads I, aVL, and V_1 to V_3. The patient's initial serum levels of creatine kinase-MB (CK-MB) and troponin T were within the normal range (5 µg/L and <0.05 µg/L, respectively). The angiography revealed an occlusion of the left anterior descending coronary artery.

Based on his initial ECG, the patient had an Anderson-Wilkins Acuteness Score of 3.6 suggesting a hyperacute stage of myocardial infarction. His Sclarovsky-Birnbaum Ischemia Grade was II.

The patient received myocardial perfusion SPECT with a perfusion tracer injected prior to opening of the coronary artery. Furthermore, the patient received CMR imaging approximately 1 week after acute coronary occlusion with addition of a T2-weighted sequence.

Ischemic myocardium:

- By myocardial perfusion SPECT: 37% of the left ventricle
- By T2-weighted CMR: 36% of the left ventricle

Infarct size:

- By CMR imaging: 0% of left ventricle

Myocardial salvage:

- By myocardial perfusion SPECT and CMR imaging: 100% of the initial ischemic area is salvaged

Figure 21–3 shows multimodal polar plot representations of the different methods assessed in this patient. Note that no myocardial infarction was seen on the late gadolinium-enhanced CMR images.

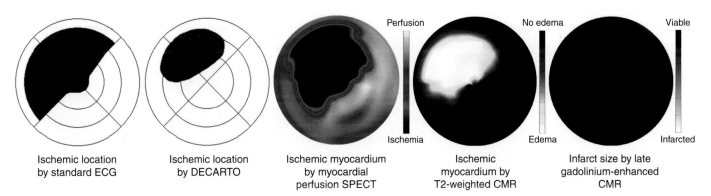

| Ischemic location by standard ECG | Ischemic location by DECARTO | Ischemic myocardium by myocardial perfusion SPECT | Ischemic myocardium by T2-weighted CMR | Infarct size by late gadolinium-enhanced CMR |

FIGURE 21–3. Multimodal polar plot representation for patient 1 of different methods for side-by-side comparison. The left polar plot shows the location of the myocardium at risk in blue as proposed by Ubachs et al.[3] The second polar plot from the left shows the location of the myocardium at risk in blue by the dipolar electrocardiotopography (DECARTO) method proposed by Bacharova et al.[1] The third polar plot with color scale represents the myocardium at risk as presented by the gold standard myocardial perfusion single photon emission computed tomography (SPECT). The dark colors represent the myocardial perfusion defect. The fourth polar plot with color scale represents the myocardium at risk as presented by T2-weighted cardiovascular magnetic resonance (CMR). The polar plot to the right shows the final infarct size by CMR imaging. In this patient, there was no infarct present on the late gadolinium-enhanced images CMR images.

This patient presented at the emergency department approximately 90 minutes after onset of chest pain. The high Anderson-Wilkins Acuteness Score (3.6) indicates that the occlusion had not remained complete for that entire 1.5 hours. The ECG myocardial perfusion SPECT and T2-weighted CMR indicate a moderate-sized ischemic region in the left anterior descending coronary artery distribution. The late gadolinium-enhanced CMR indicated a completely aborted infarction.

■ PATIENT 2: PARTIAL MYOCARDIAL SALVAGE

An 84-year-old man was admitted to the emergency department with a complaint of severe chest pain accompanied by dyspnea for approximately 4 hours. The admitting ECG showed sinus rhythm and ST-segment elevation in leads aVL and V_1 to V_4. The patient's initial serum levels of CK-MB and troponin T were within the normal range (3.5 µg/L and <0.05 µg/L, respectively). The angiography revealed an occlusion of the left anterior descending coronary artery.

Based on his initial ECG, he had an Anderson-Wilkins Acuteness Score of 2.8 and a Sclarovsky-Birnbaum Ischemia Grade of II.

The patient received myocardial perfusion SPECT with a perfusion tracer injected prior to opening of the coronary artery. Furthermore, the patient received CMR imaging approximately 1 week after acute coronary occlusion with addition of a T2-weighted sequence.

Ischemic myocardium:

- By myocardial perfusion SPECT: 39% of the left ventricle
- By T2-weighted CMR: 31% of the left ventricle

Infarct size:

- By CMR imaging: 11% of the left ventricle

Myocardial salvage:

- By myocardial perfusion SPECT and CMR imaging: 72% of the initial ischemic area is salvaged

Figure 21–4 shows multimodal polar plot representations for this patient. Note the similarities among the different methods.

This patient presented at the emergency department approximately 4 hours after pain onset. The mid-range Anderson-Wilkins Acuteness Score (2.8) indicates that the occlusion had not remained complete for those entire 4 hours. The extent of the ischemic myocardium in the left anterior descending coronary artery distribution was moderate: between 31% and 39% by the clinical modalities. Because the extent of the infarcted myocardium is much less (11%), there is "partial" myocardial salvage.

■ PATIENT 3: NO MYOCARDIAL SALVAGE BECAUSE OF LOW PROTECTION

A 74-year-old man presented to the emergency department complaining of central chest pain for approximately 2 hours. The admitting ECG showed sinus rhythm and an ST-segment elevation in leads I, aVL, and V_1 to V_6.

Based on his initial ECG, he had an Anderson-Wilkins Acuteness Score of 4.0 suggesting a hyperacute stage of myocardial ischemia/infarction; however, his Sclarovsky-Birnbaum Ischemia Grade was III, indicating poor myocardial protection. Coronary angiography performed approximately 1 hour later revealed an occlusion of the left anterior descending coronary artery, and catheter-based reperfusion was achieved approximately 90 minutes after the initial ECG. The patient received myocardial perfusion SPECT, CMR with T2-weighted imaging, and ^{18}F-FDG PET imaging during the following days.

Ischemic myocardium:

- By T2-weighted CMR: 56% of the left ventricle

Infarct size:

- By CMR imaging: 36% of the left ventricle

Myocardial salvage:

- By T2-weighted CMR and CMR imaging: 36% of the initial ischemic area is salvaged

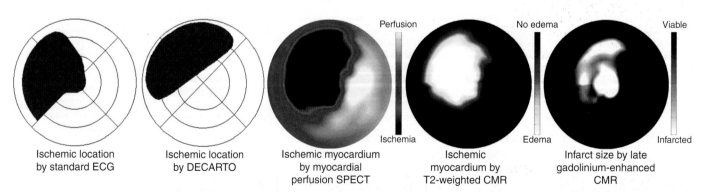

| Ischemic location by standard ECG | Ischemic location by DECARTO | Ischemic myocardium by myocardial perfusion SPECT | Ischemic myocardium by T2-weighted CMR | Infarct size by late gadolinium-enhanced CMR |

FIGURE 21–4. Multimodal polar plot representation for patient 2 of different methods for side-by-side comparison. The left polar plot shows the location of the myocardium at risk in blue as proposed by Ubachs et al.[3] The second polar plot from the left shows the location of the myocardium at risk in blue by the dipolar electrocardiotopography (DECARTO) method proposed by Bacharova et al.[1] The third polar plot with color scale represents the myocardium at risk as presented by the gold standard myocardial perfusion single photon emission computed tomography (SPECT). The dark colors represent the myocardial perfusion defect. The fourth polar plot with color scale represents the myocardium at risk as presented by T2-weighted cardiovascular magnetic resonance (CMR). The polar plot to the right shows the final infarct size by CMR imaging. In this patient, there was a final infarct size of 11%, resulting in a myocardial salvage of 72% when compared with myocardial perfusion SPECT.

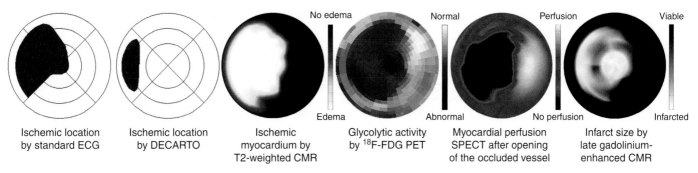

| Ischemic location by standard ECG | Ischemic location by DECARTO | Ischemic myocardium by T2-weighted CMR | Glycolytic activity by ¹⁸F-FDG PET | Myocardial perfusion SPECT after opening of the occluded vessel | Infarct size by late gadolinium-enhanced CMR |

FIGURE 21–5. Multimodal polar plot representation for patient 3 of different methods for side-by-side comparison. The left polar plot shows the location of the myocardium at risk in blue as proposed by Ubachs et al.[3] The second polar plot from the left shows the location of the myocardium at risk in blue by the dipolar electrocardiotopography (DECARTO) method proposed by Bacharova et al.[1] The third polar plot with color scale represents the myocardium at risk as presented by T2-weighted cardiovascular magnetic resonance (CMR). The fourth polar plot with color scale represents the glycolytic activity as assessed by ¹⁸F-FDG positron emission tomography (PET). The fifth polar plot with color scale represents the infarct size as assessed by myocardial perfusion single photon emission computed tomography (SPECT) where the tracer was injected after the occluded vessel was opened. The polar plot to the right shows the final infarct size by CMR imaging.

Figure 21–5 shows multimodal polar plot representations for this patient. Note the similarities among the different methods.

This patient presented at the emergency department approximately 2 hours after pain onset. On the initial ECG, the Anderson-Wilkins Acuteness Score (4.0) indicated that the ischemia/infarction process was very acute, but the Sclarovsky-Birnbaum Ischemia Grade (III) indicated absence of protection of the ischemic myocardium. The extent of the initially ischemic myocardium in the left anterior descending coronary artery distribution was estimated by T2-weighted CMR at 56% of the left ventricle, and the extent of the finally infarcted myocardium was estimated at 36% of the left ventricle. The ischemic myocardium is probably slightly overestimated due to the previously described partial volume effect, which would result in even a lower percentage of myocardial salvage. This small percentage of myocardial salvage is probably due to the rapid development of infarction in the poorly protected myocardium before reperfusion was established.

PATIENT 4: NO MYOCARDIAL SALVAGE BECAUSE OF LATE PRESENTATION AND LOW PROTECTION

A 51-year-old man presented to the emergency department with a complaint of increasing chest pain while cycling to his workplace. Since then, approximately 2 hours had passed. The admitting ECG showed sinus rhythm and an ST-segment elevation in leads aVL and V_1 to V_6. The patient's serum levels of CK-MB and troponin T approximately 6 hours after presenting at the emergency department were 780 μg/L and 14.1 μg/L, respectively. The angiography revealed an occlusion of the left anterior descending coronary artery.

Based on his initial ECG, he had an Anderson-Wilkins Acuteness Score of 3.0 and a Sclarovsky-Birnbaum Ischemia Grade of III.

The patient received myocardial perfusion SPECT, CMR imaging with T2-weighted imaging, and ¹⁸F-FDG PET imaging after the coronary artery was opened by PCI.

Ischemic myocardium:
- By T2-weighted CMR: 39% of the left ventricle

Infarct size:
- By CMR imaging: 39% of the left ventricle

Myocardial salvage:
- By T2-weighted CMR and CMR: 0% of the initial ischemic area is salvaged

Figure 21–6 shows multimodal polar plot representations for this patient. Note the similarities among the different methods.

This patient presented at the emergency department approximately 2 hours after pain onset. The mid-range Anderson-Wilkins Acuteness Score (3.0) indicated that the LAD may have remained occluded during the 2 hours following onset of chest pain, and the high Sclarovsky-Birnbaum Grade (III) indicated that the extensive (39%) region of ischemic myocardium was poorly protected. The large infarct size by CMR (39%) indicated the absence of myocardial salvage, probably because the infarction process had progressed rapidly even before the initial ECG was recorded and continued during the time before reperfusion was established.

PATIENT 5: EXTENSION OF INFARCTION BECAUSE OF INTERVENTIONAL EMBOLIZATION

A 60-year-old man presented at the emergency department with a complaint of increasing chest pain radiating to left arm and chin for approximately 60 minutes. The admitting ECG showed sinus rhythm and ST-segment elevation in leads I, aVL, and V_2 to V_5. The patient's serum levels of CK-MB and troponin T approximately 6 hours after presenting at the emergency department were 432 μg/L and 10.0 μg/L, respectively. The angiography revealed an occlusion of the left anterior descending coronary artery that was rapidly removed by PCI.

Based on his initial ECG, he had an Anderson-Wilkins Acuteness Score of 3.5 and a Sclarovsky-Birnbaum Ischemia Grade of II.

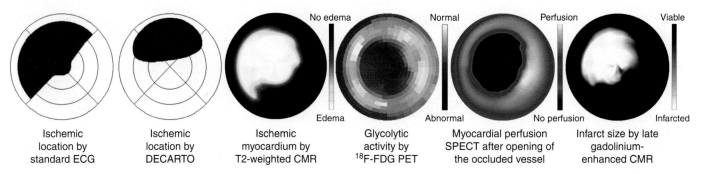

FIGURE 21–6. Multimodal polar plot representation for patient 4 of different methods for side-by-side comparison. The left polar plot shows the location of the myocardium at risk in blue as proposed by Ubachs et al.[3] The second polar plot from the left shows the location of the myocardium at risk in blue by the dipolar electrocardiotopography (DECARTO) method proposed by Bacharova et al.[1] The third polar plot with color scale represents the myocardium at risk as presented by T2-weighted cardiovascular magnetic resonance (CMR). The fourth polar plot with color scale represents the glycolytic activity as assessed by ^{18}F-FDG positron emission tomography (PET). The fifth polar plot with color scale represents the infarct size as assessed by myocardial perfusion single photon emission computed tomography (SPECT) where the tracer was injected after the occluded vessel was opened. The polar plot to the right shows the final infarct size by CMR imaging.

The patient received myocardial perfusion SPECT, CMR imaging with T2-weighted imaging, and ^{18}F-FDG PET imaging after the coronary artery was opened by PCI.

Ischemic myocardium:

• By T2-weighted CMR: 59% of the left ventricle

Infarct size:

• By CMR imaging: 51% of the left ventricle

Myocardial salvage:

• By T2-weighted CMR and CMR: 14% of the initial ischemic area is salvaged

Figure 21–7 shows multimodal polar plot representations for this patient. Note the similarities among the different methods.

This patient presented at the emergency department approximately 1 hour after pain onset, and the acuteness of the process was confirmed by the Anderson-Wilkins Acuteness Score (3.5) on the initial ECG. The Sclarovsky-Birnbaum Grade (II)

indicated the presence of protection of the extensive (59%) ischemic myocardium. Despite the early reperfusion therapy, this patient developed a large final infarct size measured by CMR (51%). This final infarct size, despite the presence of protection, can in this case be explained by a complication during the PCI.

CLINICAL RELEVANCE

Currently, patients presenting with the ST-segment changes typical of acute coronary occlusion receive primary PCI if this is logistically feasible. However, PCI is not always possible in smaller local hospitals, where these patients are treated with intravenous thrombolytic therapy. Indeed, patients with smaller, well-protected infarcts might benefit more from thrombolytic therapy instead of from PCI. The use of the polar plot representation of the ischemic region by ECG might provide support for the decision of which reperfusion treatment should be used. In centers capable of performing diagnostic methods such as

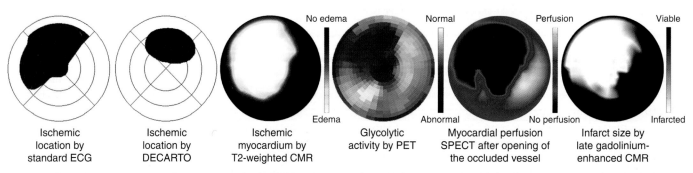

FIGURE 21–7. Multimodal polar plot representation for patient 5 of different methods for side-by-side comparison. The left polar plot shows the location of the myocardium at risk in blue as proposed by Ubachs et al.[3] The second polar plot from the left shows the location of the myocardium at risk in blue by the dipolar electrocardiotopography (DECARTO) method proposed by Bacharova et al.[1] The third polar plot with color scale represents the myocardium at risk as presented by T2-weighted cardiovascular magnetic resonance (CMR). The fourth polar plot with color scale represents the glycolytic activity as assessed by fluorine ^{18}F-FDG positron emission tomography (PET). The fifth polar plot with color scale represents the infarct size as assessed by myocardial perfusion single photon emission computed tomography (SPECT) where the tracer was injected after the occluded vessel was opened. The polar plot to the right shows the final infarct size by CMR imaging.

myocardial perfusion SPECT and magnetic resonance imaging, the polar plot provides a common format for comparing the location and extent of both the initially ischemic and finally infarcted myocardium. Furthermore, in the current era of data storage, the treating physician often has to review a great amount of files to get a clear understanding of the outcome from all the performed modalities. Polar plot representation of these modalities provides a quick visually comparable image and is therefore a potentially helpful method for patient management.

ACKNOWLEDGMENTS

The authors express their gratitude to Ljuba Bacharova, Peer Grande, Erik Hedström, Marcus Carlsson, and Håkan Arheden for assistance in performing the studies.

REFERENCES

1. Bacharova L, Mateasik A, Carnicky J, et al. The dipolar electrocardiotopographic (DECARTO)-like method for graphic presentation of location and extent of area at risk estimated from ST-segment deviations in patients with acute myocardial infarction. *J Electrocardiol*. 2009;42:172-180.
2. Galeotti L, Strauss DG, Ubachs JF, Pahlm O, Heiberg E. Development of an automated method for display of ischemic myocardium from simulated electrocardiograms. *J Electrocardiol*. 2009;42:204-212.
3. Ubachs JF, Engblom H, Hedstrom E, et al. Location of myocardium at risk in patients with first-time ST-elevation infarction: comparison among single photon emission computed tomography, magnetic resonance imaging, and electrocardiography. *J Electrocardiol*. 2009;42:198-203.
4. Heden B, Ripa R, Persson E, et al. A modified Anderson-Wilkins electrocardiographic acuteness score for anterior or inferior myocardial infarction. *Am Heart J*. 2003;146:797-803.
5. Sclarovsky S, Mager A, Kusniec J, et al. Electrocardiographic classification of acute myocardial ischemia. *Isr J Med Sci*. 1990;26:525-531.
6. Cerqueira MD, Weissman NJ, Dilsizian V, et al. Standardized myocardial segmentation and nomenclature for tomographic imaging of the heart: a statement for healthcare professionals from the Cardiac Imaging Committee of the Council on Clinical Cardiology of the American Heart Association. *J Nucl Cardiol*. 2002;9:240-245.
7. Cain PA, Ugander M, Palmer J, Carlsson M, Heiberg E, Arheden H. Quantitative polar representation of left ventricular myocardial perfusion, function and viability using SPECT and cardiac magnetic resonance: initial results. *Clin Physiol Funct Imaging*. 2005;25:215-222.
8. Strauss DG, Selvester RH. The QRS complex—a biomarker that "images" the heart: QRS scores to quantify myocardial scar in the presence of normal and abnormal ventricular conduction. *J Electrocardiol*. 2009;42:85-96.
9. Sinusas AJ, Trautman KA, Bergin JD, et al. Quantification of area at risk during coronary occlusion and degree of myocardial salvage after reperfusion with technetium-99m methoxyisobutyl isonitrile. *Circulation*. 1990;82:1424-1437.
10. Gibbons RJ, Valeti US, Araoz PA, Jaffe AS. The quantification of infarct size. *J Am Coll Cardiol*. 2004;44:1533-1542.
11. Kim RJ, Fieno DS, Parrish TB, et al. Relationship of MRI delayed contrast enhancement to irreversible injury, infarct age, and contractile function. *Circulation*. 1999;100:1992-2002.
12. Aletras AH, Tilak GS, Natanzon A, et al. Retrospective determination of the area at risk for reperfused acute myocardial infarction with T2-weighted cardiac magnetic resonance imaging: histopathological and displacement encoding with stimulated echoes (DENSE) functional validations. *Circulation*. 2006;113:1865-1870.
13. Carlsson M, Ubachs JF, Hedstrom E, Heiberg E, Jovinge S, Arheden H. Myocardium at risk after acute infarction in humans on cardiac magnetic resonance: quantitative assessment during follow-up and validation with single-photon emission computed tomography. *J Am Coll Cardiol*. 2009;2:569-576.
14. Di Carli MF, Dorbala S. Cardiac PET-CT. *J Thorac Imaging*. 2007;22:101-106.
15. Reimer KA, Lowe JE, Rasmussen MM, Jennings RB. The wavefront phenomenon of ischemic cell death. 1. Myocardial infarct size vs duration of coronary occlusion in dogs. *Circulation*. 1977;56:786-794.
16. Braunwald E, Kloner RA. The stunned myocardium: prolonged, postischemic ventricular dysfunction. *Circulation*. 1982;66:1146-1149.

CHAPTER 22
DISEASES OF THE AORTA

Igor Mamkin and John F. Heitner

AORTIC ANATOMY, PHYSIOLOGY, AND FUNCTION / 368
Anatomy of the Aorta / 368
Physiology and Function of the Aorta / 368
Imaging Considerations / 369

ANATOMIC VARIANTS AND CONGENITAL ANOMALIES / 371
Aortic Root Variants and Anomalies / 371
Aortic Arch Variants and Anomalies / 371

AORTIC DISSECTION / 372
Incidence, Etiology, and Pathophysiology / 372
Classification / 372
Diagnostic Imaging / 373
Management Strategies / 377

AORTIC INTRAMURAL HEMATOMA / 377
Incidence, Risk Factors, and Pathophysiology / 377
Diagnosis / 377

AORTIC ATHEROMATOUS DISEASE / 377
Pathophysiology / 378
Aortic Atheromatous Plaques and Atheroembolization / 378
Thrombosis and Thromboembolization / 379
Aortic Penetrating Atherosclerotic Ulcers / 380

AORTIC ANEURYSMS / 380
Thoracic Aortic Aneurysms / 380
Abdominal Aortic Aneurysms / 384

CONGENITAL AORTIC DISEASES / 385
Coarctation and Atresia of the Aorta / 385
Bicuspid AV–Associated Aortopathy / 386
Marfan Syndrome / 387

TRAUMATIC AORTIC INJURY / 388
Pathophysiology / 388
Imaging / 388

AORTIC TUMORS / 388

AORTITIS / 388
Imaging / 388
Infectious Aortitis / 389
Noninfectious Aortitis / 389

AORTIC ANATOMY, PHYSIOLOGY, AND FUNCTION

■ ANATOMY OF THE AORTA

To have an understanding of aortic diseases, it is imperative to have a good knowledge base in anatomy, physiology, and function of the normal aorta. The aorta is a large conductance blood vessel, often called *the greatest artery*, normally reaching 0.7 m in length and 3.5 cm in diameter. It arises from the heart, arches anterocranially and then posterocaudally, and descends caudally, terminating as it bifurcates into the right and left common iliac arteries. The aorta is divided into six segments: (1) the aortic root, (2) the sinotubular junction, (3) the ascending aorta, (4) the aortic arch, (5) the isthmus and descending thoracic aorta, and (6) the abdominal aorta (Fig. 22–1).

The aortic root originates at the aortic valve annulus level and extends to the sinotubular junction. Normal diameter of the aortic root (at the widest proximal portion, known as bulbous) is up to 3.5 cm. The bulbous portion of the aorta is subdivided into the sinuses of Valsalva. The site where the bulbous portion of the aorta meets the narrower tubular-shaped aorta is termed sinotubular junction. Effacement of this junction suggests annuloaortic ectasia and often is seen in patients with Marfan syndrome. The ascending aorta follows the sinotubular junction and extends to the right brachiocephalic artery. The ascending aorta is an intrapericardial structure, measuring approximately 5 cm in length and up to 3 cm in diameter. The aortic arch is extrapericardial and courses leftward anterior to the trachea and continues posterior to the left of the trachea and esophagus and gives rise to all three great vessels: the innominate artery (brachiocephalic trunk), left common carotid artery, and left subclavian artery (Fig. 22–2). The normal diameter of the aortic arch is up to 2.9 cm. Arch branch vessel variants and right-sided arches can sometimes be seen. The isthmus is the narrower portion of the aorta (by approximately 3 mm) between the left subclavian artery and ligamentum arteriosus, a remnant of the ductus arteriosus. Blunt traumatic deceleration injury, resulting in transection to the aorta often occurs at this site. The descending thoracic aorta begins at the ligamentum arteriosus and continues to the level of the diaphragm. The descending thoracic aorta gives rise to intercostal, spinal, and bronchial arteries. The abdominal aorta starts at the hiatus of the diaphragm and courses retroperitoneal to its bifurcation. Major branch vessels include celiac arteries, superior and inferior mesenteric arteries, and middle suprarenal, renal, and testicular or ovarian arteries. The diameter of the suprarenal abdominal aorta is usually up to 2 cm. The infrarenal aorta diameter should never exceed that of the suprarenal aorta.

The aorta has a trilaminar wall comprised of tunica intima, tunica media, and tunica adventitia. The tunica intima consists of an endothelium, subendothelial tissue, and an internal elastic membrane. The tunica media is composed of elastic fibers arranged as circumferential lamellae, elastin, collagen, smooth muscle cells, and ground substance. Adventitia is a thin, outermost layer of the aorta consisting of collagen; vasa vasorum, which is the vascular supply to the aorta; and nervi vascularis, which is the network of primarily adrenergic fibers.

■ PHYSIOLOGY AND FUNCTION OF THE AORTA

Elastin-to-collagen ratio in the tunica media progressively decreases from proximal aorta to distal aorta and to peripheral arteries. This architecture ensures accommodation of stroke volume (cushioning function) and storage of potential energy in systole (capacitor function) and release of kinetic energy in diastole, propelling blood forward (Windkessel phenomenon). In addition, this is responsible for progressive increase

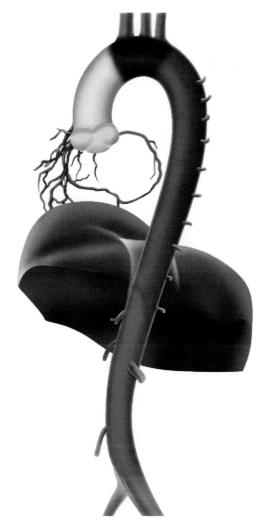

FIGURE 22-1. Segmental division of the aorta: the aortic root (light blue), the sinotubular junction (green), the ascending aorta (yellow), the aortic arch (dark blue), the isthmus and descending (thoracic) aorta (red), and the abdominal aorta (purple). This figure was published in *Aortic Diseases: Clinical Diagnostic Imaging Atlas*, Hutchinson SJ, copyright Elsevier 2009.

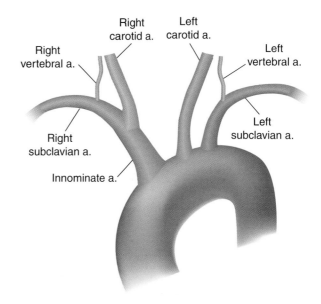

FIGURE 22-2. The most common (normal) aortic arch branching pattern found in humans has separate origins for the innominate, left common carotid, and left subclavian arteries (a). Reproduced with permission from Layton KF, et al. Bovine aortic arch variant in humans: clarification of a common misnomer. *Am J Neuroradiol.* 2006;27:1541-1542, © by American Society of Neuroradiology.

slope of the upslope and the peak are dependent on the elasticity of the vessel and the volume of blood entering the aorta. Dicrotic notch is only seen in the proximal aorta and results from the aortic valve closure. The pressure decay corresponds to diastolic pressure and is affected by peripheral resistance and reflected pressure waves (in the healthy aorta). There is a progressive decrease in mean aortic and diastolic pressures and an increase in systolic aortic pressure with increasing distance from the heart.

IMAGING CONSIDERATIONS

Chest Radiography

The aortic "knob" may be seen in the superior mediastinum, on the left side, just lateral to spinal column on the chest roentgenogram. The aortic root and proximal ascending aorta are visible as they arise from the base of the heart on the lateral chest roentgenogram. Left anterior oblique projection provides the best view of the ascending aorta and the arch. Intimal calcifications and aneurysmal dilation may be seen.

Advantages of chest radiography include wide availability, no contrast exposure, low cost, minimal radiation exposure, and the ability to be performed quickly at the bedside. Disadvantages include low spatial resolution, two-dimensional (2D) static image, and relatively poor target acquisition for aortic diseases (Table 22-1).

Echocardiography and Ultrasonography

The aortic root, sinuses of Valsalva, sinotubular junction, and proximal ascending aorta are usually well seen on a parasternal long axis view by transthoracic echocardiography (TTE).[1]

in pulse wave velocity of propagation from the proximal aorta to peripheral vessels. In the normal aorta, the pulse wave is transmitted down the aorta to its bifurcation and peripheral vasculature where it is reflected back toward the heart during diastole, contributing to diastolic pressure. These properties usually decline with aging or diseased aorta due to disruption of elastin and decreased elastin-to-collagen ratio. In the diseased aorta, the propagation wave is faster, which causes an earlier return of the reflected waves (during systole) and a summation with the systolic wave. This leads to self-perpetuation of hypertension. In addition, increased aortic stiffness has been associated with increased risk of myocardial infarction, stroke, congestive heart failure, and both cardiovascular and overall mortality.

Aortic pressure waveform can be distinguished by its four components: (1) the upslope, (2) the peak, (3) the dicrotic notch, also known as incisura, and (4) the pressure decay. The

TABLE 22–1. Comparison of Technical Specifications for Various Imaging Modalities

Variables	Chest Radiography	Echocardiography	Angiography	CT Angiography	MR Angiography
Spatial resolution	1-2 mm	~0.5-2 mm	0.16 mm	0.5-0.625 mm	1-2 mm
Temporal resolution	N/A	20-30 ms (M-mode <5 ms)	1-10 ms	83-135 ms	20-50 ms
Contrast resolution	Moderate	Low-moderate	Moderate	Low-moderate	High
Radiation	0.1 mSv	No	5-8 mSv	5.3-20 mSv	No
Target acquisition	+	++	+++	+++	+++
Contrast exposure	No	No	Yes	Yes	No
Time	<1 min	5-30 min	30-60 min	<1 min	30-40 min
Dimension	2D	2D or 3D	2D	3D	3D
Availability	+++	+++	+	++	+

Definitions: spatial resolution is the smallest distance that two targets can be separated for the system to distinguish between them; temporal resolution is the ability of the system to accurately track moving targets over time, and target acquisition is the ability of the system to accurately image the desired object.

2D, two-dimensional; 3D, three-dimensional; CT, computed tomography; MR, magnetic resonance; N/A, not applicable.

This table was published in *J Cardiovasc Comput Tomogr.*, 3, Lin E, et al. 403-408, copyright Elsevier 2009.

However, mechanical and stented bioprosthetic aortic valves produce acoustic shadows and reverberations. Distal ascending aorta and the arch are less well visualized by TTE. Suprasternal notch and supraclavicular windows offer the best views of the aorta in long and short axes. TTE allows visualization of the retrocardiac aorta in short and long axis (with clockwise rotation and lateral angulation of the transducer) on parasternal long axis view. Lateral angulation of the image plane in the apical two-chamber view can also be used to image the descending thoracic aorta. A posterior chest wall approach is particularly useful for imaging of the descending aorta in patients with large left pleural effusion. In the subcostal window, a lateral angulation of the transducer in the inferior vena cava plane allows visualization of the proximal abdominal aorta.

Transesophageal echocardiography (TEE) at 30° to 45° and 120° to 140° rotation at mid to high esophageal level is particularly helpful and less artifactual in evaluation of the aortic root, sinuses of Valsalva, sinotubular junction, and proximal ascending aorta. Withdrawing the transducer in the esophagus in the esophageal long axis plane produces more cephalad images of the ascending aorta. Medial turning and inferior angulation of transesophageal transducer at the arch level provide superior detail of the aortic arch in the long axis plane. Transesophageal transducer maybe turned around (either direction) at 0° to obtain a short axis view of the descending aorta. Rotation of the image plane to 90° allows depiction of the aorta in the long axis view, and the left subclavian artery may be located in this plane.

Ultrasonography (US) is a useful modality for abdominal aorta examination. It is commonly used for aortic disease screening, sequential monitoring for the assessment of aortic size, and evaluation of branch vessel involvement.

Advantages of echocardiography and ultrasonography include superb temporal resolution (especially with M-mode imaging), three-dimensional (3D) imaging, ability to assess functional

cardiac complications of aortic diseases, wide availability, no contrast or ionizing radiation exposure, relatively low cost, and ability to be performed quickly at the bedside. Disadvantages include suboptimal target acquisition, inability to image the entire aorta, and can be time consuming.

Computed Tomography

The aortic root, sinotubular junction, and ascending aorta have significant motion throughout the cardiac cycle, and thus are prone to significant motion artifact with non–electrocardiography (ECG)-gated imaging modalities. ECG gating is recommended when imaging these proximal structures by either computed tomography (CT) or magnetic resonance angiography (MRA). The aortic arch, isthmus, and descending aorta are subject to little motion artifact.

CT allows various postprocessing displays and generates very detailed images of the arterial wall and lumen with high spatial resolution. Pacemaker wires in the superior vena cava (SVC) and brachiocephalic vein, mechanical aortic valves, pericardial structures, and contrast dye concentrated in SVC may produce artifacts when the aortic root, ascending aorta, and aortic arch are imaged with CT. The prevalence of motion artifact on a 1-second scanning time CT is reported to be as high as 57%.[2] Multidetector CT (MDCT) technology significantly reduces respiratory artifacts and improves temporal resolution due to reduction of scanning time to 0.5 seconds. However, non–ECG-gated MDCT was reported to produce motion artifacts in 91.9% of cases.[3] Fujioka et al[4] reported a prevalence of diagnosis nonhampering motion artifact in 6.7% of cases with ECG-gated MDCT. In the absence of spinal prosthesis, CT of descending aorta produces very few artifacts.

Advantages of CT include 3D imaging, superb spatial resolution, excellent temporal resolution, very fast scanning time (<1 minute), high sensitivity and specificity for the assessment of aortic disease, postprocessing reconstruction, and wide availability. Disadvantages include ionizing radiation and contrast exposure.

Magnetic Resonance Imaging

Magnetic resonance imaging (MRI) and MRA can accurately depict the aortic lumen and the wall with minimal artifacts. The artifacts that one can encounter, however, include signal dropout from metallic clips and mechanical valves; ghosting artifacts (encountered when images are acquired during systolic phases of the cardiac cycle); insufficient dose of contrast agent (results in low signal-to-noise ratio); wraparound artifact, usually in coronal plane (aliasing due to data sampled in a discrete rather than continuous fashion); and susceptibility artifacts from concentrated contrast agent in the nearby venous structures.

MRI and MRA offer the ability to assess the aorta in both a 2D and 3D format. The number of different pulse sequences can be used to assess function and anatomy. A typical evaluation for the aorta would begin with anatomic assessment with axial, sagittal, and coronal dark blood turbo spin-echo (TSE) pulse sequence covering the entire thoracic or abdominal aorta. The dark blood TSE sequence obtains all the data for the particular slice within one heartbeat and thus allows for multiple slices without requiring the patient to hold their breath. Once the anatomic imaging is performed, cine images with a gradient echo pulse sequence are performed to assess the function of the aorta as well as the aortic valve (AV) when necessary. This image is generally performed in an oblique plane by scouting off of the dark blood TSE images. The next step in the evaluation includes typically a contrast-enhanced angiogram, which is gated to the heart (this avoids motion artifact within the proximal ascending aorta). The angiogram is a breath-hold sequence, which typically takes approximately 15 to 20 seconds to complete. If necessary, when blood flow needs to be quantified (ie, coarctation of the aorta), velocity-encoded pulse sequence is performed to assess the velocity of blood through the aorta at the level in question. This is the standard exam for the assessment of the aorta and can be tailored for each specific disease. The TSE dark blood sequence is useful in assessing the aortic wall, aortic dissection (AD), and other anatomic structures/abnormalities. If higher resolution is needed, then a single slice breath-hold TSE could be performed. This is often necessary when one wants to assess the aortic wall as in intramural hematoma or plaque assessment. The cine imaging is useful for more functional aspects of the aorta as in coarctation, AV insufficiency, and aortic distensibility. The MRA allows for a very high-resolution image of the aorta and is excellent in AD assessment and the 3D assessment of aneurysms. The benefit of 3D imaging is that the true cross-sectional diameter of an aneurysm can be easily assessed via postprocessing computer software.

Advantages of MRI include excellent temporal and spatial resolution, the wide spectrum of pulse sequences allowing for a 3D comprehensive assessment of the aorta, excellent target acquisition, and no ionizing radiation or contrast exposure. Disadvantages include lack of access at some centers, longer scanning time (can be prohibitive in patients who are hemodynamically unstable), artifacts due to respiratory motion in patients who are unable to breath-hold), inability of patients with large body habitus to fit inside the scanner, contraindication in patients with metal implants (eg, pacemakers/defibrillators, cerebral aneurysm clips), and the possibility that some patients may experience claustrophobia.

Aortography

Aortography is an invasive test during which a multiholed catheter (usually pigtail) is passed percutaneously via radial, brachial, axillary, or femoral approach into the aorta; contrast material is injected via a power injector; and multiple radiographic views (or cine) are recorded. The ascending aortogram is often performed in a moderately steep, 30° to 60° left anterior oblique view. In the past, aortography was a first-line diagnostic test for imaging the aorta; presently, it is typically reserved for guiding aortic interventions.

Advantages of aortography include superb spatial resolution, excellent target acquisition, and good temporal resolution. Disadvantages include invasiveness, exposure to ionizing radiation and contrast, lack of access in some centers, production of 2D images, and time consuming to perform.

ANATOMIC VARIANTS AND CONGENITAL ANOMALIES

■ AORTIC ROOT VARIANTS AND ANOMALIES

In approximately 1% of healthy individuals, the AV is bicuspid forming two sinuses, rather than the usual tricuspid valve with three sinuses. Quadricuspid AVs with four sinuses are a rare finding with incidence of up to 0.01%. Bicuspid AVs may be associated with various pathologies of the ascending aorta and may result in AD. Anomalies of coronary artery ostia are common. These include separate ostia for left anterior descending artery and left circumflex artery, one or more infundibular (conal) arteries arising from separate ostia, duplicated arteries, high take-off (above sinotubular junction), and ostium arising from opposite sinus or pulmonary trunk.

■ AORTIC ARCH VARIANTS AND ANOMALIES

The second most common pattern of the aortic arch is a common origin of innominate and left common carotid arteries, and a less common variant occurs when the left common carotid artery originates directly from the innominate artery. Both are commonly referred to as *bovine-type arch*. However, a true bovine aortic arch has no resemblance to any of these variations. In cattle, a single brachiocephalic trunk originates from the aortic arch and gives rise to both subclavian arteries and a bicarotid trunk, which then branches into right and left common carotid arteries. Other variants include internal mammary artery originating from the thyrocervical trunk and left vertebral artery coming off the aortic arch. Kommerell's diverticulum is a diverticulum of the proximal portion of an aberrant left subclavian artery (occurs with right-sided aortic arch) or right subclavian artery (occurs with left-sided aortic arch), potentially compressing the esophagus posteriorly. Double aortic arch

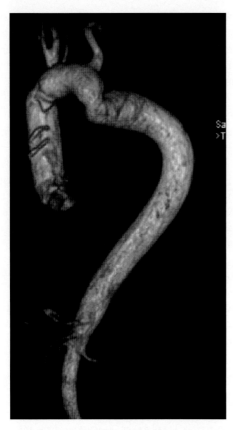

FIGURE 22–3. Magnetic resonance angiography with contrast and three-dimensional reconstruction revealing kinking and buckling of the aorta typically seen in pseudocoarctation.

is a common form of vascular ring in which the trachea and esophagus are encircled by the aortic arches (right arch tends to be larger). The most common form of right-sided aortic arch is associated with an aberrant origin of the left subclavian artery, diverticulum of Kommerell, and left-sided ligamentum arteriosum. The second most common right-sided aortic arch is associated with brachiocephalic vessels originating from the arch in mirror-image fashion with the left innominate artery. The other two types are rare. A cervical aortic arch is a rare entity, sometimes associated with other cervical vessel anomalies and commonly presenting as a pulsatile mass on either side of the neck or supraclavicular area. Aortic spindle is a circumferential bulge in the posterior aortic arch area just distal to the left subclavian artery. Pseudocoarctation develops from elongation of the aortic arch and kinking at the level of insertion of the ligamentum arteriosum without a pressure gradient across this region (Fig. 22–3). Other very rare anomalies include double dorsal aorta, subclavian artery as the first branch of the aortic arch, persistence in the fifth aortic arch, and pulmonary artery sling. The great anterior radiculomedullary artery (the artery of Adamkiewicz) is the dominant feeder of the spinal cord. Therefore, in patients with thoracoabdominal aortic aneurysms, identification of this artery is critical to minimize the risk of postoperative spinal cord ischemia. The artery of Adamkiewicz

originates from a left intercostal or lumbar artery, but in up to 75% of individuals, it arises from T9 to T12 intercostal artery. Ductus diverticulum is a focal, smooth convexity in the ventromedial aspect of proximal descending aorta. The important clinical significance of this structure lies in distinguishing it from a traumatic aortic disruption.

AORTIC DISSECTION

■ INCIDENCE, ETIOLOGY, AND PATHOPHYSIOLOGY

Acute AD is an uncommon but catastrophic aortic disease. AD may frequently be overlooked, with the diagnosis in a significant number of cases being established only postmortem. The estimated incidence is up to 3.5 per 100,000 per year, with at least 7000 cases per year in the United States.[5] Although early mortality was estimated at 1% per hour for untreated cases, the survival may be dramatically improved with timely management. In 1996, the International Registry of Acute Aortic Dissection (IRAD) was established, with the mission to better understand the presentation, diagnosis, management, and outcomes of patients presenting with acute AD. To date, IRAD has enrolled more than 2000 patients from 26 institutions and enlightened the understanding of this very important disease.[6]

Among the risk factors of AD, the most common are hypertension, advanced age, vascular atherosclerosis, preexisting aortic aneurysms, iatrogenic during cardiac surgery and percutaneous procedures, pregnancy (usually peripartum period), bicuspid AV, direct blunt trauma, Marfan syndrome, Ehlers-Danlos syndrome, inflammatory diseases, and cocaine use.

AD usually begins with an intimal tear (spontaneous due to diseased aortic wall, known as cystic medial degeneration, or iatrogenic, as a complication of various percutaneous or surgical procedures), allowing luminal blood to penetrate the medial layer, dissecting it longitudinally and forming the false lumen. Typically, the dissection extends anterogradely to or beyond common iliac arteries. The false lumen is often lateral to the true lumen in the descending aorta; however, medial or spiral (barber pole) orientations are described. AD may also be initiated with the rupture of vasa vasorum, resulting in aortic hematoma. Occasionally, the hematoma may extend distally or rupture through the intima causing an intimal tear and dissection.

■ CLASSIFICATION

Several classifications of AD have been developed, two of which, Stanford and DeBakey, are based on the aortic segment involved (Fig. 22–4). Recently, the Svensson classification was proposed and is based on the underlying pathologic process (Table 22–2). Stanford and DeBakey classifications share the same principle of grouping AD based on the involvement of ascending aorta (location of the intimal flap, irrespective of site of origin or location of the intimal tear), which in turn dictates the management and predicts the overall prognosis. ADs involving the

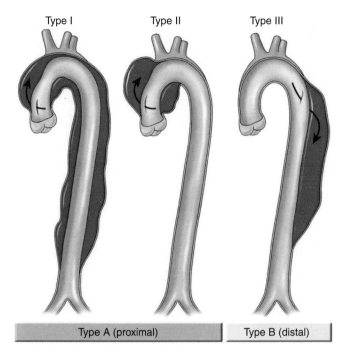

FIGURE 22–4. DeBakey and Stanford classification systems for aortic dissection (refer to Table 22–2 for definitions). This figure was published in *Braunwald's Heart Disease: A Textbook of Cardiovascular Medicine*, Libby P, et al, copyright Elsevier 2008.

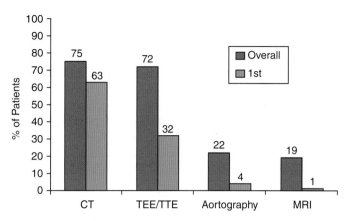

FIGURE 22–5. Overall percentage of study patients according to the imaging study of choice. CT, computed tomography; MRI, magnetic resonance imaging; TEE, transesophageal echocardiography; TTE, transthoracic echocardiography. Reproduced with permission from Moore AG, et al. Choice of computed tomography, transesophageal echocardiography, magnetic resonance imaging, and aortography in acute aortic dissection: International Registry of Acute Aortic Dissection (IRAD). *Am J Cardiol.* 2002;89:1235-1238.

ascending aorta comprise approximately two-thirds of AD, and current recommendations are to treat surgically, whereas ADs not involving the ascending aorta seem to do better with medical therapy (barring specific complications). Because the duration of AD (the time from symptom onset to presentation) also predicts the associated morbidity and mortality, AD is also classified as acute (<2 weeks) and chronic (≥2 weeks).

■ DIAGNOSTIC IMAGING

The imaging techniques for AD center on the use of CT, TEE, MRI, and aortography. The choice of diagnostic modality depends on patients' clinical status, equipment availability, and staff expertise. CT and TEE are the two most frequently used diagnostic tests, and the majority of the patients usually undergo two or more imaging tests (Fig. 22–5).

TABLE 22–2. Common Classification Systems of Thoracic Aortic Dissection

Type	Description
DeBakey	
Type I	Originates in the ascending aorta, propagates at least to the aortic arch and often beyond it distally
Type II	Originates in and confined to the ascending aorta
Type III	Originates in the descending aorta and extends distally down the aorta or, rarely, retrograde into the aortic arch and ascending aorta
Stanford	
Type A	All dissections involving the ascending aorta, regardless of the site of origin
Type B	All dissections not involving the ascending aorta
Svensson	
Class I	Classical aortic dissection with an intimal flap between true and false lumen
Class II	Medial disruption with formation of intramural hematoma
Class III	Discrete/subtle dissection without hematoma, eccentric bulge at tear site
Class IV	Plaque rupture leading to aortic ulceration, penetrating aortic atherosclerotic ulcer with surrounding hematoma, usually subadventitial
Class V	Iatrogenic and traumatic dissection

Computed Tomography

Spiral (helical) CT is the most frequently used imaging test for diagnosing acute AD around the world due to its accuracy and wide accessibility. CT provides a very detailed 3D depiction of the aorta and its branches. Earlier studies reported CT to be associated with insufficient sensitivity and specificity. However, a recent systematic review of the diagnostic accuracy of CT reported a mean sensitivity and specificity of 100% and 98%, respectively.[7] When compared with TEE and MRI, CT was also better for ruling out AD in patients at low pretest probability.[7] In addition to aiding in establishing the diagnosis of AD, CT assists in the management by providing invaluable information on the extent of the dissection, location of the intimal tear and flap, branch involvement, presence of an intramural hematoma, size of the true and false lumen, and presence of pericardial and/or pleural fluid (Fig. 22–6). Although motion artifacts of the aortic root and ascending aorta were rather common with older CT systems, contemporary 64-slice MDCT technology with ECG gating has significantly shortened scanning time, increased resolution, eliminated motion artifacts, and allowed simultaneous imaging of the aorta and coronary and pulmonary arteries.

Echocardiography

Echocardiography is well suited not only for the diagnosis of AD, but most importantly, for the evaluation of cardiac complications of acute AD such as presence and severity of aortic regurgitation, identification of pericardial effusion and tamponade, and evaluation of regional left ventricular wall motion abnormalities (in case of extension of a dissection into the coronary arteries, usually the right coronary artery). TTE has a sensitivity of 59% to 85% and a specificity of 63% to 96% for the diagnosis of AD.[8] TTE evaluation includes the standard and high parasternal windows for imaging of the ascending aorta, suprasternal notch window for the aortic arch, parasternal and apical windows for the descending aorta, and subcostal window for proximal abdominal aorta (Figs. 22–7 and 22–8).

TEE is the second most commonly used imaging test in the diagnosis of acute AD. Anatomic proximity of the esophagus

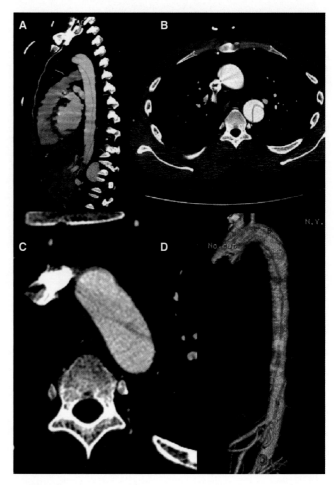

FIGURE 22–6. Contrast-enhanced computed tomography scan showing type B aortic dissection originating at the aortic arch and terminating just superior to the renal arteries. Sagittal view (**A**), transverse view of the ascending and proximal descending aorta (**B**), magnified view of the aortic arch (**C**), and three-dimensional reconstruction (**D**).

to the aorta makes it a far better technique than TTE, although proximal aortic arch is still difficult to image due to interference from the air-filled trachea and main stem bronchus (Fig. 22–9). The sensitivity of TEE for detecting AD is 98%, and

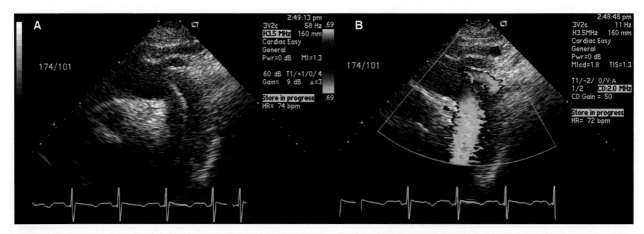

FIGURE 22–7. Transthoracic suprasternal view showing the aortic arch and descending aorta with an intimal flap (**A**) and color flow imaging demonstrating communication between the true and false lumen (**B**). With permission from Yuliya Kats, MD. See Moving Image 22–7.

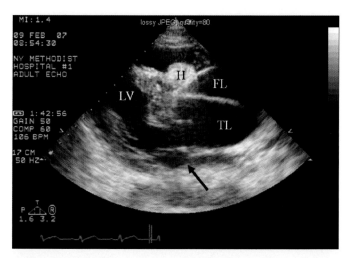

FIGURE 22–8. Transthoracic echocardiogram. Parasternal long axis view demonstrates massively dilated aorta (6.7 cm) compressing the left atrium (arrow). Type A aortic dissection with the true lumen (TL) separated from the false lumen (FL) by the intimal flap is evident. There is also evidence of the periaortic hematoma (H). LV, left ventricle.

the specificity is approximately 95%.[7] Differential flow between true and false lumens can often be visualized (Fig. 22–10). TEE does not require intravenous contrast or radiation, and advantageously in hemodynamically unstable patients, it can be performed at the bedside in 10 to 15 minutes. However, TEE may be associated with bradycardia, aspiration, hypertension, hypotension, transient atrioventricular block, and rarely, esophageal perforation, especially in patients with esophageal disease (eg, strictures, varices).

The 2003 American College of Cardiology (ACC)/American Heart Association (AHA)/American Society of Echocardiography (ASE) practice guidelines for echocardiography give a class I recommendation for TEE use in patients with AD, aortic rupture, and follow-up of AD, especially after surgical repair when complication or progression is suspected (class IIa recommendation is given to follow-up of AD after surgical repair without suspicion of complication or progression). The practice guidelines give a class IIa recommendation for TTE use in AD and class IIb recommendation for aortic rupture.[9]

Briefly, the ACC/AHA/ASE classification of recommendations is as follows: class I—conditions for which there is evidence for and/or general agreement that a given procedure or treatment is beneficial, useful, and effective; class II—conditions for which there is conflicting evidence and/or a divergence of opinion about the usefulness/efficacy of a procedure or treatment; class IIa—weight of evidence/opinion is in favor of usefulness/efficacy; class IIb—usefulness/efficacy is less well established by evidence/opinion; and class III—conditions for which there is evidence and/or general agreement that a procedure/treatment is not useful/effective and in some cases may be harmful.

Magnetic Resonance Imaging

MRI and MRA have a high mean sensitivity and specificity (98%) and yield the highest value for confirming AD in patients

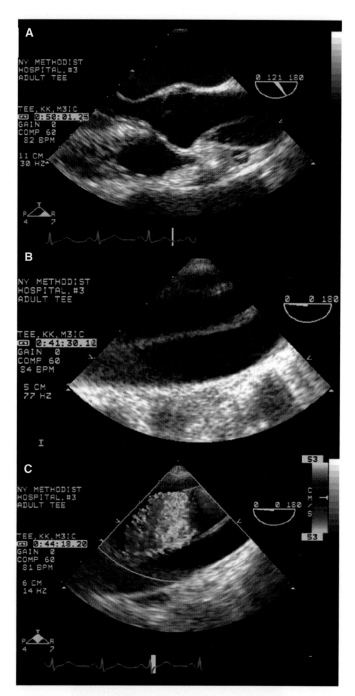

FIGURE 22–9. A transesophageal echocardiogram from a patient with acute type A aortic dissection. The intimal flap can be easily visualized in the long axis (120°) view of the aortic root and the ascending aorta (**A**) and in the long axis view (0°) of the aortic arch without (**B**) and with (**C**) Doppler color flow imaging.

with high pretest probability for AD.[7] Despite this, MRI is much less commonly used in the diagnosis of acute AD (Fig. 22–11) because of its limited availability, time delay, incompatibility with implantable devices (MRI-safe permanent pacemakers are becoming more available) and surgical clips, limited monitoring during the study, and claustrophobia.

However, MRI has certain advantages. It is not associated with radiation exposure, has a high sensitivity for type A and type B acute AD, is useful in detecting features of intramural hematoma

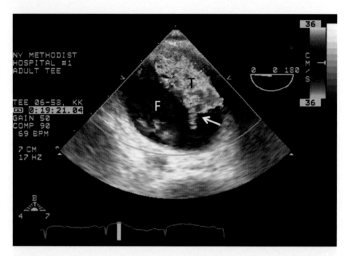

FIGURE 22–10. A transesophageal echocardiogram with Doppler color flow imaging at 0° showing the distal aortic arch in cross-section and evidence of a small communication (arrow) between the true (T) and false (F) lumen.

and penetrating aortic ulcer, and is considered the test of choice for follow-up evaluations of patients with surgically and/or medically managed aortic disease (Fig. 22–12). In addition, the safety profile of gadolinium is more favorable than that of the

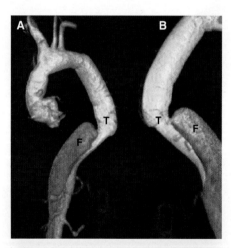

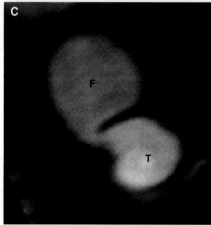

FIGURE 22–11. Magnetic resonance angiography with three-dimensional reconstruction of a descending aortic dissection (**A** and **B**) and transaxial view revealing the connection between the true (T) and false (F) lumen (**C**). See Moving Image 22–11.

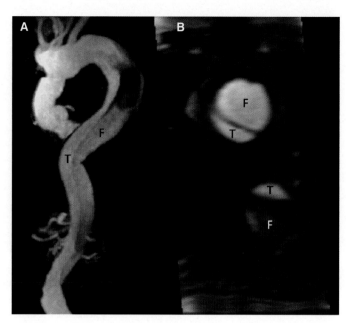

FIGURE 22–12. A. Magnetic resonance angiography of the thoracic and abdominal aorta in a patient with type A chronic aortic dissection who underwent surgery, showing the residual dissection that starts in the distal ascending thoracic aorta and involves the aortic arch and the descending thoracic aorta. **B.** Cross-sectional view of the distal ascending aorta and descending thoracic aorta, showing the dissection in these territories. Note the true (T) and false (F) lumen in the ascending and descending aorta. See Moving Image 22–12.

iodinated contrast medium used in CT, even though rare cases of nephrogenic systemic fibrosis in patients with severe renal insufficiency have been documented with gadolinium.[10]

Aortography

Retrograde aortography previously was considered the gold standard for the diagnosis of acute AD. It has largely been replaced by other widely available, noninvasive, and more accurate imaging modalities. The disadvantages of this procedure include the small risk of contrast-induced nephropathy, the risk of perforation by canalizing the false lumen, radiation exposure, and the time delay associated with the patient transfer and preparation. However, the positive aspects of aortography include its ability to assess the presence and severity of aortic regurgitation and major branch vessel and coronary artery involvement (Fig. 22–13A).

Chest Radiography

Although the chest radiogram is often abnormal in patients with AD, it is not an adequate test to either confirm or exclude the diagnosis of AD. The most common features include widening of the aortic silhouette and superior mediastinum (Fig. 22–13B). Intimal calcification ≥1 mm medial to the outer border of the aortic shadow, tracheal shift, pleural effusion (left to right), and new findings in the aortic and mediastinal silhouettes compared with a prior radiogram can also be seen. However, up to 10% to 15% of patients with acute AD have normal findings on chest radiography.[11]

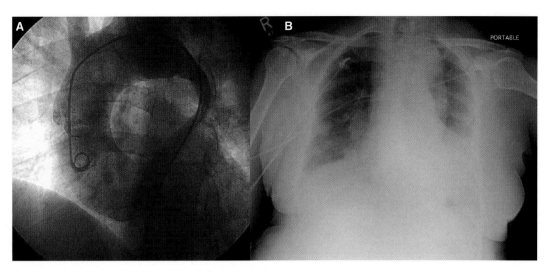

FIGURE 22–13. A. Aortogram in the left oblique projection demonstrating aortic dissection originating at the aortic arch. The true lumen was cannulated with the pigtail catheter. **B.** A portable chest radiograph showing cardiomegaly, marked widening of the aortic silhouette and the superior mediastinum due to ascending aortic dissection.

Coronary Angiography

The role of routine coronary angiography (preoperative or intraoperative) in the setting of acute type A AD to assess the presence of dissection extension into the coronary arteries or presence of coronary artery disease (CAD) (that may require surgical intervention) is not clear. Although, some reports suggest preoperative coronary angiography in all stable patients, the majority of experts recommend against it, unless there is a known history of CAD, prior coronary artery bypass graft, or evidence of ischemia on ECG.

■ MANAGEMENT STRATEGIES

No randomized trials have been conducted to date evaluating management strategies for AD. Therefore, all proposed management strategies are based primarily on registries, case reports, systematic reviews, and experts' opinion. The only society-based consensus or guidelines were published in 2001 by the European Society of Cardiology.[12]

AORTIC INTRAMURAL HEMATOMA

■ INCIDENCE, RISK FACTORS, AND PATHOPHYSIOLOGY

Aortic intramural hematoma (IMH) was first described in 1920. At present, the etiology and pathogenesis remain debatable. Traditionally, IMH was described as a hemorrhage occurring within the medial layer of the aortic wall in the setting of intact intima due to spontaneous rupture of the aortic vasa vasorum. Another, less established, explanation is an atherosclerotic ulcer penetrating into the internal elastic lamina, leading to IMH formation. The prevalence of IMH in patients with suspected AD is up to 30%.[12] The risk factors associated with IMH are similar to those seen with AD, and it is more commonly identified in the descending aorta (type B) than in the ascending aorta (type A).

■ DIAGNOSIS

Noninvasive imaging modalities (CT, MRI, and TEE) are critical in IMH diagnosis. Conventional aortography images the aortic lumen, rather than the aortic wall and, therefore, should not be used to diagnose or exclude IMH. In CT, demonstration of continuous, usually crescentic, high attenuation areas along the aortic wall without an intimal flap is characteristic before contrast injection; these areas fail to be enhanced after injection of contrast medium[13] (Fig. 22–14). Acute IMH on MRI gives a high signal on T2-weighted images and isodense signal on T1-weighted images, whereas subacute IMH produces high signal both on T1- and T2-weighted images. A typical crescentic wall thickening, which also does not enhance after the injection of contrast material, is seen on MRI. MRI is an excellent modality in detecting recurrent bleeds in the aorta wall and therefore is recommended in subacute and chronic phases. TEE is another excellent imaging modality because it allows direct observation of the aortic intima, and demonstration of flow communication is feasible with the Doppler technique.[13] According to experts' recommendations, regional circumferential or crescentic aortic wall thickness ≥7 mm (normal <3 mm) has been suggested as diagnostic of IMH. Sometimes a large echo-free space is associated with contrast enhancement in CT, possibly due to "intimal microtear," which is too small to be detected by the Doppler flow measurement. In addition to being the most operator-dependent method, TEE is of limited utility in the setting of heavily calcified aortic wall or plaques and when the identification of penetrating ulcers is required.

AORTIC ATHEROMATOUS DISEASE

Atherosclerosis is one of the most common causes of mortality and morbidity in the United States and worldwide. It is a systemic disease and affects all arterial vasculature, including the aorta. The principle clinical syndromes associated with aortic

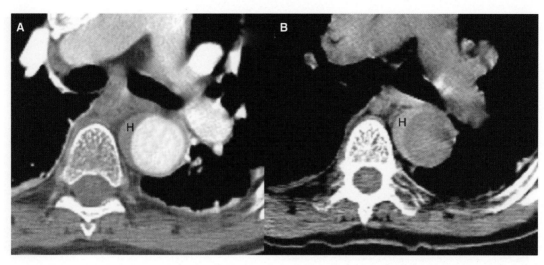

FIGURE 22–14. Intramural hematoma of the descending thoracic aorta. **A.** An axial contrast-enhanced computed tomography (CT) at the level of the pulmonary artery demonstrates crescentic dark thickening of the aortic wall (H) that does not enhance, confirming the presence of an intramural hematoma. Note that neither the size nor the shape of the aortic lumen is distorted the way it would typically be in the presence of a classic aortic dissection. **B.** On a non–contrast-enhanced CT scan, there is crescentic thickening of the aortic wall that is of increased density (H) compared with blood in the lumen, consistent with an intramural hematoma of the aorta. This figure was published in *Braunwald's Heart Disease: A Textbook of Cardiovascular Medicine*, Libby P, et al, copyright Elsevier 2008.

atherosclerosis are aortic aneurysms, IMH aortic atheromatous plaques, atheroembolization, thrombosis and thromboembolization, and aortic penetrating atherosclerotic ulcers (PAUs).

■ PATHOPHYSIOLOGY

The process of atherosclerosis usually begins early in life and involves a series of interrelated events. These include lipid abnormalities (elevated low-density lipoprotein and triglycerides and decreased high-density lipoprotein), platelet activation and thrombosis (aggregation of platelets is triggered by plaque rupture and facilitated by tissue factor and von Willebrand factor), vascular endothelial regulation and dysfunction (primarily by releasing nitric oxide, a potent vasodilator, and endothelin and angiotensin II, which antagonize the actions of nitric oxide), inflammatory process (mediated by macrophages and T cells, releasing various cytokines), oxidant stress (production of reactive oxygen species or radicals), vascular smooth muscle cell proliferation (positive and then negative remodeling), altered matrix metabolism (mainly secretion of matrix metalloproteinase), vasa vasorum, and genetic and acquired risk factors (eg, cigarette smoking, diabetes mellitus, hypertension). Atherosclerosis affects the abdominal aorta to the greatest extent, possibly due to local hemodynamic stresses, thin aortic wall, and the lack of vasa vasorum (damage or decrease in vasa vasorum is associated with plaque formation) (Fig. 22–15).

■ AORTIC ATHEROMATOUS PLAQUES AND ATHEROEMBOLIZATION

An aortic atheromatous plaque, known as aortic atheroma, is suspected to be among the leading causes of embolic stroke. Because emboli propagation is flow dependent, plaques in the ascending aorta are usually associated with stroke, whereas those in the descending aorta are associated with mesenteric, renal, or

peripheral ischemia and infarction. Aortic atheroma is characterized by irregular intimal thickening, usually protruding into the aortic lumen. Its thickness, plaque burden, and complexity (mobile debris, overlying thrombus, and ulcerations) have been shown to be associated with stroke. Other predisposing factors to atheroembolization are absence of calcifications, pedunculation, iatrogenic instrumentation, and aortocoronary bypass. Commonly, plaques ≥4 mm in thickness are classified as complex and are strongly associated with the risk of ischemic stroke.[14] Another classification based on TEE was proposed, where grade I is normal intima, grade II is minimal intimal thickening, grade III is raised irregular plaque <5 mm in thickness, and grade IV is complex protruding plaque with ≥5 mm thickness, ulceration, or calcific density.[15]

TEE is the imaging modality of choice because in addition to measuring plaque thickness, ulceration, and calcifications, it can sometimes predict the risk of embolization by visualizing mobile thrombi (Fig. 22–16). MRI with MRA is the second best imaging modality and can also visualize various plaque components, including the fibrous cap, which may be helpful in assessing plaque stability. The major advantage over TEE includes its ability to visualize the distal ascending aorta. MRI is frequently used for chronic monitoring of aortic plaques. The availability, cost, and contraindication in patients with implantable devices, however, remain problems. MDCT is widely available, noninvasive, and less costly and can be rapidly performed. However, lower sensitivity for noncalcified plaques and exposure to radiation and iodinated contrast limit its use for plaque imaging. Although not used routinely in clinical practice, fluorine 18 (^{18}F) fluorodeoxyglucose (FDG) positron emission tomography (PET) may emerge as an important imaging modality for noninvasive identification of plaques with high embolic risk, (vulnerable plaques) by assessing inflammation within the plaque.

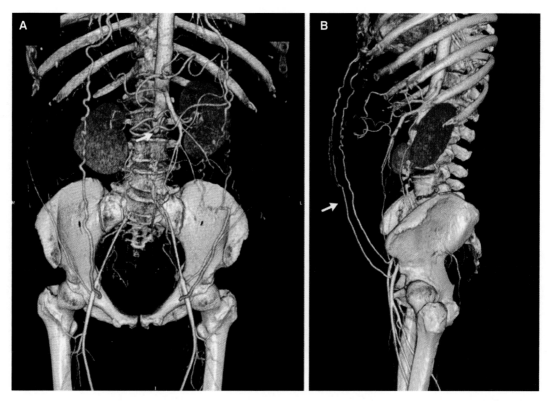

FIGURE 22–15. Computed tomography angiography showing complete occlusion of infrarenal aorta (**A**, arrow) and a lateral view showing collateral blood flow from both internal thoracic arteries through subcutaneous epigastric abdominal vessels to the external iliac arteries (**B**, arrow). Reproduced with permission from Hirsch AT, Miedema MD. Infrarenal aortic occlusion. *N Engl J Med.* 2008;359:7. Copyright 2008 Massachusetts Medical Society. All rights reserved.

■ THROMBOSIS AND THROMBOEMBOLIZATION

The aorta has been reported to be the source of thromboembolism in a minority of cases. Most commonly, thrombus formation and thromboembolism are seen in the setting of an atherosclerotic aorta with an atheroma protruding into the lumen (Fig. 22–17). The risk may even be higher with concomitant hereditary (eg, antiphospholipid antibody syndrome, hyperhomocysteinemia, prothrombin G20210A mutation, antithrombin deficiency, protein S or C deficiency) or acquired (eg, malignancy, pregnancy, recent surgery, trauma, immobility, estrogen use) hypercoagulable states, as well as with vasculitis or smoking. Rarely, aortic thrombus formation may occur spontaneously in the nonatherosclerotic aorta. Generally,

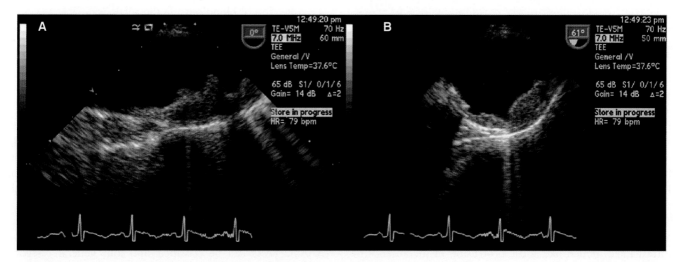

FIGURE 22–16. Transesophageal longitudinal axis (**A**) and short axis (**B**) images of a complex aortic plaque protruding into the lumen in the aortic arch and the proximal descending aorta. With permission from Yuliya Kats, MD. See Moving Image 22–16.

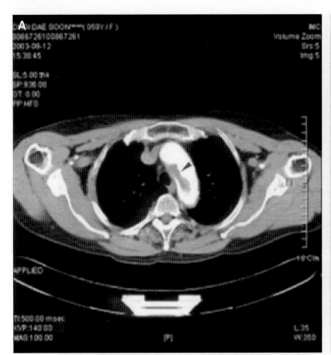
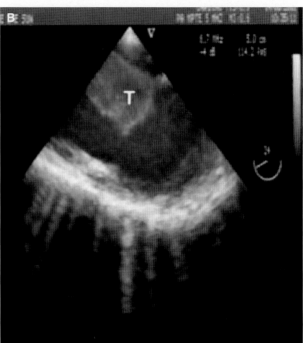

FIGURE 22–17. Computed tomography image of the floating thrombus in the aortic arch (black arrowhead) (**A**) and transesophageal echocardiographic image of a thrombus (T) in the distal aortic arch and the descending aorta (**B**). The adjacent aortic wall was thickened with diffuse atherosclerosis and focal calcific plaque. Reproduced with permission from Choi JB, et al. Floating thrombus in the proximal aortic arch. *Tex Heart Inst J.* 2004;31:432-434. Copyright 2004 by the Texas Heart Institute, Houston.

diagnostic and management strategies for aortic thrombosis and thromboembolism are similar to those of atheromatous plaques.

■ AORTIC PENETRATING ATHEROSCLEROTIC ULCERS

PAU, first recognized by Shennan in 1934 and further defined by Stanson in 1986, is an ulceration of an atherosclerotic lesion of the aorta that disrupts and penetrates the internal elastic lamina of the aortic wall. Such ulcerations typically affect the descending thoracic aorta of elderly patients with advanced atherosclerosis and may precipitate a variable amount of hematoma formation. The hematoma formed by a PAU usually remains localized but infrequently may lead to formation of frank IMH, pseudoaneurysm, AD, or rupture. Rarely, PAU may arise in the ascending aorta or the arch. Table 22–3 outlines the main characteristics of PAU, IMH, and AD.

The best estimate of incidence of PAU in patients presenting with signs and symptoms of acute AD comes from the IRAD registry and is reported to be between 2.3% and 11%. However, because a proportion of PAUs progress to IMH and AD prior to patient presentation and imaging, these numbers may be falsely low.

The clinical diagnosis of PAU is not always straightforward. Although its presentation may sometimes resemble that of acute AD, often there is a paucity of specific symptoms and signs. Previously, aortography has been used as a standard for PAU diagnosis. However, this was largely replaced by noninvasive imaging. CT and MRA accurately depict the lesion as a focal, contrast-filled, pouch-like aortic protrusion in the absence of a dissection flap or false lumen, usually surrounded by marked atherosclerosis, calcifications, and small hematoma (Figs. 22–18

and 22–19). TEE usually reveals a crater-like ulcer with jagged edges in the presence of significant atheroma, thrombus, or even dissection (Fig. 22–20).

AORTIC ANEURYSMS

The term aortic aneurysm is used to describe a pathologic dilation (>4 cm or >1.5 times larger than normal) of the aorta. Morphologically, aneurysms are described as fusiform, a symmetrical dilation involving the full circumference of the aorta, or saccular, a localized outpouching of only a portion of the aortic wall. Pseudoaneurysms or false aneurysms are better described as a collection of blood outside the aortic wall (Fig. 22–21). In addition to morphology, aortic aneurysms are classified according to their location, size, and etiology.

■ THORACIC AORTIC ANEURYSMS

Epidemiology and Classification

The true incidence of thoracic aortic aneurysms (TAAs) is not completely known due to underdetection but is estimated to be 6 to 10 cases per 100,000 patient-years. TAAs most commonly occur in the sixth and seventh decade of life and are more common in men than women (3:1). Hypertension is a contributing factor and is found in a majority of patients.

TAAs involve the ascending and descending thoracic aorta and are much less prevalent than abdominal aortic aneurysms (AAAs). TAAs can be classified into four general categories: ascending aortic aneurysm (60%), descending aortic aneurysm (40%), aortic arch aneurysm (10%), and thoracoabdominal

TABLE 22–3. Characteristics Distinguishing Penetrating Ulcer, Intramural Hematoma, and Aortic Dissection

Characteristic	Penetrating Ulcer	Intramural Hematoma	Aortic Dissection
Features	No intimal flap IMH Localized ulceration penetrating internal elastic lamina	No intimal flap No ulceration Hematoma within aortic wall	Flap with contrast filling false lumen
Typical patient	Elderly hypertensive Hypertensive	Elderly Hypertensive	Younger Hypertensive Occasional bicuspid AV Marfan syndrome
Symptoms	Severe chest pain or mid-scapular pain	Same	Same
Signs	Absent No branch vessel occlusion	Absent No branch vessel occlusion	AR (type A) Compromise of blood flow to branch vessels Pulse inequality Neurologic deficits
Location	Largely descending aorta	Largely descending aorta	Even distribution of ascending and descending aorta
Extent of lesion	Focal	Focal	Usually extensive
Atherosclerosis	Always severe	Variable	Variable, often minimal
Aortic size	Largest, ~6.2 cm	Larger, ~5.5 cm	Smaller, ~5.2 cm
Concomitant AAA	Common	Common	Occasional (except type B, common)

AAA, abdominal aortic aneurysm; AR, aortic regurgitation; AV, aortic valve; IMH, intramural hematoma.

Reprinted from *Cardiology Clinics*, 17/4, Coady MA, et al. Pathologic variants of thoracic aortic dissections: penetrating atherosclerotic ulcers and intramural hematomas, 637-657, copyright 1999, with permission from Elsevier.

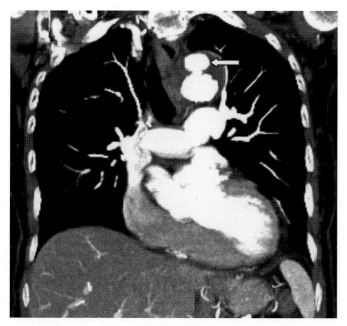

FIGURE 22–18. White arrow indicates penetrating atherosclerotic ulcer with intramural hematoma in the proximal descending thoracic aorta. Reproduced with permission from Brinster DR. Endovascular repair of the descending thoracic aorta for penetrating atherosclerotic ulcer disease. *J Card Surg*. 2009;24:203-208. Copyright by Wiley Periodicals, Inc.

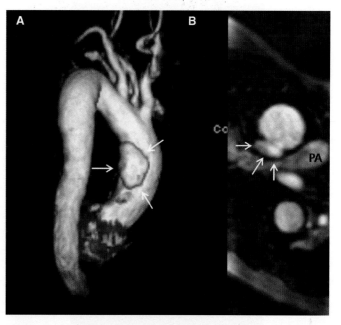

FIGURE 22–19. Magnetic resonance angiography three-dimensional reconstruction image with a large penetrating ulcer (white arrows) in the proximal ascending aorta (**A**) and cross-sectional view with the penetrating ulcer in the ascending aorta at the level of the pulmonary artery (PA) (**B**). See Moving Image 22–19.

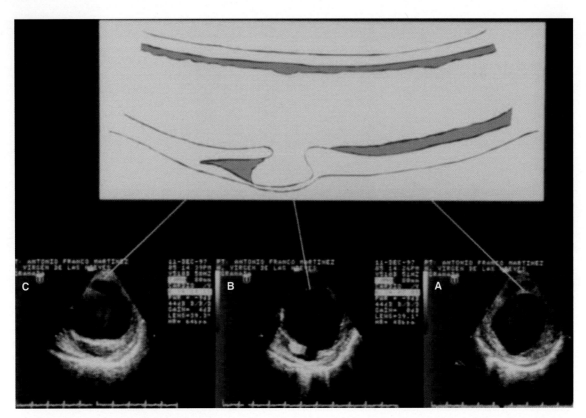

FIGURE 22–20. Schematic drawing of a longitudinal section of the aorta and transesophageal echocardiogram scans in the transverse plane showing a dissection flap secondary to an aortic ulcer. **A.** Mural thrombus. **B.** Aortic ulcer. **C.** Localized aortic dissection. Reprinted from *J Am Coll Cardiol.*, 32, Vilacosta I, et al, Penetrating atherosclerotic aortic ulcer: documentation by transesophageal echocardiography, 83-89, copyright 1998, with permission from Elsevier.

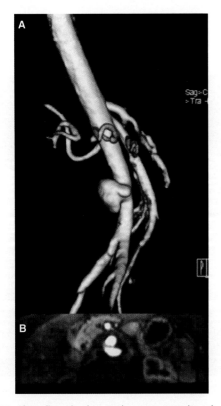

FIGURE 22–21. Three-dimensional magnetic resonance angiography reconstructed image with a pseudoaneurysm present in the distal aorta proximal to the bifurcation (**A**) and cross-sectional aorta revealing the same pseudoaneurysm (**B**).

aneurysm (10%). A categorization of ascending aortic aneurysm into supracoronary type, Marfanoid type (also termed annuloaortic ectasia), and tubular type was proposed.[16] Supracoronary type is the most common type and is associated with a normal-size aortic annulus as well as a normal aorta between the annulus and the coronary orifices. The Marfanoid type has a "flask-like" shape and is associated with dilated aortic annulus and proximal ascending aorta. The tubular type has a moderate, uniform dilation of the entire ascending aorta (Fig. 22–22). Aneurysms of the sinuses of the Valsalva are rarely seen. These aneurysms may be single (right sinus aneurysms being the most common type) or multiple and may fistulize into an adjacent chamber

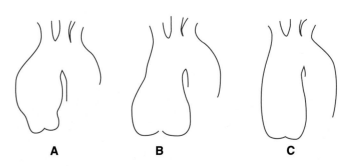

FIGURE 22–22. Three common patterns of ascending aortic aneurysm disease: supracoronary (**A**), Marfanoid or annuloaortic ectasia (**B**), and tubular (**C**). Reprinted from *Curr Probl Cardiol.*, 33, Elefteriades JA, Thoracic aortic aneurysm: reading the enemy's playbook, 203-277. Copyright 2008, with permission from Elsevier.

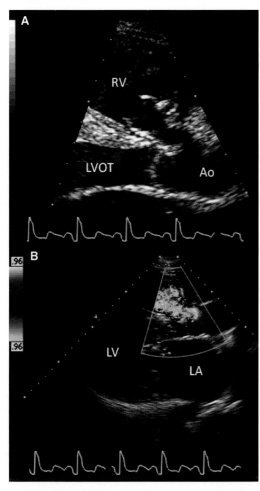

FIGURE 22–23. Transthoracic echocardiogram showing a ruptured aneurysm of the right sinus of Valsalva in magnification (**A**) and color flow imaging Doppler indicating a turbulent, high-velocity jet from the aneurysm into the right ventricle (**B**). Ao, aortic root; LA, left atrium; LV, left ventricle; LVOT, left ventricular outflow tract; RV, right ventricle. With permission from Yuliya Kats, MD. See Moving Image 22–23.

(Fig. 22–23). Thoracoabdominal aortic aneurysms contain elements of both thoracic and abdominal aneurysms and constitute only a minority of all aneurysms. Crawford classification (type I to IV), based on the extent of involvement, is used for their categorization.[17]

Pathophysiology and Risk Factors

TAAs most often result from cystic medial degeneration or necrosis that leads to the weakening of the aortic wall. Congenital and acquired causes of cystic medial necrosis are manifold. Aneurysms of the aortic root are typically associated with Marfan syndrome and bicuspid AVs. Congenital causes of ascending aortic aneurysms include Marfan syndrome, Turner syndrome, Ehlers-Danlos syndrome, bicuspid AVs, osteogenesis imperfecta, and polycystic kidney disease. Acquired causes of ascending aortic aneurysms include atherosclerosis, hypertension, various rheumatologic processes (Takayasu arteritis, giant-cell arteritis, rheumatoid arthritis, and systemic lupus erythematosus), trauma, and infections (syphilitic or mycotic). The

majority of aneurysms involving the descending thoracic aorta are atherosclerotic in etiology. Infrequently, in the setting of diffuse atherosclerosis, these may extend to the ascending aorta or the arch. Although some of the descending aortic aneurysms may rarely compress mediastinal structures, most of them are asymptomatic.

Imaging

Chest Radiography Asymptomatic aneurysms of the ascending aorta and the arch are sometimes incidentally detected on the routine chest radiography. The most common radiographic features include the finding of mediastinal widening, enlarged or prominent aortic knob, displaced intimal calcifications, or midline shift of the trachea. However, all of these are not very specific and cannot distinguish an aneurysm from the normal variant or tortuous aorta.

Echocardiography TTE has an important role in imaging of the aortic root and proximal ascending aorta, and in the current 2003 ACC/AHA practice guidelines, it is given a class I recommendation for imaging of aortic aneurysms, particularly aortic root, and aortic root dilation in Marfan or other connective tissue syndromes.[9] However, its use is limited in imaging the arch and the descending aorta. Therefore, TEE is preferred in the imaging of the thoracic aorta (except the upper ascending aorta and the arch due to the artifacts created by a column of air in the trachea) and also carries a class I recommendation[9] (Fig. 22–24). The 2008 ACC/AHA guidelines on valvular heart disease recommend an

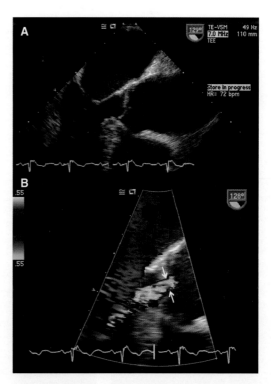

FIGURE 22–24. Two-dimensional transesophageal echocardiographic view of the dilated ascending aorta (**A**) associated with significant aortic regurgitation (vena contracta is indicated by arrows) as seen with color flow Doppler imaging (**B**). With permission from Yuliya Kats, MD. See Moving Image 22–24.

initial assessment of the aortic root and ascending aorta diameters with TTE in patients with known bicuspid AVs.[18] Importantly, both TTE and TEE are commonly used for diagnosis of complications such as aortic insufficiency. Given that TEE is semi-invasive, CT and MRI are usually preferred for the diagnosis or chronic follow-up in clinically stable patients.

CT and MRI   Contrast-enhanced CT and MRA can very accurately depict the size and location of TAA, as well as branch vessel or mediastinal structure involvement (Fig. 22–25). Recent advances, such as 3D reconstruction, allow accurate measurement of the aortic diameter in cases of very tortuous aorta when axial images alone are insufficient (axial images often overestimate the aortic diameter because it transects the aorta off axis). Aneurysms involving the aortic root are much better imaged with MRI than with CT. The 2008 ACC/AHA valvular heart disease practice guidelines give a class I recommendation for CT or MRI use in patients with bicuspid AVs when morphology of the aortic root or ascending aorta cannot be assessed accurately with echocardiography.[18] Serial annual evaluations with echocardiography, CT, or MRI are also recommended in patients with bicuspid AV and >4.0-cm aortic root or ascending aorta diameter (lower value for patients of small stature).[18]

Aortography   Retrograde aortography had long been the preferred method for aneurysm evaluation. It provides very accurate information regarding the aortic anatomy and branch vessel involvement. However, it is being increasingly replaced by the noninvasive imaging modalities described earlier due to its inability to discern extraluminal aneurysmal size and the procedure-associated risks.

ABDOMINAL AORTIC ANEURYSMS

Epidemiology and Classification

Similar to TAA, the true prevalence of AAA is not completely known due to various diagnostic criteria (usually when anteroposterior diameter of the aorta is ≥3.0 cm), various imaging modalities used, and underdetection. However, it is known that AAA is 5 to 10 times more common in men than women and that its incidence rises dramatically in the sixth and seventh decades. Generally, the prevalence of AAA of 2.9 to 4.9 cm in diameter ranges from 1.3% for men age 45 to 54 years to up to 12.5% for men age 75 to 84 years. Comparable prevalence figures for women are 0% and 5.2%, respectively.[19] AAA is the thirteenth leading cause of death and third leading cause of sudden death among men over the age of 60 in the United States, which translates into approximately 15,000 deaths annually. Some estimate that the actual rate may be as high as 30,000 deaths per year. AAAs are much more prevalent than TAAs. Most are fusiform, and the minority are saccular. AAAs are classified as suprarenal aneurysms, affecting the aortic segment containing the superior mesenteric and celiac arteries; juxtarenal aneurysms, arising distal to the renal arteries but in very close proximity to them; pararenal aneurysms, involving the origin of one or both renal arteries; and infrarenal aneurysms, occurring below the renal arteries (95% of cases).

Pathophysiology and Risk Factors

Elastin and collagen comprise the aortic extracellular matrix, which plays a critical role in maintaining the aortic shape and integrity. Degradation of these important proteins may weaken the aortic wall and lead to formation of the aneurysm. Although, there is still some controversy regarding the factors degrading elastin and collagen, an inflammatory process appears to be the most accepted. Inflammatory cells (in particular macrophages and T cells) and endothelial and smooth muscle cells produce proteolytic enzymes, such as matrix metalloproteinases, plasmin, and cathepsin S and K, which degrade the extracellular matrix. The early experimental reports of inhibition of matrix metalloproteinases with hydroxymethylglutaryl-coenzyme A (HMG-CoA) reductase inhibitors and tetracyclines in animal models are promising.

Among the factors that may contribute to the aortic wall inflammation, smoking appears to be the most important one, followed by sex, family history (first-degree relative) of AAA, age, hypertension, and atherosclerosis. The risk of AAA in heavy smokers is six to seven times that of nonsmokers. AAA >4.0 cm occurs up to 10 times more frequently in men compared with women. Women, however, may be at higher risk of rupture. Approximately 15% to 28% of patients with AAA have first-degree relatives affected with aneurysms.

Imaging

Ultrasonography   US is an accurate and inexpensive modality used for screening and surveillance of infrarenal aneurysms. It has an excellent diagnostic sensitivity and specificity of 92% to

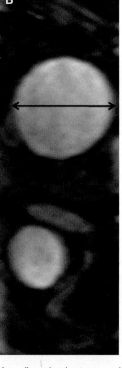

FIGURE 22–25. A. Magnetic resonance angiography three-dimensional reconstructed image of a supracoronary ascending aneurysm (black double arrow) with "bovine arch" (the left common carotid artery originates directly from the innominate artery, white arrow). **B.** Cross-sectional image of the aneurysm. See Moving Image 22–25.

99% and 100%, respectively, and can image an aneurysm in the transverse and longitudinal planes. However, US is less reliable for imaging of juxtarenal or suprarenal aneurysms. Because of this limitation, it is usually insufficient alone for preoperative evaluation of patients undergoing surgical repair. The 2005 ACC/AHA guidelines give a class I recommendation for AAA screening with a physical exam and US in men ≥60 years of age who are either the siblings or offspring of patients with AAA and class IIa recommendation (grade B* recommendation from the US Preventive Services Task Force[20]) for AAA screening with a physical exam or one-time US in men who are 65 to 75 years of age who have ever smoked.[19]

CT and MRA CT and MRA are highly accurate imaging modalities in assessing the size and location of the aneurysm, as well as the extent of disease, presence of mural thrombus and calcification, adjacent fluid, and iliofemoral and renal artery involvement. These modalities are preferred over US for suprarenal aneurysm imaging. However, CT tends to overestimate the size of the aneurysm by as much as 0.94 ± 0.69 cm.[21] In addition, intramural calcifications may result in less accurate evaluation of the peripheral arteries with CT, so either retrograde arteriography or MRA may be required. Presently, there is no consensus to indicate the superiority of MRA versus CT.

Aortography Although aortography is an excellent modality for assessment of the size and location of AAA, as well as branch vessel involvement, it is presently used only in selected cases due to its invasiveness, cost, limited availability, and exposure to intravenous contrast and radiation. Because contrast non-enhancing mural thrombus is nearly always associated with an AAA, aortography may also underestimate the true size of the aneurysm.

CONGENITAL AORTIC DISEASES

The proportion of individuals with congenital vascular diseases surviving into adulthood is rapidly rising. Therefore, familiarity with these diseases is essential. This section will focus on the major congenital aortic malformations, such as coarctation and atresia of the aorta, bicuspid valve–associated aortopathy, and Marfan syndrome–associated aortopathy, which account for a significant proportion of congenital vascular malformations.

■ COARCTATION AND ATRESIA OF THE AORTA

Incidence, Etiology, and Pathophysiology

Coarctation of the aorta was described pathologically at autopsy by Morgagni in 1760 and was clinically recognized in the early 1900s. It is usually a discrete narrowing (rarely involves a long segment) of the thoracic aorta just distal to the ligamentum arteriosum (juxtaductal) resulting in at least a 20-mm Hg gradient across the coarctation (Fig. 22–26A). Less frequently, coarctation

---

*Grade B: The USPSTF [US Preventive Services Task Force] recommends that clinicians provide [the service] to eligible patients. The USPSTF found at least fair evidence that [the service] improves important health outcomes and concludes that benefits outweigh harms.

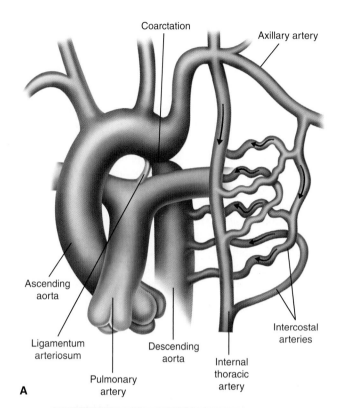

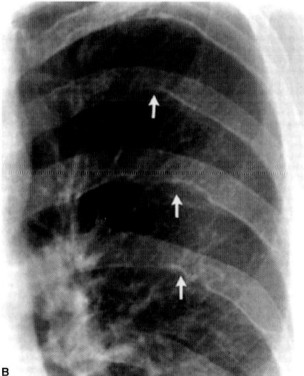

FIGURE 22–26. A. Coarctation causes severe obstruction of blood flow in the descending thoracic aorta. The descending aorta and its branches are perfused by collateral channels from the axillary and internal thoracic arteries through the intercostal arteries (arrows). Reproduced with permission from Brickner ME, et al. Congenital heart disease in adults. First of two parts. *N Engl J Med*. 2000;342:256-263. Copyright © 2000 Massachusetts Medical Society. All rights reserved. **B.** The chest radiogram from a patient with aortic coarctation showing marked rib notching (arrows). Reproduced with permission from Bruce CJ, et al. Images in clinical medicine. Aortic coarctation and bicuspid aortic valve. *N Engl J Med*. 2000;342:249. Copyright © 2000 Massachusetts Medical Society. All rights reserved.

occurs proximal to the left subclavian artery. Previous categorization as preductal (infantile) and postductal (adult) is misleading and should not be used. It is a common malformation responsible for up to 8% of all cardiovascular congenital defects and occurs two to five times more frequently in males than females. Simple coarctation is the most common form detected de novo in adults and is not associated with other intracardiac lesions. Complex coarctation has a frequent association with bicuspid AV (50%-80% of cases), ventricular septal defect, patent ductus arteriosus, subvalvular aortic stenosis, parachute mitral stenosis, and circle of Willis cerebral artery aneurysm (berry aneurysm; 10% of cases). The etiology of aortic coarctation is not known. The reduction of antegrade intrauterine blood flow causing underdevelopment of the aortic arch (flow theory), constriction of ductal tissue extending into the thoracic aorta (ductal theory), and a primary defect of the aortic wall are the proposed theories for the development of congenital aortic coarctation. Acquired causes include inflammatory processes, such as Takayasu arteritis, and severe atherosclerosis.

Aortic atresia, complete interruption of the aorta, is usually lethal unless it is treated surgically within the first month of life and can be classified based on the segment involved: type A, interruption of the aortic arch distal to the left subclavian artery; type B, between the left subclavian artery and the left carotid artery (most common); or type C, between the innominate artery and the left carotid artery.[22]

Aortic pseudocoarctation is a rare congenital anomaly of an excessive elongated aorta, resulting in its kinking and buckling. Pseudocoarctation is not associated with an aortic gradient (see Fig. 22-3).

Imaging

Chest Radiography Prominent ascending aortic shadow, absence of the proximal descending aortic arch shadow, a "3 sign" (indentation at the coarctation site), and notching on the underside of the ribs (from dilated collateral vessels) may be seen on anteroposterior chest radiogram (Fig. 22–26B).

Echocardiography According to 2008 ACC/AHA guidelines, TTE, including suprasternal notch acoustic windows, is useful for initial imaging and hemodynamic evaluation in suspected aortic coarctation (class I).[23] Discrete area of narrowing with increased turbulence and velocities in the proximal descending aorta, characteristic forward diastolic flow, and decreased pulsatility and absence of early diastolic flow reversal in the abdominal aorta can be documented with color flow imaging and continuous wave spectral Doppler examination (Fig. 22–27). Abnormal flow in the dilated and tortuous collateral vessels may also be detected. TEE is rarely needed because suprasternal images from TTE usually provide excellent evaluation of the involved aorta.

CT and MRA According to 2008 ACC/AHA guidelines, every patient with coarctation (repaired or not) should have at least one cardiovascular MRI or CT scan for complete evaluation of the thoracic aorta and intracranial vessels (class I).[23] CT angiography and gadolinium-enhanced MRA are excellent techniques for the evaluation of anatomic details, precise location and severity of coarctation, and the status of a ductus arteriosus and extent of collateralization. The velocity-encoded phase-contrast magnetic resonance protocol allows accurate assessment of a gradient across the coarctation.

Aortography Although CT and MRI are the preferred methods of imaging, diagnostic aortography is an excellent technique to delineate the location and extent of a coarctation, as well as the associated vascular malformations, and should be performed when noninvasive imaging modalities are inconclusive or unavailable or if catheter-based intervention is to be performed. Anterograde catheterization via radial approach maybe preferred over the retrograde catheterization via femoral artery due to absent or markedly diminished femoral pulse.

■ BICUSPID AV–ASSOCIATED AORTOPATHY

Incidence, Etiology, and Pathophysiology

Bicuspid AV is the most common congenital cardiac malformation, occurring in up to 2% of the general population, with a

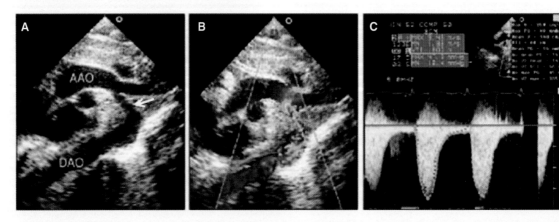

FIGURE 22–27. Echocardiographic findings in a 3-month-old child with moderate aortic coarctation and hypoplasia of the arch. **A.** Two-dimensional echocardiographic view of the aortic arch shows a moderate aortic coarctation (arrow). **B.** Color Doppler image showing turbulence in the arch due to the coarctation. **C.** Continuous wave Doppler across the arch estimates the gradient across the narrowing to be almost 48 mm Hg. Note the diastolic run-off indicating the severity of the coarctation. AAO, ascending aorta; DAO, descending aorta. Reproduced with permission from Agarwala BN, et al. Clinical manifestations and diagnosis of coarctation of the aorta. In: UpToDate, Basow DS, ed, UpToDate, Waltham, MA, 2009. Copyright 2009 UpToDate, Inc. For more information, visit www.uptodate.com.

male-to-female ratio of ≥3:1. It has an autosomal dominant with incomplete penetrance inheritance and is strongly associated with Turner syndrome and coarctation of aorta. Individuals with bicuspid valve (including those with normal AV function) have significantly a larger aortic root and ascending aorta than those with tricuspid AV, which translates into nine-fold higher incidence of AD. The prevalence of bicuspid AV–associated ascending aortic aneurysm was estimated to be approximately 7.5% to 59% at the annulus, 16% to 78% at the sinus of Valsalva, 15% to 79% at the sinotubular junction, and 35% to 68% at the proximal ascending aorta.[24] This process of aortic dilation is due to aortopathy and is independent of valvular and hemodynamic abnormalities.

Imaging

For patients with known bicuspid AV, the 2008 ACC/AHA valvular heart disease guidelines recommend an initial TTE to assess the diameters of the aortic root and ascending aorta (class I).[18] In individuals with large body habitus, TEE may offer an incremental yield. CT or MRI is only indicated when the aortic morphology cannot be assessed accurately by echocardiography (class I).[18] Furthermore, if the root diameter is >4.0 cm, an annual echocardiogram, MRI, or CT should be performed (class I).[18] Three-dimensional MRA and CT are the most accurate for aortic size measurement, whereas steady-state free precession MRI pulse sequence is commonly used for AV functional assessment (eg, visualization of an eccentric systolic jet and assessment of leaflet number) (Fig. 22–28). The flow velocity pulse sequence by MRI is also a very useful tool to assess the functional bicuspid valves by assessing the flow of blood through the opening of the AV. The appearance of a functionally bicuspid AV has an elliptical or "fish mouth" appearance rather than a triangular appearance with the functional tricuspid valve. At times, it can be a challenge to distinguish a tricuspid valve from a bicuspid valve with a prominent raphe. In diastole, there may not be any difference between these two valves, but it becomes evident during systole when the raphe does not open on either short axis TTE/TEE or on cine/flow velocity short axis MRI. If the raphe is partially fused, then classification can be quite challenging. In addition, on the long axis view by echocardiography and cine MRI, the valve will often have a doming appearance. In the case of severely calcified bicuspid AV, chest radiography may reveal increased perivalvular radiopacity.

■ MARFAN SYNDROME

Incidence, Etiology, and Pathophysiology

Marfan syndrome is a connective tissue disease affecting 1 in 3000 individuals and is autosomal dominant with spontaneous mutation observed in up to 30% of subjects. It is a systemic disease affecting central nervous, cardiovascular, pulmonary, and musculoskeletal systems. Cardiovascular abnormalities in Marfan syndrome include aortic root (sinuses of Valsalva) and ascending aorta dilation (70% of cases), mitral valve prolapse with mitral regurgitation (up to 80% of cases), TAAs and AAAs, AD (90% are type A), and IMH. In IRAD, 5% of patients with acute AD had Marfan syndrome (with an incidence of 50% among those who were <40 years of age, compared with only 2% among older patients). Various mutations involving fibrillin-1 (*FBN1*) (most commonly) and transforming growth factor-β (*TGF-β*) genes are typically responsible for the phenotype of Marfan syndrome. These mutations result in fragmentation of the elastic lamellae, cystic medial necrosis, and loss of smooth muscle cells within the aortic wall.

Imaging

The current strategy to screen for Marfan syndrome–associated aortopathy is echocardiographic assessment of the aorta, in particular the aortic root and ascending aorta. TTE is recommended as

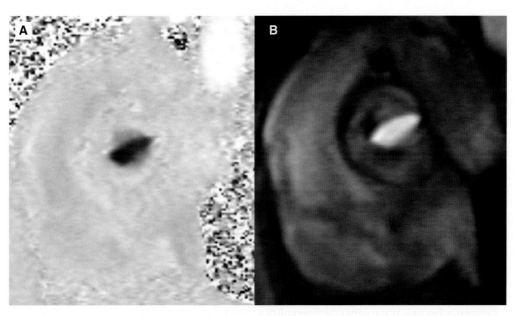

FIGURE 22–28. This flow velocity pulse sequence (**A**) and the magnitude image (**B**) at the level of the aortic valve were obtained from the same patient with bicuspid aortic valve and ascending aortic aneurysm (see Fig. 22–25) and show the typical "fish mouth" appearance of the aortic valve.

a first-line screening test for thoracic aortic disease in the affected individuals and their first-degree relatives (class I).[9] Annual routine reimaging of the aorta is also reasonable. In addition, echocardiography and MRI can detect increased aortic wall stiffness and decreased distensibility, which are correlated with higher pulse wave and blood velocity in the aorta. If there is a suggestion or confirmation of aortic dilation, then 3D MRA or CT angiography should be performed for more complete assessment.

TRAUMATIC AORTIC INJURY

Traumatic aortic injury (TAI) is an infrequent complication of blunt chest trauma. However, it is responsible for 16% of injury-related deaths and is the second most common cause of fatality in motor vehicular accidents. Up to 80% of individuals die at the accident site.[25] Aortic disruption may be complete (transection), a catastrophic event that almost always results in instantaneous death, or partial incomplete disruption of media and/or adventitia that contain the rupture.

■ PATHOPHYSIOLOGY

TAI usually follows an abrupt deceleration (most often) during automobile crashes, most commonly in a head-on impact. It has been proposed that most blunt aortic injuries involve one or more of the following forces. The isthmus is located in the proximal descending aorta, tethered by the ligamentum arteriosum in a relatively immobile position and, therefore, is subjected to the most stretching, torsional, and inertial forces with sudden deceleration or acceleration. A majority (95%) of TAI cases occur at this site. Other hypotheses involve a "water-hammer" effect, an instantaneous elevation in aortic blood pressure against a simultaneously occluded aorta, and the "osseous pinch," an entrapment of the aorta between the anterior chest wall and the vertebral column. Minimal aortic injuries affect only the intima of the vessel wall and occur approximately 10% of the time. A penetrating injury to thoracic aorta may also result from a fractured rib or vertebral body. The minority (5%) of TAIs involve the ascending and subdiaphragmatic aorta.

■ IMAGING

Widened aortic silhouette and superior mediastinum may occasionally be seen on the chest radiogram. However, a significant proportion of patients with blunt traumatic injury have normal mediastinal shadow on chest radiography. Because CT is widely available, can be performed in a timely fashion, and has very high sensitivity for detecting TAI, it has become the imaging test of choice. A normal CT essentially rules out TAI. CT findings associated with blunt aortic injury frequently include traumatic pseudoaneurysm, contained rupture, intimal flap, periaortic hematoma, a focal bulge, abnormal aortic contour, and sudden change in aortic caliber (Fig. 22–29). In addition, CT has a crucial role in the diagnosis of minimal aortic injuries. It was reported that 50% of minimal aortic injuries identified by helical CT are missed by conventional aortography. Aortography has been considered as a gold standard for TAI identification

for decades. However, given its invasiveness, limited availability, and the time delay associated with its performance, it has largely been replaced by CT. Frequently, retrograde aortography is performed preoperatively for better aortic contour and branch vessel involvement delineation in patients with already known TAI (Fig. 22–30). Echocardiography (particularly TEE) can also be used to visualize traumatic disruption of the aorta. MRA is an alternative methodology; however, in the acute setting, CT angiography is a better choice due to the faster imaging time.

AORTIC TUMORS

Primary malignancies of the aorta are extremely rare. Sarcomas represent the majority of cases, with malignant fibrous histiocytoma being the most common subtype. Other less common subtypes include malignant endothelioma, angiosarcoma, and leiomyosarcoma. Except for leiomyosarcoma, which tends to grow outward into the adjacent structures, the majority of tumors involve the intimal layer and grow into the aortic lumen.

Clinical symptoms of malignant aortic tumors include locally occlusive aortic disease, peripheral emboli, or mesenteric emboli.[26] Unlike retrograde aortography, echocardiography, MRI, and CT allow imaging of the aortic wall and, therefore, are preferred modalities for the evaluation of aortic tumors. In addition, CT and MRI are capable of surveying the whole body for the presence of metastatic disease. Given the rarity of the aortic tumors, the diagnosis, unfortunately, is frequently established only with surgical exploration or necropsy. Because distant metastases to bone, kidneys, liver, the adrenal glands, and lungs are common, oncologic approaches are frequently only palliative, and the overall prognosis remains very poor.

AORTITIS

Aortitis may have infectious (bacterial and syphilitic) or noninfectious (systemic inflammatory disorders) etiology. Infections of the aorta are most commonly caused by direct seeding of the aortic wall (frequently diseased or traumatized) by circulating bacteria. Less common etiologies include a septic embolus from bacterial endocarditis, contiguous spread of infection from adjacent structures, impaired immunity, and infection of the vasa vasorum. Systemic rheumatologic diseases, such as Takayasu disease, giant-cell aortitis, rheumatoid arthritis, and systemic lupus erythematosus, can often affect the aorta to various degrees.

■ IMAGING

^{18}F-FDG PET is an excellent modality to define increased aortic wall metabolism due to inflammation. Given a very high sensitivity of PET, it may emerge as a gold standard for arteritis diagnosis, as well as assessment of response to therapy. MRI/MRA has also been used for detection of aortic wall thickening and branch vessel occlusion. The morphologic pulse sequence with black blood TSE is used to assess the aortic wall thickness. Different weighting with T1, T2, or proton density, combined with fat saturation, and contrast enhancement can

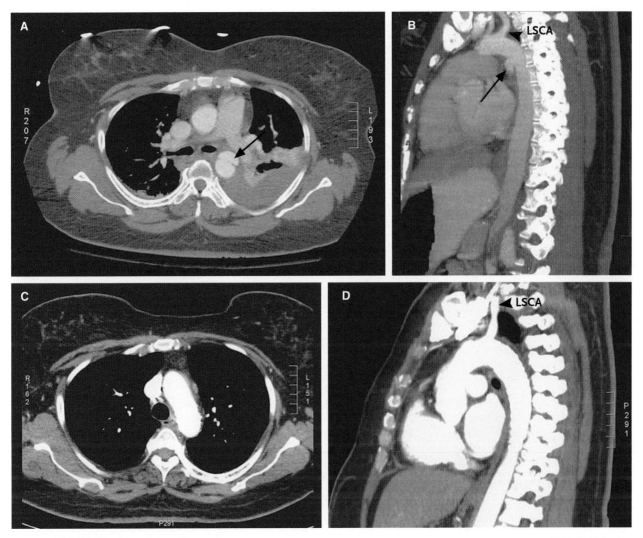

FIGURE 22–29. Computed tomography performed with contrast material shows an aortic injury with an associated pseudoaneurysm (**A**, arrow), which is highlighted in a three-dimensional reconstruction (**B**, arrow) near the left subclavian artery (LSCA) (arrowhead). A postoperative scan shows a patent endograft with resolution of the pseudoaneurysm (**C**), with a three-dimensional reconstruction (**D**). Reproduced with permission from Neschis DG, et al. Blunt aortic injury. *N Engl J Med*. 2008;359:1708-1716. Copyright 2008 Massachusetts Medical Society. All rights reserved.

help delineate aortitis from intramural hematoma and mural thrombus. MRA is also used to assess the luminal consequences of stenosis and, at times, dilation. CT and echocardiography are also reasonable initial diagnostic tests and may uncover luminal narrowing, aneurysms, and wall thickening.

INFECTIOUS AORTITIS

Diseased aortic wall segments (eg, atherosclerotic aneurysm, healed dissection, iatrogenic trauma, repair site) are prone for bacterial infections. *Staphylococcus aureus* and *Salmonella* species are the two most common pathogens responsible for infectious or mycotic aneurysms. In addition to adhering to atheromatous aortic segments, *Salmonella* infrequently may affect normal endothelium. *Mycobacterium tuberculosis*, *Streptococcus pneumoniae*, and *Treponema pallidum* once accounted for a significant number of cases but are now rare with the advent of antibiotics. Because *T. pallidum* invades the aortic wall via vaso vasorum,

it primarily causes inflammation and aneurysm formation in the ascending aorta and the arch (abdominal aorta has minimal amount of vaso vasorum). Other organisms that were reported to rarely cause mycotic aneurysms are fungi, *Pseudomonas*, *Klebsiella*, *Bacteroides fragilis*, and *Neisseria gonorrhoeae*.

The diagnosis of infectious aneurysm may be suspected on imaging studies. However, isolation of the organism by microbiologic (blood cultures) or serologic (VDRL or FTA-ABS) investigations is often important. Therapeutic options include parenteral antibiotic therapy alone or often in combination with surgical exploration or endovascular therapy.

NONINFECTIOUS AORTITIS

Takayasu Disease

Takayasu disease, Takayasu arteritis, or pulseless disease is a chronic large-vessel vasculitis that primarily affects the aorta

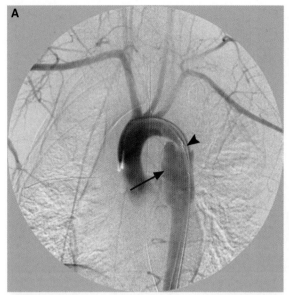

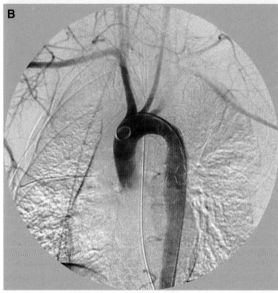

FIGURE 22–30. A. Aortography performed during surgery for blunt aortic injury. An aortic pseudoaneurysm (arrow) is visible with a first endograft component in position before deployment (arrowhead). **B.** An aortogram obtained after completion of the procedure shows the patent endograft and successful exclusion of the pseudoaneurysm. Reproduced with permission from Neschis DG, et al. Blunt aortic injury. *N Engl J Med.* 2008;359:1708-1716. Copyright 2008 Massachusetts Medical Society. All rights reserved.

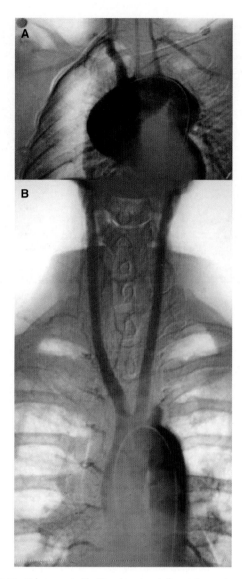

FIGURE 22–31. Takayasu arteritis. Granulomatous inflammation and medial destruction has led to marked aortic root dilation (**A**) in a 17-year-old female high school student who developed symptoms of congestive heart failure and exertional angina. She also had diffuse narrowing of the left common carotid artery and irregular dilation of the innominate artery. Occlusion of both subclavian arteries has led to leg pressures being the only reliable measure of central aortic pressure (**B**). This figure was published in *Braunwald's Heart Disease: A Textbook of Cardiovascular Medicine*, Libby P, et al, 2008, copyright Elsevier 2008.

and its main branches, causing arterial stenoses (more common) and aneurysms. In 90% of cases, it affects women in their second and third decades of life. Although Asians have the highest prevalence of the disease (approximately 150 new cases are diagnosed annually in Japan), cases have been reported in all races and ethnicities. The incidence of Takayasu disease is estimated at approximately 2.6 cases per 1 million persons in the United States. The initial lesions commonly occur in the left subclavian artery. As Takayasu arteritis progresses, the great vessels, including the coronary, pulmonary, iliac, and visceral arteries, may be affected (Fig. 22–31). Peripheral arterial pulses are commonly diminished and often asymmetrical. Systemic hypertension is

common due to stiffening and scarring of the aorta (secondary to chronic inflammation) and the involvement of renal arteries. Other findings include aortic insufficiency (due to aortic root dilation), congestive heart failure, acute coronary syndromes, or sudden cardiac death (in cases of coronary involvement).

Giant-Cell Arteritis

Giant-cell arteritis (GCA) is also known to cause sterile inflammation of medium- and large-sized vessels. In the United States, it has a prevalence of approximately 18 per 100,000 cases among individuals older than 50 years of age. Women are slightly more commonly affected than men. The most common clinical features of GCA include severe headache (60%-90%) and temporal artery tenderness (40%-70%). Unlike Takayasu arteritis, GCA causes clinically relevant aortitis associated with aortic aneurysms only in a minority of affected individuals (15%-20%). However, necropsy studies have suggested that these numbers might underestimate the true prevalence of GCA.

Other Noninfectious Aortitides

A rapidly progressive aortic valvulitis and less often aortitis and aortic aneurysms have been described in association with rheumatoid arthritis. Aortitis with associated aortic insufficiency can sometimes be seen in patients with systemic lupus erythematosus. Aortic root disease with associated valvular regurgitation has been found in a significant number of patients with ankylosing spondylitis as well. Rarely, aortitis may be observed with Behcet syndrome, Crohn disease, and sarcoidosis.

Moving Images
All moving images are located on the complementary DVD.

REFERENCES

1. Otto C. *Textbook of Clinical Echocardiography*. Philadelphia, PA: Saunders; 2004.
2. Qanadli SD, El Hajjam M, Mesurolle B, et al. Motion artifacts of the aorta simulating aortic dissection on spiral CT. *J Comput Assist Tomogr*. 1999;23:1-6.
3. Ko SF, Huang CC, Ng SH, et al. MDCT angiography for evaluation of the complete vascular tree of hemodialysis fistulas. *AJR Am J Roentgenol*. 2005;185:1268-1274.
4. Fujioka C, Horiguchi J, Kiguchi M, Yamamoto H, Kitagawa T, Ito K. Survey of aorta and coronary arteries with prospective ECG-triggered 100-kV 64-MDCT angiography. *AJR Am J Roentgenol*. 2009;193:227-233.
5. Meszaros I, Morocz J, Szlavi J, et al. Epidemiology and clinicopathology of aortic dissection. *Chest*. 2000;117:1271-1278.
6. Tsai TT, Trimarchi S, Nienaber CA. Acute aortic dissection: perspectives from the International Registry of Acute Aortic Dissection (IRAD). *Eur J Vasc Endovasc Surg*. 2009;37:149-159.
7. Shiga T, Wajima Z, Apfel CC, Inoue T, Ohe Y. Diagnostic accuracy of transesophageal echocardiography, helical computed tomography, and magnetic resonance imaging for suspected thoracic aortic dissection: systematic review and meta-analysis. *Arch Intern Med*. 2006;166:1350-1356.
8. Libby P, Bonow R, Mann DL, et al. *Braunwald's Heart Disease: A Textbook of Cardiovascular Medicine*. Philadelphia, PA: Saunders; 2008.
9. Cheitlin MD, Armstrong WF, Aurigemma GP, et al. ACC/AHA/ASE 2003 guideline update for the clinical application of echocardiography: summary article: a report of the American College of Cardiology/American Heart Association Task Force on Practice Guidelines (ACC/AHA/ASE Committee to Update the 1997 Guidelines for the Clinical Application of Echocardiography). *Circulation*. 2003;108:1146-1162.
10. Ramanath VS, Oh JK, Sundt TM 3rd, Eagle KA. Acute aortic syndromes and thoracic aortic aneurysm. *Mayo Clin Proc*. 2009;84:465-481.
11. Nienaber CA, Fattori R, Mehta RH, et al. Gender-related differences in acute aortic dissection. *Circulation*. 2004;109:3014-3021.
12. Erbel R, Alfonso F, Boileau C, et al. Diagnosis and management of aortic dissection. *Eur Heart J*. 2001;22:1642-1681.
13. Song JK. Diagnosis of aortic intramural haematoma. *Heart*. 2004;90:368-371.
14. Amarenco P, Cohen A, Tzourio C, et al. Atherosclerotic disease of the aortic arch and the risk of ischemic stroke. *N Engl J Med*. 1994;331:1474-1479.
15. Vaduganathan P, Ewton A, Nagueh SF, Weilbaecher DG, Safi HJ, Zoghbi WA. Pathologic correlates of aortic plaques, thrombi and mobile "aortic debris" imaged in vivo with transesophageal echocardiography. *J Am Coll Cardiol*. 1997;30:357-363.
16. Elefteriades JA. Thoracic aortic aneurysm: reading the enemy's playbook. *Curr Probl Cardiol*. 2008;33:203-277.
17. Crawford ES, Crawford JL, Safi HJ, et al. Thoracoabdominal aortic aneurysms: preoperative and intraoperative factors determining immediate and long-term results of operations in 605 patients. *J Vasc Surg*. 1986;3:389-404.
18. Bonow RO, Carabello BA, Chatterjee K, et al. 2008 focused update incorporated into the ACC/AHA 2006 guidelines for the management of patients with valvular heart disease: a report of the American College of Cardiology/American Heart Association Task Force on Practice Guidelines (Writing Committee to revise the 1998 guidelines for the management of patients with valvular heart disease). Endorsed by the Society of Cardiovascular Anesthesiologists, Society for Cardiovascular Angiography and Interventions, and Society of Thoracic Surgeons. *J Am Coll Cardiol*. 2008;52:e1-e142.
19. Hirsch AT, Haskal ZJ, Hertzer NR, et al. ACC/AHA 2005 guidelines for the management of patients with peripheral arterial disease (lower extremity, renal, mesenteric, and abdominal aortic): executive summary—a collaborative report from the American Association for Vascular Surgery/Society for Vascular Surgery, Society for Cardiovascular Angiography and Interventions, Society for Vascular Medicine and Biology, Society of Interventional Radiology, and the ACC/AHA Task Force on Practice Guidelines (Writing Committee to Develop Guidelines for the Management of Patients With Peripheral Arterial Disease) endorsed by the American Association of Cardiovascular and Pulmonary Rehabilitation; National Heart, Lung, and Blood Institute; Society for Vascular Nursing; TransAtlantic Inter-Society Consensus; and Vascular Disease Foundation. *J Am Coll Cardiol*. 2006;47:1239-312.
20. US Preventice Services Task Force. Screening for abdominal aortic aneurysm: recommendation statement. *Ann Intern Med*. 2005;142:198-202.
21. Sprouse LR 2nd, Meier GH 3rd, Lesar CJ, et al. Comparison of abdominal aortic aneurysm diameter measurements obtained with ultrasound and computed tomography: is there a difference? *J Vasc Surg*. 2003;38:466-471; discussion 71-72.
22. Davutoglu V, Soydinc S, Sirikci A, Dinckal H, Akdemir I. Interrupted aortic arch in an adolescent male. *Can J Cardiol*. 2004;20:1367-1368.
23. Warnes CA, Williams RG, Bashore TM, et al. ACC/AHA 2008 guidelines for the management of adults with congenital heart disease: a report of the American College of Cardiology/American Heart Association Task Force on Practice Guidelines (writing committee to develop guidelines on the management of adults with congenital heart disease). *Circulation*. 2008;118:e714-e833.
24. Tadros TM, Klein MD, Shapira OM. Ascending aortic dilatation associated with bicuspid aortic valve: pathophysiology, molecular biology, and clinical implications. *Circulation*. 2009;119:880-890.
25. Neschis DG, Scalea TM, Flinn WR, Griffith BP. Blunt aortic injury. *N Engl J Med*. 2008;359:1708-1716.
26. Bohner H, Luther B, Braunstein S, Beer S, Sandmann W. Primary malignant tumors of the aorta: clinical presentation, treatment, and course of different entities. *J Vasc Surg*. 2003;38:1430-1433.

CHAPTER 23

PERIPHERAL VASCULAR DISEASE

Rajan Hundal, Anthony DeFrance, and Peter S. Fail

INTRODUCTION / 392

CASE 1: CAROTID ARTERY DISEASE / 392
Case Discussion / 392
Key Points / 394

CASE 2: CAROTID ARTERY DISEASE / 394
Case Discussion / 394
Key Points / 396

CASE 3: AORTIC ANEURYSM / 396
Case Discussion / 396

CASE 4: AORTIC ANEURYSM / 397
Case Discussion / 398
Key Points / 399

CASE 5: LOWER EXTREMITY PERIPHERAL ARTERIAL DISEASE / 399
Case Discussion / 399
Key Points / 400

INTRODUCTION

Peripheral vascular disease continues to be a leading cause of death and disability in the United States and the Western world.[1] Advancements in imaging modalities have enhanced our ability to better understand both the anatomy and pathophysiology of vascular diseases. Health care practitioners with a clear understanding of the available imaging modalities and their utilization will be better positioned to optimize outcomes in patients with peripheral vascular diseases.

In this chapter, we present carotid, aortic, and lower extremity atherosclerotic peripheral vascular disease cases with computed tomography angiography (CTA) images that illustrate key points in diagnosis and treatment.

The recent and rapid advancement of computed tomography (CT) scanners from single-row to multidetector-row scanners has greatly enhanced our ability to image the body's vasculature. Wider detector arrays allow for more rapid image acquisition, using less contrast and less radiation dose. Improved spatial resolution of the new generation of scanners also provides more details of the vascular anatomy including plaque morphology characterization. Postprocessing of these rapidly acquired images with three-dimensional (3D) workstations allows viewing of images in multiple planes and with multiple viewing techniques.

CTA imaging has several advantages in peripheral arterial disease: (1) excellent spatial resolution; (2) exceptional sensitivity

and specificity; (3) ability to assess postocclusion anatomy; (4) short examination time; (5) ability to accurately assess vasculature that has been revascularized (stented or bypassed); (6) imaging in multiple planes; (7) lack of interference with metal, including cardiac devices; and (8) patient preference and comfort. There is also the added benefit that CTA and magnetic resonance (MR) can potentially allow for the diagnosis of nonvascular abnormalities that may be clinically significant.

The main disadvantages potentially include: (1) nephrotoxic contrast agents; (2) exposure to radiation; and (3) potential "blooming" (partial volume) artifact from excessive calcium in the vascular system.

CASE 1: CAROTID ARTERY DISEASE

A 68-year-old man presents to the office of his primary care physician after experiencing several episodes of transient right hand paresthesias that last for less than 1 hour. He has a history of hypertension, dyslipidemia, and known coronary artery disease with three-vessel bypass 5 years prior to presentation. Physical exam is without focal neurologic deficits but does reveal bilateral carotid bruits. Blood pressure is 95/55 mm Hg. A duplex ultrasound (DUS) of the neck is ordered for evaluation.

Carotid DUS shows a "possible complete occlusion" of the left common carotid artery and "mild" disease within the right carotid system. The patient is referred to cardiology, and a CTA of the neck is ordered for further clarification. See Figs. 23–1 to 23–3.

■ CASE DISCUSSION

Stroke is the third leading cause of death in the United States, with an estimated 610,000 new strokes and 185,000 recurrent strokes diagnosed each year.[1,2] Strokes are costly to diagnose and treat, with cost estimates of $73 billion for 2010.[1] An estimated 15% to 30% of all strokes are related to atherosclerotic disease within the carotid bifurcation.[3] The atherosclerotic process is postulated to be similar to that of coronary atherosclerotic disease involving areas of low shear stress, inflammation, lipid accumulation, and activation of enzymatic processes.[4] The two main mechanisms of transient ischemic attack (TIA) or stroke caused by atherosclerotic disease within the carotid system are embolization and reduced blood flow in the setting of inadequate collateral circulation or impaired vasoreactivity.[5]

The patient is a 68-year-old man with several risk factors for stroke and carotid disease who appears to be suffering TIAs in the form of stuttering focal right hand paresthesias. The neurologic symptoms that suggest TIA or stroke related to carotid artery disease are focal and typically involve the ipsilateral middle cerebral artery. TIAs are defined as transient episodes of neurologic dysfunction that are caused by a disruption of blood flow to the central nervous system that does not cause permanent injury and resolve within 24 hours. In the United States, the incidence of TIA is estimated at 200,000 to 500,000, and the prevalence is approximately 2.3%, or close to 5,000,000 people.[6] At least 15% of all strokes are preceded by a TIA, underscoring the importance of patients and clinicians pursuing an aggressive evaluation and

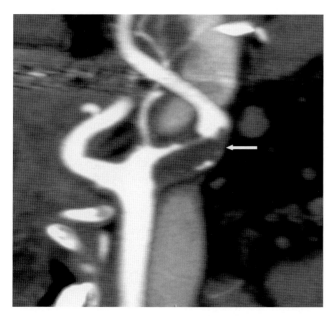

FIGURE 23–1. Left carotid system. Maximum intensity projection view of stenosis (arrow) of the left internal carotid artery with a large plaque burden. The average Hounsfield units of 27 within the plaque indicate low-density lipid-laden plaque.

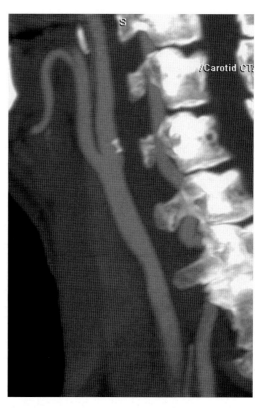

FIGURE 23–3. Small calcified plaque at the right carotid bulb.

management strategy.[7] The risk of stroke is highest in the 30-day period following a TIA, with the North American Symptomatic Carotid Endarterectomy Trial (NASCET) demonstrating a 20% stroke risk at 90 days, and other studies showing a 1-year

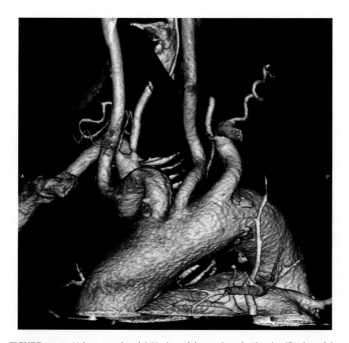

FIGURE 23–2. Volume-rendered (VR) view of the aortic arch. The classification of the arch is important when exploring an invasive strategy. This is a class II arch with the innominate, left carotid, and subclavian arteries slightly below the apex of the arch. The vertical distance from the origin of the innominate artery to the top of the arch determines the arch type. Type 1 is less than one time the diameter of the common carotid artery (CCA), type 2 is one to two times the diameter of the CCA, and type 3 is greater than two times the diameter of the CCA. Also note the tortuosity for the innominate artery.

mortality of 25%.[8,9] These studies demonstrate the need for relatively urgent imaging for risk stratification in patients who have recently experienced TIAs. Factors that predict an upcoming stroke in patients experiencing a TIA are age >60 years, diabetes mellitus, focal weakness or speech impairment, and symptoms that last for longer than 10 minutes.[10]

TIAs related to carotid disease are usually caused by embolization of debris from the carotid arch or can be caused by low cerebral perfusion as a result of a significant carotid stenosis in the setting of inadequate collateral circulation and impaired vasoreactivity. Clinically, the low flow states usually present with brief symptomatic episodes, whereas embolic phenomena generally result in more prolonged symptoms. The risk of low flow TIAs resulting from total occlusion of the internal carotid is generally greatest at the time of occlusion but can also occur weeks to months later due to thrombotic embolization of the occlusive material, resulting in a delayed stroke.

The risk of stroke caused by carotid plaque is directly correlated with the degree of carotid stenosis.[11] Carotid disease is progressive; patients with high-grade stenosis should be followed up every 6 months, and patients with moderate stenosis should be followed up annually. Plaque characteristics such as ulceration, degree of fibrous cap formation, and inflammatory factors also play a role. Active thrombotic plaque is usually found in patients who have suffered a stroke, whereas plaque from patients suffering TIAs or who are asymptomatic are much less likely to show active thrombus.[12] Another important finding was that active thrombus was still found on plaques that were removed almost a year after symptom onset.

The patient's symptom of stuttering right arm paresthesias is a common and typical presentation of systemic hypotension leading to reduced cerebral perfusion in a patient with poor collateral circulation, although this could also have been a result of embolic phenomena. The patient was noted to have bilateral carotid bruits. Although assessment of bruits is recommended, the presence or absence of a bruit is a poor predictor of future stroke or significant carotid disease in asymptomatic patients.[13] Bruits represent a hemodynamically significant lesion 30% of the time; however, in patients with hemodynamically significant lesions, a bruit was detected in only 50% of patients.[14]

The use of invasive arteriography and digital subtraction angiography is considered the gold standard when evaluating carotid artery disease. The incidence of stroke during the procedure is greater than 1% in most series, and there are additional morbidities such as access site complications, contrast nephropathy, and the exposure of patients and operators to radiation.[15] Given these limitations, noninvasive imaging has taken on a larger role for screening and preoperative assessment of carotid disease. In this case, the initial imaging modality chosen was carotid DUS. The assessment is performed by evaluating peak systolic and end-diastolic velocities proximal and distal to the stenosis. The limitation of DUS is that its effectiveness is operator and patient dependent, with some studies estimating a misclassification rate as high as 25%.[16] In general, it is felt that DUS is similar to MR and CT imaging in detecting complete occlusions but less effective in evaluating nonocclusive lesions.[16] For stenoses in the 70% to 99% range, the sensitivity and specificity for DUS are 83% and 89%, respectively.[17] The limitation of DUS in differentiating between complete and severe occlusions is important because procedural treatment is not indicated in complete occlusions. Given this, alternative confirmatory imaging modalities such as MR angiography (MRA) and CTA play a large role in patients who are likely to undergo carotid surgical or intravascular intervention. In the case presented, a CTA was chosen. This modality has a sensitivity of 80% to 95% and a specificity of 92% to 99% for lesions in the 70% to 99% range, with greater sensitivity and specificity noted in studies using multirow scanners.

In summary, CTA offers an excellent platform when carotid duplex is ambiguous, permitting visualization of aortic arch or high bifurcation pathology, reliable differentiation of total and subtotal occlusion, and assessment of ostial and tandem stenosis. Screening of the general population with imaging studies is not recommended but may be indicated in some patients with a higher prevalence of disease.

In our case, the CT showed the left internal carotid artery (ICA) to be severely stenotic but not occluded. The DUS showed a "possible complete occlusion," which is an absolute contraindication for surgical or interventional treatment approaches. Given the findings of CTA, our patient was referred for carotid endarterectomy (CEA).

■ KEY POINTS

- Carotid artery atherosclerotic disease is a major cause of TIA and stroke in symptomatic and asymptomatic individuals.

- The risk of stroke is correlated with the degree of carotid stenosis.

- TIAs are a warning sign of future stroke; therefore, imaging and evaluation should take place promptly after a patient experiences symptoms.

- DUS is an effective screening test. Limitations include high variability, operator dependence, and difficulty in distinguishing whether there is a complete occlusion or severe stenosis.

- Screening for carotid artery disease is not recommended for the general public but can be helpful in risk stratifying high-risk individuals.

- CTA is an excellent modality to evaluate the carotid arteries that is both highly sensitive and specific.

CASE 2: CAROTID ARTERY DISEASE

The patient is a 67-year-old man with a history of coronary artery disease and multivessel percutaneous coronary intervention several years ago. He is sent for a DUS of his carotid arteries following the complaint of visual changes in his left eye, which shows a left carotid artery stenosis of 80% to 99%.

A CTA is ordered for confirmation and to help guide management. See Figs. 23–4 and 23–5.

The patient undergoes an endarterectomy of the left ICA, but his postoperative course is complicated by right-sided weakness. He returns to the operating department, where a large dissection is noted along the length of the left ICA. Attempts to repair are unsuccessful, and the patient is started on Plavix, aspirin, and Coumadin. He is transferred to the catheterization laboratory for urgent angiography, which verifies the dissection.

CTA of the neck is performed. See Figs. 23–6 and 23–7.

No intervention is performed, and he subsequently has marked improvement in his right-sided motor deficits after 2 weeks. At 8 months, he again experiences right-sided weakness. A CTA is performed. See Fig. 23–8.

The patient undergoes successful stenting of the left ICA. See Fig. 23–9. Three weeks later, he has a recurrent event. CTA reveals a separation of the stents. See Fig. 23–10. The stent separation is treated with repeat stenting with excellent results.

■ CASE DISCUSSION

This is a complex case of a 67-year-old man who is asymptomatic but undergoes CEA because of a severe left ICA stenosis discovered on a DUS screening test. CEA is the gold standard treatment for patients with symptomatic or asymptomatic carotid stenosis, with several randomized control trials showing reduction in ipsilateral stroke. The NASCET trial randomized patients who were symptomatic with >70% stenosis to CEA or medical management. At 18 months, the risk of stroke was 9% in the CEA arm and 25% in the medical management arm,[8] with even greater benefit with more severe stenoses. A second cohort also found benefit in patients with 50% to 69% stenosis but no statistically significant difference in patients with less than 50% stenosis. The Asymptomatic Carotid Atherosclerosis

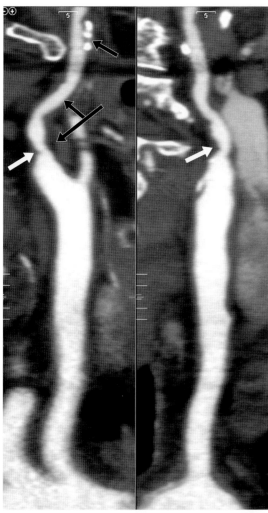

FIGURE 23–4. Coronal and sagittal multiplaner reformation images of the Left carotid prior to the endarterectomy. Notice the significant diffuse plaque that lines the entire left internal carotid artery (black arrows). Moderate stenosis (white arrow).

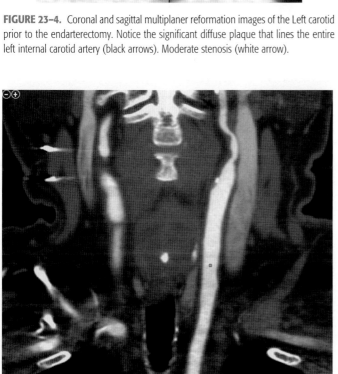

FIGURE 23–5. Axial view before carotid endarterectomy.

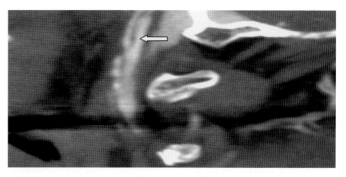

FIGURE 23–6. Computed tomography angiography showing carotid artery dissection (arrow).

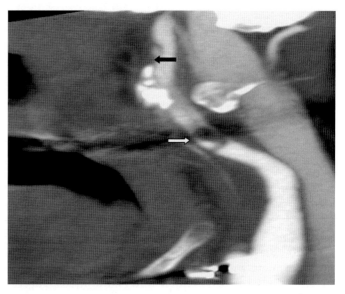

FIGURE 23–7. Dissection with probable thrombus, with Hounsfield units of 74 (white arrow). There is also thrombus present at the origin of the dissection (black arrow).

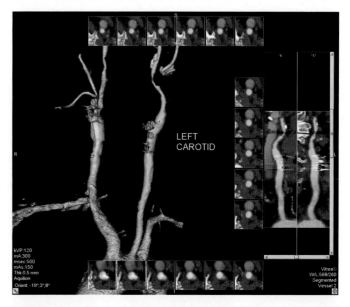

FIGURE 23–8. Volume-rendered image before stenting indicating severe stenosis of the left internal carotid artery.

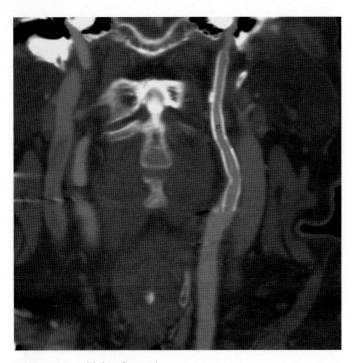

FIGURE 23–9. Axial view after stenting.

Study (ACAS) evaluated asymptomatic patients with stenosis ranging from 60% to 99% and randomized them to CEA or medical management.[18] At 5 years, the risk of stroke was 5% in the CEA arm and 11% in the medical arm.[18] The European Carotid Surgery Trial (ECST) also showed benefit in treating asymptomatic patients with relatively severe stenosis.[19]

The Stenting and Angioplasty with Protection in Patients at High Risk for Endarterectomy (SAPPHIRE) trial compared carotid artery stenting (with mandatory distal protection) and CEA. This trial demonstrated noninferiority of CAS in high-risk patients who were asymptomatic or symptomatic.[19] Stent fracture is a relatively rare complication that, in this case, was diagnosed with CTA. It was treated with repeat stenting with good result. In general, CTA is preferred over MR with stents that are newly placed.

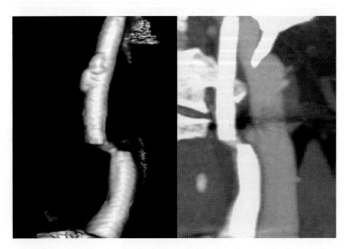

FIGURE 23–10. Volume-rendered and "thick slab" view of stent separation.

■ KEY POINTS

- CEA is indicated in patients with symptomatic carotid stenosis of >50% with greater benefit seen in patients with greater degrees of stenosis (NASCET), if the operative risk is less than 6%.
- CEA showed benefit in asymptomatic patients with stenosis >60% (ACAS).
- Carotid artery stenting is a safe and reasonable alternative to CEA and is preferred in patients who represent a high surgical risk.
- CTA is an excellent and safe modality to evaluate stent architecture and patency.

CASE 3: AORTIC ANEURYSM

An 80-year-old man with a history of coronary artery disease, tobacco dependence, and hypertension is referred for evaluation of a pulsating mass in his abdomen. There is no history of pulmonary or renal disease. He denies family history of aneurysm. Physical examination is suggestive of a large abdominal aortic aneurysm (AAA) with findings of a pulsatile mass in the abdomen. An abdominal CTA is ordered. See Figs. 23–11 and 23–12.

■ CASE DISCUSSION

Aortic aneurysm remains an important clinical entity, with an estimated 15,000 deaths annually in the United States.[20] An aneurysm is defined as a focal dilatation of the three aortic layers that is 1.5 times greater than that of the normal lumen. They are thought to be caused by collagen and elastin breakdown that is mitigated by inflammatory factors, eventually leading to weakening and distortion of the aortic wall. It is estimated that

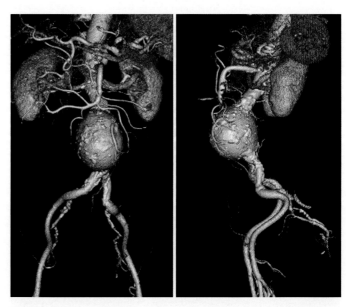

FIGURE 23–11. Coronal and sagittal volume-rendered reconstruction images of a large abdominal aortic aneurysm.

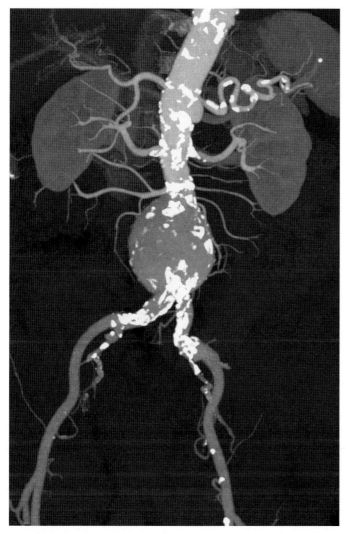

FIGURE 23–12. Maximum intensity projection image of extensive calcification and large abdominal aortic aneurysm.

25% of aortic aneurysms are thoracic and 75% are abdominal.[20] The prevalence estimates of AAA are 4% to 7% in the US adult population, with a male-to-female ratio of at least 5:1.[21] It is the tenth most common cause of death in patients older than age 55 years. Aneurysms are characterized as fusiform if the dilatation is relatively symmetrical and circumferential or as saccular if the outpouching of the aortic wall is focal. Thoracic and abdominal aneurysms are usually asymptomatic until the time of rupture, which is usually fatal. AAAs are further classified as suprarenal, juxtarenal, pararenal, or infrarenal. Juxtarenal aneurysms are in close proximity to the renal arteries, and pararenal aneurysms involve the origin of one or both renal arteries. The vast majority of AAAs are infrarenal.

Multiple imaging modalities can be used to image the aorta. CTA is particularly useful when endovascular intervention is being considered. Noninvasive imaging by CTA has become the mainstay for evaluating patients for endovascular aortic reconstruction (EVAR), allowing the clinician to "size" a particular device for a given anatomy.

The patient is an 80-year-old man who presented with a pulsating mass noted on physical exam, with subsequent CTA imaging showing a 7.5-cm infrarenal aortic aneurysm. Palpation of the abdomen for AAA has a sensitivity of 50%, with a specificity of 90% in a high-risk population.[22] His risk factors are age, smoking, male sex, hypertension, and previous history of atherosclerotic disease. The risk of AAA in patients who smoke is six to seven times that of nonsmokers.[23] The patient does not have a family history of AAA, but some studies show that 25% of those diagnosed with AAA will have a first-degree relative that is affected.[20] The prevalence of AAA in patients 75 to 84 years of age is estimated at 12%.[20] The large size of the aneurysm in this patient places him in a high-risk category for rupture, thromboembolic complications, or morbidity related to erosion of adjacent structures. For aneurysms greater than 5 cm, the 5-year risk of rupture is estimated at 25% to 40%, and for aneurysms in the 7- to 8-cm range, the 1-year rate of rupture is greater than 25%.[24] Larger aneurysms can expand as much as 6 to 8 mm/year.[24] In addition, his hypertension and continued use of tobacco independently increase the risk of rupture. The chance of surviving aortic rupture is estimated at 10%, with more than 75% dying before reaching the operating table.[25]

Treatment options include an open surgical approach, endovascular stenting, and watchful waiting on appropriate medical management. Despite understanding these risks, the patient opted for medical management. Control of blood pressure, lipids, and smoking cessation is imperative. It is a class I recommendation that AAA greater that 5.5 cm be surgically repaired to reduce the risk of rupture.[20]

CASE 4: AORTIC ANEURYSM

A 71-year-old woman with a history of hypertension and family history of AAA is sent for a screening ultrasound, which shows a 4.8-cm AAA. A follow-up CT scan is ordered 6 months later for evaluation. See Fig. 23–13.

A decision is made to treat the patient medically with β-blockers and observation. Six months later, she presents to

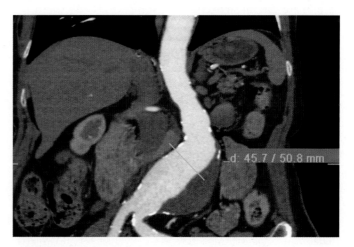

FIGURE 23–13. Abdominal aortic aneurysm that measures 51 mm.

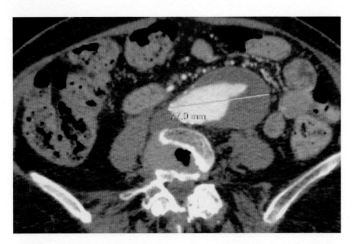

FIGURE 23–14. Axial image showing erroneous measurement.

the emergency room because of a recent fall and lower back pain. A CTA done at this time reveals an AAA measured at 70 mm. Side-by-side review of the two CT scans shows no appreciable difference. This discrepancy occurs when the AAA is measured off axis in an axial view as opposed to centerline. See Fig. 23–14.

During her hospitalization, the patient reconsiders her treatment options and undergoes EVAR. See Fig. 23–15.

The patient remains asymptomatic, but a follow-up surveillance CTA at 6 months reveals a type II endoleak with an increase in the AAA diameter. See Fig. 23–16.

■ CASE DISCUSSION

The patient is a 71-year-old woman with hypertension, a significant smoking history, and a first-degree relative with an AAA. She was appropriately sent for a screening ultrasound, which showed a 4.9-cm AAA. A CT showed a 5.1-cm AAA. Although she met criteria for elective repair, she opted for medical management at that time. Class I recommendations include surveillance imaging with CT or ultrasound every 6 to 12 months for infrarenal aneurysms measuring 4 to 5 cm.[20] Ultrasound screening is recommended in patients older than 60 who have a first-degree relative with an AAA or men age 65 to 75 who have been or are current smokers.

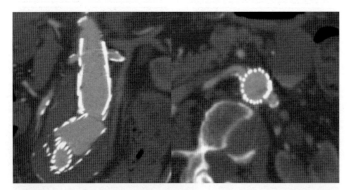

FIGURE 23–15. Axial and coronal views after endovascular aortic reconstruction. Good apposition with suprarenal fixation.

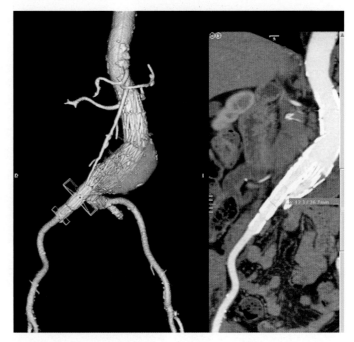

FIGURE 23–16. Volume-rendered and maximum intensity projection images showing a type II endoleak.

Six months later, the patient presented to the emergency room with a recent fall and back pain, and CT imaging at that time erroneously reported a 7.1-cm AAA. The source of error is the off-axis measurement of the AAA in the axial plane (axial slice artifact), which commonly overestimates the aortic diameter. The patient at this juncture decided to proceed to EVAR. A stent graft was placed through a femoral approach with excellent result. In EVAR, a graft is inserted into the aorta at the site of the aneurysm and deployed forming a seal with the aorta acting as a conduit for blood that excludes the aneurysm. After a period of time, the aneurysm will thrombose with eventual shrinking of the aneurysmal sac. Selection of appropriate patients for endovascular repair is based on risk of AAA rupture in comparison to operative risk, life expectancy, anatomic considerations, comorbidities, and patient preference. Unsuitable anatomy alone excludes as many as 50% of all AAAs for potential EVAR. Mortality estimates for elective open surgical repair are between 2.5% and 6%.[25] The 2005 American College of Cardiology/American Heart Association guidelines recommend open repair for patients at low surgical risk and EVAR for high-risk patients. According to the guideline, EVAR may be considered in low-risk patients, although with less established evidence of benefit. A meta-analysis published in 2008 that included the Dutch Randomised Endovascular Aneurysm Management (DREAM) and EVAR studies evaluated 21,000 patients who underwent either open surgical or endovascular repair. There was a clear benefit shown in the EVAR group for 30-day mortality and postoperative complications and in long-term aneurysm-related mortality.[25]

After EVAR, the patient was placed on surveillance protocol with CT scans at 1, 6, and 12 months. Unfortunately, at 6 months, the surveillance CT showed a type II endoleak. Endoleaks are a result of persistent blood flow into the aneurysmal sac after device placement. Type I endoleaks occur at the proximal or distal attachment site and are a result of inadequate graft apposition with the aorta. Type II endoleaks result from flow into the aneurysmal sac from branch vessels. They are the most common form of endoleak. Type III and type IV endoleaks are the result of breakdown, leaks, or tears within the endograft. CTA imaging is an excellent tool to evaluate AAAs for potential EVAR repair as well as in surveillance protocols post-EVAR to assess for endoleaks. At the 1 year mark, the endoleak persists but the aneurysm has not increased.

■ KEY POINTS

- Aortic aneurysms are clinically very important, with high mortality rates if left untreated.
- Aneurysms can be clinically silent, and clinicians must have a high clinical suspicion and have a command of the best use of imaging technology for early diagnosis.
- CTA imaging of the aorta is highly sensitive and specific.
- CTA imaging is the imaging modality of choice for evaluating aortic aneurysms that may potentially undergo surgical or endovascular repair.

CASE 5: LOWER EXTREMITY PERIPHERAL ARTERIAL DISEASE

The patient is a 66-year-old woman with a 25-year history of diabetes who presents with a nonhealing wound on her right foot that was sustained following minimal trauma. Physical exam revealed a 3-cm nonhealing ulcer on her right heal. There was a weak right femoral pulse and an absent popliteal pulse. The ankle-brachial index (ABI) was 0.6.

A CTA is ordered of the peripheral vasculature. See Figs. 23–17 to 23–19.

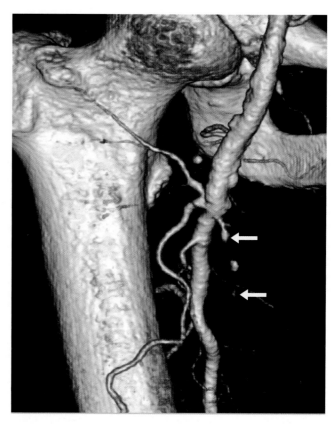

FIGURE 23–18. Volume-rendered image of the occlusion.

■ CASE DISCUSSION

Lower extremity peripheral arterial disease (PAD) is a common and growing problem. The Intersociety Consensus for the Management of Peripheral Arterial Disease (TASC II)

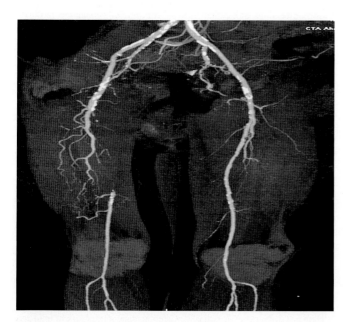

FIGURE 23–17. Maximum intensity projection view of 100% occlusion of right superficial femoral artery with reconstitution at the popliteal.

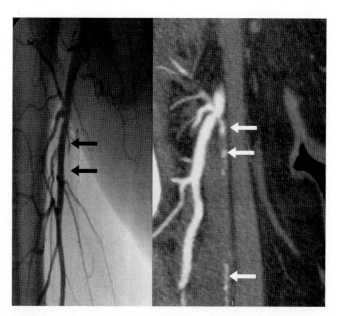

FIGURE 23–19. Comparison of off-axis maximum intensity projection (MIP) and angiogram of 100% occlusion. Off-axis MIP view shows the entrance point as well as minimal collateral flow in the proximal segment.

consensus document estimates that 27 million patients are affected in the United States and Europe.[26] The prevalence increases with age, with an estimated 10% to 14% of people above the age of 70 having an ABI of less than 0.9.[26] Classic symptoms include rest pain and claudication. One study estimates that 3% to 6% of American men older than age 60 will experience intermittent claudication due to obstructive disease of the aortoiliac and lower extremities.[27] Imaging methods used to assess lower extremity PAD include invasive angiography, DUS, MRA, and CTA. The rapid evolution of CTA technology has led to a dramatic increase in its use to evaluate disease and as a guide to treatment. Many physicians use CTA to determine a management strategy *after* PAD is diagnosed with physical exam or with noninvasive DUS. For interventionalists, CTA has become an important modality for mapping vascular anatomy and delineating location and severity of stenosis. This information is of paramount importance in selecting patients who are candidates for endovascular or surgical revascularization. Additional information including presence of aneurysms, popliteal entrapment, and cystic adventitial disease are also provided by CTA. In this group of patients, multidetector CT is noted to have high sensitivity (96%) and specificity (97%) and excellent interobserver agreement when compared with digital subtraction angiography (DSA) as the gold standard.[28,29] One disadvantage can be the overestimation of the stenosis, which is seen with heavily calcified plaque due to partial volume artifact (blooming). In many cases, this can be overcome by using thin slice multiplanar reformation (MPR) images and routinely adjusting window and leveling setting in the presence of calcium. In addition, postprocessing filters (kernels) can be used, which improve edge detection at the cost of increased image noise.

Image acquisition with run-off studies may be challenging because the large areas covered by wide detector arrays can cause one to "outrun" the bolus. In essence, this means that the CT images are acquired before the contrast has had time to arrive at the area of interest. Routine rescan of the run-off vessels (popliteal trunk and anterior and posterior tibial and peroneal vessels) can be programmed into the run-off protocol on most machines to minimize the likelihood of this occurring.

Sensitivity of CTA for detection of stenosis more than 50% in the lower extremity including inflow and distal crural arteries is in the order of 90%. Another potential limitation of CTA is difficulty in analyzing the distal peroneal, anterior tibial, and posterior tibial vessels, especially in the presence of severe calcification. This information is very important when bypasses to these vessels are being considered. In this situation, MRA has been shown to be useful. In the authors' experience, these limitations can usually be overcome with good acquisition parameters and the utilization of 3D workstations that allow multiplanar imaging and thin slice MPR. CTA offers the clinician the ideal platform for analyzing postsurgical or catheter-based patients who present with a sudden change in their claudication symptoms.

■ KEY POINTS

- MDCT provides nonvascular tissue and organ images and is the preferred modality when deciding on a treatment strategy.
- CTA is less invasive and faster, with less exposure to ionizing radiation, when compared with conventional DSA.
- CTA is the preferred modality in the presence of surgical clips, metal implants, and pacemakers.
- Limitations to run-off CTA include mistimed contrast and heavily calcified vessels below the knee.

REFERENCES

1. Hirsch AT, Haskal ZJ, Hertzer NR, et al. ACC/AHA 2005 practice guidelines for the management of patients with peripheral arterial disease (lower extremity, renal, mesenteric, and abdominal aorta): a collaborative report from the American Association for Vascular Surgery/Society for Vascular Surgery, Society for Cardiovascular Angiography and Interventions, Society for Vascular Medicine and Biology, Society of Interventional Radiology, and the ACC/AHA Task Force on Practice Guidelines (Writing Committee to Develop Guidelines for the Management of Patients With Peripheral Arterial Disease): endorsed by the American Association of Cardiovascular and Pulmonary Rehabilitation; National Heart, Lung, and Blood Institute; Society for Vascular Nursing; TransAtlantic Inter-Society Consensus; and Vascular Disease Foundation. *Circulation*. 2006;113:e463-e654.
2. Lloyd-Jones D, Adams R, Carnethon M, et al. Heart Disease and stroke statistics–2009 update. A report from the American Heart Association Statistics Committee and Stroke Statistics Subcommittee. *Circulation*. 2009;119: e21-e181.
3. Hollander M, Bots ML, Del Sol AI, et al. Carotid plaques increase the risk of stroke and subtypes of cerebral infarction in asymptomatic elderly: the Rotterdam study. *Circulation*. 2002;105:2872-2877.
4. Stork S, van den Beld AW, von Schacky C, et al. Carotid artery plaque burden, stiffness, and mortality risk in elderly men: a prospective, population-based cohort study. *Circulation*. 2004;110:344-348.
5. Silvestrini M, Vernieri F, Pasqualetti P, et al. Impaired cerebral vasoreactivity and risk of stroke in patients with asymptomatic carotid artery stenosis. *JAMA*. 2000;283:2122-2127.
6. Rosamond W, Flegal K, Furie K, et al. Heart disease and stroke statistics–2008 update. A report from the American Heart Association Statistics Committee and Stoke Statistics Subcommittee. *Circulation*. 2008;117: e25-e146.
7. Hankey GJ. Impact of treatment of people with transient ischemic attack on stroke incidence and public health. *Cerebrovasc Dis*. 1996;6(Suppl 1):26-33.
8. Barnett HJ, Taylor DW, Eliasziw M, et al. Benefit of carotid endarterectomy in patients with symptomatic moderate or severe stenosis. North American Symptomatic Carotid Endarterectomy Trial Collaborators (NASCET). *N Engl J Med*. 1998;339:1415-1425.
9. Kleindorfer D, Panagos P, Pancioli A, et al. Incidence and short-term prognosis of transient ischemic attack in a population-based study. *Stroke*. 2005;36:720-723.
10. Johnston SC, Gress DR, Browner WS, Sidney S. Short-term prognosis after emergency department diagnosis of TIA. *JAMA*. 2000;284:2901-2906.
11. Ferguson GG, Eliasziw M, Barr HW, et al. The North American Symptomatic Carotid Endarterectomy Trial: surgical results in 1415 patients. *Stroke*. 1999;30:1751-1758.
12. Spagnoli LG, Mauriello A, Sangiorgi G, et al. Extracranial thrombotically active carotid plaque as a risk factor for ischemic stroke. *JAMA*. 2004;292:1845-1852.
13. Rea T. The role of carotid bruit in screening for carotid stenosis. *Ann Intern Med*. 1997;127:657-658.
14. Ratchford EV, Jin Z, Di Tullio MR, et al. Carotid bruit for detection of hemodynamically significant carotid stenosis: the Northern Manhattan Study. *Neurol Res*. 2009;31:748-752.
15. Hankey GJ, Warlow CP, Sellar RJ. Cerebral angiographic risk in mild cerebrovascular disease. *Stroke*. 1990;21:209-222.

16. Sabeti S, Schillinger M, Mlekusch W, et al. Quantification of internal carotid artery stenosis with duplex US: comparative analysis of different flow velocity criteria. *Radiology*. 2004; 232:431-439.

17. Tsuruda JS, Saloner D, Anderson C. Noninvasive evaluation of cerebral ischemia. Trends for the 1990s. *Circulation*. 1991;83(Suppl):I176.

18. Executive Committee for the Asymptomatic Carotid Atherosclerosis Study. Endarterectomy for asymptomatic carotid artery stenosis. *JAMA*. 1995;273:1421-1428.

19. European Carotid Surgery Trialists' Collaborative Group. MRC European Carotid Surgery Trial: interim results for symptomatic patients with severe (70-99%) or with mild (0-29%) carotid stenosis. *Lancet*. 1991;337:1235-1243.

20. Isselbacher EM. Thoracic and abdominal aortic aneurysms. *Circulation*. 2005;111:816-828.

21. Singh K, Bonaa KH, Jacobsen BK, et al. Prevalence of and risk factors for abdominal aortic aneurysms in a population-based study: the Tromso Study. *Am J Epidemiol*. 2001;154:236-244.

22. Simon G, Nordgren D, Connelly S, Shultz PJ. Screening for abdominal aortic aneurysms in a hypertensive patient population. *Arch Intern Med*. 1996;156:2081-2084.

23. Lederle FA, Johnson GR, Wilson SE, Chute EP. The aneurysm detection and management study screening program: validation cohort and final results. Aneurysm Detection and Management Veterans Affairs Cooperative Study Investigators. *Arch Intern Med*. 2000;160:1425-1430.

24. Gadowski GR, Pilcher DB, Ricci MA. Abdominal aortic aneurysm expansion rate: effect of size and beta-adrenergic blockade. *J Vasc Surg*. 1994;19:727-731.

25. Lovegrove RE, Javid M, Magee TR, Galland RB. A meta-analysis of 21,178 patients undergoing open or endovascular repair of abdominal aortic aneurysm. *Br J Surg*. 2008;95:677-684.

26. Norgren L, Hiatt WR, Dormandy JA, et al. Inter-Society Consensus for the Management of Peripheral Arterial Disease (TASC II). *J Vasc Surg*. 2007;45(Suppl):S5.

27. Hirsch AT, Criqui MH, Treat-Jacobson D, Regensteiner JG. Peripheral arterial disease detection, awareness, and treatment in primary care. *JAMA*. 2001;286:1317-1324.

28. Romano M, Mainenti PP, Imbriaco M, et al. Multidetector row CT angiography of the abdominal aorta and lower extremities in patients with peripheral arterial occlusive disease: diagnostic accuracy and interobserver agreement. *Eur J Radiol*. 2004;50:303-308.

29. Met R, Bipat S, Legemate DA. Diagnostic performance of computed tomography angiography in peripheral arterial disease: a systematic review and meta-analysis. *JAMA*. 2009;301:415-424.

CHAPTER 24
PULMONARY VASCULAR DISEASE

Stephen F. Crawley and Andrew J. Peacock

IDIOPATHIC PULMONARY ARTERIAL HYPERTENSION / 402
Background / 402
Clinical Presentation / 402
Imaging / 402
Management / 405
Case Study / 406

CHRONIC THROMBOEMBOLIC PULMONARY HYPERTENSION / 408
Background / 408
Clinical Presentation / 408
Imaging / 408
Management / 411
Case Study / 412

PULMONARY ARTERIOVENOUS MALFORMATIONS / 412
Background / 412
Clinical Presentation / 412
Imaging / 414
Management / 416
Case Study / 416

IDIOPATHIC PULMONARY ARTERIAL HYPERTENSION

■ BACKGROUND

Idiopathic pulmonary arterial hypertension (IPAH) represents pulmonary arterial hypertension in its purest form. By definition, IPAH exists when an underlying cause of the pulmonary arterial hypertension (PAH) cannot be identified. It is a rare disease with a poor prognosis and is characterized by luminal obliteration of small pulmonary arteries. The overall result is increased resistance to pulmonary blood flow, increasing pulmonary artery pressure (PAP), and ultimately, right ventricular failure and death.

Women are affected more commonly than men, with a female-to-male ratio of approximately 1.7:1. Cruelly, there is a predilection for IPAH to affect otherwise normal young women of childbearing age. The mean age for developing the condition is approximately 40 years, but it can occur at any age. Elderly patients often have other coexisting cardiac and respiratory disease, making the diagnosis of pure IPAH more challenging.

■ CLINICAL PRESENTATION

Most patients with IPAH present with exertional dyspnea, developing over months or years. This classical, although nonspecific, symptom is thought to be due to the inability of the right heart to raise output on exertion. Chest pain, syncope, and peripheral edema are more common in advanced IPAH and indicate right ventricular failure.[1,2]

The clinical signs of IPAH include right ventricular heave, loud pulmonary component of the second heart sound, a pansystolic murmur of tricuspid regurgitation, and a right ventricular third sound. Jugular venous distension, hepatomegaly, peripheral edema, ascites, and cold extremities indicate patients in a more advanced state with right ventricular failure at rest. Central cyanosis may also be present in advanced cases.

Unfortunately, the absence of findings on clinical examination and nonspecific symptoms frequently lead to a delay in referral to the appropriate specialist center and, subsequently, a delay in diagnosis and treatment. Symptoms are often initially attributed to poor physical fitness, especially in overweight patients, and the diagnosis only becomes apparent with the development of chest pain, syncope, or edema.

■ IMAGING

Chest Radiograph

The chest radiograph may give the first clue to the presence of IPAH, providing invaluable information on the heart size, the lung parenchyma, and the pulmonary vasculature.

The main chest radiograph features of IPAH consist of enlargement of the main pulmonary arteries and rapid tapering of the vessels as they extend to the periphery of the lungs, giving rise to peripheral oligemia. The heart, particularly the right-sided chamber, is usually enlarged but may be of normal size (Fig. 24–1).

Ventilation/Perfusion Scan

In IPAH, the ventilation/perfusion scan is usually normal or shows heterogeneous perfusion.[3] Occasionally, larger mismatch perfusion defects may be seen in IPAH, thought to be as a result of thrombosis in situ.

Computed Tomography

The key features of IPAH on computed tomography (CT) are as follows:

1. Enlargement of the main pulmonary artery (Fig. 24–2). In one study, a main pulmonary artery diameter of ≥29 mm had a positive predictive value of >95% for PAH.[4]

2. Right ventricular dilatation and hypertrophy and enlargement of the right atrium (Fig. 24–3). Flattening or "bowing" of the interventricular septum can also be observed.

3. Reflux of contrast from the right atrium into the inferior vena cava when CT pulmonary angiogram is performed. This occurs as a result of tricuspid regurgitation, and the extent of reflux correlates with mean PAP; however, it can be observed in normal patients.[5]

4. The presence of pericardial effusions.

5. Small centrilobular ground-glass nodules.

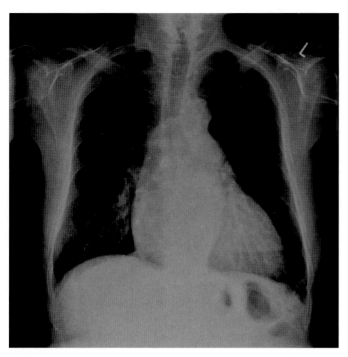

FIGURE 24–1. Chest radiograph of a patient with idiopathic pulmonary arterial hypertension. Cardiomegaly, prominent pulmonary arteries, and peripheral oligemia are present.

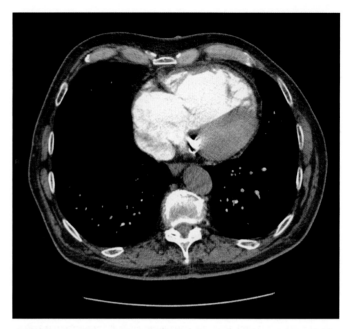

FIGURE 24–3. Computed tomography pulmonary angiogram in a patient with idiopathic pulmonary arterial hypertension demonstrating dilatation of the right ventricle and right atrium and right ventricular hypertrophy.

Electrocardiogram

The electrocardiogram (ECG) may demonstrate right ventricular hypertrophy and strain and right atrial dilatation in IPAH.

Pulmonary Function Tests

Pulmonary function tests in IPAH often reveal normal spirometry but reduced diffusion capacity for carbon monoxide.

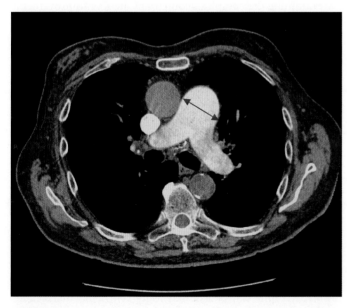

FIGURE 24–2. Computed tomography pulmonary angiogram demonstrating enlargement of the main pulmonary artery (arrow) in a patient with idiopathic pulmonary arterial hypertension.

Echocardiography

The use of echocardiography in the assessment of IPAH focuses on detection of elevated PAP, evaluation of the right ventricle, and exclusion of other possible differential diagnoses.

In IPAH, chronic progressive pressure loading results in right ventricular (RV) remodeling, particularly RV hypertrophy and later RV dilatation. RV dilatation can result in tricuspid annular dilatation, often causing significant tricuspid regurgitation. As IPAH progresses, there is impaired RV diastolic function and increased RV end-diastolic pressure, with displacement or "bowing" of the interventricular septum toward the left ventricle.

PAH can be suggested by abnormalities on a number of echocardiographic views:

1. Parasternal long axis view: The RV will appear dilated (Fig. 24–4), and in severe cases, there is compression of the left ventricular cavity with "bowing" of the interventricular septum.

2. Short axis view: The RV is again dilated, with the characteristic D-shaped left ventricle visible (Fig. 24–5).

3. Apical four-chamber view: There is dilatation and hypertrophy of the RV and often hypertrophy of the moderator band (Fig. 24–6). Tricuspid regurgitation jets will be visible in the majority of patients with pulmonary hypertension, and application of continuous wave Doppler mapping on this jet allows calculation of the tricuspid regurgitation velocity (Fig. 24–7). This velocity represents the RV to right atrial pressure difference and can be used to estimate pulmonary artery systolic pressure (PASP) through the Bernoulli equation: PASP = RV systolic pressure = $4 (V_{TR})^2$ + RAP, where

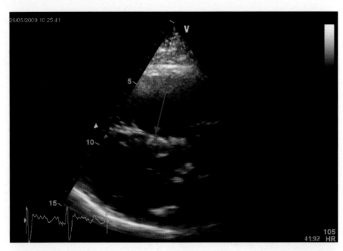

FIGURE 24–4. Echocardiogram. Parasternal long-axis view of a patient with idiopathic pulmonary arterial hypertension demonstrating right ventricular (RV) dilatation (arrow), with RV diameter of 5 cm.

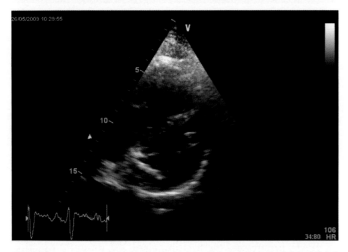

FIGURE 24–5. Echocardiogram. Short axis view of same patient with idiopathic pulmonary arterial hypertension as seen in Fig. 24–4. There is right ventricular dilatation and D-shaping of the left ventricle

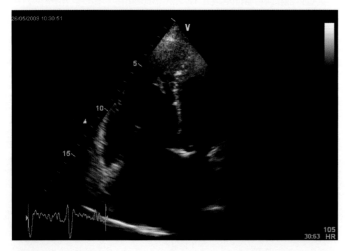

FIGURE 24–6. Echocardiogram. Apical chamber view of patient with idiopathic pulmonary arterial hypertension seen in Figs. 24–4 and 24–5. There is marked dilatation of the right-sided cardiac chambers, with interventricular septal bowing.

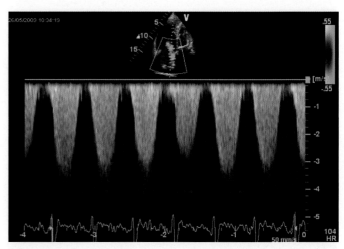

FIGURE 24–7. Application of continuous wave Doppler mapping to the tricuspid regurgitant jet observed in Fig. 24–6. The tricuspid regurgitation velocity is approximately 4 m/s, giving a pulmonary artery systolic pressure of 64 mm Hg + right atrial pressure.

V_{TR} is tricuspid regurgitant velocity and RAP is right atrial pressure.

4. Tricuspid annular plane systolic excursion (TAPSE): TAPSE represents the basal to apical shortening of the RV during systole. TAPSE will be reduced when there is impaired RV systolic function, and a TAPSE of less than 1.5 cm is associated with poor prognosis in PAH.[6]

5. A pericardial effusion may be visible on a number of views, and the size of the effusion has prognostic importance in IPAH.

Cardiac Magnetic Resonance Imaging

Cardiac magnetic resonance (CMR) imaging is ideally suited for examining the complex geometry of the RV. Improvements in CMR technology have reduced the length of breath-holds required to obtain high-quality images, particularly important in patients with IPAH who are often dyspneic on minimal exertion.[7]

A diagnosis of IPAH is supported the following CMR abnormalities:

• Increased RV end-diastolic volume (RVEDV)

• Reduced RV ejection fraction, stroke volume, and cardiac output

• Poor left ventricular filling, observed as a low left ventricular end-diastolic volume (LVEDV)

• Bowing of the interventricular septum toward the left ventricle (Fig. 24–8)

• RV hypertrophy, occurring as a result of the increased pulmonary afterload (Fig. 24–9)

RV hypertrophy can be assessed using ventricular mass index (VMI), which is the ratio of RV mass to LV mass. VMI has been shown to correlate closely with mean PAP obtained at right heart catheterization.[8] Studies have also shown that an increased

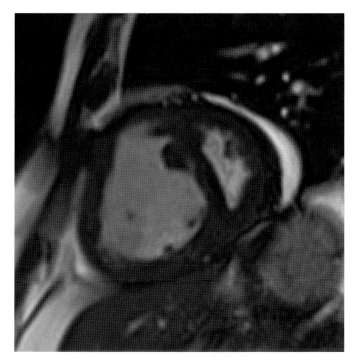

FIGURE 24–8. Cardiac magnetic resonance imaging. Short axis view of a patient with idiopathic pulmonary arterial hypertension demonstrating a dilated, hypertrophied right ventricle; marked interventricular septal bowing; and a pericardial effusion.

RVEDV, poor left ventricular filling, and low stroke volume are associated with poor prognosis in IPAH.[9]

Velocity-encoded CMR imaging is another approach for assessing the patient with suspected IPAH. This technique allows us to quantify blood flow within the main pulmonary artery and calculate peak and average pulmonary artery flow velocities and

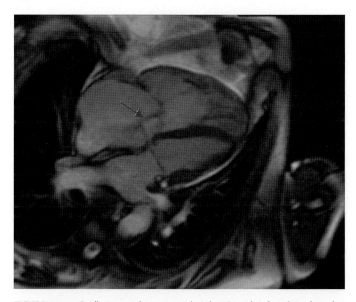

FIGURE 24–9. Cardiac magnetic resonance imaging. Four-chamber view of another patient with idiopathic pulmonary arterial hypertension. There is gross dilatation of the right atrium and right ventricle, increased right ventricular trabeculation, and a visible tricuspid regurgitant jet (arrow).

provides an alternative method for estimating stroke volume and cardiac output. Pulmonary artery distensibility can also be measured by CMR and has been found to be significantly lower in PAH patients compared with normal subjects.[10]

Right Heart Catheterization

Right heart catheterization remains the gold standard for the diagnosis of IPAH. Patients typically have a markedly elevated mean PAP, usually ≥50 mm Hg (normal, <25 mm Hg). A low cardiac output and high pulmonary vascular resistance (PVR) indicate severe disease and poorer prognosis. If PAP is high, then vasoreactivity testing in an expert center should be done because a successful response mandates different therapy.

■ MANAGEMENT

There is as yet no cure for IPAH, so management is usually divided into general measures, disease-targeted therapy, and surgical intervention.[11,12]

General Measures

- **Oxygen:** Acute oxygen therapy can improve pulmonary hemodynamics in hypoxic and normoxic patients. Patients with resting partial pressure of oxygen in arterial blood (PaO_2) of <8 kPa may be prescribed oxygen for at least 15 h/d.

- **Anticoagulation:** IPAH is associated with abnormalities in coagulation and fibrinolytic pathways and impaired platelet function. Anticoagulation may prevent vascular thrombotic lesions and pulmonary embolism.[13,14]

- **Diuretics:** In IPAH, there is excessive afterload, resulting in RV dilatation and right heart failure. Diuretic therapy, often at high doses, may benefit patients with significant fluid overload.

- **Arrhythmia management:** Tachyarrhythmias are poorly tolerated and often manifest with worsening dyspnea, syncope, or right heart failure.[15,16] The use of β-blockers is contraindicated in IPAH because it limits the ability to raise cardiac output by tachycardia.

Disease-Targeted Therapy

In the last 10 to 15 years, a number of new disease-targeted therapies for PAH have been developed. These treatments are expensive and have significant adverse effects; however, they have been shown to improve symptoms and exercise capacity in IPAH, and some have been shown to improve survival.

The main classes of disease-targeted therapy for IPAH are as follows:

- **Prostanoids:** Prostanoids are analogs of prostacyclin and are available in intravenous (epoprostenol), nebulized (iloprost), and subcutaneous (treprostinil) forms. They are the treatment of choice for patients with severe (class IV) disease, and epoprostenol has been shown to improve survival in IPAH.[17,18]

- **Phosphodiesterase-5 (PDE-5) inhibitors:** PDE-5 inhibitors are oral agents that act by inhibiting the breakdown of cyclic guanosine monophosphate, thereby increasing the effect of locally produced nitric oxide. This results in inhibition of smooth muscle growth and pulmonary vasodilation. Sildenafil is the most widely used PDE-5 inhibitor at present.[19]

- **Endothelin antagonists:** Increased circulating levels of endothelin-1, a potent vasoconstrictor are observed in IPAH. Several oral agents are now available that can modify the endothelin system.[20,21] Bosentan is a nonspecific endothelin antagonist, whereas ambrisentan and sitaxsentan are specific endothelin-A receptor blockers. Approximately 10% of patients on bosentan will have an elevation in hepatic transaminases, although the incidence is lower with the other endothelin antagonists.

It is now common practice to use combination therapy for patients with IPAH who have deteriorated despite targeted monotherapy. The rationale is that using multiple agents will be more effective in targeting the different pathophysiologic pathways that have been identified in IPAH. Approximately 30% of patients with IPAH are receiving combination therapy at present.

Surgical Intervention

Atrial septostomy is thought to be of benefit in patients with IPAH who are in World Health Organization (WHO) functional class IV with right heart failure refractory to medical therapy.[22] Atrial septostomy can decompress the RV, increase left ventricular preload, and increase cardiac output, particularly during exercise. This improves systemic oxygen transport despite the arterial oxygen desaturation.

Despite the development of disease-targeted therapy, there are still a significant number of patients who deteriorate on medical treatment, and these patients should be referred for transplantation.[23] In the United Kingdom, current practice is for patients with IPAH requiring transplantation to receive bilateral lung transplantations. Recent changes in surgical technique, perioperative care, and immunosuppression have significantly improved outcome following transplantation, with survival rates of 86% at 1 year, 75% at 5 years, and 66% at 10 years now described in patients who undergo transplantation for IPAH.[24]

Follow-Up

Imaging modalities, particularly echocardiography and cardiac magnetic resonance imaging (MRI), are becoming increasingly important in the follow-up of patients with IPAH, both in the setting of clinical trials and everyday clinical practice. Physicians have previously been reliant on WHO functional class, 6-minute walk test, biologic markers (such as N-terminal prohormone brain natriuretic peptide), and right heart catheterization to monitor response to treatment, all of which have acknowledged limitations.

Echocardiography is an attractive follow-up modality given that it is widely available, inexpensive, and safe. However, it is relatively operator dependent, and images may be suboptimal in patients with tachycardia, obesity, or poor acoustic windows. Cardiac MRI is now gaining widespread acceptance as the ideal marker in IPAH, providing abundant information regarding RV morphology and function in a safe, reproducible manner (Fig. 24–10). Extensive investigations are now under way to determine whether changes in CMR-derived RV functional parameters correspond to patient outcome.

■ CASE STUDY

A 33-year-old woman presented with an 18-month history of progressively worsening exertional dyspnea.

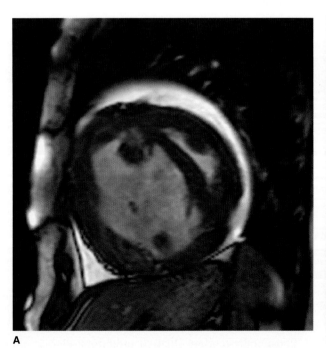
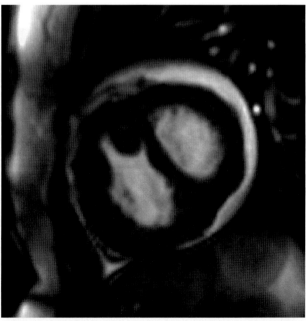

A   **B**

FIGURE 24–10. Short axis views of a patient with idiopathic pulmonary arterial hypertension at the time of diagnosis (**A**) and after 12 months of epoprostenol and sildenafil (**B**). Note the reduction in right ventricular dilatation, improved left ventricular filling, and resolution of the interventricular septal bowing.

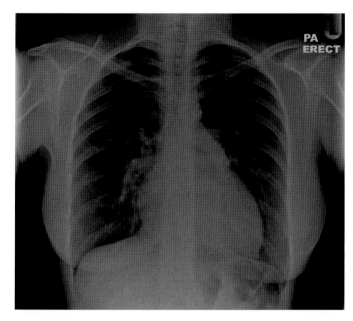

FIGURE 24–11. Chest radiograph of 33-year-old woman with worsening exertional dyspnea. Note the cardiomegaly and prominent central pulmonary arteries but rapid tapering of these vessels.

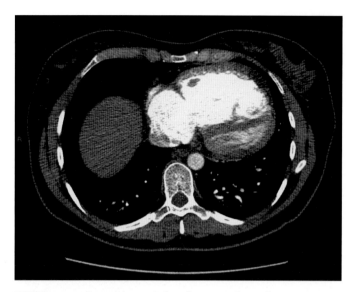

FIGURE 24–13. Computed tomography pulmonary angiogram in a young woman suspected of having idiopathic pulmonary arterial hypertension. The right atrium and right ventricle are grossly dilated.

Clinical examination revealed a loud second heart sound and a tricuspid regurgitation murmur. ECG demonstrated right axis deviation and RV hypertrophy. Chest radiograph revealed cardiomegaly, prominent pulmonary arteries, and peripheral oligemia (Fig. 24–11).

Her echocardiogram showed marked dilatation of the right-sided cardiac chambers and tricuspid regurgitation (Fig. 24–12). Her estimated PASP was 85 mm Hg. CT pulmonary angiogram revealed no evidence of pulmonary thromboembolic disease, but there was an enlarged main pulmonary artery and a dilated right heart (Fig. 24–13). Cardiac MRI demonstrated interventricular septal bowing and RV dilation, and planimetric evaluation revealed a markedly increased RVEDV, low LVEDV, and low stroke volume (Fig. 24–14).

She proceeded to right heart catheterization, where her mean PAP was elevated at 50 mm Hg, PVR was elevated at 12 Wood units, and cardiac output was low at 3.0 L/min. No other cause of PAH could be identified, so she was diagnosed as having IPAH. The patient was commenced on anticoagulation and the endothelin antagonist bosentan.

After 12 months of disease-targeted therapy, she had noticed a reduction in dyspnea, her 6-minute walk test had improved, and

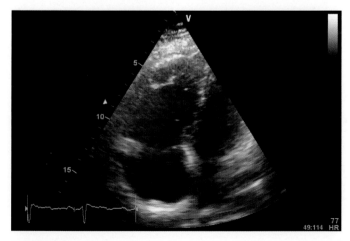

FIGURE 24–12. Apical four-chamber view of 33-year-old woman showing marked right ventricular and right atrial dilatation.

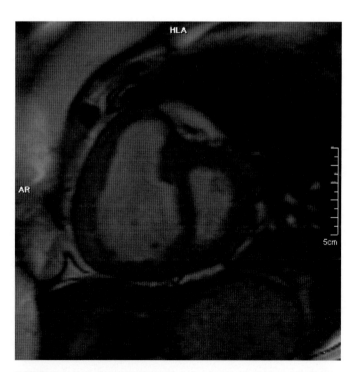

FIGURE 24–14. Cardiac magnetic resonance imaging. Short axis view of the 33-year-old woman with exertional dyspnea. There is right ventricular dilatation and hypertrophy and interventricular septal bowing.

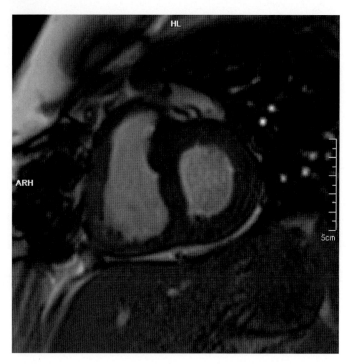

FIGURE 24–15. Cardiac magnetic resonance imaging. Short axis view performed after 12 months of bosentan therapy for idiopathic pulmonary arterial hypertension. Note the reduction in right ventricular dilatation and resolution of the interventricular septal bowing.

repeat cardiac MRI demonstrated an improvement in stroke volume and cardiac output, with a reduction in RV dilatation (Fig. 24–15).

CHRONIC THROMBOEMBOLIC PULMONARY HYPERTENSION

■ BACKGROUND

Chronic thromboembolic pulmonary hypertension (CTEPH) results from an obstruction of the pulmonary vessels with organized blood clots. It is estimated that 3.8% of patients suffering an acute pulmonary embolus will develop CTEPH.[25] However, a significant proportion of CTEPH cases may originate from asymptomatic venous thromboembolism.[26].

Patients at greatest risk include those with previous episodes of venous thromboembolism, massive and submassive pulmonary embolism, an elevated PASP on admission, or elevated pressure 2 months after initial presentation. Additional risk factors for CTEPH include the presence of ventriculoatrial shunts for the treatment of hydrocephalus, low-grade malignancy, splenectomy, chronic osteomyelitis, inflammatory bowel disease, and thyroid replacement therapy.[27,28]

The pathophysiology of CTEPH is related to increased resistance to flow through the pulmonary arteries, initially from obstruction of pulmonary arteries (usually main to subsegmental levels) by organized thromboembolic material and subsequently from vascular remodeling in smaller unobstructed vessels.[29] The vascular remodeling arises in response to increased flow and consequent shear stress in the distal unobstructed pulmonary arterial vascular bed.

■ CLINICAL PRESENTATION

The most common symptoms of CTEPH are exertional dyspnea and fatigue, although chest pain, syncope, hemoptysis, and vertigo are also observed. The clinical course is initially episodic, with long "honeymoon periods" of only mild or no symptoms. If CTEPH is left untreated, there is a progressive increase in PVR, RV dysfunction, and death.

The diagnosis of CTEPH is made based on radiologic investigations performed during the assessment of pulmonary hypertension.

■ IMAGING

Chest Radiograph

The characteristic findings on chest radiograph in CTEPH are enlargement of the RV and prominence of the central pulmonary arteries. If thrombosis or embolism occurs in the central pulmonary arteries, then asymmetrical and/or bulging vessels may be present. Another feature of CTEPH is decreased vascularity termed *mosaic oligemia*.[30] These areas of decreased vascularity on plain radiographs can be confirmed on pulmonary angiography to be associated with chronic emboli (Fig. 24–16). "Peripheral pruning" or discordance in caliber between central and peripheral pulmonary arteries is a distinct feature of PAH regardless of the underlying etiology and thus will often be visible in CTEPH.

Ventilation/Perfusion Scan

The role of ventilation/perfusion scintigraphy is to distinguish IPAH from CTEPH. With CTEPH, the ventilation/perfusion scan is usually high probability, showing multiple mismatch

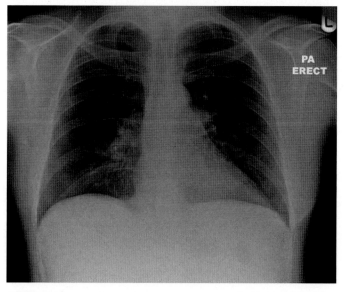

FIGURE 24–16. Plain chest radiograph in chronic thromboembolic pulmonary hypertension demonstrating prominent pulmonary arteries and peripheral pruning.

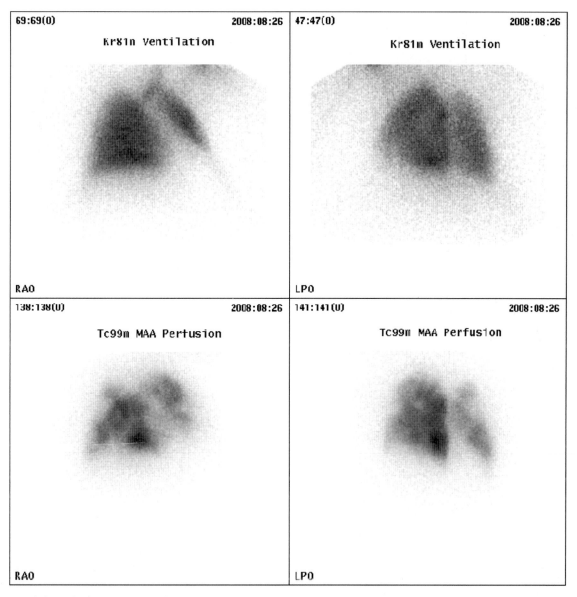

| 69:69(0) | 2008:08:26 | 47:47(0) | 2008:08:26 |

FIGURE 24–17. Ventilation/perfusion scan in patient with chronic thromboembolic pulmonary hypertension showing multiple mismatched perfusion defects. Kr81m, krypton-18m; MAA, macroaggregated albumin; Tc99m, technetium-99m.

segmental or larger perfusion defects (Fig. 24–17). A normal or low probability scan effectively excludes CTEPH.[31,32] In patients who have intermediate- or high-probability scans, the diagnosis of CTEPH can usually be confirmed by CT pulmonary angiography (CTPA).

Although ventilation/perfusion scintigraphy is a safe and highly sensitive test for suspected CTEPH, large mismatch perfusion defects may arise in other processes that result in obliteration of the central arteries and veins. These "CTEPH mimics" include large-vessel vasculitis, pulmonary artery sarcoma, extrinsic compression due to cancer, lymphadenopathy, fibrosing mediastinitis, and pulmonary veno-occlusive disease.[33]

Computed Tomography

The hallmark of CTEPH on CTPA is the absence or sudden loss of contrast-filled vessels. Abnormalities in the main pulmonary

artery may be highly suggestive of CTEPH, with the most common finding being the eccentric location of thrombus, resulting in a crescentic filling defect adjacent to the vessel wall[34] (Fig. 24–18). Other vascular signs of CTEPH that are visible on CT are recanalization within intraluminal fillings and arterial webs (Fig. 24–19) and stenoses.

Bronchial artery hypertrophy occurs in approximately half of patients with CTEPH and only rarely in IPAH.[35] It occurs most commonly in chronic inflammatory diseases of the airways and when there is chronic pulmonary hypoperfusion, when the bronchial arteries act as a collateral blood supply to the pulmonary parenchyma. Bronchial artery hypertrophy is defined as curvilinear mediastinal vessels >1.5 mm in diameter, seen along the course of the proximal bronchial tree and is best identified on coronal reformatted projections (Fig. 24–20). In CTEPH, the distal circulation may be morphologically normal and therefore

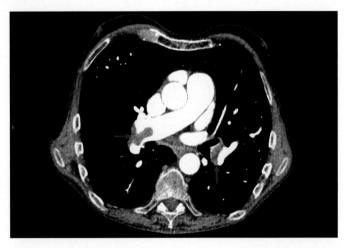

FIGURE 24–18. Computed tomography pulmonary angiogram demonstrating bilateral filling defects due to laminated thrombus in the right and left pulmonary arteries (arrows).

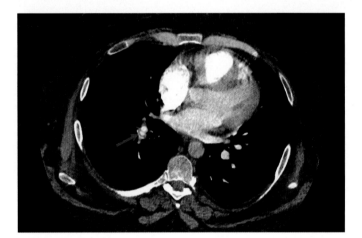

FIGURE 24–19. Computed tomography pulmonary angiogram demonstrating an arterial web in the right middle lobe pulmonary artery (arrow).

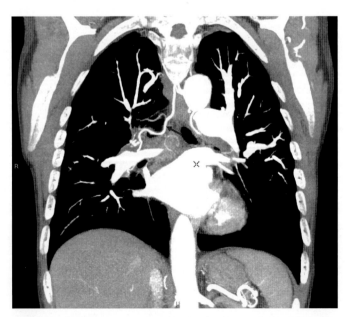

FIGURE 24–20. Computed tomography pulmonary angiogram with coronal reformatted projection showing bronchial artery hypertrophy (arrow) in a patient with chronic thromboembolic pulmonary hypertension.

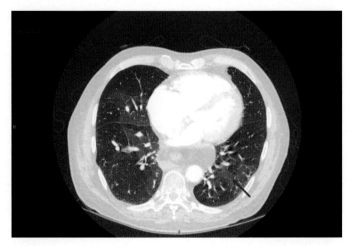

FIGURE 24–21. High-resolution computed tomography scan of chest showing subtle areas of mosaic oligemia (arrows) in a patient with chronic thromboembolic pulmonary hypertension.

able to accommodate this increased collateral supply, whereas in IPAH, the plexogenic arteriopathy is centered at arteriolar level.

In CTEPH, there is mosaic oligemia visible on high-resolution scanning, caused by obliteration of parts of the vascular bed (Fig. 24–21). This results in hypoperfusion with arteries of diminished size in some areas and with normal or increased perfusion and enlarged arteries in other areas.

Peripheral lung parenchymal opacities are another common finding in CTEPH[36,37] (Fig. 24–22). They represent pulmonary infarcts due to occlusion of segmental and smaller pulmonary arteries and therefore occur more commonly in "peripheral-type" CTEPH than "central-type."

Pulmonary Angiography

At present, pulmonary angiography remains the definitive investigation for the diagnosis and assessment of surgically correctable CTEPH. The typical findings include vascular cut-offs representing complete occlusion of the vessel (Fig. 24–23) and vascular

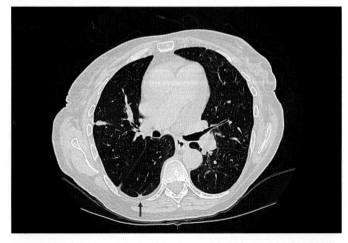

FIGURE 24–22. High-resolution computed tomography showing multiple peripheral lung opacities (arrows) in a patient with distal chronic thromboembolic pulmonary hypertension.

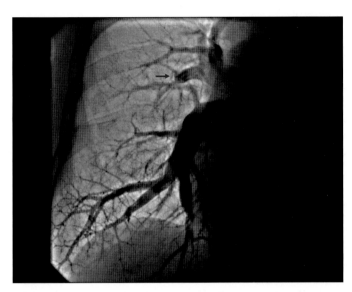

FIGURE 24-23. Conventional pulmonary angiogram in a patient with chronic thromboembolic pulmonary hypertension demonstrating abrupt cut-off of the right middle lobe pulmonary artery (arrow) and a paucity of vessels in the right mid zone.

webs that result from organization of thromboembolic material in the vessel lumen with subsequent scar formation. Smaller pulmonary arteries can appear tortuous and taper rapidly, particularly in patients with distal inoperable CTEPH (Fig. 24–24).

Other Investigations

The ECG and echocardiographic abnormalities observed in CTEPH are similar to those seen in IPAH, which have been discussed earlier in this chapter.

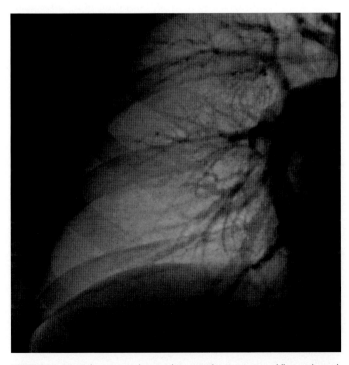

FIGURE 24-24. Pulmonary angiogram demonstrating tortuous, rapidly tapering pulmonary arteries and a generalized paucity of vessels in the right lower zone of a patient with distal inoperable chronic thromboembolic pulmonary hypertension.

Magnetic resonance angiography (MRA) does not require exposure to radiation or nephrotoxic contrast agents and is becoming increasingly important in the diagnosis, assessment, and long-term follow-up of patients with CTEPH. In experienced centers, images produced with MRA are comparable to those acquired using conventional pulmonary angiography.

All patients with suspected CTEPH should undergo right heart catheterization to confirm the presence of pulmonary hypertension (mean PAP >25 mm Hg), to measure cardiac output (usually by thermodilution technique), and to calculate PVR. Right heart catheterization and pulmonary angiography are often performed as a single procedure.

■ MANAGEMENT

Surgical Intervention

It is widely recognized that the definitive treatment for CTEPH is pulmonary endarterectomy (PEA). It is the only proven treatment to give prognostic and symptomatic benefit. PEA is performed on cardiopulmonary bypass via a median sternotomy and involves the removal of organized and incorporated fibrous obstructive tissues from the pulmonary arteries. Completion of the endarterectomy procedure is usually possible within a 20-minute period of circulatory arrest for each lung.

PEA is a major undertaking, often performed in patients with significant RV dysfunction, and should only be carried out at a specialized center by a PEA-experienced surgeon. The decision as to whether PEA is feasible will depend on the abnormalities seen on CT and conventional angiography, on the hemodynamics observed at right heart catheterization, and on whether the patient has other significant comorbidities. Patients with proximal disease have a much better risk-to-benefit ratio from surgery than patients with more distal disease. Patients with a PVR >1200 dyne/s/cm have a higher risk of mortality with attempted PEA.[38,39] In patients with a PVR disproportionately higher than the segmental obstruction visible by imaging, there is less benefit from PEA and a much higher risk of mortality. There are very few absolute contraindications to surgery, and good results have even been achieved in patients over age 80 years.

Despite the complexity of the procedure, PEA is associated with mortality rates of only 5% to 10%.[37] Severe preoperative RV dysfunction and residual postoperative pulmonary hypertension are both associated with poor outcome after PEA. In many cases, RV and pulmonary hemodynamics will return to normal within hours of the procedure. Following a successful PEA, the occurrence of reperfusion lung injury is common, with up to a third of patients requiring prolonged ventilatory support, and is a key factor in determining perioperative morbidity and mortality.[40] Shorter cardiac arrest periods, the use of cooling jackets to the head, and antegrade cerebral perfusion techniques have reduced the occurrence of cerebral injury associated with PEA.

Medical Therapies

All patients with CTEPH should receive lifelong anticoagulation with warfarin in the therapeutic international normalized ratio range between 2 and 3. It is common practice to insert an inferior vena cava filter in patients with CTEPH undergoing PEA surgery to reduce the risk of thromboembolism in the early postoperative period until full anticoagulation is reestablished.

The natural history of untreated CTEPH is dismal; <20% of patients survive for 2 years if the mean PAP is >50 mm Hg at the time of presentation.[41] Although PEA is a realistic option for cure, unfortunately, up to 50% of patients are judged inoperable.[42]

In recent years, there has been increasing use of PAH-specific medical therapies in CTEPH. They have been used in a number of settings, including to provide hemodynamic stability prior to surgery, in patients with persisting or recurrent pulmonary hypertension despite PEA, and in patients who have distal inoperable disease.[43-45] Use of the endothelin receptor antagonist bosentan in patients with inoperable CTEPH was associated with improvements in pulmonary hemodynamics, although not all studies report improvements in exercise capacity.[46,47] There are currently ongoing studies examining the potential use of endothelin receptor antagonists, PDE-5 inhibitors, prostanoids, and other novel agents in CTEPH.

CASE STUDY

An overweight 38-year-old woman, with a background of inhaler-controlled asthma, was referred with 18 months of worsening breathlessness. She had no past history of deep vein thrombosis or pulmonary embolism and no significant family history. On examination, she was cyanosed, with resting oxygen saturation of 90%, and had bilateral pitting ankle edema.

Her ECG showed right axis deviation and RV hypertrophy. Chest radiograph demonstrated prominent pulmonary arteries and some peripheral pruning (Fig. 24–25). On echocardiogram,

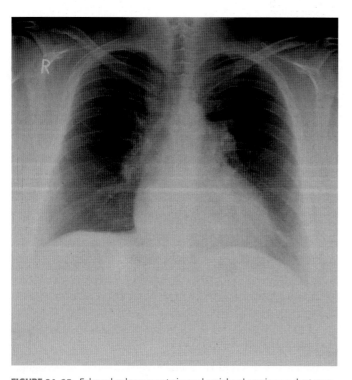

FIGURE 24–25. Enlarged pulmonary arteries and peripheral pruning on chest x-ray.

she had a severely dilated RV with poor systolic function, dyskinetic septal motion, and elevated estimated PASP. The bubble contrast study was negative.

The patient had a high-probability ventilation/perfusion scan, with bilateral mismatched perfusion defects (Fig. 24–26). CTPA demonstrated a dilated main pulmonary artery (Fig. 24–27), dilated right-sided cardiac chambers (Fig. 24–28), multiple filling defects, cut-off of the right interlobar artery, and a paucity of vessels in the right lower lobe. There was also evidence of a left interlobar artery web (Fig. 24–29). CT also showed multiple peripheral lung parenchymal opacities (Fig. 24–30) and mosaic oligemia (Fig. 24–31).

She proceeded to right heart catheterization, which confirmed severe pulmonary hypertension (mean PAP, 58 mm Hg; cardiac index, 1.9 L/min/m²; PVR, 8.7 Wood units). Conventional pulmonary angiography was performed and confirmed the abnormalities identified at CTPA, namely the right-sided cut-off and a paucity of vessels in the lower lobes, particularly on the right (Fig. 24–32). The diagnosis of CTEPH was confirmed.

The patient was then anticoagulated, commenced on the PDE-5 inhibitor sildenafil as disease-targeted therapy to improve pulmonary hemodynamics, and referred to the national PEA center for consideration of PEA.

PULMONARY ARTERIOVENOUS MALFORMATIONS

BACKGROUND

Pulmonary arteriovenous malformations (PAVMs) are abnormal communications between pulmonary arteries and pulmonary veins, resulting in right-to-left shunting and subsequent hypoxemia. The vast majority of PAVMs (at least 80%) occur in the context of hereditary hemorrhagic telangiectasia (HHT), although these are radiologically and histologically indistinguishable from idiopathic PAVMs. When PAVMs occur in the setting of HHT, they are more likely to be multiple and bilateral.[48-50]

CLINICAL PRESENTATION

The most frequent presenting symptom of PAVM is exertional dyspnea,[51] often related to the severity of right-to-left shunting. However, many patients have very little dyspnea and good exercise tolerance due to low PVR, facilitating increased cardiac output on exertion.[52] Other symptoms include hemoptysis and chest pain, whereas clinical examination may reveal cyanosis, finger clubbing, and telangiectasia. Classical orthodeoxia (a reduction in oxygen saturation when rising from the supine position), present in a minority of patients with large PAVM, has limited diagnostic value.

The diagnosis of PAVM may be precipitated by one of the potentially severe infectious or embolic complications of the condition. Right-to-left shunting that bypasses the pulmonary capillary bed allows bacteria and thrombotic emboli into the systemic and often cerebral circulation. Cerebral abscesses occur in approximately 10% of patients with HHT and PAVM[53] and

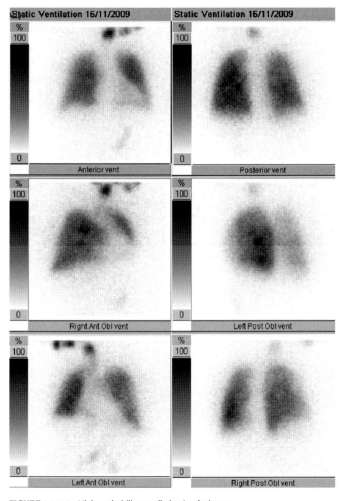

FIGURE 24–26. High probability ventilation/perfusion scan.

are often due to multiple anaerobic organisms. Extracerebral infection can result in abscesses within soft tissue, knee, liver, kidney, and spinal cord, as well as causing endocarditis, meningitis, and septicaemia.[54] These extracerebral infections are

usually due to *Staphylococcus aureus*. As a result of passage of thrombotic emboli into the cerebral circulation, PAVMs are associated with an increased risk of ischemic stroke and transient ischemic attack.[49] Severe hemorrhagic complications can

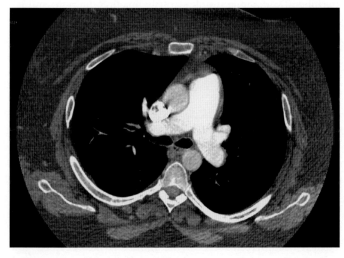

FIGURE 24–27. Dilated main pulmonary artery on computed tomography pulmonary angiogram.

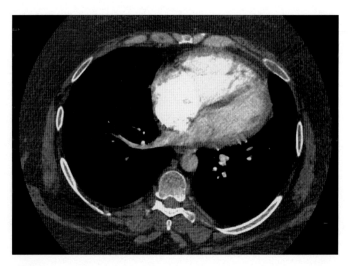

FIGURE 24–28. Dilated right ventricle and right atrium on computed tomography pulmonary angiogram.

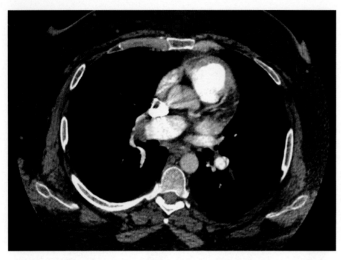

FIGURE 24–29. Right-sided filling defect and left pulmonary artery web (arrow).

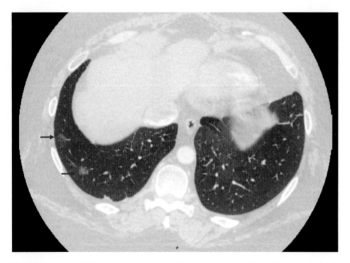

FIGURE 24–30. High-resolution computed tomography of chest showing multiple peripheral pulmonary opacities (arrows).

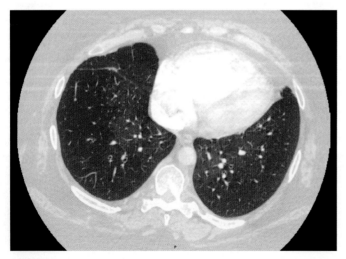

FIGURE 24–31. High-resolution computed tomography of chest demonstrating a subtle area of mosaic oligemia (arrow).

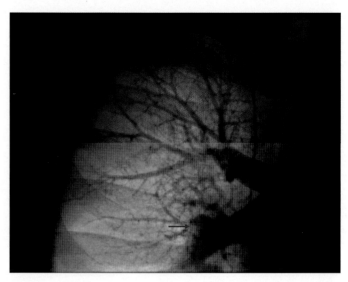

FIGURE 24–32. Right interlobar artery cut-off on conventional pulmonary angiogram (arrow).

also occur, including intrabronchial or intrapleural rupture of PAVM, but thankfully, these are rare.

■ IMAGING

Chest Radiograph

Chest radiograph can detect large PAVM, often visible as a rounded 1- to 5-cm opacity with sharply defined borders and feeding vessels[55] (Fig. 24–33); however, small PAVMs or those located at the costodiaphragmatic angles are not easily identifiable.

Contrast Echocardiography

Transthoracic contrast echocardiography is the screening test of choice, with a sensitivity of greater than 90% for the detection of PAVM in HHT patients.[56] It is performed by injecting 4 to 5 mL of agitated saline solution with 0.5 mL room air into a peripheral vein while simultaneously imaging the right and left atria with two-dimensional echocardiography. This technique allows the right-to-left shunt to be directly visualized and helps distinguish intracardiac shunting (contrast enhancement of left atrium within one to three cardiac cycles) from the intrapulmonary shunting observed in PAVM (delay of four to eight cardiac cycles, or 2 to 5 seconds).

However, it has been noted that contrast echocardiography may be positive in patients with no PAVM visible on chest CT and that contrast echocardiography remains positive after endovascular treatment of PAVM in up to 90% of patients.[57] This may be due to microscopic and diffuse PAVM causing genuine right-to-left shunting or is simply a false-positive test result.

Computed Tomography

Helical multidetector CT of the thorax is the accepted gold standard for the diagnosis of PAVM, identifying a nodular or rounded opacity of variable size, with both afferent and efferent

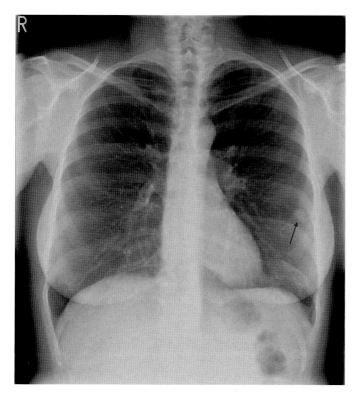

FIGURE 24–33. Chest radiograph demonstrating a 1-cm soft tissue density opacity in the left mid zone (arrow) that was subsequently found to be a pulmonary arteriovenous malformation.

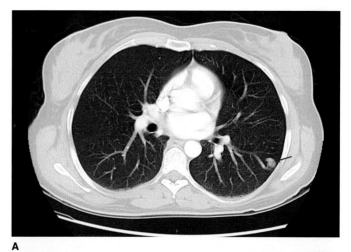

A

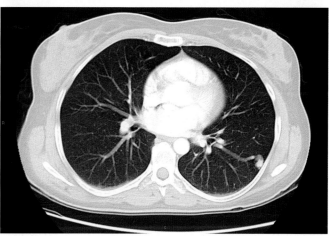

B

FIGURE 24–34. Computed tomography of thorax demonstrating a pulmonary arteriovenous malformation situated peripherally in the apical segment of the left lower lobe (arrow). The feeding artery (**A**) and vein (**B**) are clearly visualized (arrowheads).

vessels[58] (Fig. 24–34). Additional intravenous injection of contrast shows enhancement of the PAVM, allowing differentiation from other nodules. CT of the thorax even allows for identification of thrombosed or very small PAVMs that may be missed using conventional pulmonary angiography and is overall a highly sensitive modality for the diagnosis of PAVM (>95%).[59]

Magnetic Resonance Imaging

A variety of MRI techniques have been studied in the evaluation of PAVM; however, it remains an expensive modality with limited availability and, at present, is not as efficient as CT.

Radionuclide Perfusion Lung Scanning

Radionuclide perfusion lung scanning has been found to be useful in the diagnosis of PAVM. In normal patients without PAVM, intravenous injection of radionuclide-labeled albumin particles results in filtering of these particles by the capillaries of the lung. However, in patients with PAVM, the intrapulmonary shunts allow passage of these large particles through the lungs, with eventual filtering by capillary beds in the other organs such as the brain or kidneys.

Shunt Fraction Measurement

Most patients with clinically significant PAVM have an elevation in the fraction of cardiac output that bypasses the pulmonary capillaries, the shunt fraction. This can be assessed using the 100% oxygen method, which involves measurement of PaO_2

and arterial oxygen saturation after breathing 100% oxygen through a mouthpiece or airtight mask for 15 to 20 minutes (with a deep inspiration every minute). A shunt fraction of more than 5% is considered abnormal.

Despite its high specificity (98%), shunt fraction assessment has inadequate sensitivity (60% to 65%) for diagnosis of PAVM,[56] and it is now mostly used for the quantification of right-to-left shunting rather than as a screening modality.

Screening for Pulmonary Hypertension

Pulmonary hypertension can complicate PAVM in two very distinct forms. The more common form occurs when there is high-output cardiac failure as a result of coexisting systemic AVM, mostly in the liver. In this context, right heart catheterization will show moderately elevated mean PAP and high cardiac output but normal PVR. The rarer form is when PAH occurs with PAVM in HHT. The hemodynamic profile at right heart catheterization shows markedly elevated mean PAP, reduced cardiac output, normal pulmonary artery occlusion pressure, and elevated PVR.

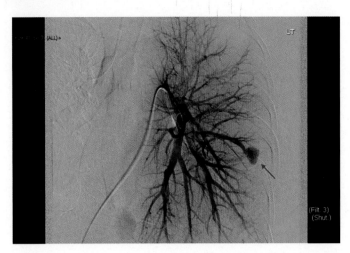

FIGURE 24–35. Pulmonary angiogram demonstrates a moderate arteriovenous malformation (arrow) in the lateral left mid zone with a single feeding arterial vessel.

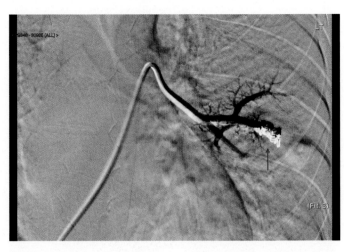

FIGURE 24–36. The lesion in Fig. 24–35 was then successfully embolized with 2 × 4 mm and 2 × 3 mm tightly packed coils (arrow).

Doppler echocardiography is a useful screening tool when assessing patients with PAVM for pulmonary hypertension. Patients with elevated Doppler-derived estimates of PASP should proceed to right heart catheterization.

Pulmonary Angiography

Standard pulmonary angiography is no longer performed as an initial diagnostic procedure, but it is sensitive for the detection of PAVM amenable to embolization and is used to accurately define the architecture of individual lesions (Fig. 24–35). Pulmonary angiography is usually performed on all portions of the lungs at the time of embolotherapy to look for other PAVM, and all lesions are examined for intra- and extrathoracic vascular communications.

■ MANAGEMENT

Untreated PAVMs are associated with significant morbidity and mortality. Most deaths are related to stroke, cerebral abscess, hemoptysis, or hemothorax. The risk of neurologic complications increases with age and with the number of PAVMs. Untreated PAVMs gradually enlarge, usually at approximately 0.3 to 2 mm/y.[60]

Transcatheter embolotherapy is now the current standard treatment for PAVM[61] and is recommended for PAVM when the feeding vessel(s) is (are) ≥3 mm in diameter, even in asymptomatic patients. This procedure involves direct catheter placement of embolic material (usually steel coils) into the feeding artery of the PAVM until blood flow ceases (Fig. 24–36). PAVMs with very large feeding vessels may require specific devices such as Amplatzer occluders or detachable balloons in order to prevent paradoxical embolization of material. Multiple PAVM can be embolized in a single session, although additional sessions may be required if additional PAVMs remain perfused.

The most common complication of embolotherapy is benign self-limited pleuritic chest pain, affecting 5% to 10% of patients.[62] More serious but rare complications include stroke, transient ischemic attack, pulmonary infarction, and systemic migration of the closure device. Infections related to the procedure are prevented by the use of prophylactic antibiotics. Caution is warranted when performing embolotherapy in patients with PAVM and PAH. PAVM effectively unloads the RV, so embolization could theoretically lead to an increase in RV afterload and precipitate right heart failure.[63]

Several long-term series have demonstrated excellent procedural success and long-term efficacy (80%) for occlusion of PAVM.[62,64] Decrease in right-to-left shunting can occur immediately, resulting in improved arterial blood gases and reduced dyspnea. The reperfusion rate for occluded PAVM is reported to be in the range 10% to 17%,[65] so early and long-term follow-up is necessary to identify PAVMs that require repeat embolization. Similarly, many patients will have small detectable residual PAVMs that should be monitored and embolized when significant. Most centers now recommend CT of the thorax as the modality of choice for follow-up of PAVM.

Surgical intervention for PAVM is usually only necessary with lesions that are not technically amenable to embolotherapy or for patients with untreatable allergy to contrast material.

■ CASE STUDY

A 31-year-old man, with a background of recurrent epistaxis and a family history of hereditary hemorrhagic telangiectasia, had a routine preoperative chest radiograph performed. It demonstrated a right mid-zone abnormality (Fig. 24–37). Clinical examination revealed oral telangiectasia. He underwent a CT scan of the chest, which showed a 28 × 20 mm PAVM in the apical segment of the right lower lobe. There was a clearly defined feeding artery and draining vein visible (Fig. 24–38). This was an isolated PAVM, and there was no evidence of hepatic malformations. A subsequent contrast echocardiogram was positive, with late entry of saline contrast into the left heart (Fig. 24–39).

Right heart catheterization was performed to exclude any coexisting pulmonary hypertension, and conventional pulmonary angiography helped confirm the location and anatomy of the abnormality (Fig. 24–40). The PAVM was then

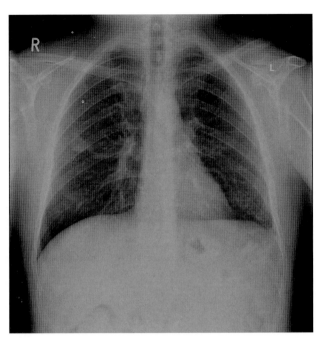

FIGURE 24–37. Chest radiograph demonstrating a 3-cm right mid-zone opacity (arrow), with visible feeding vessel.

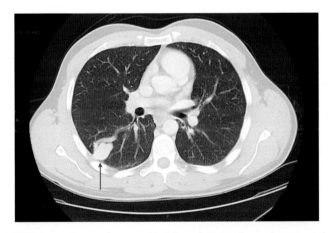

FIGURE 24–38. Computed tomography of thorax demonstrating a pulmonary arteriovenous malformation measuring 28 × 20 mm situated peripherally in the apical segment of the right lower lobe (arrow). A large clearly defined feeding artery can be seen.

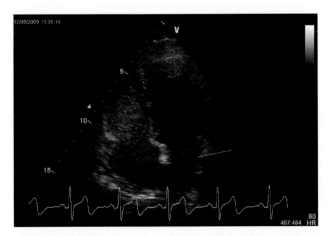

FIGURE 24–39. Transthoracic contrast echocardiogram demonstrating late contrast enhancement of the left atrium.

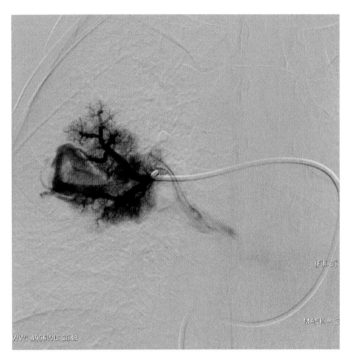

FIGURE 24–40. Pulmonary angiogram demonstrated that the lesion was in fact a complex pulmonary arteriovenous malformation with several small feeding vessels in addition to the single large one.

successfully embolized using multiple coils and an Amplatzer plug (Fig. 24–41). The patient will be followed up at his local pulmonary vascular unit and was also referred for genetic counseling.

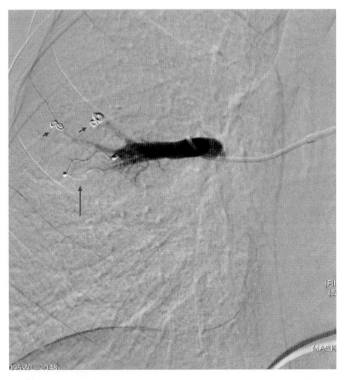

FIGURE 24–41. Embolization of the pulmonary arteriovenous malformation was achieved using multiple coils (arrowheads) and an Amplatzer plug occluder (arrow).

REFERENCES

1. Rich S, Dantzker DR, Ayres SM, et al. Primary pulmonary hypertension. A national prospective study. *Ann Intern Med.* 1987;107:216-223.

2. Gaine SP, Rubin LJ. Primary pulmonary hypertension. *Lancet.* 1998;352:719-725.

3. Worsley DF, Palevski HI, Alavi A. Ventilation-perfusion lung scanning in the evaluation of pulmonary hypertension. *J Nucl Med.* 1994;35:793-796.

4. Tan RT, Kuzo R, Goodman LR, et al. Utility of CT scan evaluation for predicting pulmonary hypertension in patients with parenchymal lung disease. *Chest.* 1998;113:1250-1256.

5. Groves AM, Win T, Charman SC, et al. Semi-quantitative assessment of tricuspid regurgitation on contrast-enhanced multidetector CT. *Clin Radiol.* 2004;59:715-719.

6. Forfia PR, Fisher MR, Mathai SC, et al. Tricuspid annular displacement predicts survival in pulmonary hypertension. *Am J Respir Crit Care Med.* 2006;174:1034-1041.

7. McLure LE, Peacock AJ. Cardiac magnetic resonance imaging for the assessment of the heart and pulmonary circulation in pulmonary hypertension. *Eur Respir J.* 2009;33:1454-1466.

8. Saba TS, Foster J, Cockburn M, et al. Ventricular mass index using magnetic resonance imaging accurately estimates pulmonary artery pressure. *Eur Respir J.* 2002;20:1519-1524.

9. Van Wolferen SA, Marcus JT, Boonstra A, et al. Prognostic value of right ventricular mass, volume, and function in idiopathic pulmonary arterial hypertension. *Eur Heart J.* 2007;28:1250-1257.

10. Bogren HG, Klipstein RH, Mohiaddin RH, et al. Pulmonary artery distensibility and blood flow patterns: a magnetic resonance study of normal subjects and of patients with pulmonary arterial hypertension. *Am Heart J.* 1989;118:990-999.

11. National Pulmonary Hypertension Centers of the UK and Ireland. Consensus statement on the management of pulmonary hypertension in clinical practice in the UK and Ireland. *Thorax.* 2008;63(Suppl II):ii1-ii41.

12. The Task Force for the Diagnosis and Treatment of Pulmonary Hypertension of the European Society of Cardiology (ESC) and European Respiratory Society (ERS). Guidelines for the diagnosis and treatment of pulmonary hypertension. *Eur Heart J.* 2009;30:2493-2537.

13. Fuster V, Steele PM, Edwards WD, et al. Primary pulmonary hypertension: natural history and the importance of thrombosis. *Circulation.* 1984;70:580-587.

14. Herve P, Humbert M, Sitbon O, et al. Pathobiology of pulmonary hypertension: the role of platelets and thrombosis. *Clin Chest Med.* 2001;22:451-458.

15. Tongers J, Schwerdtfeger B, Klein G, et al. Incidence and clinical relevance of supraventricular tachyarrhythmias in pulmonary hypertension. *Am Heart J.* 2007;153:127-132.

16. Rich S, Seidlitz M, Dodin E, et al. The short-term effects of digoxin in patients with right ventricular dysfunction from pulmonary hypertension. *Chest.* 1998;114:787-792.

17. Barst RJ, Rubin LJ, Long WA, et al. A comparison of continuous intravenous epoprostenol (prostacyclin) with conventional therapy for primary pulmonary hypertension. The Primary Pulmonary Hypertension Study Group. *N Engl J Med.* 1996;334:296-302.

18. McLaughlin VV, Shillington A, Rich S. Survival in primary pulmonary hypertension: the impact of epoprostenol therapy. *Circulation.* 2002;106:1477-1482.

19. Galie N, Ghofrani HA, Torbicki A, et al. The Sildenafil Use in Pulmonary Arterial Hypertension (SUPER) Study Group. Sildenafil citrate therapy for pulmonary arterial hypertension. *N Engl J Med.* 2005;353:2148-2157.

20. Rubin LJ, Badesch DB, Barst RJ, et al. Bosentan therapy for pulmonary arterial hypertension. *N Engl J Med.* 2002;346:896-903.

21. Galie N, Olschewski H, Oudiz RJ, et al. Ambrisentan for the treatment of pulmonary arterial hypertension. Results of the ambrisentan in pulmonary arterial hypertension, randomized, double-blind, placebo-controlled, multicenter, efficacy (ARIES) study 1 and 2. *Circulation.* 2008;117:3010-3019.

22. Kurzyna M, Dabrowski D, Bielecki D, et al. Atrial septostomy in treatment of end-stage right heart failure in patients with pulmonary hypertension. *Chest.* 2007;131:977-983.

23. Orens JB, Estenne M, Arcasoy S, et al. International guidelines for the selection of lung transplant candidates: 2006 update—a consensus report from the Pulmonary Scientific Council of the International Society for Heart and Lung Transplantation. *J Heart Lung Transplant.* 2006;25:745-755.

24. Trulock EP, Edwards LB, Taylor DO, et al. Registry of the International Society for Heart and Lung Transplantation: twenty third official adult lung and heart lung transplantation report–2006. *J Heart Lung Transplant.* 2006;25:880-892.

25. Pengo V, Lensing W, Prins MH, et al. Incidence of chronic thromboembolic pulmonary hypertension after pulmonary embolism. *N Eng J Med.* 2004;350:2257-2264.

26. Dartevelle P, Fadel E, Mussot S, et al. Chronic thromboembolic pulmonary hypertension. *Eur Respir J.* 2004;23:637-648.

27. Bonderman D, Skoro-Sajer N, Jakowitsch J, et al. Predictors of outcome in chronic thromboembolic pulmonary hypertension. *Circulation.* 2007;115:2153-2158.

28. Bonderman D, Jakowitsch J, Adlbrecht C, et al. Medical conditions increasing the risk of chronic thromboembolic pulmonary hypertension. *Thromb Haemost.* 2005;93:512-516.

29. Moser KM, Bloor CM. Pulmonary vascular lesions occurring in patients with chronic major vessel thromboembolic pulmonary hypertension. *Chest.* 1993;103:685-692.

30. Woodruff WW, Hoeck BE, Chitwood WR, et al. Radiographic findings in pulmonary hypertension from unresolved embolism. *AJR Am J Roentgenol.* 1985;144:681-686.

31. Tunariu N, Gibbs SJ, Win Z, et al. Ventilation-perfusion scintigraphy is more sensitive than multidetector CTPA in detecting chronic thromboembolic pulmonary disease as a treatable cause of pulmonary hypertension. *J Nucl Med.* 2007;48:680-684.

32. Hoeper MM, Mayer E, Simonneau G, et al. Chronic thromboembolic pulmonary hypertension. *Circulation.* 2006;113:2011-2020.

33. Widera E. Pulmonary artery sarcoma misdiagnosed as chronic thromboembolic pulmonary hypertension. *Mt Sinai J Med.* 2005;72:360-364.

34. Roberts HC, Kauczor HU, Schweden F, et al. Spiral CT of pulmonary hypertension and chronic thromboembolism. *J Thorac Imaging.* 1997;12:118-127.

35. Shimizu H, Tanabe N, Terada J, et al. Dilatation of bronchial arteries correlates with extent of central disease in patients with chronic thromboembolic pulmonary hypertension. *Circ J.* 2008;72:1136-1141.

36. Heinrich M, Uder M, Tscholl D, et al. CT findings in chronic thromboembolic pulmonary hypertension: predictors of haemodynamic improvement after pulmonary thromboendarterectomy. *Chest.* 2005;127:1606-1613.

37. Jamieson SW, Kapelanski DP, Sakakibara N, et al. Pulmonary endarterectomy: experience and lessons learned in 1500 cases. *Ann Thorac Surg.* 2003;76:1457-1462.

38. Thistlethwaite PA, Mo M, Madani MM, et al. Operative classification of thromboembolic disease determines outcome after pulmonary endarterectomy. *J Thorac Cardiovasc Surg.* 2002;124:1203-1211.

39. Kim NH, Fesler P, Channick RN, et al. Preoperative partitioning of pulmonary vascular resistance correlates with early outcome after thromboendarterectomy for chronic thromboembolic pulmonary hypertension. *Circulation.* 2004;109:18-22.

40. Auger WR, Kim KM, Kim HN, et al. Chronic thromboembolic pulmonary hypertension. *Circulation.* 2006;22:453-466.

41. Riedel M, Stanek V, Widimsky J, et al. Long-term follow-up of patients with pulmonary thromboembolism. Late prognosis and evolution of haemodynamic and respiratory data. *Chest.* 1982;81:151-158.

42. Lang IM, Klepetko W. Chronic thromboembolic pulmonary hypertension: an updated review. *Curr Opin Cardiol.* 2008;23:555-559.

43. Kerr KM, Rubin LJ. Epoprostenol therapy as a bridge to pulmonary thromboendarterectomy for chronic thromboembolic pulmonary hypertension. *Chest.* 2003;123:319-320.

44. Condliffe R, Kiely DG, Gibbs JS, et al. Improved outcomes in medically and surgically treated chronic thromboembolic pulmonary hypertension. *Am J Respir Crit Care Med.* 2008;177:1122-1127.

45. Ghofrani HA, Schermuly RT, Rose F, et al. Sildenafil for long-term treatment of nonoperable chronic thromboembolic pulmonary hypertension. *Am J Respir Crit Care Med.* 2003;167:1139-1141.

46. Hoeper MM, Kramm T, Wilkens H, et al. Bosentan therapy for inoperable chronic thromboembolic pulmonary hypertension. *Chest.* 2005;128: 2363-2367.

47. Hughes R, George P, Parameswar J, et al. Bosentan improves inoperable chronic thromboembolic pulmonary hypertension. *Eur Respir J.* 2006;28:138-143.

48. Cottin V, Chinet T, Lavole A, et al. Pulmonary arteriovenous malformations in hereditary haemorrhagic telangiectasia: a series of 126 patients. *Medicine.* 2007;86:1-17.

49. Swanson KL, Prakash UB, Stanson AW. Pulmonary arteriovenous fistulas: Mayo Clinic experience, 1982-1997. *Mayo Clin Proc.* 1999;74:671-680.

50. Moussouttas M, Fayad P, Rosenblatt M, et al. Pulmonary arteriovenous malformations: cerebral ischaemia and neurologic complications. *Neurology.* 2000;55:959-964.

51. Shovlin CL, Letarte M. Hereditary haemorrhagic telangiectasia and pulmonary arteriovenous malformations: issues of clinical management and review of pathogenic mechanisms. *Thorax.* 1999;54:714-729.

52. Whyte MK, Hughes JM, Jackson JE, et al. Cardiopulmonary response to exercise in patients with intrapulmonary vascular shunts. *J Appl Physiol.* 1993;75:321-328.

53. Post MC, Letteboer TG, Mager JJ, et al. A pulmonary right-to-left shunt in patients with hereditary haemorrhagic telangiectasia is associated with an increased prevalence of migraine. *Chest.* 2005;128:2485-2489.

54. Dupuis-Girod S, Giraud S, Decullier E, et al. Hemorrhagic hereditary telangiectasia (Rendu-Osler disease) and infectious diseases: an underestimated association. *Clin Infect Dis.* 2007;44:841-845.

55. Jaskolka J, Wu L, Chan RP, et al. Imaging of hereditary hemorrhagic telangiectasia. *AJR Am J Roentgenol.* 2004;183:307-314.

56. Cottin V, Plauchu H, Bayle JY, et al. Pulmonary arteriovenous malformations in patients with hereditary hemorrhagic telangiectasia. *Am J Respir Crit Care Med.* 2004;169:994-1000.

57. Lee WL, Graham AF, Pugash RA, et al. Contrast echocardiography remains positive after treatment of pulmonary arteriovenous malformations. *Chest.* 2003;123:351-358.

58. Cottin V, Dupuis-Girod S, Lesca G, et al. Pulmonary vascular manifestations of hereditary hemorrhagic telangiectasia (Rendu-Osler disease). *Respiration.* 2007;74:264-275.

59. Remy J, Remy-Jardin M, Giraud F, et al. Angioarchitecture of pulmonary arteriovenous malformations: clinical utility of three-dimensional helical CT. *Radiology.* 1994;191:657-664.

60. Vase P, Holm M, Arendrup H. Pulmonary arteriovenous fistulas in hereditary hemorrhagic telangiectasia. *Acta Med Scand.* 1985;218:105-109.

61. Faughnan ME, Granton JT, Young LH. The pulmonary vascular complications of hereditary haemorrhagic telangiectasia. *Eur Respir J.* 2009;33:1186-1194.

62. Mager JJ, Overtoom TT, Blauw H, et al. Embolotherapy of pulmonary arteriovenous malformations: long-term results in 112 patients. *J Vasc Interv Radiol.* 2004;15:451-456.

63. Shovlin CL, Tighe HC, Davies RJ, et al. Embolisation of pulmonary arteriovenous malformations: no consistent effect on pulmonary artery pressure. *Eur Respir J.* 2008;32:162-169.

64. Lee DW, White RI Jr, Egglin TK, et al. Embolotherapy of large pulmonary arteriovenous malformations: long-term results. *Ann Thorac Surg.* 1997;64:930-939.

65. Pollak JS, Saluja S, Thabet A, et al. Clinical and anatomic outcomes after embolotherapy of pulmonary arteriovenous malformations. *J Vasc Interv Radiol.* 2006;17:35-44.

CHAPTER 25
ATRIAL FIBRILLATION

Rob MacLeod and J. J. E. Blauer

INTRODUCTION / 420
Clinical Profile of AF / 420
Mechanisms of AF / 420
Imaging and AF / 421

OVERVIEW OF CURRENT IMAGING MODALITIES / 421
Fluoroscopy / 421
Electroanatomic Mapping and Imaging / 422
Echocardiography/Ultrasound / 422
Anatomic MRI/Multislice CT / 422
Merging of Modalities / 423

MRI-BASED EVALUATION OF ATRIAL TISSUE / 423
Evaluation of Postablation Scar Formation / 423
Evaluation of AF Substrate / 423

REAL-TIME MRI FOR ABLATION OF AF / 424
Catheter Ablation of AF / 425
MRI-Compatible Catheters / 426
Visualization of Imaging Results / 426
Real-Time Detection of Lesion Formation / 427

SUMMARY / 427

INTRODUCTION

Atrial fibrillation (AF) is the most common form of cardiac arrhythmia, so a review of the role imaging in AF is a natural topic to include in this book. Further motivation comes from the fact that the treatment of AF probably includes more different forms of imaging, often merged or combined in a variety of ways, than perhaps any other clinical intervention. A typical clinical electrophysiology lab for the treatment of AF usually contains no less than six and often more than eight individual monitors, each rendering some form of image-based information about the patient undergoing therapy. There is naturally great motivation to merge different images and different imaging modalities in the setting of AF, but this is also very challenging as a result of a host of factors, including the small size, extremely thin walls, large natural variation in atrial shape, and the fact that fibrillation is occurring so atrial shape is changing rapidly and irregularly. Thus, the use of multimodal imaging has recently become a very active and challenging area of image processing and analysis research and development, driven by an enormous clinical need to understand and treat a disease that affects approximately five million Americans alone, a number that is predicted to increase to almost 16 million by 2050.[1]

In this chapter, we attempt to provide an overview of the large variety of imaging modalities and their uses in the management and understanding of AF, with special emphasis on the most novel applications of magnetic resonance imaging (MRI) technology. To provide clinical and biomedical motivation, we outline the basics of the disease together with some contemporary hypotheses about its etiology and management. We then describe briefly the imaging modalities in common use in the management and research of AF, and then focus on the use of MRI for all phases of the management of patients with AF and indicate some of the major engineering challenges that can motivate further progress.

■ CLINICAL PROFILE OF AF

AF is a growing problem in modern societies, with an enormous impact on both short-term quality of life and long-term survival.[2] Approximately 0.5% of people age 50 to 59 years have AF, and 9% of people age 80 to 89 years have AF, and these prevalences are increasing.[1,3] Although many people with the condition go untreated, AF is associated with an almost twofold increase in the risk of mortality. AF patients experience a dramatically increased rate of stroke (from 1.5% for those aged 50 to 59 years to 23.5% for those between age 80 and 89),[4] a risk that, by contrast, decreases with age in the normal population. Treatment of AF represents a significant health care burden, with the annual costs estimated at approximately seven billion US dollars.[5]

Restoring and maintaining normal sinus rhythm remains one of the major goals in treating patients with AF. One treatment modality is a combination of cardioversion and antiarrhythmic drugs[6]; however, only 40% to 60% of the AF population is maintained in regular rhythm 1 year after such treatment. The treatment itself may also have serious adverse effects[7-9] and must usually continue for the lifetime of the patient. In contrast, maintaining sinus rhythm without the use of antiarrhythmic drugs seems to be associated with increased survival.[10] The inadequacies of drug-based treatments for AF have long been the major motivation for finding a truly curative approach, that is, to maintain sinus rhythm and suppress AF.

■ MECHANISMS OF AF

The mechanisms underlying AF have been the topic of extensive research over many years, and there is consensus that the disease, like most cardiac arrhythmias, has two components, the tissue substrate and some initiating electrical events or triggers. Perhaps the most complete description of the substrate of AF comes from Wijffels et al, who first postulated that the longer the atria spend in the state of fibrillation, the more difficult it becomes to reverse the condition (ie, "Atrial fibrillation begets atrial fibrillation").[11] Their conclusions were based largely on animal studies in which rapid pacing of the heart induced AF through a continuous process of electrical and then structural remodeling, a transition that is initially reversible but then becomes essentially permanent. Rapid pacing of the heart does not, of course, occur spontaneously, and the etiology of the disease in humans is thought to be closely linked to the gradual and inevitable increase in fibrosis in the atria that comes with age[12,13] and that predisposes a heart to AF whether or not associated conditions such as heart failure are present.[14] In animals subjected to the rapid pacing protocols developed to induce AF, treatment with a drug that suppresses the formation of fibrosis reduced the likelihood of developing AF compared with control animals,[15] hence the clear link between fibrosis and the AF substrate. As we will discuss later, one application of imaging, especially MRI, is directed at identifying and quantifying the extent of fibrosis in the left atrium and thus identifying the progression of the disease substrate.

The role of triggers in AF is also motivation for novel imaging approaches. With electrical and electroanatomic mapping (ie, recording electrical activity from a number of known sites on a surface the heart), it is possible to identify the sites of triggers and thus also localize causes of induction of AF. Leaders in mapping triggers of AF are Haissaguerre and coworkers,[16-19] who identified trigger sites both in the atria and especially within the pulmonary veins of the left atrium. Once identified and localized, it is possible to electrically isolate these triggers, which was the unknown consequence of an earlier surgical technique for AF management, known as the Cox maze procedure, first performed in 1988.[20] This operation isolates not only the pulmonary veins but also different regions of the atria by creating a "maze," a tortuous path for electrical conduction in the atria, reducing the ability of triggers to interact with a substrate that could sustain arrhythmias. Modern, catheter-based *ablation* approaches seek to achieve similar goals by applying very focused energy to the endocardial surface of the atria to isolate the triggers known to exist in the pulmonary veins[17] and create the same maze of broken conduction in the left atrium.[16,21,22] The electroanatomic mapping approaches necessary to guide such interventions are, however, invasive and often time consuming, so there remains a pressing need to develop noninvasive imaging approaches to localize trigger sites. Current research in AF management seeks to develop imaging based on MRI,[23-25] ultrasound,[26] and computed x-ray tomography[27] to visualize the ablation lesions and thus direct the intervention.

■ IMAGING AND AF

We outline in subsequent sections the use of a broad range of imaging modalities in AF management and then focus on a comprehensive approach to the management of AF using MRI for all phases of evaluation and intervention. The most novel approaches to imaging in AF are in the areas of merging multiple modalities and in the rapid expansion of the use of MRI. The rationale for this growth is that, unlike other modalities, MRI is naturally suited to detect changes in soft tissue characteristics and hence capable of revealing the progress of substrate in AF and in visualizing the creation of lesions during ablation. These capabilities, combined with the ability to reveal atrial anatomy at high resolutions, make MRI the natural adjunct to all phases of management of AF patients.

OVERVIEW OF CURRENT IMAGING MODALITIES

The use of imaging is ubiquitous in clinical electrophysiology, especially in interventions that require remote access to the heart by means of catheters. On one hand, imaging is required to guide the catheter, and on the other hand, the catheter itself often captures and conveys functional and diagnostic information that must be integrated into the procedure. Figure 25–1 summarizes the most common modes of displaying information in a typical electrophysiology study, and we describe here briefly these modalities. The focus of subsequent, more detailed discussion will be MRI, the modality that is now the topic of extensive research and development.

■ FLUOROSCOPY

Fluoroscopy is an x-ray–based modality that has been a mainstay of cardiac catheterization procedures from their inception. Like all x-ray–based imaging, fluoroscopy can reveal dense materials like bone and metallic objects (eg, electrodes, devices, catheters) but, without contrast agents, is not capable of visualizing soft tissue or blood. In catheter ablation, fluoroscopy serves primarily to guide catheter navigation and to direct the transseptal puncture of the atrial septum that is necessary to access the left atrium. With contrast agent injection, it is also possible to visualize vessels and cardiac chambers using fluoroscopy. Significant

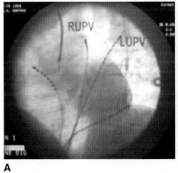
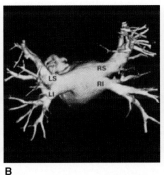
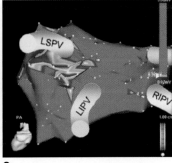
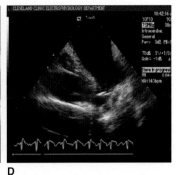

A   **B**   **C**   **D**

FIGURE 25–1. Overview of imaging modalities in common use for atrial fibrillation evaluation and ablation. The figure shows examples of fluoroscopy (**A**), computed tomography (**B**), electroanatomic mapping (**C**), and intracardiac echocardiography (**D**) as they are used for guiding ablation of atrial arrhythmias. LI, left inferior; LIPV, left inferior pulmonary vein; LS, left superior; LSPV, left superior pulmonary vein; LUPV, left upper pulmonary vein; RI, right inferior; RIPV, right inferior pulmonary vein; RS, right superior; RUPV, right upper pulmonary vein.

strengths of fluoroscopy include the ability to perform real-time imaging at frame rates of tens per second, the simplicity provided by very evolved technology, and ready availability. Acknowledged weaknesses include the poor soft tissue contrast and the cumulative exposure to ionizing radiation. More fundamentally, fluoroscopy is a two-dimensional modality so that revealing three-dimensional cardiac shape is challenging.

Modern fluoroscopy systems seek to address these limitations by providing multiple, orthogonally oriented cameras (biplane fluoroscopy) and rotational angiography systems for full, three-dimensional reconstructions of venous and cardiac shape during catheterization procedures,[28,29] all at the lowest possible field strengths. The anatomic models obtained by rotational angiography systems approach the resolution and accuracy of computed tomography (CT) and MRI images. Furthermore, because imaging occurs intraprocedurally, the resulting models can be better aligned to the coordinate system in which the procedure occurs and are less vulnerable to intravascular volume changes and shifts in body position and shape that may limit the accuracy of remotely acquired MRI and CT images.[30,31] Acquisition of geometric information in the same reference frame and at the same time of procedures significantly aids the integration of imaging modalities by obviating the need for registration.[32]

ELECTROANATOMIC MAPPING AND IMAGING

Electroanatomic mapping (EAM) is an essential component of cardiac ablation procedures that has been used widely since the mid-1990s.[33-38] All such systems produce a patient-specific geometric model of the endocardium together with electrograms at numerous sites on that surface. There are two competing EAM technologies, CARTO from Biosense Webster (Diamond Bar, CA)[39] and EnSite from St Jude Medical (St. Paul, MN),[33] which differ in the manner by which they generate the electrical signals on the endocardium. CARTO measures potentials directly by touching a manually steered catheter sequentially to the heart surface and can thus be used on both the endocardial and epicardial surfaces. Its major weakness is the time required to sample enough points to create true maps of electrical activity, which can present challenges when the underlying arrhythmias are unstable and poorly tolerated by the patient. The EnSite technology differs in that it is based on simultaneous recording from an inflatable catheter containing 80 electrodes that is placed inside the chamber of interest. The system solves the resulting bioelectric field inverse problem in terms of endocardial potentials from a single heartbeat, reducing the burden on patients with unstable arrhythmias.

More recently, clinicians have adopted EAM for evaluation and guidance during ablation of AF,[34-36] but here, the goal is often simpler—to measure only the amplitude of electrical activity in the posterior wall of the left atrium and thus evaluate the success of ablation. In the setting of MRI-guided AF ablation, the role of EAM will likely change as the MRI itself can provide direct evidence of the extent of ablation lesion so that mapping of voltage will become of secondary importance.

ECHOCARDIOGRAPHY/ULTRASOUND

Various modalities of ultrasound-based echocardiography are used in the management of AF. Transthoracic echocardiography (TTE), transesophageal echocardiography (TEE), and intracardiac echocardiography (ICE) are routinely used before, during, and after catheter ablation of AF, always with the goal of providing detailed and fine-scale anatomic information. We will briefly describe the context in which each of these modalities is commonly used.

Transthoracic Echocardiography

TTE is routinely used for screening and evaluation purposes in the management of AF, typically to screen for underlying heart disease, including heart failure, valvular heart disease, and left ventricular hypertrophy.[40] Additionally, TTE can be used to assess left atrium size and anatomy.[41] Postablation TTE can be used to detect pericardial effusion and to evaluate left atrial function and size.[42] Although other imaging modalities outperform TTE in these tasks, TTE remains an effective, readily available, noninvasive, and relatively inexpensive modality.

Transesophageal Echocardiography

TEE has shown high sensitivity and specificity for the detection of left atrial thrombus before ablation treatment.[43] It is also useful for assessment of the location and number of pulmonary veins when CT and MRI are not feasible. Due to patient discomfort (the probe must be placed in the esophagus at the level of the heart) and need for airway management, TEE has not traditionally been used intraprocedurally.[42]

Intracardiac Echocardiography

ICE has become a standard imaging utility in most modern electrophysiology laboratories because of its high spatial and temporal resolution, achieved in part from the immediate proximity of the sensor and the heart. ICE is capable of visualizing the anatomy of the left atrium, including the pulmonary veins and appendage, as well as other local anatomy including the aorta, mitral valve, and esophagus. In AF ablation procedures, the ultrasound catheter is navigated intravenously to the right atrium and is used to guide transseptal punctures, navigate ablation catheters, confirm electrode-tissue contact, and titrate energy delivery.[44-47] Additionally, ICE plays a critical role in the prevention and detection of complications by monitoring the formation of thrombus or coagulum, pericardial effusion and tamponade, and flow acceleration indicative of pulmonary vein stenosis.[48-51] Limitations of ICE include the requirement for additional intravenous access and confinement to two-dimensional imaging.

ANATOMIC MRI/MULTISLICE CT

Multislice CT (MSCT) and MRI-based angiography are routinely performed before ablation to define left atrial and pulmonary vein anatomy and size. Models of the relevant cardiac anatomy, generated from these images, are created to help guide intraprocedural navigation and tissue targeting.[52-54] Trade-offs exist between the selection of MSCT or MRI for angiography. MSCT-based angiography is faster and has higher spatial resolution, whereas MRI does not require exposure to ionizing radiation. Most patients with pacemakers or implantable cardiac defibrillators are also ineligible for MRI. High-fidelity representations of the anatomy can be generated from both modalities, and consequently, both are considered acceptable for this purpose. Both modalities are also used after ablation to identify complications such as pulmonary vein stenosis, atrioesophageal fistula, and reverse remodeling (ie, decrease in atrial volume).[42,55-59] MRI and MSCT have also been successfully used to identify surrounding structures that may be at risk of collateral injury during AF ablation, including coronary vessels and the esophagus.[60-62]

MERGING OF MODALITIES

Clearly, no imaging modality is a panacea for all of the requirements inherent in the assessment and treatment of a disease with such diverse and complex imaging needs as AF. Often a merging of modalities is necessary or at least desirable to achieve the necessary coverage of anatomic and functional information to manage the disease. The challenges presented by merging imaging modalities include the need to align or register images acquired in different coordinate systems and different resolutions and then to present them to the operator in a way that is flexible and intuitive enough to be useful.

The centerpiece of contemporary integrated image merging systems tends to be the EAM system, which includes the necessary merging, registration, and visualization hardware and software. The goal of such systems is almost always to use a previously acquired angiography (by MRI or MSCT) to provide a geometric substrate for the subsequent EAM of the heart.[63-69] This registration step usually relies on operator identification of landmarks common to both the angiography and the EAM to rigidly align them in the coordinate system of the EAM system. Further refinements of the alignment are then updated as more points are sampled for the EAM. Much of the mismatch that remains can be attributed to the differences in the MSCT and MRI data acquired sometimes days before the procedure. Other sources of error in the match of MRI and MSCT models to intraprocedure anatomy include respiration, patient movement, and changes in cardiac rhythm.[70,71] Real-time integration of ICE imaging with the EAM system has recently emerged as a means to allow intraprocedural generation and updating of anatomic models, further improving navigational accuracy.[72,73]

MRI-BASED EVALUATION OF ATRIAL TISSUE

Cardiac MRI has become the gold standard for imaging and analysis of numerous cardiac conditions. Generally, MRI is limited by comparatively slow image acquisition and reconstruction times, low resolution, susceptibility to noise, and magnetic field incompatibility of some patients. However, the two primary benefits of MRI are soft tissue contrast and absence of ionizing radiation. These two strengths come to bear significantly in the arena of AF management. First, AF is known to influence cardiac structural properties in a process known as remodeling. Second, the stated goal of AF ablation is to modify, isolate, or abolish arrhythmogenic tissues. In both cases, the soft tissue contrast available in MRI provides insight for physicians into the entrenchment of AF and success of scar formation, respectively. Finally, modern ablation procedures still rely heavily on fluoroscopy for procedural guidance. The introduction of AF ablation procedures into the MRI environment opens the door for the departure of ionizing radiation from the management of AF.

Late gadolinium-enhanced (LGE) MRI is used to evaluate alterations in tissue structure associated with numerous cardiomyopathies.[74,75] To acquire LGE images, a dose of chelated gadolinium contrast agent is administered intravenously as would be done for standard magnetic resonance angiography. Following the injection, the gadolinium is allowed time to wash clear of normal myocardium, and an inversion-recovery prepared gradient echo pulse sequence is applied to detect regions of tissue where the contrast agent remains sequestered. Any region in which perfusion has decreased or extracellular space has increased will appear bright in LGE images due to enhanced concentrations of gadolinium relative to surrounding tissues.[76]

EVALUATION OF POSTABLATION SCAR FORMATION

The first reported use of LGE-MRI of atrial tissue to assess ablation lesions came from Peters et al.[77] In this prospective study, contrast enhancement was found in the left atrium and pulmonary vein ostia of all patients who had undergone radiofrequency (RF) ablation of AF 1 to 3 months previously. These findings were supported by McGann et al,[78] who quantified the extent of enhancement observed in the left atrial wall 3 months after ablation using the methods outlined in Fig. 25–2 and compared extent of scar to procedural outcomes. In this study, patients who experienced a recurrence of AF were found to have less enhancement (12.4 ± 5.7%) compared with patients who did not experience recurrence (19.3 ± 6.7%, $P = .004$).[78] Subsequent studies have expanded on these initial findings to show that lesion remodeling stabilizes by 3 months after ablation and that the extent and continuity of lesions encompassing the pulmonary veins play an important role in preventing recurrences.[79-81]

The ability to noninvasively assess the lesion sets created in AF ablation procedures can provide valuable feedback to electrophysiologists searching for the optimal ablation strategy. Although freedom from AF after a single intervention will remain the goal for procedural success, LGE-MRI can help explain how and why a particular lesion set succeeds or fails at terminating AF and provide direction in subsequent ablation procedures.

EVALUATION OF AF SUBSTRATE

As previously noted, AF is associated with structural remodeling of the left atrium. Motivated by the success of LGE-MRI in identifying structural heart disease and, in particular, fibrosis,

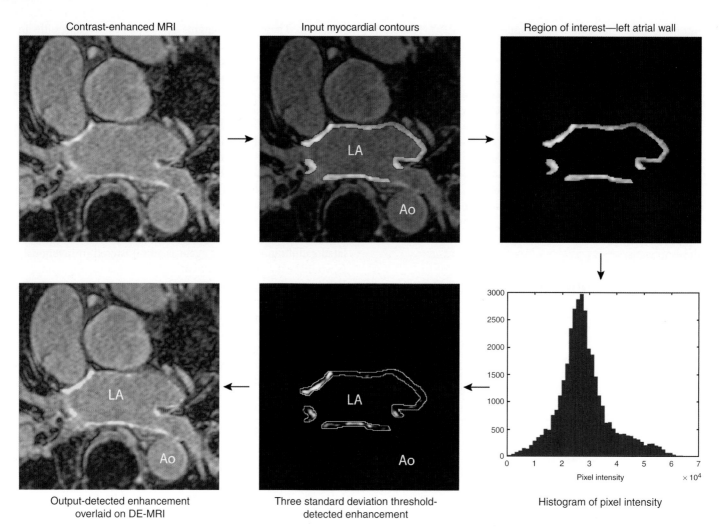

Contrast-enhanced MRI

Input myocardial contours

Region of interest—left atrial wall

Output-detected enhancement overlaid on DE-MRI

Three standard deviation threshold-detected enhancement

Histogram of pixel intensity

FIGURE 25–2. Algorithm for quantification of postablation scar burden in the left atrium (LA). The wall of the LA in late gadolinium-enhanced magnetic resonance imaging scans (top left) is segmented on a slice-by-slice basis (top center). Once isolated (top right), a histogram of the LA wall pixel intensities is generated (bottom right), and the rising phase of the primary mode is used to predict normal tissue pixel intensities. Pixel intensities three standard deviations above the mean of normal tissue is marked as scar (bottom center). Overlays of pixels marked as scar onto original images shows good correlation with hyperenhancement. Ao, aorta; DE-MRI, delayed-enhanced magnetic resonance imaging.

Oakes et al[82] analyzed LGE-MRI scans from a cohort of 81 AF patients and six normal volunteers to explore the relationship between contrast enhancement and AF structural remodeling. This study revealed a positive correlation between low-voltage tissue regions in EAMs (bipolar voltage amplitude ≤ 0.5 mV) and left atrial wall enhancement ($r^2 = 0.61$, $P < .05$). Furthermore, patients with mild (<15%, n = 43), moderate (15%-35%, n = 30), and extensive (>35%, n = 8) amounts of left atrial wall enhancement were found to have significantly different rates of AF recurrence at a mean follow-up of 9.6 months (14%, 43%, and 75%, respectively). These findings suggest that the degree of left atrial wall enhancement, which is assumed to reflect extent of fibrosis in the atrial tissue, is a predictor of failure for ablation. Based in part on these results, a staging system for determining the amount of enhancement has been proposed. Figure 25–3 shows the Utah staging system, with examples of LGE-MRI scans from each of the four stages. Under this system, patients with Utah stage III or IV

enhancement are not considered to be ideal candidates for ablation therapy.

The utility of the Utah AF stages is currently under extensive evaluation, both at our institution and through a multicenter clinical study involving major AF centers from around the world.

REAL-TIME MRI FOR ABLATION OF AF

As outlined in the Introduction, catheter-based ablation of the left atrium represents the most common intervention to cure or at least suppress the symptoms of AF. To carry out ablation requires considerable imaging support in order to identify anatomy, evaluate substrate, and determine success of the intervention. Conventional approaches to AF ablation make use of fluoroscopy, CT, intracardiac ultrasound, and EAM. Not only is MRI used as a preprocedural method to generate anatomic images, but also its broader use represents the leading

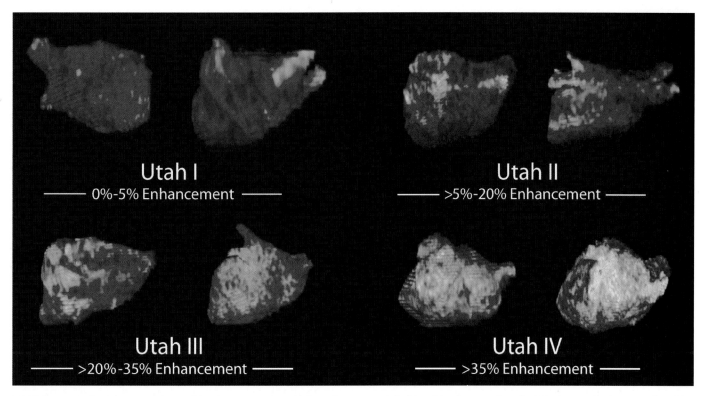

FIGURE 25-3. Utah staging system for stratifying the amount of preablation enhancement of the left atrial wall. Images in each of the four panels show examples of late gadolinium-enhanced magnetic resonance images, with enhanced regions color coded in green and normal tissues colored in blue.

edge of research in real-time imaging to support the guidance of catheters and the evaluation of lesion formation in a three-dimensional form. The need to combine anatomic and functional information continues to drive the development of novel merging and registration approaches.[34]

■ CATHETER ABLATION OF AF

The past decades have seen significant progress in understanding the underlying mechanisms of AF that sustain its persistence,[11,17] and this knowledge has led to the treatment paradigm of AF ablation, which is the targeted destruction of tissue predominantly in the left atrium in order to isolate electrical triggers and reduce the ability of the atrium to sustain rapid activation. AF ablation, typically based on RF energy delivery through a venous catheter, has already produced encouraging results and is the topic of innumerable research reports, but it has yet to reach its full potential. Despite the fact that ablation, when successful, allows the patient to discontinue the use of antiarrhythmics and anticoagulants, the success rate of ablation in maintaining regular sinus rhythm without the use of such medications is still only 60% to 80%.[83] Moreover, the penetration of ablation, although difficult to measure with accuracy, appears to lie well below the need; there are fewer ablations carried out each year than there are new cases of AF. In an effort to increase the penetration of this potentially curative approach, there have been many modifications to the ablation procedure aimed at improving

outcome and hence promoting the adoption of the ablation approach.[16,34,72,84-89] Despite such progress, daunting technical challenges to carrying out successful ablation remain, and many of these are related to imaging.

Currently, AF ablation is performed using catheters that can be visualized under fluoroscopy and/or projected onto a three-dimensional virtual shell acquired through EAM during the procedure.[34] There are multiple challenges associated with these approaches. First, it is impossible for the operator to visualize the catheter tip/tissue interface; hence, delivery of RF energy is based on guidance from the morphology of local electrogram or by using the virtual shell from EAM to assure that the catheter tip is in contact with the atrial wall. However, both of these approaches have known errors that can exceed 1 cm,[90] leading to frequent delivery of inappropriate lesions that may only partially damage the atrial tissue, promoting tissue recovery and hence reoccurrence of the arrhythmia. Moreover, this lack of visualization of the catheter tip can result in localized heating of blood, thus leading to char formation, a major cause of embolic stroke during the ablation procedure.[91] Defining a technology or a system that would allow accurate visualization of the catheter tip/tissue interface would overcome this major problem for the operator. Another major challenge of the ablation procedure is the lack of an imaging modality that allows immediate assessment of tissue damage as the RF energy is applied. MRI is the most obvious and perhaps only imaging system that could overcome this problem.

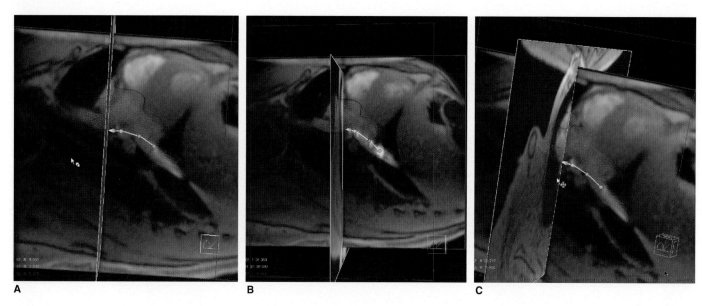

A   B   C

FIGURE 25–4. Visualization of catheter during real-time magnetic resonance imaging (MRI). Each panel shows a slightly different view of the MRI-compatible catheter superimposed on the local MRI image together with a rendered mesh of the right atrium and superior and inferior vena cava from this animal.

Although MRI has the inherent capability of visualizing soft tissue and thus providing both anatomic and functional guidance for RF ablation of AF, there are challenges to creating a viable MRI-based approach. First, it is necessary to develop an MRI-compatible catheter and associated software that allows visualization of the catheter during navigation and energy delivery within the atrial chamber. This catheter and software must be part of a system that tightly integrates the diverse instrumentation required to complete a clinical atrial ablation procedure. The system must exploit the benefits of soft tissue contrast unique to MRI (near real-time visualization of myocardial interfaces and ablation lesions) while providing a smooth workflow for the physician and technicians. Recent reports showing progress toward these ends by our and other groups[23-25] suggest that a full MRI-guided AF ablation procedure in humans, although still very challenging, is likely to represent the future of this methodology.

■ MRI-COMPATIBLE CATHETERS

The development of an MRI-guided system for AF ablation is completely novel in terms of the devices and support systems that are required to create a working system. MRI-compatible catheters have just begun to appear in the literature[23,33,52,92] but are still prototypes and have not been used in any human ablation studies. Similarly, the real-time MRI guidance systems required to place the catheters in the appropriate locations are in their infancy, with only sparse reports of placing an MRI-compatible catheter in the human heart under MRI guidance.[52] MRI-compatible versions of most of the other elements of the contemporary AF ablation instruments—the lasso catheter, the coronary sinus catheter, and the needle required to carry out transseptal punctures—are also only just under initial development and have yet to receive approval for use in humans.

We have participated in the development of catheters that are MRI compatible, steerable in a way similar to standard clinical catheters, and capable of both delivering RF energy and recording endocardial electrograms.[25] It is possible to track the location of the catheters and to display their position superimposed on the real-time MRI images and with a geometric shell model of the atria and great vessels that we create from volumetric MRI scans recorded in the early phases of the procedure. Figure 25–4 shows an example of MRI images recorded during a real-time ablation procedure in which the catheter is visible superimposed on the orthogonal MRI images. Also visible in the image is a polygonal surface or shell of the right atrium and inferior and superior vena cava, created by segmenting a previously acquired high-resolution scan of the animal's atrial anatomy.

■ VISUALIZATION OF IMAGING RESULTS

Scientific visualization is an essential step in using imaging data, and the unique and challenging needs of AF ablation continue to drive new approaches. For example, EAM requires the integration of spatial information describing the shape of the endocardial surface with time signals, that is, electrograms recorded from that surface, and parameters extracted from the electrograms. In addition, there is volumetric information from MRI and CT that can be visualized as a sequence of two-dimensional images but is much richer when rendered in a three-dimensional form. Naturally, there is a need to merge these two (and other) forms of anatomic and functional information, and novel visualization technology continues to improve such merging in a setting of interactive manipulation and rendering.[34]

We have developed techniques that combine not only visualization of volume- and surface-based approaches but also projection of the information from the volume to the surface. Figure 25–5 shows an example of such a visualization in which Fig. 25–5A shows an EAM from an animal experiment showing three clusters of lesions performed under fluoroscopy guidance; the red dots in panel A show the lesion sites. Figure 25–5B shows

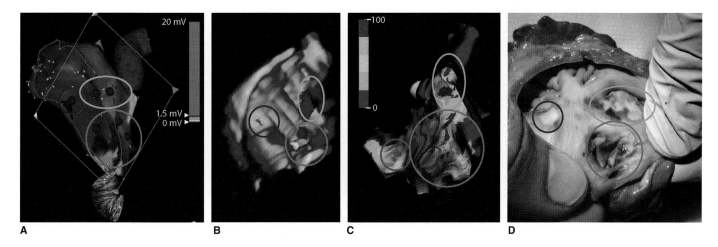

FIGURE 25–5. Multimodal visualization of ablation lesions from an experiment using magnetic resonance imaging (MRI) during and after lesion formation. The images show the results of electroanatomic mapping (**A**), late gadolinium-enhanced MRI (**B** and **C**), and gross dissection of the right atrium from an animal experiment (**D**).

the LGE rendering of the same heart, performed in the MRI scanner directly after the ablation procedure. We then used segmentation of the volume images to define the endocardial surface and projected the information from the MRI scan onto that surface, shown in Fig. 25–5C. Confirmation of the actual lesion locations is evident from dissection documented in Fig. 25–5D.

The motivation of such projection approaches is to present information from multiple modalities (in this case, EAM of electrogram amplitude and MRI tissue changes) in a common reference frame (in this case, the endocardial surface). Such merging of information provides for quantitative analysis and comparisons and also a means of conveying information in a form that is familiar to the clinicians (in this case, electrophysiologists who are highly conversant in the conventions of endocardial and epicardial mapping).

■ REAL-TIME DETECTION OF LESION FORMATION

The most significant advantage of MRI-guided ablation is its potential to obtain rapid feedback on tissue changes during the ablation procedure—to watch the lesions form. There is no viable modality at this time that can determine the effectiveness of ablation; even electrical mapping approaches only measure depressed electrical activity in the endocardium that may return within weeks of the ablation and cause a recurrence of AF. MRI, on the other hand, has the potential to visualize changes in tissue structure related to permanent cell damage following the application of energy and thus establish the presence and depth in the atrial wall of terminally destructive lesions. Visualization of lesion formation and extent would improve the effectiveness and the safety of RF ablation procedures.

To visualize lesion formation with MRI requires acquisition of high-quality images in rapid sequence in order to achieve adequate spatial and temporal resolution. As with all imaging modalities, there is a trade-off in MRI between the time needed to acquire the image and the quality of that image. Furthermore, real-time imaging of the heart is driven both by the need to capture information rapidly enough to avoid blurring due to

cardiac and respiratory motion and the desire to optimize image quality to see small changes within structures that are only a few millimeters thick. Another challenge specific to ablation is the need to see changes quickly enough to allow the operator to control the time and the energy dose in order to create lesions that are deep enough, but not so deep as to degrade the structural integrity of the heart wall.

In animal studies within our group, we have achieved image refresh rates of up to 5.5 frames per second based on customized MRI scan sequences and have been able to visualize lesion formation within 10 to 15 seconds of onset of RF energy.[25,93] Figure 25–6 shows just one example of such a case, in which catheter placement is documented in Fig. 25–6A, followed by a sequence of images (using a different MRI scan sequence) that reveal the formation of the lesion in Fig. 25–6B to 25–6F. Figure 25–6G shows a postmortem image in the same plane, and Fig. 25–6H contains a photographic record of the lesion seen immediately after the experiment. To our knowledge, this is the first report of visualizing lesion formation as it occurs in any tissues of the heart. We have also compared lesion sizes measured from MRI imaging with those determined through postmortem dissection and shown excellent agreement.[25]

SUMMARY

Imaging has always been an essential component of the management of all forms of cardiac arrhythmias, and its use will continue to expand in pace with improvements in the imaging acquisition technology, the image processing and analysis, and the integrating software that can efficiently support the clinical workflow. In the setting of AF, the use of MRI is making particular advances as its utility in all phases of the disease becomes evident. Preablation imaging provides a means to stage patients and determine their best treatment options; the emergence of the Utah AF staging system suggests a very specific means by which image analysis and quantification can indicate disease status and risk. Similar techniques provide a means of noninvasively determining the

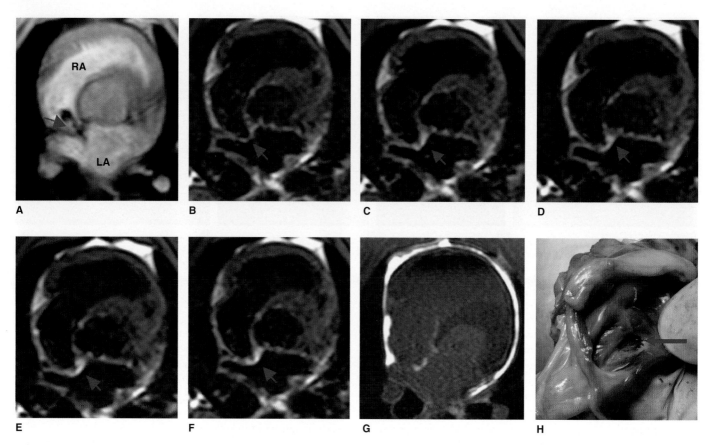

FIGURE 25–6. Detection of acute atrial lesion. **A.** Image from a three-dimensional scan to locate the catheter tip. **B-F.** T2-weighted dark blood images acquired before ablation (**B**) and after ablation at 20 seconds (**C**), 50 seconds (**D**), 2.5 minutes (**E**), and 8 minutes (**F**). **G.** Postmortem, high-resolution, delayed-enhancement magnetic resonance image. **H.** Photo of excised heart. Blue arrow indicates the position of the catheter tip at septal wall. Red arrows indicate the location where the lesion was created using a 30-second ablation with 30 W. LA, left atrium; RA, right atrium.

outcome of AF ablation by mapping the formation of scar to both evaluate interventional success and to guide subsequent interventions, should they be necessary. The Comprehensive Arrhythmia Research and Management Center has carried out over 600 scans on over 250 patients to date and is now collaborating with similar laboratories around the world in multicenter trials of these MRI-based approaches. The results of these studies could completely transform the way that AF is treated when it arises and even enable preventative measures that are simply impossible without a means of tracking the tissue changes that preface the onset of electrical symptoms.

The potential for imaging, especially MRI in the treatment of patients with AF is equally exciting and bright. We have carried out over 30 animals studies in developing the prototype MRI-guided navigation system and are focused on developing and testing such a system for use in humans. We have created lesions both under fluoroscopy and real-time MRI guidance in the atria and ventricles of anesthetized dogs and swine and then carried out detailed imaging both of the entire animal thorax and of the excised preserved heart. In the process, we have made advances in MRI-compatible catheter design, exploitation of novel sensing coils, incorporation of tracking coils into catheter housings, improvement in pulse sequence design for rapid acquisition, integrated interactive display of images and devices, and image processing and analysis tools for postprocedure evaluation of results. Other groups have made similar progress, and there is little doubt that the first human studies are immanent.

A major initial goal of these studies was to ensure that it is indeed possible to visualize lesions soon after ablation, despite the thin atrial walls and small extent of RF lesions. Figure 25–6 shows an example of such a result in which we sampled from the same slice before, during, and repeatedly after application of the RF energy.[93]

ACKNOWLEDGMENTS

The authors are deeply indebted to the contributions of the other members of Comprehensive Arrhythmia Research and MAnagement (CARMA) Center at the University of Utah for this material (www. carmacenter.org). The mission of CARMA is to provide worldwide pioneering leadership in advancing clinical treatments and research for cardiac arrhythmias, especially atrial fibrillation. We also thank the Cardiovascular Research and Training Institute (CVRTI) for their support in experiments of MRI-guided ablation.

Support for this research comes from the NIH NCRR Center for Integrative Biomedical Computing (www.sci.utah.edu/cibc),

NIH NCRR Grant No. 5P41-RR012553-10 at the Scientific Computing and Imaging (SCI) Institute and from research grants from Surgivision Inc. and Siemens Healthcare.

REFERENCES

1. Miyasaka Y, Barnes ME, Gersh BJ, et al. Secular trends in incidence of atrial fibrillation in Olmsted County, Minnesota, 1980 to 2000, and implications on the projections for future prevalence. *Circulation.* 2006;114:119-125.

2. Calkins H, Brugada J, Packer DL, et al. HRS/EHRA/ECAS expert consensus statement on catheter and surgical ablation of atrial fibrillation: recommendations for personnel, policy, procedures and follow-up. *Europace.* 2007;9:335-379.

3. Benzinger GR, Kyle JW, Blumenthal KM, Hanck DA. A specific interaction between the cardiac sodium channel and site-3 toxin anthopleurin B. *J Biol Chem.* 1998;273:80-84.

4. Kannel WB, Wolf PA, Benjamin EJ, Levy D. Prevalence, incidence, prognosis, and predisposing conditions for atrial fibrillation: population-based estimates. *Am J Cardiol.* 1998;82(8A):2N-9N.

5. Coyne KS, Paramore C, Grandy S, Mercader M, Reynolds M, Zimetbaum P. Assessing the direct costs of treating nonvalvular atrial fibrillation in the United States. *Value Health.* 2006;9:348-356.

6. Falk RH. Atrial fibrillation. *N Engl J Med.* 2001;344:1067-1078.

7. Brodsky MA, Allen BJ 3rd, Walker CJ, Casey TP, Luckett CR, Henry WL. Amiodarone for maintenance of sinus rhythm after conversion of atrial fibrillation in the setting of a dilated left atrium. *Am J Cardiol.* 1987;60:572-575.

8. Crijns HJ, Van Gelder IC, Van der Woude HJ, et al. Efficacy of serial electrical cardioversion therapy in patients with chronic atrial fibrillation after valve replacement and implications for surgery to cure atrial fibrillation. *Am J Cardiol.* 1996;78:1140–1144.

9. Van Gelder IC, Crijns HJ, Tieleman RG, et al. Chronic atrial fibrillation. Success of serial cardioversion therapy and safety of oral anticoagulation. *Arch Intern Med.* 1996;156:2585-2592.

10. Corley SD, Epstein AE, DiMarco JP, et al. Relationships between sinus rhythm, treatment, and survival in the Atrial fibrillation Follow-Up Investigation of Rhythm Management (AFFIRM) study. *Circulation.* 2004;109:1509-1513.

11. Wijffels MC, Kirchhof CJ, Dorland R, Allessie MA. Atrial fibrillation begets atrial fibrillation. A study in awake chronically instrumented goats. *Circulation.* 1995;92:1954-1968.

12. Boldt A, Wetzel U, Lauschke J, et al. Fibrosis in left atrial tissue of patients with atrial fibrillation with and without underlying mitral valve disease. *Heart.* 2004;90:400-405.

13. Nattel S, Shiroshita-Takeshita A, Cardin S, Pelletier P. Mechanisms of atrial remodeling and clinical relevance. *Curr Opin Cardiol.* 2005;20:21-25.

14. Cha TJ, Ehrlich JR, Zhang L, et al. Dissociation between ionic remodeling and ability to sustain atrial fibrillation during recovery from experimental congestive heart failure. *Circulation.* 2004;109:412-418.

15. Lee KW, Everett TH, Rahmutula D, et al. Pirfenidone prevents the development of a vulnerable substrate for atrial fibrillation in a canine model of heart failure. *Circulation.* 2006;114:1703-1712.

16. Haissaguerre M, Jais P, Shah DC, et al. Electrophysiological end point for catheter ablation of atrial fibrillation initiated from multiple pulmonary venous foci. *Circulation.* 2000;101:1409-1417.

17. Haissaguerre M, Jais P, Shah DC, et al. Spontaneous initiation of atrial fibrillation by ectopic beats originating in the pulmonary veins. *N Engl J Med.* 1998;339:659-666.

18. Takahashi Y, Hocini M, O'Neill MD, et al. Sites of focal atrial activity characterized by endocardial mapping during atrial fibrillation. *J Am Coll Cardiol.* 2006;47:2005-2012.

19. Takahashi Y, Sanders P, Jais P, et al. Organization of frequency spectra of atrial fibrillation: relevance to radiofrequency catheter ablation. *J Cardiovasc Electrophysiol.* 2006;17:382-388.

20. Cox JL, Schuessler RB Jr, D'Agostino HJ, et al. The surgical treatment of atrial fibrillation. III. Development of a definitive surgical procedure. *J Thorac Cardiovasc Surg.* 1991;101:569-583.

21. Jais P, Haissaguerre M, Shah D, et al. Staged approach for paroxysmal atrial fibrillation ablation. *PACE.* 1996;19:I-265.

22. Marrouche NF, Dresing T, Cole C, et al. Circular mapping and ablation of the pulmonary vein for treatment of atrial fibrillation: impact of different catheter technologies. *J Am Coll Cardiol.* 2002;40:464-474.

23. Dukkipati SR, Mallozzi R, Schmidt EJ, et al. Electroanatomic mapping of the left ventricle in a porcine model of chronic myocardial infarction with magnetic resonance-based catheter tracking. *Circulation.* 2008;118:853-862.

24. Schmidt EJ, Mallozzi RP, Thiagalingam A, et al. Electroanatomic mapping and radiofrequency ablation of porcine left atria and atrioventricular nodes using magnetic resonance catheter tracking. *Circ Arrhythm Electrophysiol.* 2009;2:695-704.

25. Vergara GR, Vijayakumar S, Kholmovski EG, et al. Real time MRI guided radiofrequency ablation and visualization of lesion formation at 3 tesla. Poster session presented at Heart Rhythm Society Scientific Sessions 2010, Denver.

26. Wright M, Harks E, Deladi S, et al. Catheter assessment of lesion quality using a novel ultrasound radiofrequency ablation catheter. *Heart Rhythm Soc.* 2010;(Suppl):S86.

27. Girard-Hughes E, Fahrig R, Moore T, Boese J, Lauritsch G, Al-Ahmad A. Visualization of radiofrequency ablation lesions with iodine contrast-enhanced cardiac dynact. *Heart Rhythm Soc.* 2010;(Suppl):S85.

28. Kriatselis C, Tang M, Roser M, Fleck E, Gerds-Li H. A new approach for contrast-enhanced x-ray imaging of the left atrium and pulmonary veins for atrial fibrillation ablation: rotational angiography during adenosine-induced asystole. *Europace.* 2009;11:35-41.

29. Li JH, Haim M, Movassaghi B, et al. Segmentation and registration of three-dimensional rotational angiogram on live fluoroscopy to guide atrial fibrillation ablation: a new online imaging tool. *Heart Rhythm.* 2009;6:231-237.

30. Nolker G, Gutleben KJ, Marschang H, et al. Three-dimensional left atrial and esophagus reconstruction using cardiac C-arm computed tomography with image integration into fluoroscopic views for ablation of atrial fibrillation: accuracy of a novel modality in comparison with multislice computed tomography. *Heart Rhythm.* 2008;5:1651-1657.

31. Thiagalingam A, Manzke R, d'Avila A, et al. Intraprocedural volume imaging of the left atrium and pulmonary veins with rotational x-ray angiography: implications for catheter ablation of atrial fibrillation. *J Cardiovasc Electrophysiol.* 2008;19:293-300.

32. Burkhardt JD, Natale A. New technologies in atrial fibrillation ablation. *Circulation.* 2009;120:1533-1541.

33. Beatty GE, Remole SC, Johnston MK, Holte JE, Benditt DG. Non-contact electrical extrapolation technique to reconstruct endocardial potentials. *PACE.* 1994;17:765.

34. Dong J, Dickfeld T, Dalal D, et al. Initial experience in the use of integrated electroanatomic mapping with three-dimensional MR/CT images to guide catheter ablation of atrial fibrillation. *J Cardiovasc Electrophysiol.* 2006;17:459-466.

35. Marrouche NF, Verma A, Wazni O, et al. Mode of initiation and ablation of ventricular fibrillation storms in patients with ischemic cardiomyopathy. *J Am Coll Cardiol.* 2004;43:1715-1720.

36. Paul T, Windhagen-Mahnert B, Kriebel T, et al. Atrial reentrant tachycardia after surgery for congenital heart disease: endocardial mapping and radiofrequency catheter ablation using a novel, noncontact mapping system. *Circulation.* 2001;103:2266-2271.

37. Smeets J, Haim SB, Rodriguez L, Timmermans C, Wellens H. New method for nonfluoroscopic endocardial mapping in humans. *Circulation.* 1998;97:2426-2432.

38. Thiagalingam A, Wallace EM, Boyd AC, et al. Noncontact mapping of the left ventricle: insights from validation with transmural contact mapping. *Pacing Clin Electrophysiol.* 2004;27:570-578.

39. Callans DJ, Ren JF, Michele J, Marchlinski FE, Dillon SM. Electroanatomic left ventricular mapping in the porcine model of healed anterior myocardial infarction. Correlation with intracardiac echocardiography and pathological analysis. *Circulation.* 1999;100:1744-1750.

40. Nieuwlaat R, Capucci A, Camm AJ, et al. Atrial fibrillation management: a prospective survey in ESC member countries: the Euro Heart Survey on Atrial fibrillation. *Eur Heart J.* 2005;26:2422-2434.

41. Lang RM, Bierig M, Devereux RB, et al. Recommendations for chamber quantification: a report from the American Society of Echocardiography's Guidelines and Standards Committee and the Chamber Quantification Writing Group, developed in conjunction with the European Association of Echocardiography, a branch of the European Society of Cardiology. *J Am Soc Echocardiogr.* 2005;18:1440-1463.

42. Calkins H, Brugada J, Packer DL, et al. HRS/EHRA/ECAS expert consensus statement on catheter and surgical ablation of atrial fibrillation: recommendations for personnel, policy, procedures and follow-up. A report of the Heart Rhythm Society (HRS) task force on catheter and surgical ablation of atrial fibrillation. *Heart Rhythm.* 2007;4:816-861.

43. Pearson AC, Labovitz AJ, Tatineni S, Gomez CR. Superiority of transesophageal echocardiography in detecting cardiac source of embolism in patients with cerebral ischemia of uncertain etiology. *J Am Coll Cardiol.* 1991;17:66-72.

44. Epstein LM, Smith T, TenHoff H. Nonfluoroscopic transseptal catheterization: safety and efficacy of intracardiac echocardiographic guidance. *J Cardiovasc Electrophysiol.* 1998;9:625-630.

45. Marrouche NF, Martin DO, Wazni O, et al. Phased-array intracardiac echocardiography monitoring during pulmonary vein isolation in patients with atrial fibrillation: impact on outcome and complications. *Circulation.* 2003;107:2710-2716.

46. Mitchel JF, Gillam LD, Sanzobrino BW, Hirst JA, McKay RG. Intracardiac ultrasound imaging during transseptal catheterization. *Chest.* 1995;108:104-108.

47. Verma A, Marrouche NF, Natale A. Pulmonary vein antrum isolation: intracardiac echocardiography-guided technique. *J Cardiovasc Electrophysiol.* 2004;15:1335-1340.

48. Jongbloed MRM, Bax JJ, van der Wall EE, Schalij MJ. Thrombus in the left atrial appendage detected by intracardiac echocardiography. *Int J Cardiovasc Imaging.* 2004;20:113-116.

49. Ren J-F, Marchlinski FE, Callans DJ. Left atrial thrombus associated with ablation for atrial fibrillation: identification with intracardiac echocardiography. *J Am Coll Cardiol.* 2004;43:1861-1867.

50. Ren J-F, Marchlinski FE, Callans DJ, Zado ES. Intracardiac Doppler echocardiographic quantification of pulmonary vein flow velocity: an effective technique for monitoring pulmonary vein ostia narrowing during focal atrial fibrillation ablation. *J Cardiovasc Electrophysiol.* 2002;13:1076-1081.

51. Saad EB, Cole CR, Marrouche NF, et al. Use of intracardiac echocardiography for prediction of chronic pulmonary vein stenosis after ablation of atrial fibrillation. *J Cardiovasc Electrophysiol.* 2002;13:986-989.

52. Mansour M, Holmvang G, Sosnovik D, et al. Assessment of pulmonary vein anatomic variability by magnetic resonance imaging: implications for catheter ablation techniques for atrial fibrillation. *J Cardiovasc Electrophysiol.* 2004;15:387-393.

53. Marom EM, Herndon JE, Kim YH, McAdams HP. Variations in pulmonary venous drainage to the left atrium: implications for radiofrequency ablation. *Radiology.* 2004;230:824-829.

54. Scharf C, Sneider M, Case I, et al. Anatomy of the pulmonary veins in patients with atrial fibrillation and effects of segmental ostial ablation analyzed by computed tomography. *J Cardiovasc Electrophysiol.* 2003;14:150-155.

55. Lemola K, Sneider M, Desjardins B, et al. Effects of left atrial ablation of atrial fibrillation on size of the left atrium and pulmonary veins. *Heart Rhythm.* 2004;1:576-581.

56. Packer DL, Keelan P, Munger TM, et al. Clinical presentation, investigation, and management of pulmonary vein stenosis complicating ablation for atrial fibrillation. *Circulation.* 2005;111:546-554.

57. Qureshi AM, Prieto LR, Latson LA, et al. Transcatheter angioplasty for acquired pulmonary vein stenosis after radiofrequency ablation. *Circulation.* 2003;108:1336-1342.

58. Saad EB, Rossillo A, Saad CP, et al. Pulmonary vein stenosis after radiofrequency ablation of atrial fibrillation: functional characterization, evolution, and influence of the ablation strategy. *Circulation.* 2003;108:3102-3107.

59. Tsao H-M, Wu M-H, Huang B-H, et al. Morphologic remodeling of pulmonary veins and left atrium after catheter ablation of atrial fibrillation: insight from long-term follow-up of three-dimensional magnetic resonance imaging. *J Cardiovasc Electrophysiol.* 2005;16:7-12.

60. Lemola K, Sneider M, Desjardins B, et al. Computed tomographic analysis of the anatomy of the left atrium and the esophagus: implications for left atrial catheter ablation. *Circulation.* 2004;110:3655-3660.

61. Tops LF, Krishnan SC, Schuijf JD, Schalij MJ, Bax JJ. Non-coronary applications of cardiac multidetector row computed tomography. *JACC Cardiovasc Imaging.* 2008;1:94-106.

62. Tops LF, Schalij MJ, Bax JJ. Imaging and atrial fibrillation: the role of multi-modality imaging in patient evaluation and management of atrial fibrillation. *Eur Heart J.* 2010;31:542-551.

63. Dong J, Calkins H, Solomon SB, et al. Integrated electroanatomic mapping with three-dimensional computed tomographic images for real-time guided ablations. *Circulation.* 2006;113:186-194.

64. Dong J, Dickfeld T, Dalal D, et al. Initial experience in the use of integrated electroanatomic mapping with three-dimensional MR/CT images to guide catheter ablation of atrial fibrillation. *J Cardiovasc Electrophysiol.* 2006;17:459-466.

65. Kistler PM, Earley MJ, Harris S, et al. Validation of three-dimensional cardiac image integration: use of integrated CT image into electroanatomic mapping system to perform catheter ablation of atrial fibrillation. *J Cardiovasc Electrophysiol.* 2006;17:341-348.

66. Kistler PM, Rajappan K, Jahngir M, et al. The impact of CT image integration into an electroanatomical mapping system on clinical outcomes of catheter ablation of atrial fibrillation. *J Cardiovasc Electrophysiol.* 2006;17:1093-1101.

67. Mikaelian BJ, Malchano ZJ, Neuzil P, et al. Images in cardiovascular medicine. Integration of 3-dimensional cardiac computed tomography images with real-time electroanatomic mapping to guide catheter ablation of atrial fibrillation. *Circulation.* 2005;112:e35-e36.

68. Rubenstein J, Kadish A. Three-dimensional image integration: a first experience with guidance of atrial fibrillation ablations. *J Cardiovasc Electrophysiol.* 2006;17:467-468.

69. Tops LF, Bax JJ, Zeppenfeld K, et al. Fusion of multislice computed tomography imaging with three-dimensional electroanatomic mapping to guide radiofrequency catheter ablation procedures. *Heart Rhythm.* 2005;2:1076-1081.

70. Daccarett M, Segerson NM, Golker J, et al. Blinded correlation study of three-dimensional electro-anatomical image integration and phased array intra-cardiac echocardiography for left atrial mapping. *Europace.* 2007;9:923-926.

71. Noseworthy PA, Malchano ZJ, Ahmed J, Holmvang G, Ruskin JN, Reddy VY. The impact of respiration on left atrial and pulmonary venous anatomy: implications for image-guided intervention. *Heart Rhythm.* 2005;2:1173-1178.

72. den Uijl DW, Tops LF, Tolosana JM, et al. Real-time integration of intracardiac echocardiography and multislice computed tomography to guide radiofrequency catheter ablation for atrial fibrillation. *Heart Rhythm.* 2008;5:1403-1410.

73. Packer DL, Johnson SB, Kolasa MW, Bunch TJ, Henz BD, Okumura Y. New generation of electro-anatomic mapping: full intracardiac ultrasound image integration. *Europace.* 2008;10(Suppl 3):iii35-iii41.

74. Ordovas K, Reddy G, Higgins C. MRI in nonischemic acquired heart disease. *J Magn Reson Imaging.* 2008;27:1195-1213.

75. Weinsaft JW, Klem I, Judd RM. MRI for the assessment of myocardial viability. *Cardiol Clin.* 2007;25:35-56.

76. Moon J, Reed E, Sheppard M, et al. The histologic basis of late gadolinium enhancement cardiovascular magnetic resonance in hypertrophic cardiomyopathy. *J Am Coll Cardiol.* 2004;43:2260-2264.

77. Peters DC, Wylie JV, Hauser TH, et al. Detection of pulmonary vein and left atrial scar after catheter ablation with three-dimensional navigator-gated delayed enhancement MR imaging: initial experience. *Radiology.* 2007;243:690-695.

78. McGann CJ, Kholmovski EG, Oakes RS, Blauer JJE, et al. New magnetic resonance imaging-based method for defining the extent of left atrial wall injury after the ablation of atrial fibrillation. *J Am Coll Cardiol.* 2008;52:1263-1271.

79. Badger TJ, Adjei-Poku YA, Burgon NS, et al. Initial experience of assessing esophageal tissue injury and recovery using delayed-enhancement MRI after atrial fibrillation ablation. *Circ Arrhythm Electrophysiol.* 2009;2:620-625.

80. Peters DC, Wylie JV, Hauser TH, et al. Recurrence of atrial fibrillation correlates with the extent of post-procedural late gadolinium enhancement: a pilot study. *JACC Cardiovasc Imaging.* 2009;2:308-316.

81. Reddy VY, Schmidt EJ, Holmvang G, Fung M. Arrhythmia recurrence after atrial fibrillation ablation: can magnetic resonance imaging identify gaps in atrial ablation lines? *J Cardiovasc Electrophysiol.* 2008;19:434-437.

82. Oakes RS, Badger TJ, Kholmovski EG, et al. Detection and quantification of left atrial structural remodeling with delayed-enhancement magnetic resonance imaging in patients with atrial fibrillation. *Circulation.* 2009;119:1758-1767.

83. Cappato R, Calkins H, Chen SA, et al. Updated worldwide survey on the methods, efficacy and safety of catheter ablation for human atrial fibrillation. *Circ Arrhythm Electrophysiol.* 2010;3:32-38.

84. Badger TJ, Oakes RS, Daccarett M, et al. Temporal left atrial lesion formation after ablation of atrial fibrillation. *Heart Rythm J*. 2009;6:161-168.

85. Chen MS, Marrouche NF, Khaykin Y, et al. Pulmonary vein isolation for the treatment of atrial fibrillation in patients with impaired systolic function. *J Am Coll Cardiol*. 2004;43:1004-1009.

86. Gillinov AM, Bakaeen F, McCarthy PM, et al. Surgery for paroxysmal atrial fibrillation in the setting of mitral valve disease: a role for pulmonary vein isolation? *Ann Thorac Surg*. 2006;81:19-26; discussion 27-28.

87. Gillinov AM, McCarthy PM, Blackstone EH, et al. Surgical ablation of atrial fibrillation with bipolar radiofrequency as the primary modality. *J Thorac Cardiovasc Surg*. 2005;129:1322-1329.

88. Kilicaslan F, Verma A, Saad E, et al. Transcranial Doppler detection of micro-embolic signals during pulmonary vein antrum isolation: implications for titration of radiofrequency energy. *J Cardiovasc Electrophysiol*. 2006;17:495-501.

89. Pappone C, Rosanio S, Oreto G, et al. Circumferential radiofrequency ablation of pulmonary vein ostia: a new anatomic approach for curing atrial fibrillation. *Circulation*. 2000;102:2619-2628.

90. Fahmy TS, Mlcochova H, Wazni OM, et al. Intracardiac echo-guided image integration: optimizing strategies for registration. *J Cardiovasc Electrophysiol*. 2007;18:276-282.

91. Wazni OM, Rossillo A, Marrouche NF, et al. Embolic events and char formation during pulmonary vein isolation in patients with atrial fibrillation: impact of different anticoagulation regimens and importance of intracardiac echo imaging. *J Cardiovasc Electrophysiol*. 2005;16:576-581.

92. Kolandaivelu A, Lardo AC, Halperin HR. Cardiovascular magnetic resonance guided electrophysiology studies. *J Cardiovasc Magn Reson*. 2009;11:21.

93. Vijayakumar S, Kholmovski EG, MacLeod RS, et al. Visualizing acute RF ablation lesions in the heart using non-contrast MRI at 3T. Poster Presentation. International Society for Magnetic Resonance in Medicine, Honolulu, HI, 2009.

INDEX

NOTE: Page numbers followed by *f* and *t* indicates figures and tables.

A

abdominal aortic aneurysms, 384–385
  classification of, 384
  epidemiology of, 384
  imaging of, 384–385
    aortography, 385
    computed tomography, 379
    magnetic resonance angiography, 388
    ultrasonography, 384–385
  pathophysiology of, 384
  risk factors for, 384
ACAS. *See* Asymptomatic Carotid
    Atherosclerosis Study
ACC/AHA/ASE guidelines
  acute coronary syndromes, 34
  arrhythmias, 22–23
  cardiomyopathy, 20, 33
  cardiovascular screening, 38
  chest pain, 34
  dyspnea, 20
  edema, 20
  heart murmur, 28
  hypertension, 21
  mitral valve prolapse, 25
  neurologic events, 26
  palpitations, 22–23
  pericardial disease, 35
  syncope, 28
  valve endocarditis, 36
  valvular stenosis, 30–31
ACS. *See* acute coronary syndrome
activation and propagation mapping
    (three-dimensional contact
    mapping system), 163, 165*f*
acute coronary syndrome (ACS), 34, 104
  ACC/AHA/ASE guidelines for, 34
  infarct evolution, 105, 106*f*, 107, 107*f*
  myocardium at risk, 105
acute myocardial infarction, 361*f*
  cardiovascular magnetic resonance, 360
  clinical relevance, 366
  electrocardiogram, 360–362
    Anderson-Wilkins Acuteness Score,
      363, 363*f*
    localizing myocardial ischemia,
      361–362
    Sclarovsky-Birnbaum Ischemia
      Grading System, 361
  myocardial perfusion SPECT, 360
  myocardial salvage and, 364
  patients, 362–366
    complete myocardial salvage-aborted
      infarction, 363–364, 363*f*

acute myocardial infarction, patients
    (*Cont.*):
    infarct extension because of
      interventional embolization,
      365–366, 366*f*
    no myocardial salvage because of late
      presentation and low protection,
      365, 366*f*
    no myocardial salvage because of low
      protection, 364–365, 365*f*
    partial myocardial salvage, 364, 364*f*
    positron emission tomography, 365
acute pulmonary embolism, 78
adenosine stress test, 56
AF. *See* atrial fibrillation
ALCAPA. *See* anomalous origin of LCA
    from pulmonary artery
American College of Cardiology (ACC).
    See ACC/AHA/ASE guidelines
American Heart Association (AHA).
    See ACC/AHA/ASE guidelines
American Society of Echocardiography
    (ASE). *See* ACC/AHA/ASE
    guidelines
anatomic magnetic resonance imaging,
    236–237, 236*f*
  atrial fibrillation and, 420–421
Andersen-Tawil syndrome,
    arrhythmogenesis in tissue model
    of, 186–187, 187*f*
Anderson-Wilkins Acuteness Score,
    360, 360*f*
aneurysms, aortic, 380–384, 383*f*, 396–399,
    396*f*–398*f*
  abdominal, 384–385
    classification of, 384
    epidemiology of, 384
    imaging of, 384–385
    pathophysiology of, 384
    risk factors for, 384
  thoracic, 380–384
    classification of, 380–383, 382*f*, 383*f*
    epidemiology of, 380–383, 382*f*, 383*f*
    imaging of, 383–384
    pathophysiology of, 383
    risk factors of, 383
angiography
  coronary
    of aortic dissection, 377
    complications with, 72
    contraindications for, 71
    indications for, 71
    multimodal imaging and, 78

angiography, coronary (*Cont.*):
    physical requirements for, 71
    technique, 71
  pulmonary
    of chronic thromboembolic
      pulmonary hypertension, 408–411
    pulmonary arteriovenous
      malformations and, 412
anomalous origin of LCA from pulmonary
    artery (ALCAPA), 75
anomalous origin of RCA from pulmonary
    artery (ARCAPA), 75
anterior ST elevation myocardial infarction,
    angiographic factors determining
    ECG changes in, 77
anticoagulants, idiopathic pulmonary
    arterial hypertension and, 405
aorta
  anatomic variants of, 371–372
    aortic arch, 371–372, 372*f*
    aortic root, 371
  anatomy of, 368, 369*f*
  aneurysms of, 380–384, 382*f*, 396–400,
    396*f*–399*f*
    abdominal, 384–385
    thoracic, 380–384
  aortitis, 388–391
    imaging of, 388–389
    infectious, 389
    noninfectious, 389–391
  atheromatous disease of, 377–378
    aortic penetrating atherosclerotic
      ulcers, 380, 381*f*, 381*t*, 382*f*
    atheroembolization, 378, 379*f*
    pathophysiology of, 378, 379*f*
    plaques, 378, 379*f*
    thromboembolization,
      379–380, 380*f*
    thrombosis, 379–380, 380*f*
  congenital anomalies of, 371–372
    aortic arch, 371–372, 374*f*
    aortic root, 371
    bicuspid AV-associated aortopathy,
      387–388
  congenital disease of, 385–388
    atresia of aorta, 385–386
    coarctation of aorta, 385–387
    Marfan syndrome, 387–388
  dissection of, 35, 35*f*, 372–377
    classification, 372–373, 373*f*, 373*t*
    diagnostic imaging, 373–377, 373*f*
    etiology, 372
    incidence, 372

aorta, dissection of (*Cont.*):
  management strategies, 377
  pathophysiology, 372
function of, 368–369
imaging considerations of, 369
  aortography, 371
  chest radiography, 369, 370*t*
  computed tomography, 370–371
  echocardiography, 369–370
  magnetic resonance imaging, 371
  ultrasonography, 369–370
intramural hematoma
  diagnosis of, 377, 378*f*
  incidence of, 377
  pathophysiology of, 377
  risk factors for, 377
physiology of, 368–369
regurgitation of, 24
  chronic, 31–32, 31*f*, 32*t*
stenosis of, 29–31, 29*f*, 30*f*
  severity of, 31*t*
traumatic injury of, 388
  imaging of, 388, 389*f*, 390*f*
  pathophysiology of, 388
tumors of, 388
aortitis, 388–391
  imaging of, 388–389
  infectious, 389
  noninfectious, 389–391
    giant-cell arteritis, 390–391
    Takayasu disease, 389–390, 390*f*
aortography, 371
  of abdominal aortic aneurysms, 385
  of aorta, dissection, 376, 377*f*
  of atresia of aorta, 386
  of coarctation of aorta, 386
  of thoracic aortic aneurysm, 384
apical five-chamber view, 11, 12*f*, 13*t*
apical four-chamber view, 11, 12*f*, 12*t*
apical three-chamber view, 11, 13*f*, 13*t*
apical two-chamber view, 11, 13*f*, 13*t*
ARCAPA. *See* anomalous origin of RCA
    from pulmonary artery
arrhythmia management, idiopathic
    pulmonary arterial hypertension
    and, 405
arrhythmias, 22–23
  atrial fibrillation, 23
  ventricular, 23
arrhythmogenesis
  during acute ischemia and reperfusion,
    180–183, 182*f*, 183*f*
  in tissue model of Andersen-Tawil
    syndrome, 186–187, 187*f*
arrhythmogenic right ventricular dysplasia
    (ARVD), 21*t*, 23, 176, 176*f*, 177*f*,
    346, 346*f*–347*f*, 348, 349*f*, 350*f*
ARVD. *See* arrhythmogenic right
    ventricular dysplasia

Asymptomatic Carotid Atherosclerosis
    Study (ACAS), 394–396
atheroembolization, 378, 379*f*
atheromatous disease, aorta, 377–379
  aortic penetrating atherosclerotic ulcers,
    380, 381*f*, 381*t*, 382*f*
  atheroembolization, 378, 379*f*
  pathophysiology of, 378, 379*f*
  plaques, 378, 380*f*
  thromboembolization, 379–380, 380*f*
  thrombosis, 379–380, 380*f*
atherosclerotic lesions, ancillary methods to
    study, 77–78
  intravascular ultrasound, 78
  novel invasive imaging modalities, 78
  stenotic lesions, physiologic significance
    of, 78
athletes, student, 37–38
atresia of aorta, 385–386
  etiology of, 385–386, 385*f*
  imaging of, 386
    aortography, 386
    chest radiography, 386
    computed tomography, 386
    echocardiography, 386, 386*f*
    magnetic resonance angiography, 386
  incidence of, 385–386, 385*f*
  pathophysiology of, 385–386, 385*f*
atrial fibrillation (AF), 23, 23*f*, 24*f*, 26
  ablation of, realtime MRI for, 424–427
    catheter, 425–426
    image results visualization,
      426–427, 427*f*
    MRI-compatible catheters, 426, 426*f*
    real-time detection of lesion
      formation, 427, 428*f*
  cardioversion for, 23
  clinical profile of, 420
  imaging modalities and, 421, 421*f*
    anatomic MRI, 422–423
    echocardiography/ultrasound, 422
    electroanatomic mapping and
      imaging, 422
    fluoroscopy, 421–422
    merging of, 423
    multiple computed tomography,
      422–423
  mechanisms of, 420–421
  MRI-based evaluation of, 423–424
    AF substrate evaluation, 423–424, 426*f*
    postablation scar formation
      evaluation, 423, 424*f*
  radiofrequency ablation for, 23
atrial septal defects, 26–27, 27*f*
  in congenital heart disease, 342
atrioventricular conduction axis,
    308, 309*f*
atrioventricular insulating planes,
    310, 311*f*

atrioventricular nodal re-entry, optical
    mapping, of electrical activity,
    187–188, 188*f*
atrioventricular node, 306–308, 307*f*, 308*f*
atrioventricular ring tissues, 309–310, 309*f*
atrioventricular septal defect (AVSD)
  anatomy of, 315–320, 316*f*
    imaging of, 315–320
  challenges of, 315
  electroanatomic relationships in, 320
  electrophysiology of, 318–320
    body surface maps, 318, 319*f*
    conduction system, 320
    epicardial mapping, 319–320
    vectorcardiogram, 318
atrioventricular valve complex, 320
atrioventricular valve function,
    atrioventricular septal defect and,
    317–318, 318*f*
AVSD. *See* atrioventricular septal defect

B

BARI. *See* Bypass Angioplasty
    Revascularization Investigators
beat-by-beat heart rate tachograms
    information, 290–296, 293*f*
  erratic sinus rhythm identification,
    295–296, 295*f*
  sleep period identification, 290, 293*f*
  sleep-disordered breathing identification,
    290–294, 294*f*, 295
bed and wake times, heart rate patterns,
    graphical analysis of, 286–288,
    287*f*, 289
benign cardiac neoplasms, 92
  fibroma, 92
  hemangiomas, 92
  lipoma, 92
  myxoma, 92
  papillary fibroelastoma, 92
  rhabdomyoma, 92
  teratomas, 92
Bernoulli equation, 29–30
β-blockers, stress test and, 56
bicuspid AV-associated aortopathy,
    386–387
  etiology of, 386–387
  imaging of, 387, 387*f*
  incidence of, 386–387
  pathophysiology of, 386–387
bidomain equations, 243–244
body surface maps, atrioventricular septal
    defect and, 318, 319*f*
body surface potential mapping (BSPM),
    205–207, 206*f*, 207*f*
BSPM. *See* body surface potential mapping
Bull's eye image, 51, 51*f*
Bypass Angioplasty Revascularization
    Investigators (BARI), 72

C

CAD. *See* coronary artery disease
caffeine, stress test and, 56–57
calcific aortic stenosis. *See* aorta
calcium blockers, stress test and, 56
calculated epicardial potentials,
 electrocardiography of
 body surface potential mapping,
 205–207, 206*f*, 207*f*
 in clinical electrophysiology, 209–214
 forward problem of, 207
 inverse problem of, 209
 patient-specific torso model generation,
 207–209, 208*f*, 209*f*
 three-dimensional mapping, 210
canine ventricles
 failing, 229–230, 229*f*
 normal, 228–229, 228*f*, 229*f*
carcinoid heart disease, in congenital heart
 disease, 343
cardiac anatomy, model construction of,
 236–239
 fibrous architecture assignment, 241–243
 experimentally derived, 241–242
 histologically derived, 242
 image processing, 237–240
 segmentation and feature extraction,
 237–238
 tissue classification and voxel tagging,
 238–240, 239*f*
 mesh generation, 240
 meshing software, 240
 results of, 240
 multimodal image acquisition, 236–237
 anatomic magnetic resonance imaging,
 236–237, 236*f*
 diffusion tensor MRI, 237
 postprocessing, 240–241, 241*f*
cardiac bioelectric activity stimulation, 243
 governing equations, 243–244
 bidomain equations, 243–244
 monodomain equations, 244
 numerical solution, 248–249
 linear systems solving, 249
 Purkinje network simulation,
 244–246, 244*f*
 geometrical model, 245
 mathematical basis, 245–246, 245*f*
 in silico experiments, 249–253
 model setup, 252–253, 253*f*
 spatial discretization, 247–248
 temporal discretization, 246–247
 ionic model computation techniques,
 246–247
cardiac catheterization, phonocardiography
 and, 48
cardiac computed tomography, 82*f*.
 See also multidetector computed
 tomography

cardiac computed tomography (*Cont.*):
 applications for, 86–93
 cardiac masses, 91–93
 congenital heart disease, 89
 coronary artery evaluation, 86–87
 pericardial disease, 89–91
 pulmonary vein evaluation, 86–89
 case examples and, 98, 99*f*
 multimodal applications, 97–98
 cardiac structure and function
 secondary assessment, 98
 congenital cardiovascular disease,
 97–98
 coronary artery disease, 97
 myocardial evaluation, 94
 chamber size and functions, 94
 ischemia, 95–96, 96*f*
 viability, 94–95, 95*f*
 valvular heart disease, 96–97
 infective endocarditis, 97, 97*f*
 native valves, 96–97, 96*f*
 prosthetic valves, 97, 97*f*
cardiac computed tomography (CCT),
 right ventricular multidetector,
 338, 338*f*
cardiac cycle selection, in gating
 process, 172
cardiac echocardiography Doppler
 examination, 9–14
 standard imaging views, 9–14, 10*f*
cardiac heart failure, resynchronization in,
 176–178, 177*f*
cardiac masses, 91–93, 91*f*
 benign cardiac neoplasms, 92
 fibroma, 92
 hemangiomas, 92
 lipoma, 92
 myxoma, 92
 papillary fibroelastoma, 92
 rhabdomyoma, 92
 teratomas, 92
 CT characteristics features of, 91*t*
 malignant cardiac neoplasms, 92–93
 lymphomas, 93
 metastatic disease, 92
 sarcomas, 92–93
 pseudotumors
 normal cardiac structures, 93
 thrombi, 93
 vegetation, 93, 94*f*
cardiac positron emission tomography,
 152, 153*f*
cardiac resynchronization therapy (CRT),
 21, 222, 223
 cardiac electromechanical modeling and,
 223–224
cardiac simulation, for education, 266
 forward problem, matrix formulation of,
 269–270, 269*f*

cardiac simulation, for education (*Cont.*):
 source model, 266–269
 equivalent double layer, 266–267, 267*f*
 thorax model, 269
cardiomyopathies, 20
 ACC/AHA/ASE guidelines for, 20, 33
 arrhythmogenic RV dysplasia, 21*t*
 dilated, 21, 21*f*, 21*t*, 22*f*
 hypertrophic, 21*t*
 restrictive, 21*t*
 right ventricular, 341–350
 arrhythmogenic RV cardiomyopathy/
 dysplasia, 346, 346*f*–348*f*, 349,
 349*f*, 350*f*
 congenital heart disease, 342–343
 dysfunction secondary to LV
 dysfunction, 340
 general approach (algorithm), 340, 341*f*
 infarction, 340
 pericardial constriction, 345
 pressure overload, 343–345, 345*f*
 Uhl anomaly, 350
 volume overload, 342, 343
 Takotsubo, 78
 WHO classification of, 21*t*
cardiovascular magnetic resonance (CMR)
 imaging, 149–152, 150*f*, 151*f*
 acute myocardial infarction and, 362
 computed tomography and, 149–151,
 150*f*, 151*f*
 contrast agents, 109–110
 intravascular, 110
 nephrogenic systemic fibrosis, 110
 paramagnetic, 109–110, 110*f*
 of idiopathic pulmonary arterial
 hypertension, 404–405, 405*f*
 with implanted cardiac devices,
 151–152
 late Gd enhancement and,
 electrocardiography compared with,
 137, 142, 142*f*–144*f*
 for left ventricular scar mapping, 152
 myocardial perfusion MRI, 119–121
 stress function with high-dose
 dobutamine, 120–121, 121*f*
 stress perfusion with adenosine or
 dipyridamole, 119–120, 120*f*
 myocardium at risk, 110–112
 contrast-enhanced SSFP MRI, 111, 112*f*
 endocardial extent of infarction,
 111–112, 113*f*
 T2-weighted MRI, 110–111, 111*f*
 noninvasive coronary angiography,
 121, 122*f*
 right ventricular, 336–338
 black blood, static imaging,
 336, 336*f*
 myocardial delayed contrast
 enhancement, 336*f*, 338

cardiovascular magnetic resonance (CMR)
    imaging, right ventricular (*Cont.*):
    ttagging sequences, 338
    white wood, cine imaging,
        336–338, 337*f*
    viability and infarct imaging, 112–119
        extracellular MR contrast dynamics,
            112–113, 116*f*
        first-pass dynamics, 115
        inversion time, 116–117, 118*f*
        late Gd enhancement CMR, 116, 117*f*,
            118–119
        late Gd enhancement MRI, 112,
            113*f*–115*f*
        microvascular obstruction,
            115–116, 117*f*
        phase-sensitive LGE, 117–118, 118*f*, 119*f*
cardiovascular screening, ACC/AHA/ASE
    guidelines for, 38
cardioversion, for atrial fibrillation, 23
carotid artery disease, 392–394, 393*f*,
    395*f*, 396*f*
case studies
    arrhythmias, 22–23
    athletes, student, 37–38
    cerebrovascular accident, 25–28
    chest pain, 33–35
    chronic thromboembolic pulmonary
        hypertension, 414, 414*f*–416*f*
    congestive heart failure, 20–21
    heart murmurs, 28–33
    hypertension, 21–22
    infective endocarditis, 36–37, 37*f*
    mitral regurgitation, 24–25
    pericarditis, acute, 35–36
    pulmonary arteriovenous malformations,
        416–417, 417*f*
    routine screening, 37–38
    syncope, 25–28
CASS. *See* Coronary Artery Surgery Study
catheter, realtime MRI for ablation of atrial
    fibrillation, 424–425
catheterization, of right heart, idiopathic
    pulmonary arterial hypertension
    and, 405
CCT. *See* cardiac computed tomography
cerebrovascular accident, 25–28
    cardiac sources of emboli causing, 26*t*
chest pain, 33–35
    ACC/AHA/ASE guidelines for, 34
    cardiovascular causes of, 34*t*
    "low risk" acute, SPECT/PET and,
        61, 62*f*
children, heart sounds in, 41–42
chronic ischemia, 107–109, 108*t*
    hibernating myocardium, 109
    repetitive stunning, 108–109
    stress-induced, 108
    stunned myocardium, 108

chronic thromboembolic pulmonary
    hypertension (CTEPH)
    background of, 408
    case study, 412, 412*f*–414*f*
    clinical presentation of, 408
    imaging of, 408–411
        chest radiograph, 408, 408*f*
        computed tomography, 409–410, 410*f*
        magnetic resonance angiography, 411
        pulmonary angiography, 410–411
        ventilation/perfusion scan,
            408–409, 409*f*
    management of, 411–412
        medical therapies, 411–412
        surgical intervention, 411
cine angiography, right ventricular invasive
    imaging techniques, 338–339, 339*f*
Clinical Outcomes Utilizing
    Revascularization and Aggressive
    Drug Evaluation (COURAGE)
    trial, 64
CMR imaging. *See* cardiovascular magnetic
    resonance imaging
coarctation of aorta, 385–387
    etiology of, 385–386, 385*f*
    imaging of, 386
        aortography, 386
        chest radiography, 386
        computed tomography, 386
        echocardiography, 386, 386*f*
        magnetic resonance angiography, 386
    incidence of, 385–386, 385*f*
    pathophysiology of, 385–386, 385*f*
collateral circulation, 74*f*, 76
color flow Doppler, 9, 9*f*
computational cardiac electrophysiology
    future perspectives of, 235–236
    modeling advances, 234–235
    use of silico approaches, 233–234
computed tomography (CT)
    of abdominal aortic aneurysms, 385
    of aorta, 370–371
        dissection, 374, 374*f*
    of atresia of aorta, 386
    atrial fibrillation and, 423–424
    cardiac. *See* cardiac computed
        tomography
    cardiac magnetic resonance imaging and,
        149–151, 150*f*, 151*f*
    of chronic thromboembolic pulmonary
        hypertension, 409–411, 410*f*
    of coarctation of aorta, 386
    hybrid imaging with
        positron emission tomography and,
            58, 60, 60*f*
        single photon emission computed
            tomography and, 58, 60, 60*f*
    of idiopathic pulmonary arterial
        hypertension, 402, 403*f*

computed tomography (CT) (*Cont.*):
    of ischemic heart disease, 355–358, 357*f*,
        358*f*–358*f*
    of pulmonary arteriovenous
        malformations, 414–415, 415*f*
    of thoracic aortic aneurysm, 384
conduction system, atrioventricular septal
    defect and, 320
conduction tissues, development of,
    305–310, 305*f*
    atrioventricular conduction axis,
        308, 309*f*
    atrioventricular insulating planes,
        310, 311*f*
    atrioventricular node, 306–308,
        307*f*, 308*f*
    atrioventricular ring tissues, 309–310,
        309*f*
    interatrial myocardium, 308
    outflow tracts, myocardium of, 310, 311*f*
    pulmonary venous myocardial
        sleeves, 310
    sinus node, 306, 306*f*–307*f*
    ventricular conducting tissues, 308–309
congenital anomalies, of aorta, 371–372
    aortic arch, 371–372, 372*f*
    aortic root, 371
    bicuspid AV-associated aortopathy,
        386–387
    Marfan syndrome, 387–388
congenital disease, of aorta, 385–388
    atresia of aorta, 385–386
    coarctation of aorta, 385–387
congenital heart disease, 89, 89*f*,
    342–343
    atrial septal defect, 342
    atrioventricular septal defect
        anatomy of, 315–320, 316*f*
        challenges of, 315
        electroanatomic relationships in, 320
        electrophysiology of, 318–320
    carcinoid heart disease, 343
    Ebstein anomaly, 342
    patent ductus arteriosus, 342
    pericardium absence, 342
    tetralogy of Fallot with pulmonary
        regurgitation, 342, 343*f*–344*f*
congenital pericardial lesions, 91
congestive heart failure, 20–21
continuity equation, 30
contraction chronology, using temporal
    Fourier analysis, 172–173, 173*f*
contrast coronary CTA
    bypass grafts assessment, 87, 87*f*
    coronary anomalies, 86–87
    coronary artery disease, 86
    stent patency assessment, 87, 87*f*
contrast echocardiography, of pulmonary
    arteriovenous malformations, 414

conventional Doppler techniques, echocardiography, right ventricular, 328–329, 329*f*
conventional phonocardiography, 41, 42*f*
coronary angiography
   of aorta, dissection, 377
   complications with, 72
   contraindications for, 71
   indications for, 71
   multimodal imaging and, 78
   physical requirements for, 71
   technique, 71
coronary artery
   anomalies, 75–76
      anomalous origin of LCA from pulmonary artery, 75
      anomalous origin of RCA from pulmonary artery, 75
      bridging, 75–76
      fistulae, 76
   evaluation of, 86–87
      contrast coronary CTA, 86–87, 87*f*
      noncontrast CT for calcium scoring, 86, 86*f*
coronary artery disease (CAD)
   angiographic, 75
   athletes and, 38
Coronary Artery Surgery Study (CASS), 72
coronary flow, angiographic assessment of, 76
coronary occlusion
   ischemic cascade in, 131, 131*f*
   transmural ischemia due to, 132–133, 132*f*, 132*t*
coronary stenosis
   fractional flow reserve and, 78
   physiologic significance of, SPECT/PET and, 61, 62*f*
COURAGE trial. *See* Clinical Outcomes Utilizing Revascularization and Aggressive Drug Evaluation trial
CRT. *See* cardiac resynchronization therapy
CT. *See* computed tomography
CTEPH. *See* chronic thromboembolic pulmonary hypertension

D

DECARTO. *See* dipolar electrocardiotopography imaging
decartogram normal values, 192–193, 194*f*
defibrillation therapy, optimizing, modeling methodology applications, 253–255
   defibrillation threshold lowering, 255–256
   low-voltage defibrillation theoretical considerations, 256–257, 257*f*
DHF. *See* dyssynchronous heart failure
diffusion tensor MRI (DT-MRI), 237
digital phonocardiography, 41

dilated cardiomyopathy, 21, 21*f*, 21*t*, 22*f*
dipolar electrocardiotopography (DECARTO) imaging
   ECG-based graphical methods and, 196–197, 197*t*
   imaging cardiac pathophysiology using, 194–195
      myocardial infarction, 194–195, 195*f*, 196*f*
      ventricular hypertrophy, 196
   limitations of, 200
   method description, 191–193, 193*f*
      decartogram normal values, 192–193, 194*f*
      vectorcardiography, 191, 192*f*
   non-ECG methods and, 197–198, 198*f*
   superimposition of, onto three-dimensional images, 198–200, 199*f*
dipyridamole stress test, 56
dissection, of aorta, 35, 35*f*, 372–377
   classification, 372–373, 373*f*, 373*t*
   diagnostic imaging, 373–377, 373*f*
   etiology, 372
   incidence, 372
   management strategies, 377
   pathophysiology, 372
diuretics, idiopathic pulmonary arterial hypertension and, 405
Dobutamine stress test, 56
Doppler
   cardiac echocardiography examination, standard imaging views, 9–14, 10*f*
   principles, 8–9, 9*f*
Doppler, Christian, 8
Doppler imaging, tissue, right ventricular echocardiography, 329–332, 330*f*–334*f*
Doppler recording, fetal heart sounds, phonocardiography *vs.*, 47
Doppler shift principle, 8–9, 9*f*
Doubutamine stress echocardiography. *See* stress echocardiography
dyspnea, ACC/AHA/ASE guidelines for, 20
dyssynchronous heart failure (DHF), 222–223
   image-based reconstruction of geometry and structure of, 224–226, 224*f*
      fiber and sheet mapping, 225–226, 226*f*
      infarct segmentation, 224
      mesh generation, 224–225, 225*f*
      suspension medium removal, 224
      ventricle separation from atria, 224

E

Ebstein anomaly, in congenital heart disease, 342
ECG. *See* electrocardiography
ECGSIM, 270–271, 270*f*. *See also* cardiac simulation

ECGSIM (*Cont.*):
   direct current recordings, ST-T changes, 281–282, 282*f*
   normal EGG, 271–273, 271*f*, 272*f*
   potential field at S_h, 273, 273*f*, 274*f*
   T wave, 275–278, 277*f*
   timing parameters statistics, 273–274, 274*f*–276*f*
   transmembrane potential parameters change, 278–281, 279*f*–281*f*
echocardiography. *See also* cardiac echocardiography Doppler examination
   of aorta, 369–370
      dissection, 374–375, 374*f*–376*f*
   of atresia of aorta, 386, 386*f*
   atrial fibrillation and, 422
   atrioventricular septal defect and, 315–317, 317*f*
   of coarctation of aorta, 386, 386*f*
   contrast, of pulmonary arteriovenous malformations, 414
   of idiopathic pulmonary arterial hypertension, 403–404, 404*f*
   phonocardiography and, 48
   right ventricular, 325–336
      conventional Doppler techniques, 328–329, 329*f*
      one-dimensional (M-mode), 325, 326*f*–327*f*
      three-dimensional, 332–335, 333*f*–334*f*, 335*t*
      tissue Doppler imaging, 329–332, 330*f*–332*f*
      transesophageal, 335
      two-dimensional, 325, 327*f*, 328*f*
   stress, 19–20, 20*f*, 35
      biphasic response, 19–20
      classification, 20
      guidelines, 20
      of ischemic heart disease, 355
      ischemic response, 19
      normal response, 19
      of thoracic aortic aneurysm, 383–384, 383*f*
   transthoracic. *See* transthoracic echocardiography
echocardiography systems, 7–8, 8*f*, 9*f*
ECST. *See* European Carotid Surgery Trial
edema, ACC/AHA/ASE guidelines for, 20
EDL. *See* equivalent double layer
electroanatomic mapping and imaging, atrial fibrillation and, 422
electrocardiogram
   for acute myocardial infarction, 360–362
      Anderson-Wilkins Acuteness Score, 360, 361*f*
      localizing myocardial ischemia, 361–362

electrocardiogram, for acute myocardial
    infarction (*Cont.*):
  Sclarovsky-Birnbaum Ischemia
      Grading System, 361
  of idiopathic pulmonary arterial
      hypertension, 403
electrocardiogram triggering. *See* gated
      single photon emission computed
      tomography
electrocardiography (ECG)
  of calculated epicardial potentials
    body surface potential mapping,
        205–207, 206*f*, 207*f*
    in clinical electrophysiology, 209–214
    forward problem of, 207
    inverse problem of, 209
    patient-specific torso model
        generation, 207–209, 208*f*, 209*f*
    three-dimensional mapping, 210
  of ischemic heart disease, 130
  of myocardial infarction, 133–134
  of myocardial ischemia, 131–133
    acuteness (time-course), 134–135, 135*t*
    characterization, 135–137, 136*f*, 137*f*
    compared with LGE CMR, 137, 142,
        142*f*–144*f*
    compared with myocardial perfusion
        SPECT, 137, 138*f*–141*f*
    location, size, and severity in, 134, 134*f*
  phonocardiography and, 48
electromechanical delay (EMD)
      evaluation, 228
electrophysiologic mapping
  multimodal imaging, 152–167
    ablation and impedance mapping,
        160–161, 160*f*
    activation and propagation mapping
        (three-dimensional contact
        mapping system), 163, 165*f*
    cardiac MRI, CT and, 162
    catheter guidance without exposure to
        ionizing radiation, 167
    catheter mapping of tachycardia, 158
    characterizing focal (automatic or
        triggered) arrhythmias,
        159–160, 159*f*
    characterizing macro-re-entrant
        arrythmias, 158–159
    conduction intervals, activation
        sequence, and refractory periods,
        156–158
    data analysis, 155–156
    EGM interpretation, 156
    EGM recording, 153, 155, 155*f*
    electronic stimulator and fluoroscopy,
        155, 155*f*–157*f*
    electrophysiology laboratory, 153, 154*f*
    intracardiac echocardiography,
        161–162, 161*f*, 162*f*

electrophysiologic mapping, multimodal
      imaging (*Cont.*):
    limitations of, 165
    remote catheter navigation systems,
        167–168, 167*f*
    tachycardia mechanism and location,
        156, 157*f*
    three-dimensional contact mapping,
        162–163, 163*f*
    three-dimensional electroanatomic
        mapping (three-dimensional
        noncontact mapping system),
        165, 166*f*
    three-dimensional transesophageal
        echocardiography, 161, 161*f*
    voltage mapping (three-dimensional
        contact mapping system), 163, 164*f*
  postprocedural evaluation, 167–168
    cardiac MRI for assessment of ablated
        tissue, 167–168, 168*f*
    cardiac PET, 168, 169*f*
    esophageal evaluation, 167
    pulmonary vein evaluation, 167, 168*f*
  preprocedural evaluation, 146–152
    arrhythmia substrate, 147–148
    cardiac MRI, 149–152, 150*f*, 151*f*
    cardiac positron emission
        tomography, 152, 153*f*
    patient history, 146, 147*f*
    transesophageal echocardiography,
        149, 149*f*
    transthoracic echocardiography,
        148–149, 149*f*
    12-lead ECG in arrhythmia, 146–147,
        148*f*
    wide QRS complex tachycardia, 148
electrophysiology, nuclear cardiology
      applied to
  arrhythmogenic right ventricular
      dysplasia, 176, 176*f*, 177*f*
  cardiac cycle selection in gating
      process, 172
  contraction chronology using temporal
      Fourier analysis, 172–173, 173*f*
  gating principle, 171, 172*f*
  innervation, 171
  mean and standard deviation, 173,
      173*f*, 174*f*
  mechanical function, 171
  myocardial sympathetic heterogeneity
      assessment, 178
  myocardial sympathetic innervation
      imaging using MIBG, 174,
      174*f*, 175*f*
  perfusion, 171
  phase histogram descriptive values, 173,
      173*f*, 174*f*
  planar and three-dimensional right
      ventricular imaging, 172, 172*f*

electrophysiology, nuclear cardiology
      applied to (*Cont.*):
    resynchronization in cardiac heart
        failure, 176–178, 177*f*
    viability, 171
    Wolff-Parkinson-White syndrome,
        174–175, 175*f*
emboli, cerebrovascular accident and, 26*t*
EMD. *See* electromechanical delay
      evaluation
endocarditis
  infective, 36–37, 37*f*
  valve, 36
endothelin antagonists, idiopathic
      pulmonary arterial hypertension
      and, 406
epicardial mapping, atrioventricular septal
      defect and, 318, 319
equivalent double layer (EDL), cardiac
      simulation for education,
      266–267, 267*f*
  dipolar approximations of, 269
  generalization of, 267–268
  potentials generated by, 268–269, 268*f*
erratic sinus rhythm identification,
      295–296, 295*f*
European Carotid Surgery
      Trial (ECST), 396
exercise stress test, 55

F

fetal heart sounds, Doppler recording,
      phonocardiography *vs.*, 47
^{18}F-FDG. *See* ^{18}F-2-deoxy-2-fluoro-D-
      glucose
FFR. *See* fractional flow reserve
fibromas, 92
5-minute averaged heart rate patterns,
      284–285, 285*f*, 286*f*
fluoroscopy
  of atrial fibrillation, 421–422
  of ischemic heart disease, 354
fractional flow reserve (FFR), coronary
      stenosis and, 78
fractional shortening, 15, 17*f*
Framingham Heart Study, 22
^{18}F-2-deoxy-2-fluoro-D-glucose
      (^{18}F-FDG), 57

G

gadolinium (Gd), 110
gastrointestinal tracer activity, on
      myocardial perfusion imaging, 66
gated single photon emission computed
      tomography, 51–53, 53*f*, 54*f*, 67
GCA. *See* giant-cell arteritis
Gd. *See* gadolinium
generalized singular value decomposition
      (GSVD), 218–219

giant-cell arteritis (GCA), 390–391
GISSI-I. *See* Gruppo Italiano per lo Studio della Streptochinasi nell'Infarto Miocardico I study
governing equations, cardiac bioelectric activity stimulation, 243–244
  bidomain equations, 243–244
  monodomain equations, 244
Gruppo Italiano per lo Studio della Streptochinasi nell'Infarto Miocardico I study (GISSI-I), 105
GSVD. *See* generalized singular value decomposition

H

$H_2{}^{15}O$. *See* oxygen 15-labeled water
heart
  anatomy of, 72–75, 72f–75f. *See also* cardiac anatomy
    fibrous architecture assignment, 241–243
    model construction of, 236–239
    postprocessing, 240–241, 241f
  catheterization of, idiopathic pulmonary arterial hypertension and, 407
  development of, 299–300, 300f, 301f
    atrial chamber formation, 302–305, 302f–304f
    conduction tissues, 305–310, 305f
    postnatal conduction tissues morphologic recognition, 300–301, 301f, 302f
  failure of. *See also* congestive heart failure
    diastolic, elements of, 22
    with preserved LV systolic function, 22
  murmurs of, 41
  myxomas of, 27–28, 28f
  stimulating electromechanical activity in, 226–228
    bi-V pacing implementation, 227–228
    electrical and mechanical tissue properties, 227
    electromechanical delay evaluation, 228
    left bundle branch block implementation, 227–228
    multiscale electromechanical model structure and modules, 226–227, 226f, 227f
    sinus rhythm implementation, 227–228
    species-specific ionic and myofilament model choice, 227, 227f
heart disease, congenital, 89, 89f
  atrioventricular septal defect
    anatomy of, 315–320, 316f
    challenges of, 315
    electroanatomic relationships in, 320
    electrophysiology of, 318–320

heart murmurs, 28–33
  ACC/AHA/ASE guidelines for, 28
heart rate patterns, graphical analysis of, for cardiac autonomic function assessment, 284
  beat-by-beat heart rate tachograms information, 290–296, 293f
  bed and wake times, 286–288, 287f, 289
  5-minute averaged heart rate patterns, 284–285, 285f, 286f
  heart failure portion abnormalities, 288
  HRV patterns abnormal organization, 288–290
  Poincaré plots information, 290, 291f, 292f
  power spectral analysis, 285–286
  sleep-disordered breathing heart rate patterns, 288
heart rate variability (HRV)
  graphical, 296, 297
  multiple plots, 296–297
heart sounds. *See also* phonocardiography
  analysis of, 41–47
    in adults, 42, 42f
    in children, 41–42
    examples, 42–43, 43f–47f
    in telemedicine, 47
hemangiomas, 92
hematoma, aortic intramural. *See* intramural hematoma
hibernating myocardium, 109
HRV. *See* heart rate variability
hypertension, 21–22, 22f
hypertrophic cardiomyopathy, 21t, 33, 34f

I

ICE. *See* intracardiac echocardiography
idiopathic pulmonary arterial hypertension (IPAH)
  background of, 402
  case study, 406–408, 407f, 408f
  clinical presentation of, 402
  imaging of, 402
    cardiac magnetic resonance imaging, 404–405, 405f
    chest radiography, 402, 403f
    computed tomography, 402, 403f
    echocardiography, 403–404, 404f
    electrocardiogram, 403
    pulmonary function tests, 403
    right heart catheterization, 405
    ventilation/perfusion scan, 402
  management of, 405
    anticoagulants, 405
    arrhythmia management, 405
    disease-targeted therapy, 405–406
    diuretics, 405
    endothelin antagonists, 406
    follow-up, 406

idiopathic pulmonary arterial hypertension (IPAH), management of (*Cont.*):
    oxygen, 405
    phosphodiesterase-5 inhibitors, 405–406
    prostanoids, 405
    surgical intervention, 406
IHD. *See* ischemic heart disease
IMH. *See* intramural hematoma
^{123}I-mIGB. *See* radiolabeled 123-meta-iodobenzylguanidine imaging
infarction, right ventricular, 340
infectious aortitis, 389
infective endocarditis, 36–37, 37f
inferior ST elevation myocardial infarction, angiographic factors determining ECG changes in, 77
interatrial myocardium, 308
International Registry of Acute Aortic Dissection (IRAD), 372
intracardiac echocardiography (ICE)
  electrophysiologic mapping, 161–162, 161f, 162f
  right ventricular invasive imaging techniques, 341
intramural hematoma (IMH)
  diagnosis of, 377, 378f
  incidence of, 377
  pathophysiology of, 377
  risk factors for, 377
intravascular contrast agents, 110
intravascular ultrasound (IVU), atherosclerotic lesions and, 78
IPAH. *See* idiopathic pulmonary arterial hypertension
IRAD. *See* International Registry of Acute Aortic Dissection
ischemia
  assessment of, with prior revascularization, SPECT/PET and, 62, 63f
  on cardiac computed tomography, 95–96, 96f
  chronic, 107–109, 108t
    hibernating myocardium, 109
    repetitive stunning, 108–109
    stress-induced, 108
    stunned myocardium, 108
  single photon emission computed tomography detection of
    cardiac MRI *vs.*, 67
    perfusion contrast echocardiography *vs.*, 67
    stress echocardiography *vs.*, 67
ischemic cascade, 104, 105f
ischemic heart disease (IHD)
  categorization of, 354, 355f, 355t
  computed tomography, 355–357, 356f, 357f–358f

ischemic heart disease (IHD) (*Cont.*):
  electrocardiography of, 130
  fluoroscopy, 354
  invasive imaging methods, 359
  magnetic resonance imaging, 358
  nuclear cardiology, 358
  pathophysiology, 104
  primary diagnosis of, SPECT/PET and,
    60–61, 60*f*, 61*f*
  radiography, 354
  stress echocardiography, 355
  ultrasound, 354–355
ischemic myocardium, single photon
    emission computed tomography
    and, 63–64, 64*f*
ISIS-2. *See* Second International Study of
    Infarct Survival
isovolumic relaxation time (IVRT), 15
IVRT. *See* isovolumic relaxation time
IVU. *See* intravascular ultrasound

L

Laplace-Dirichlet method, 242
late Gd enhancement (LGE)
  electrocardiography compared with, 137,
    142, 142*f*–144*f*
  viability and infarct imaging
    CMR, 116, 117*f*, 118–119
    MRI, 112, 113*f*–115*f*
lateral ST elevation myocardial infarction,
    angiographic factors determining
    ECG changes in, 77
LBBB. *See* left bundle branch block
left bundle branch block (LBBB), single
    photon emission computed
    tomography and, 65, 65*f*
left heart disease, pulmonary hypertension
    due to, in right ventricular pressure
    overload, 345
left ventricular diastolic function,
    assessment of, 15–19
  abnormal, 17, 19*f*
  diastasis period, 15
  early rapid filling, 15
  end-diastole phase, 16
  inflow patterns, 16, 18*f*
  isovolumic relaxation time, 15
  normal, 16–17, 19*f*
  tissue Doppler imaging, 18–19, 19*f*
  Valsalva maneuver, 17
left ventricular mural thrombus, 26, 26*f*
left ventricular systolic function, assessment
    of, 14–15
  contrast enhancement, 15, 15*f*
  quantitative methods, 15, 17*f*
  regional wall motion scoring, 15,
    16*f*, 16*t*
  visual inspection, 15, 15*t*
LGE. *See* late Gd enhancement

lipomas, 92
lone atrial fibrillation, 23
Look-Locker sequence, 110
lower extremity peripheral arterial disease,
    399–400, 399*f*
low-flow/low-gradient aortic stenosis, 30
lymphomas, 93

M

MACE. *See* major adverse
    cardiovascular event
magnetic resonance angiography (MRA)
  of abdominal aortic aneurysms, 385
  of atresia of aorta, 386
  of chronic thromboembolic pulmonary
    hypertension, 411
  of coarctation of aorta, 386
magnetic resonance imaging (MRI)
  anatomic, 236–237, 236*f*
  of aorta, 371
    dissection, 375–376, 376*f*
  atrial fibrillation and, 422–423
  cardiac. *See* cardiovascular magnetic
    resonance imaging
  of ischemic heart disease, 358
  phonocardiography and, 48
  of pulmonary arteriovenous
    malformations, 415
  of thoracic aortic aneurysm, 384
major adverse cardiovascular event
    (MACE), 63, 64
malignant cardiac neoplasms, 92–93
  lymphomas, 93
  metastatic disease, 92
  sarcomas, 92–93
Marfan syndrome, 387–388
  etiology of, 387
  imaging of, 387–388
  incidence of, 387
  pathophysiology of, 387
MDCT. *See* multidetector computed
    tomography
meta-iodobenzyl guanidine (MIBG), 171
  myocardial sympathetic innervation
    imaging using, 174, 174*f*, 175*f*
MIBG. *See* meta-iodobenzyl guanidine
minimum distance algorithm, 242
mitral regurgitation, 24–25, 24*f*, 26*f*
  severity of, 25*t*
mitral stenosis, 32–33, 32*f*, 33*f*
  severity of, 33*t*
mitral valve prolapse, 25, 25*f*
  ACC/AHA/ASE guidelines for, 25
MMI. *See* multimodal imaging
modeling methodology, applications of
    optimizing defibrillation therapy,
    253–255
    defibrillation threshold lowering,
    255–256

modeling methodology, applications of,
    optimizing defibrillation therapy
    (*Cont.*):
    low-voltage defibrillation theoretical
      considerations, 256–257, 257*f*
    postinfarction ventricular tachycardias
      simulations, 260–261, 261*f*
    Purkinje network role, 257–260,
      258*f*, 259*f*
monodomain equations, 244
MPI SPECT. *See* myocardial perfusion
    imaging single photon emission
    computed tomography
MRA. *See* magnetic resonance angiography
MRI. *See* magnetic resonance imaging
MUGA. *See* multigated acquisition
    equilibrium scans
multidetector computed tomography
    (MDCT)
  contrast administration, 84, 85
  ECG signal for synchronization
    during, 82
  image quality, 85–86
  motion artifacts, 85
  post processing, 84, 84*f*, 85*f*
  prospective triggering, 82, 82*f*, 83*t*
  radiation considerations, 85
  retrospective triggering, 82, 83*f*, 83*t*
  right ventricular, 339, 339*f*
  scanner design, 81
  spatial resolution, 83
  temporal resolution, 82–83, 83*f*
multigated acquisition (MUGA)
    equilibrium scans, 335
multimodal image acquisition, 236–237
  anatomic magnetic resonance imaging,
    236–237, 236*f*
  diffusion tensor MRI, 237
multimodal imaging (MMI),
    electrophysiologic mapping.
    See electrophysiologic mapping
murmurs, 41
myocardial blood flow, angiographic
    assessment of, 76
myocardial bridging, 72
myocardial infarction. *See also* acute
    myocardial infarction
  dipolar electrocardiotopography
    imaging, 194–195, 195*f*, 196*f*
  ECG changes and, 133
  electrocardiography of, 133–134
  pathologic Q wave and, 133
  pathophysiology of, 133
myocardial ischemia, 50–51. *See also*
    ischemic heart disease
  decreased blood supply and, 131
  electrocardiography of, 131–133
    acuteness (time-course), 134–135, 135*t*
    characterization, 135–137, 136*f*, 137*f*

myocardial ischemia, electrocardiography of (*Cont.*):
  compared with LGE CMR, 137, 142, 142*f*–144*f*
  compared with myocardial perfusion SPECT, 137, 138*f*–141*f*
  location, size, and severity in, 134, 134*f*
  localizing, 361–362
myocardial perfusion imaging, 50–51
  gastrointestinal tracer activity on, 66
  over reporting in, 65
  positron emission tomography technique. *See* positron emission tomography
  triple-vessel disease on, 66, 66*f*–68*f*
myocardial perfusion imaging single photon emission computed tomography (MPI SPECT), 364
  right ventricular nuclear cardiology, 335
myocardial salvage
  acute myocardial infarction and, 362
  partial, in acute myocardial infarction patients, 364, 364*f*
myocardial salvage because of late presentation and low protection, no, in acute myocardial infarction patients, 365, 366*f*
myocardial salvage because of low protection, no, in acute myocardial infarction patients, 364–365, 365*f*
myocardial salvage-aborted infarction, complete, in acute myocardial infarction patients, 363–364, 363*f*
myocardial sympathetic heterogeneity assessment, 178
myocardial sympathetic innervation imaging, using MIBG, 174, 174*f*, 175*f*
myxomas, of heart, 27–28, 28*f*, 92

N

neoplasms
  benign cardiac, 92
    fibroma, 92
    hemangiomas, 92
    lipoma, 92
    myxoma, 92
    papillary fibroelastoma, 92
    rhabdomyoma, 92
    teratomas, 92
  malignant cardiac, 92–93
    lymphomas, 93
    metastatic disease, 92
    sarcomas, 92–93
nephrogenic systemic fibrosis (NSF) contrast agent, 110
neurologic events, ACC/AHA/ASE guidelines for, 26
^{13}NH$_3$, 57, 58

nitrates, stress test and, 56
non-ST-segment elevation, angiographic factors determining ECG changes in, 77
no-reflow phenomenon, 76
NSF. *See* nephrogenic systemic fibrosis contrast agent
nuclear cardiology
  applied to electrophysiology
    arrhythmogenic right ventricular dysplasia, 176, 176*f*, 177*f*
    cardiac cycle selection in gating process, 172
    contraction chronology using temporal Fourier analysis, 172–173, 173*f*
    gating principle, 171, 172*f*
    innervation, 171
    mean and standard deviation, 173, 173*f*, 174*f*
    mechanical function, 171
    myocardial sympathetic heterogeneity assessment, 178
    myocardial sympathetic innervation imaging using MIBG, 174, 174*f*, 175*f*
    perfusion, 171
    phase histogram descriptive values, 173, 173*f*, 174*f*
    planar and three-dimensional right ventricular imaging, 172, 172*f*
    resynchronization in cardiac heart failure, 176–178, 177*f*
    viability, 171
    Wolff-Parkinson-White syndrome, 174–175, 175*f*
  of ischemic heart disease, 358
  right ventricular, 335–336
    equilibrium-gated RNA, 335
    first-pass radionuclide angiography, 335
    myocardial perfusion imaging single photon emission computed tomography, 335
    radiolabeled 123-meta-iodobenzylguanidine imaging, 335
nuclear imaging. *See also* nuclear cardiology
  in arrhythmias, 171

O

one-dimensional (M-mode) echocardiography, right ventricular, 325, 326*f*–327*f*
optical mapping, of electrical activity, 180*f*
  applications of, 188–189
  arrhythmogenesis during acute ischemia and reperfusion, 180–183, 182*f*, 183*f*
  arrhythmogenesis in tissue model of Andersen-Tawil syndrome, 186–187, 187*f*

optical mapping, of electrical activity (*Cont.*):
  atrioventricular nodal re-entry, 187–188, 188*f*
  electrophysiologic heterogeneity across ventricular wall, 179–180, 181*f*
  limitations of, 188–189
  spontaneous arrhythmias in tissues recovered from ischemia, 183, 184*f*
outflow tracts, myocardium of, 310, 311*f*
oxygen, idiopathic pulmonary arterial hypertension and, 405
oxygen 15-labeled water (H$_2$^{15}O), 57, 58

P

palpitations, ACC/AHA/ASE guidelines for, 22–23
papillary fibroelastoma, 92
paramagnetic contrast agent, 109–110, 110*f*
parasternal long axis view, 10, 10*f*, 10*t*
parasternal short axis view, 11, 11*f*, 12*t*
patent ductus arteriosus, in congenital heart disease, 342
patent foramen ovale, 26–27, 27*f*
PAVMs. *See* pulmonary arteriovenous malformations
PDE-5. *See* phosphodiesterase-5 inhibitors
pericardial constriction, 345
pericardial disease, 89–91
  ACC/AHA/ASE guidelines for, 35
  acute pericarditis, 90
  congenital pericardial lesions, 91
  constrictive pericarditis, 90, 90*f*
  pericardial effusion, 90
  pericardial masses, 90–91
pericardial effusion, 35, 35*f*, 36*f*, 36*t*, 90
pericardial tamponade, 35–36, 36*f*
pericardiocentesis, 36
pericarditis
  acute, 35–36, 90
  constrictive, 90, 90*f*
pericardium absence, in congenital heart disease, 342
peripheral arterial disease, lower extremity, 399–400, 399*f*
peripheral vascular disease, 394–400
  aortic aneurysm, 396–399, 396*f*–398*f*
  carotid artery disease, 392–396, 393*f*, 395*f*, 396*f*
  lower extremity peripheral arterial disease, 399–400, 399*f*
PET. *See* positron emission tomography
pharmacologic stress test, 55–56
  adenosine, 56
  dipyridamole, 56
  dobutamine, 56
  regadenoson, 56

phonocardiography
　cardiac catheterization and, 48
　clinical auscultation, 41, 47
　conventional, 41, 42*f*
　digital, 41
　echocardiography and, 48
　electrocardiography and, 48
　fetal heart sound Doppler
　　　recording *vs.*, 47
　future of, 48
　laser Doppler vibrometry *vs.*, 47–48
　limitations of, 43, 47
　magnetic resonance imaging and, 48
　spectral, 47
phosphodiesterase-5 inhibitors (PDE-5),
　　idiopathic pulmonary arterial
　　hypertension and, 405–406
PISA. *See* proximal isovelocity surface area
　　method
planar and three-dimensional right
　　ventricular imaging, 172, 172*f*
plaques, of aorta, 378, 379*f*
Poincaré plots information, 290,
　　291*f*, 292*f*
polar plot image, 51, 51*f*
positron emission tomography (PET)
　acquisition, 55
　acute myocardial infarction and, 362
　attenuation corrections, 55
　cardiac. *See* cardiac positron emission
　　tomography
　data analysis, 58, 59*f*
　diagnostic accuracy of, 63–64
　hybrid imaging with CT, 58, 60, 60*f*
　indications for, 60–63
　　coronary stenosis, physiologic
　　　significance of, 61, 62*f*
　　ischemia assessment with prior
　　　revascularization, 62, 63*f*
　　ischemic heart disease, primary
　　　diagnosis of, 60–61, 60*f*, 61*f*
　　"low risk" acute chest pain, 61, 62*f*
　　risk assessment before major surgery, 62
　　viability testing, 62–63
　ischemia detection with
　　cardiac MRI *vs.*, 67
　　perfusion contrast
　　　echocardiography *vs.*, 67
　　stress echocardiography *vs.*, 67
　ischemic myocardium amount,
　　63–64, 64*f*
　left ventricular function on, 67
　myocardial infarction and, 64
　outcome of, 63–64
　protocols, 58
　risk assessment, 63–64
　stable angina and, 64
　suspected acute coronary syndrome
　　and, 64

positron emission tomography (PET) (*Cont.*):
　tracers
　　¹⁸F-2-deoxy-2-fluoro-D-glucose, 57
　　¹³NH₃, 57, 58
　　oxygen 15-labeled water, 57, 58
　　⁸²Rb, 57, 58
　viability assessment with, 67
postablation scar formation evaluation, in
　　atrial fibrillation, 423, 424*f*
postinfarction ventricular tachycardias
　　simulations, modeling methodology
　　applications, 260–261, 261*f*
power spectral analysis, heart rate patterns,
　　graphical analysis of, 285–286
pressure half-time (PHT), 33, 33*f*
prostanoids, idiopathic pulmonary arterial
　　hypertension and, 405
proximal isovelocity surface area (PISA)
　　method, 24–25, 24*f*
pseudotumors
　normal cardiac structures, 93
　thrombi, 93
　vegetation, 93, 94*f*
pulmonary arterial hypertension, in right
　　ventricular pressure overload,
　　343–344
pulmonary arteriovenous malformations
　　(PAVMs)
　background of, 412
　case study, 416–417, 417*f*
　clinical presentation of, 412–414
　imaging of, 414–416
　　chest radiograph, 414, 415*f*
　　computed tomography, 414–415, 415*f*
　　contrast echocardiography, 414
　　magnetic resonance imaging, 415
　　pulmonary angiography, 416
　　pulmonary hypertension screening,
　　　415–416
　　radionuclide perfusion lung
　　　scanning, 415
　　shunt fraction measurement, 415
　management of, 416, 416*f*
pulmonary embolism, acute, 78
pulmonary function tests, for idiopathic
　　pulmonary arterial
　　hypertension, 403
pulmonary hypertension
　due to left heart disease, in right
　　ventricular pressure overload, 344
　screening, pulmonary arteriovenous
　　malformations and, 415–416
pulmonary vein, evaluation of, 87–89,
　　88*f*, 89*f*
pulmonary venous myocardial sleeves, 310
Purkinje myocytes, 308
Purkinje network role, modeling
　　methodology applications, 257–260,
　　258*f*, 259*f*

Purkinje network simulation, cardiac
　　bioelectric activity stimulation,
　　244–246, 244*f*
　geometrical model, 245
　mathematical basis, 245–246, 245*f*

Q

QRS infarct scoring, 135–137, 136*f*, 137*f*

R

radiofrequency ablation, for atrial
　　fibrillation, 23
radiography
　of aorta, 369, 370*t*
　　dissection, 377
　of atresia of aorta, 386
　of chronic thromboembolic pulmonary
　　hypertension, 408, 408*f*
　of coarctation of aorta, 386
　of idiopathic pulmonary arterial
　　hypertension, 402, 403*f*
　of ischemic heart disease, 354
　of pulmonary arteriovenous
　　malformations, 414, 415*f*
　of thoracic aortic aneurysm, 383
radiolabeled 123-meta-
　　iodobenzylguanidine imaging
　　(¹²³I-mIGB), right ventricular
　　nuclear cardiology, 335
radionuclide angiography (RNA)
　equilibrium-gated, right ventricular
　　nuclear cardiology, 335
　right ventricular nuclear cardiology, 335
radionuclide perfusion lung scanning,
　　of pulmonary arteriovenous
　　malformations, 417
⁸²Rb, 57, 58
regadenoson stress test, 56
remote catheter navigation systems,
　　167–168, 167*f*
restrictive cardiomyopathy, 21*t*
reverse piezoelectricity, 7, 8*f*
rhabdomyoma, 92
right heart catheterization, idiopathic
　　pulmonary arterial hypertension
　　and, 405
right ventricular (RV), 322, 323*f*, 324*f*
　anatomy of, 322–325
　cardiomyopathies, 340–351
　　arrhythmogenic RV cardiomyopathy/
　　　dysplasia, 346, 346*f*–348*f*, 349*f*, 350*f*
　　congenital heart disease, 342–343
　　dysfunction secondary to LV
　　　dysfunction, 340
　　general approach (algorithm), 340,
　　　341*f*
　　infarction, 340
　　pericardial constriction, 345
　　pressure overload, 343–345, 345*f*

right ventricular (RV), anatomy of (*Cont.*):
Uhl anomaly, 350
volume overload, 342, 343
dysfunction, secondary to LV
dysfunction, 340
inflow view, 10, 11*f*, 11*t*
invasive imaging techniques, 338
cine angiography, 338–339, 339*f*
intracardiac echocardiography, 340
noninvasive imaging techniques,
325–339
CMR imaging, 336–338
echocardiography, 325–336
multidetector cardiac computed
tomography, 338, 338*f*
nuclear cardiology, 335–336
physiology of, 322–325
wall motion abnormalities
incidence, 323*t*
right ventricular pressure overload
(RVPO), 343–345, 345*f*
pulmonary arterial hypertension,
344–345
pulmonary hypertension due to left heart
disease, 344
RNA. *See* radionuclide angiography
routine screening, 37–38
RV. *See* right ventricular
RVPO. *See* right ventricular pressure
overload

S

salvagability time window, 363
SAPPHIRE. *See* Stenting and Angioplasty
with Protection in Patients at High
Risk for Endarterectomy
sarcomas, 92–93
Sclarovsky-Birnbaum Ischemia Grading
System, 361
SDNNIDX. *See* standard deviation of
5-minute N-N intervals
SDS. *See* summed difference score
Second International Study of Infarct
Survival (ISIS-2), 105
sestamibi, 57
shunt fraction measurement, pulmonary
arteriovenous malformations
and, 417
Simpson method, 15, 17*f*
single photon emission computed
tomography (SPECT), 51–55,
51*f*–53*f*
attenuation correction, 54–55, 54*f*
diagnostic accuracy of, 63–64
gated, 51–53, 53*f*, 54*f*, 67
hybrid imaging with CT, 58, 60, 60*f*
indications for, 60–63
coronary stenosis, physiologic
significance of, 61, 62*f*

single photon emission computed
tomography (SPECT), indications
for (*Cont.*):
ischemia assessment with prior
revascularization, 62, 63*f*
ischemic heart disease, primary
diagnosis of, 60–61, 60*f*, 61*f*
"low risk" acute chest pain, 61, 62*f*
risk assessment before major
surgery, 62
viability testing, 62–63
left bundle branch block and, 65, 65*f*
left ventricular function on, 67
myocardial infarction and, 64
new detector technology for, 54
outcome of, 63–64
protocols, 57–58
risk assessment, 63–64
stable angina and, 64
suspected acute coronary syndrome
and, 64
tracers
sestamibi, 57
99mTc-labeled tetrofosmin, 57, 58
thallium 201, 57, 58
viability assessment with, 67
sinus node, 306, 306*f*–307*f*
sleep period identification, 290, 293*f*
sleep-disordered breathing
heart rate patterns, 288
identification, 290–294, 294*f*, 295
sound, 7
wave, 7, 8*f*
frequency of, 7
reflection, 7, 8*f*
spatial discretization, 247–248
SPECT. *See* single photon emission
computed tomography
spectral phonocardiography, 47
SRS. *See* summed rest score
SSFP. *See* Steady-state free precession
SSS. *See* summed stress score
ST elevation myocardial infarction
(STEMI), angiographic factors
determining ECG changes in
anterior, 77
inferior, 77
lateral, 77
standard deviation of 5-minute N-N
intervals (SDNNIDX), 296
steady-state free precession (SSFP), 111, 112*f*
STEMI. *See* ST elevation myocardial
infarction
Stenting and Angioplasty with Protection
in Patients at High Risk for
Endarterectomy (SAPPHIRE), 396
stress echocardiography, 19–20, 20*f*, 35
biphasic response, 19–20
classification, 20

stress echocardiography (*Cont.*):
guidelines, 20
of ischemic heart disease, 357
ischemic response, 19
normal response, 19
stress test
caffeine and, 56–57
exercise, 55
inadequate, 65
medication discontinuation before,
56–57
pharmacologic, 55–56
adenosine, 56
dipyridamole, 56
dobutamine, 56
regadenoson, 56
stress-induced chronic ischemia, 108
ST-segment deviation, 132–133, 132*t*
stunned myocardium, 108
subxiphoid view, 14, 14*f*, 14*t*
sudden death, ventricular arrhythmias
and, 23
summed difference score (SDS), 63
summed rest score (SRS), 63
summed stress score (SSS), 63
suprasternal notch view, 14, 14*f*, 14*t*
syncope, 25–28
ACC/AHA/ASE guidelines for, 28
SYNTAX score, 75

T

T wave, 275–278, 277*f*
TAA. *See* thoracic aortic aneurysm
Takayasu disease, 389–390, 390*f*
Takotsubo cardiomyopathy, 78
TAPSE. *See* tricuspid annular plane systolic
excursion
99mTc-labeled tetrofosmin, 57, 58
TEE. *See* transesophageal echocardiography
temporal discretization, ionic model
computation techniques, 246–247
teratomas, 92
tetralogy of Fallot with pulmonary
regurgitation, in congenital heart
disease, 342, 343*f*–344*f*
thallium 201 (201Tl), 57, 58
201Tl. *See* thallium 201
thoracic aortic aneurysm (TAA),
380–386
classification of, 380–383, 382*f*, 383*f*
epidemiology of, 380–383, 382*f*, 383*f*
imaging of, 383–384
aortography, 384
chest radiography, 383
computed tomography, 384
echocardiography, 383–384, 383*f*
magnetic resonance imaging, 384
pathophysiology of, 383
risk factors of, 383

three-dimensional echocardiography, right ventricular, 333–336, 333f–334f, 335t

three-dimensional electroanatomic mapping (three-dimensional noncontact mapping system), 165, 166f

thromboembolization, 379–380, 380f

Thrombolysis in Myocardial Infarction (TIMI), 76

thrombosis, aortic, 379–380, 380f

Tikhonov regularization scheme, 219–220

TIMI. *See* Thrombolysis in Myocardial Infarction

transducer positions, for standard transthoracic echocardiography, 10f
    apical five-chamber, 11, 12f, 13t
    apical four-chamber, 11, 12f, 12t
    apical three-chamber, 11, 13f, 13t
    apical two-chamber, 11, 13f, 13t
    parasternal long axis, 10, 10f, 10t
    parasternal short axis, 11, 11f, 12t
    right ventricular inflow, 10, 11f, 11t
    subxiphoid, 14, 14f, 14t
    suprasternal notch, 14, 14f, 14t

transesophageal echocardiography (TEE), right ventricular, 335

transmembrane potential parameters change, ECGSIM and, 278–281

transthoracic echocardiography, transducer positions for, 10–14, 10f

traumatic aortic injury, 388
    imaging of, 388, 389f, 390f
    pathophysiology of, 388

tricuspid annular plane systolic excursion (TAPSE), 325

triple-vessel disease, on myocardial perfusion imaging, 66, 66f–68f

tumors, of aorta, 390

two-dimensional echocardiography, right ventricular, 325, 327f, 328f

U

UDL. *See* uniform double layer

ultrasonography
    of abdominal aortic aneurysms, 384–385
    of aorta, 369–370

ultrasound
    atrial fibrillation and, 422
    of ischemic heart disease, 354–355

uniform double layer (UDL). *See* equivalent double layer

unstable coronary artery disease. *See* acute coronary syndrome

V

Valsalva maneuver, 17

valve endocarditis, ACC/AHA/ASE guidelines for, 36

valvular heart disease, 96–97
    infective endocarditis, 97, 97f
    native valves, 96–97, 96f
    prosthetic valves, 97, 97f

valvular regurgitation, ACC/AHA/ASE guidelines for, 24

valvular stenosis, ACC/AHA/ASE guidelines for, 30–31

vectorcardiogram, for atrioventricular septal defect, 318

vectorcardiography, 191, 192f

velocity, 7

ventilation/perfusion scan
    of chronic thromboembolic pulmonary hypertension, 408–409, 409f
    of idiopathic pulmonary arterial hypertension, 402

ventricular arrhythmias, 23

ventricular conducting tissues, 308–309

ventricular hypertrophy, dipolar electrocardiotopography imaging, 196

voltage mapping (three-dimensional contact mapping system), 163, 164f

volume overload, right ventricular, 342, 343

W

wall motion score index (WMSI), 15, 16t

WHO. *See* World Health Organization

WMSI. *See* wall motion score index

Wolff-Parkinson-White syndrome, nuclear cardiology, applied to electrophysiology, 174–175, 175f

World Health Organization (WHO), 20